ATOPIC DERMATITIS

edited by

Thomas Bieber
University of Bonn
Bonn, Germany

Donald Y. M. Leung
National Jewish Medical and Research Center
Denver, Colorado

MARCEL DEKKER, INC.   NEW YORK · BASEL

ISBN: 0-8247-0742-7

This book is printed on acid-free paper.

Headquarters
Marcel Dekker, Inc.
270 Madison Avenue, New York, NY 10016
tel: 212-696-9000; fax: 212-685-4540

Eastern Hemisphere Distribution
Marcel Dekker AG
Hutgasse 4, Postfach 812, CH-4001 Basel, Switzerland
tel: 41-61-261-8482; fax: 41-61-261-8896

World Wide Web
http://www.dekker.com

The publisher offers discounts on this book when ordered in bulk quantities. For more information, write to Special Sales/Professional Marketing at the headquarters address above.

Preface

Atopic dermatitis is one of the most common skin conditions found in the general population. Patients afflicted with skin disease suffer greatly as it adversely affects their quality of life. This book offers a new, integrating view of all aspects relevant to the complex pathophysiology of this disorder. Each chapter provides a comprehensive and up-to-date review of a particular field of research and also considers links to other pathomechanisms of this disease. All aspects—especially the newest immunoallergological and biochemical concepts—are thoroughly discussed with regard to established, experimental, and potential new therapeutical strategies.

The book is divided into several parts to make a clear presentation of the various aspects of this disease. Part I examines the impact of atopic dermatitis, addressing the epidemiological, psychological, and socioeconomic effects of this disease. A distinction is also made between allergic vs. non-allergic atopic dermatitis. Part II provides an overview of the general mechanisms with in-depth discussions on the immunogenetics, risk factors, skin barrier function, and immunologic basis of atopic dermatitis including the pathophysiology of itching, which is the most prominent feature of this skin disease. Part III focuses on the individual cell types that contribute to atopic dermatitis and therefore provides potential therapeutic targets for intervention. Part IV reviews the immunologic triggers (foods, inhalants, bacteria, and fungi) that aggravate atopic dermatitis, and discusses how to prevent them from becoming such a problem. The final part of the book deals with management. How should skin care be approached? What is the current state of the art in treatment and what new treatments are on the horizon?

As atopic dermatitis is a highly prevalent skin disease and provides important insights into mechanisms of allergic skin immune responses, clinicians from many specialties, including dermatologists, allergists, family practitioners, and pediatricians as well as medical students and experimental investigators will benefit from this work, which gives the information necessary for understanding the modern management of atopic dermatitis.

Thomas Bieber
Donald Y. M. Leung

Contents

v

Part III: CELLULAR ASPECTS

Part IV: IMMUNOLOGICAL TRIGGERS AND INTERVENTION

Part VI: THE FUTURE

Contributors

Werner Aberer   Department of Dermatology, University of Graz, Graz, Austria

Cezmi A. Akdis   Swiss Institute of Allergy and Asthma Research (SIAF), Davos, Switzerland

Mübeccel Akdis   Swiss Institute of Allergy and Asthma Research (SIAF), Davos, Switzerland

Hiroaki Aoyama   Department of Dermatology, Tohoku University School of Medicine, Sendai, Japan

Thomas Bieber   Department of Dermatology and Allergology, University of Bonn, Bonn, Germany

Kurt Blaser   Swiss Institute of Allergy and Asthma Research (SIAF), Davos, Switzerland

Christine Bodemer   Service de Dermatologie, Hôpital Necker Enfants Malades, Paris, France

Mark Boguniewicz   National Jewish Medical and Research Center, and Department of Pediatrics, University of Colorado School of Medicine, Denver, Colorado

Burkhard Brosig Department of Psychosomatic Dermatology, Justus Liebig University Giessen, Giessen, Germany

Carolyn R. Charman Department of Dermatology, Queen's Medical Centre, University Hospital, Nottingham, United Kingdom

Kevin D. Cooper Department of Dermatology, University Hospitals of Cleveland, and Case Western Reserve University, Cleveland, Ohio

Ulf G. Darsow Department of Dermatology and Allergy Biederstein, Technical University Munich, Munich, Germany

Yves de Prost Service de Dermatologie, Hôpital Necker Enfants Malades, Paris, France

Peter M. Elias Department of Dermatology, University of California, San Francisco, California

Kate Elliott Murdoch Childrens Research Institute, Melbourne, Australia

Lisa Ellman-Grunther Department of Allergy and Immunology, Mount Sinai School of Medicine, New York, New York

Elizabeth A. Erwin Department of Internal Medicine, University of Virginia, Charlottesville, Virginia

Susan Forrest Murdoch Childrens Research Institute, Melbourne, Australia

Alberto Giannetti Department of Dermatology, University of Modena and Reggio Emilia, Modena, Italy

Uwe Gieler Department of Psychosomatic Medicine, Justus Liebig University Giessen, Giessen, Germany

Giampiero Girolomoni Second Division of Dermatology and Laboratory of Immunology, Istituto Dermopatico dell'Immacolata, IRCCS, Rome, Italy

Gerald J. Gleich* Department of Immunology, Mayo Clinic and Mayo Foundation, Rochester, Minnesota

---

* *Current affiliation*: Department of Dermatology, University of Utah, Salt Lake City, Utah.

Udo Herz Department of Clinical Chemistry and Molecular Diagnostics, Philipps University Marburg, Marburg, Germany

Anne-Marie Irani Division of Pediatric Allergy, Immunology, and Rheumatology, Department of Pediatrics, Virginia Commonwealth University, Richmond, Virginia

Naotomo Kambe Department of Internal Medicine, Virginia Commonwealth University, Richmond, Virginia

Kefei Kang Department of Dermatology, University Hospitals of Cleveland, and Case Western Reserve University, Cleveland, Ohio

Alexander Kapp Department of Dermatology and Allergology, Hannover Medical University, Hannover, Germany

Philip E. Kerr Department of Dermatology, Brown Medical School, Providence, Rhode Island

Caroline S. Koblenzer Department of Dermatology, University of Pennsylvania, and Faculty, Philadelphia Association for Psychoanalysis, Philadelphia, Pennsylvania

Jean Thomas Krutmann Environmental Health Institute at the Heinrich Heine University Düsseldorf, Düsseldorf, Germany

Candace S. Lapidus Department of Dermatology, Brown Medical School, Providence, Rhode Island

Kristin M. Leiferman* Department of Dermatology, Mayo Clinic and Mayo Foundation, Rochester, Minnesota

Donald Y. M. Leung Division of Allergy and Immunology, National Jewish Medical and Research Center, Denver, Colorado

Thomas A. Luger Department of Dermatology and Boltzmann Institute for Cell and Immunobiology of the Skin, University of Muenster, Muenster, Germany

---

* *Current affiliation*: Department of Dermatology, University of Utah, Salt Lake City, Utah.

Akimichi Morita   Department of Dermatology, Nagoya City University Medical School, Nagoya, Japan

Volker Niemeier   Clinic for Psychosomatic Medicine and Psychotherapy, Justus Liebig University Giessen, Giessen, Germany

Mikiko Okada*   Department of Dermatology, Tohoku University School of Medicine, Sendai, Japan

Saveria Pastore   Laboratory of Immunology, Istituto Dermopatico dell'Immacolata, IRCCS, Rome, Italy

Douglas A. Plager   Department of Dermatology, Mayo Clinic and Mayo Foundation, Rochester, Minnesota

Thomas A. E. Platts-Mills   Department of Internal Medicine, University of Virginia, Charlottesville, Virginia

Ehrhardt Proksch   Department of Dermatology, University of Kiel, Kiel, Germany

Ulrike Raap   Department of Clinical Chemistry and Molecular Diagnostics, Philipps University Marburg, Marburg, Germany

Haydee M. Ramirez   Department of Dermatology, University Hospitals of Cleveland, and Case Western Reserve University, Cleveland, Ohio

John R. Reed   Departments of Dermatology and Immunology, Royal Free Hospital, London, United Kingdom

Sakari Reitamo   Department of Dermatology, Hospital for Skin and Allergic Diseases, University of Helsinki, Helsinki, Finland

Harald Renz   Department of Clinical Chemistry and Molecular Diagnostics, Philipps University Marburg, Marburg, Germany

Johannes Ring   Department of Dermatology and Allergy Biederstein, Technical University Munich, Munich, Germany

---

* *Current affiliation*: Department of Dermatology, Sendai Shakaihoken Hospital, Sendai, Japan.

Malcolm H. A. Rustin   Department of Dermatology, Royal Free Hospital, London, United Kingdom

Hugh A. Sampson   Department of Pediatrics, Mount Sinai School of Medicine, New York, New York

Luis F. Santamaria   Pharmacology Department, Almirall Prodesfarma S.A., Barcelona, Spain

Peter Schmid-Grendelmeier*   Swiss Institute for Allergy and Asthma Research (SIAF), Davos, Switzerland

Lawrence B. Schwartz   Division of Allergy, Immunology, and Rheumatology, Department of Internal Medicine, Virginia Commonwealth University, Richmond, Virginia

Sonja Ständer   Department of Dermatology, University of Muenster, Muenster, Germany

Martin Steinhoff   Department of Dermatology, University of Muenster, Muenster, Germany

Seth R. Stevens   Department of Dermatology, University Hospitals of Cleveland, and Case Western Reserve University, Cleveland, Ohio

Hachiro Tagami   Department of Dermatology, Tohoku University School of Medicine, Sendai, Japan

Tadashi Terui   Department of Dermatology, Tohoku University School of Medicine, Sendai, Japan

Axel Trautmann   Swiss Institute of Allergy and Asthma Research (SIAF), Davos, Switzerland

Erika von Mutius   Department of Pulmonology and Allergology, University Children's Hospital, Munich, Germany

Thomas Werfel   Department of Dermatology and Allergology, Hannover Medical University, Hannover, Germany

---

* *Current affiliation*: Allergy Unit, Department of Dermatology, University Hospital, Zurich, Switzerland.

Hywel C. Williams   Department of Dermatology, Queen's Medical Centre, University Hospital, Nottingham, United Kingdom

Klaus Wolff   Department of Dermatology, University of Vienna, Vienna, Austria

Andreas Wollenberg   Department of Dermatology and Allergology, University of Munich, Munich, Germany

Brunello Wüthrich   Allergy Unit, Department of Dermatology, University Hospital, Zurich, Switzerland

ATOPIC DERMATITIS

1
Definition and Diagnosis of Intrinsic Versus Extrinsic Atopic Dermatitis

Brunello Wüthrich
University Hospital, Zurich, Switzerland

Peter Schmid-Grendelmeier*
Swiss Institute for Allergy and Asthma Research (SIAF), Davos, Switzerland

I. HISTORICAL ASPECTS—THE CONCEPT OF ATOPY AND THE DISCOVERY OF IgE

In 1923 Coca and Cooke (1) introduced the term "atopy" to designate phenomena of hypersensitivity in humans. Atopy was adapted from the Greek word meaning "out of place" or "strange disease." Atopy in the concept of Coca and Cooke is (1) hereditary, (2) limited to a small group of human beings, (3) different from anaphylaxis, referring to a lack of protection, and allergy, meaning an altered reactivity, both of which can also be induced experimentally in humans and in animals, (4) qualitatively an abnormal response occurring only in particular individuals (atopics), (5) clinically characterized by hay fever and bronchial asthma, and (6) associated with immediate-type (flare-and-wheal) skin reactions. The authors wanted to describe a familial or hereditary tendency—which does not occur in normals—to become sensitized in a natural way to certain substances in the environment, e.g., house dust, pollen, or food, and to develop hypersensitivity reactions such as hay fever and asthma, which are associated with immediate-type (flare-and-wheal) skin reactions. At this time Coca and Cooke were evidently unaware of the work of Prausnitz and Küstner (2), published in 1921, about the passive transfer of immediate hypersensitivity in humans by serum. However, 2 years later Coca and Grove (3) defined the "atopic reagins" as the specifically

---

* *Current affiliation*: University Hospital, Zurich, Switzerland.

1

reacting substances in the serum of atopic individuals that can be demonstrated by the Prausnitz-Küstner test. In their original definition of atopy, Coca and Cooke included only allergic rhinitis and bronchial asthma. Wise and Sulzberger (4) discussed in the *1933 Year Book of Dermatology and Syphilogy* the conditions of eczema, neurodermatitis, lichenification, and "prurigo diathésiques" described by the French dermatologists Besnier (5) and Brocq (6) and stated in a footnote that:

> Of all these forms of more or less confused and confusing types of localized and generalized lichenification, at least one is emerging as a fairly distinct and clear-cut entity. This is probably best called atopic dermatitis, but is generally known as generalized neurodermitis or diffuse pruritus with lichenification. This is characterized by the following cardinal qualities: (1) atopic family history; (2) antecedent infantile eczema; (3) localization in antecubital and popliteal spaces, the anterior portions of the neck and chest and the face, particularly the eye-lids; (4) the presence of a grayish or brownish coloration of the skin; (5) the absence of true vesicles, clinically and histologically; 6) vasomotor instability or irritability; (7) the usual negative patch test with many contact allergens; (8) many positive reactions of immediate wheal type to scratch or intradermal testing and (9) the presence of many reagins in the blood serum.

Many population studies, particularly those conducted by Schwartz (7) and by Schnyder (8), and follow-up studies of children first seen with infantile eczema (9,10) supported the close association of bronchial asthma, hay fever, perennial rhinitis, atopic dermatitis, and some forms of food allergies with classic atopic disease. Late in the 1960s, Ishizaka and Ishizaka (11) and Johansson (12) identified a new class of immunoglobulins, the IgE antibodies, as carrier of reaginic activity, raised in atopic individuals, and, therefore, a characteristic of the atopic condition. Shortly after the discovery of the IgE molecule it was shown that serum IgE levels in atopic dermatitis are increased on average (13–15) and that this serum IgE increase in related to the increase of specific IgE against several environmental allergens (16–18). Furthermore, it was shown that the severity of the atopic dermatitis was highly correlated to the levels of serum IgE (19–22). However, it was also observed that in moderate or mild forms and even in few cases of severe atopic dermatitis without a coexistent bronchial asthma or allergic rhinitis, the IgE values were in the normal ranges (20–22).

In the following years, however, it clearly appeared that the initial criteria for defining atopy according to Coca and Cooke could no longer be accepted because (1) atopic diseases can also be nonfamilial, (2) "intrinsic" asthma also has a hereditary background (7), (3) animals can also suffer from hay fever, asthma, and atopic dermatitis and produce reaginic antibodies (23), and (4) reagins are not qualitatively abnormal responses. In 1976, Spector and Farr (24) discussed the different immunological and pharmacological characteristics of atopic individuals and of asthmatic subjects, such as elevated IgE levels, impaired T-cell function, decreased β-adrenergic receptor responsiveness, etc. They thought that there was a need for a more realistic definition of the terms allergy and atopy and for a more disciplined use of terminology. In 1979 Lowell (25) proposed redefining atopy to include the respiratory syndromes of asthma and rhinitis, allergic (IgE-mediated) or nonallergic, which share a genetic predisposition, eosinophilia, hyperreactivity to an α-adrenergic agent, and responsiveness to steroids. However, this author, like Coca and Cooke, had omitted to include atopic dermatitis in the definition of atopy.

II. DEFINITION AND CLINICAL FEATURES OF ATOPIC DERMATITIS

As recently as the late 1970s at least 12 synonyms for atopic dermatitis were used, and it is unclear whether these names depicted the same clinical concept (26). The Hanifin and Rajka consensus criteria marked in 1980 an important milestone in listing the main clinical features of atopic dermatitis and are those most often referred to and widely applied with regard to the diagnosis of atopic dermatitis (atopic eczema) (27) (Table 1). They stated that ''at the present time increased serum IgE can only be considered as one of the features of the disease, possibly reflecting dysfunctional control of immunoglobulin producing cells. As a practical test serum IgE levels offer little aid to either diagnosis or prognosis in clinical situations.'' Other diagnostic criteria were elaborated in Germany by Diepgen and coworkers (28) and in the United Kingdom by Williams and co-workers (26,29) more for epidemiological purposes to use by nondermatologists in population-based studies. They do not consider raised IgE levels and positive immediate type skin reactivity as an absolute prerequisite for diagnose atopic dermatitis. The Lillehammer Criteria of 1994 (30) (Table 2) are based on the idea that the distribution of the atopic dermatitis may differ in the infantile, childhood, and adult phases:

1. The clinical criteria concentrate upon dermatitis of larger characteristic areas.
2. For simplifying and didactic reasons the anamnestic criteria are identical in the three phases.
3. The laboratory criteria for IgE and skinprick test have been placed separately.
4. The criteria comprise a certain duration of the disease.

Besides full-blown atopic dermatitis, there are minor or atypical disease manifestations. The description of these forms can be attributed primarily to French authors in the middle of the 1960s and the beginning of the 1970s (31–

Table 1   Guidelines for the Diagnosis of Atopic Dermatitis

Must have three or more basic features:
1. Pruritus
2. Typical morphology and distribution:
   Flexural lichenification or linearity in adults
   Facial or extensor involvement in infants and children
3. Chronic or chronically relapsing dermatitis
4. Personal or family history of atopy (asthma, allergic rhinitis, atopic dermatitis)

Plus three or more minor features:
1. Xerosis
2. Ichthyosis/palmar hyperlinearity/keratosis pilaris
3. Immediate (type I) skin test reactivity
5. Elevated serum IgE
6. Early age of onset
7. Tendancy toward repeated cutaneous infections (especially *Staphylococcus aureus* and Herpes simplex)/impaired cell-mediated immunity
8. Tendancy toward nonspecific hand or foot dermatitis
9. Nipple eczema
10. Cheilitis
11. Recurrent conjunctivitis
12. Dennie-Morgan infraorbital fold
13. Keratoconus
14. Anterior subcapsular cataracts
15. Orbital darkening
16. Facial pallor/facial erythema
17. Pityriasis alba
18. Anterior neck folds
19. Itch when sweating
20. Intolerance to wool and lipid solvents
21. Perifollicular accentuation
22. Food intolerance
23. Current influenced by environmental/emotional factors
24. White dermographism/delayed blanch

Source: Ref. 27.

33) and to Herzberg (34) in the German-speaking sphere. These special forms and minimal variants can occur alone, together, or alternate with the more typical eczematous, lichenoid, pruriginous, and seborrheic forms, whose occurrence is related to age, individual predisposition, and disease duration—indicative of their status as atopic skin manifestations. The special forms of presentation attract attention because they are clinical and morphological variants and because of their particular sites of location, such as the eyelids, lips, nipples, vulva, fin-

Table 2 The Lillehammer Criteria for Diagnosing Atopic Dermatitis

I. The infantile phase (age <2 years)
A. Clinical
    1. Eczema over the face or neck
    2. Eczema on the trunk
    3. Eczema on the arms or legs (extensor or flexurar sites)
    4. Itching or scratch effects, including lichenification or impetigo
B. Anamnestic
    5. A history of relapsing course or seasonal variation
    6. A history of dry skin
    7. A history of itching when sweating or wool intolerance
    8. A history of respiratory atopy or positive family history of atopy in first-degree relatives
C. Laboratory
    9. Elevated serum IgE or positive skin prick tests
D. Duration
    10. Duration of more than 6 weeks
II. The childhood phase (age 2–12 years)
A. Clinical
    1. Eczema over the face or neck
    2. Eczema in the elbows or the kneefolds
    3. Eczema at the wrists or ankles
    4. Eczema on the hands or feet, including dermatitis plantaris sicca
    5. Pityriasis alba or reversed eczema above (below) elbows/knees or toilet seat dermatitis
    6. Itching or scratch effects, including lichenification or impetigo
B. Anamnestic
    7. A history of relapsing course or seasonal variation
    8. A history of dry skin
    9. A history of itching when sweating or wool intolerance
    10. A history of respiratory atopy or positive family history of atopy in first-degree relatives
C. Laboratory
    11. Elevated serum IgE or positive skin prick tests
D. Duration
    12. Duration of more than 3 months
III. The adult phase (age >12 years)
A. Clinical
    1. Eczema over the face or neck
    2. Eczema in the elbows or the kneefolds
    3. Eczema at the wrists or ankles
    4. Eczema on the hands or feet, including dermatitis plantaris sicca
    5. Pityriasis alba or nummular eczema on the arms or legs, or eczema on the upper trunk, including nipple eczema
    6. Itching or scratch effects, including lichenification or impetigo
B. Anamnestic
    7. A history of relapsing course or seasonal variation
    8. A history of dry skin
    9. A history of itching when sweating or wool intolerance
    10. A history of respiratory atopy or positive family history of atopy in first-degree relatives
C. Laboratory
    11. Elevated serum IgE or positive skin prick tests
D. Duration
    12. Duration of more than 3 months

Diagnostic criteria: Visible eczema in at least one of the regions (A), and at least one positive of the anamnestic or laboratory criteria (B, C), and at least three of the clinical, anamnestic, or laboratory criteria (A, B, C) fulfilled. In addition, as a fourth criterion, the skin disease should always have a duration of at least 6 weeks in the infantile phase or 3 months in the childhood and the adult phases.
Source: Adapted from Ref. 30.

Table 3 Features of Atopic Skin Diathesis

Constitutional stigmata of atopy
Dry skin
Hyperlinear palms/soles
Morgan's infraorbital fold
Orbital darkening
Hertoghe's sign
A-minima manifestations and sequelae
Patchy pityriasiform lichenoid eczema
Pityriasis alba
Pulpitis sicca
Winter feet
Nipple eczema
Dirty neck
Associated conditions
Ichthyosis vulgaris
Keratosis pilaris
Lingua geographica
Juvenile plantar dermatosis
Keratosis punctata
Lichen striatus

Source: Adapted from Ref. 36.

gerpads, and toes (35). Besides different manifestations and sequelae of atopic dermatitis, physical findings can be considered as constitutional stigmata or markers of atopic skin manifestation (36) (Table 3). Furthermore, a heterogeneous group of diseases has been found to be related to atopic dermatitis, but these conditions cannot be interpreted as direct manifestations or sequelae of atopic diseases (36).

III. SUBTYPES OF ATOPIC DERMATITIS

The Danish authors Mygind et al. wrote in their handbook in the chapter on Atopic diseases (37) that: (1) "when atopic subjects are exposed to the minute amounts of allergens in ambient air, they respond with a persistent production of IgE antibody," (2) "the atopic status of a person can be determined by skin testing with a battery of common aero-allergens," and (3) "the most important atopic diseases are atopic dermatitis, allergic rhinitis and asthma." Further: "while allergic rhinitis and asthma are IgE-mediated diseases, atopic dermatitis is, in most cases, merely IgE-associated. In other words, allergic rhinitis and asthma are atopic and allergic diseases in which symptoms are the result of allergen exposure, while atopic dermatitis is an atopic disease but not allergic disease, for symptoms are not, or only to a minor degree, caused by allergen exposure. It is confusing that an atopic disease can be both allergic and non-allergic.''

Indeed, not all patients with the clinical phenotype of atopic dermatitis are sensitized to allergens. There is clear evidence that a clinical subtype of atopic dermatitis exists without elevated IgE production and negative skin tests of the immediate type. For this type one of the authors (BW) proposed the term ''intrinsic'' atopic dermatitis in analogy to the intrinsic type of asthma (38–40). From the clinical point of view, a ''pure'' type of atopic dermatitis without associated respiratory symptoms, like rhinitis and asthma, and a ''mixed'' type with concomitant respiratory allergies can be separated; in the latter an almost polyvalent IgE sensitization to inhalants and foodstuffs is mandatory. On the basis of an allergological work-up, the ''pure'' type of atopic dermatitis can further be subdivided into an ''extrinsic'' and an ''intrinsic'' type. (Fig. 1). The ''intrinsic'' type is characterized by the following criteria: (1) clinical phenotype of atopic dermatitis, according to Hanifin and Rajka (27); (2) absence of other atopic diseases such as rhinoconjunctivitis, asthma, acute urticaria, or food allergy; (3) negative skin prick and intracutaneous tests to common aero- and food allergens; (4) total serum IgE levels in the normal ranges for infants, children, and adults (41–43); (5) negative in vitro screening for specific IgE to common aero- and food aller-

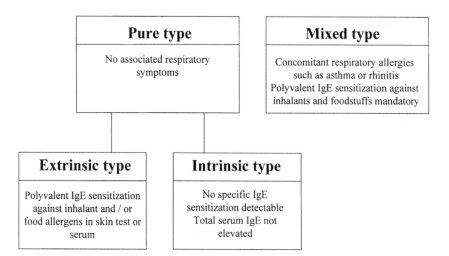

Figure 1 Subtypes of atopic dermatitis according to the presence or not of respiratory allergies and an IgE sensitization to inhalant or food allergens. (Adapted from Refs. 38, 40.)

gens (e.g., Phadiatop or SX_1, a multi-RAST containing eight known inhalant allergens, namely house dust mites, timothy, rye, birch and mugwort pollen, cat and dog epithelia as well as *Cladosporium* mold, FX_5, a food mix containing milk, egg white, wheat, fish, peanut, and soy).

In the following we emphasize various aspects of this particular subtype of atopic dermatitis. The discrimination between the two types is not just academic. The classification of atopic dermatitis into an extrinsic type with specific sensitization to allergens and into an intrinsic type without specific sensitization appears to be useful because specific sensitization significantly correlates with more severe skin condition and disease course (44). The clinician and the patient have to know if allergen avoidance and secondary prevention might be useful, as in the extrinsic type. In case of the intrinsic type, a subsequent onset of respiratory disease is quite improbable (44); a pharmacological prevention of asthma, e.g., with long-term treatment using cetirizine, an H_1-histamine antagonist with anti-inflammatory properties, is not indicated (45,46). Finally, researchers should study intrinsic atopic dermatitis particularly because the clinical and immunological findings are only related to the skin manifestation of atopy and not to the associated respiratory diseases. The key to the pathogenesis of this fascinating disease should be found in this subgroup (40). Also in genetic studies, this separation of patients with atopic dermatitis alone (with or whithout specific IgE) from those with additional atopic manifestations is of value since one explanation could be sharing of disease-susceptibility genes.

IV. EPIDEMIOLOGY AND CLINICAL FEATURES OF INTRINSIC ATOPIC DERMATITIS

The percentage of atopic dermatitis patients presenting with the intrinsic type varies among the different study populations from 10% to nearly 50% depending on the age group, hospital recruitment or epidemiological survey, and the methods used to assess the allergic sensitization (skin tests only and/or serology) (see Table 4). In our clinical-immunological studies, based on adult inpatients who underwent extensive allergological investigation, the frequency of the intrinsic type among all atopic dermatitis patients varied between 10 and 40% (46–48,52). While the overall prevalence of extrinsic atopic dermatitis in preschool children—assessed by means of skin prick tests with six common aeroallergens (birch, grass, mugwort pollen, housedust mite, cat dander, and *Cladosporium*) and two food allergens (hens' eggs, cows' milk)—was not different between eastern (4.9%; $n = 1926$) and western Germany (4.8%; $n = 2076$), the prevalence of the intrinsic type was found to be almost twice as high in eastern (8.5%) than western (4.7%) Germany (55). This indicates that factors other than allergic sensitization contribute to the manifestations of the disease. In a recent large

Table 4 Epidemiological Data of Intrinsic Atopic Dermatitis (IAD) in Various Studies

Ref.	No. of patients	Patients with IAD	Age (mean, range)	Female:Male in IAD	Mean total serum IgE(kU/l)
Kalinke et al., 1997 (44)	40 (1989)	15 (30%)	1–5 yr		<85
	22 (1997)	4 (18%)	9–13 yr		
Walker et al., 1993 (47)	25	5 (20%)	28 yr (17–56)		134 ± 39
Kägi et al., 1994 (48)	33	14 (42%)	35.5 yr (19–55)	12:2	77.7 ± 88.6
Cabon et al., 1996 (49)	59	27 (45%)	5.2 yr (0–12)		89.3
Wedi et al., 1997 (50)	21	9 (43%)	39 ± 17 yr		22.2
Schaefer et al., 1999 (51)	2201	726 (25%)	5–14 yr		76.7
Akdis et al., 1999 (52)	1151	117 (10%)	36 yr		<150
Fabrizi et al., 1999 (53)	72	8.01 ± 6.14			Skin prick tests only
Wüthrich, 1999 (46)	93	17 (18%)	37 yr		<150
Oppel et al., 2000 (54)	69	7 (10%)	Adults	7:0	76.7 ± 28.4
Schäfer et al., 2000 (55)	2057 in WG[a]	49.6%	5–6 yr		Skin prick tests only
	1926 in EG[a]	63.5%	5–6 yr		
Bradley et al., 2000 (56)	1097[b]	28%	4–84 yr		sIgE (Sx1, fx5)

[a] Population samples in preschool children (cross-sectional studies).
[b] With AD affected siblings in 481 different families.

genetic study seeking to identify susceptibility genes for atopic dermatitis by linkage analysis of 1097 affected siblings (median age 29 years; range 4–84 years) from 481 different families, 74% had raised total and/or allergen-specific IgE serum levels (56). Thus, 26% belonged to the intrinsic type.

Clinically, patients with intrinsic atopic dermatitis tend to have a late onset of the disease, but otherwise family history and disease duration seem to be similar (57). As is generally seen in atopic dermatitis, a female predominance has also been observed in intrinsic atopic dermatitis (51,53). Distribution and clinical features of the skin lesions do not differ. A more common "head-and-neck type" distribution has also been shown by some studies, which is characteristic of atopic dermatitis associated with sensitization to fungi, mainly *Pityrosporum ovale* (58,59). Because *P. ovale* is not routinely tested in SPT and standardized extracts are not available, this could be a cause of the missed IgE sensitization. Histological differences are not observed. The typical features of spongiosis and lymphocytic infiltration in acute stage lesions and acanthosis in the more chronic stages are similar in both forms of atopic dermatitis.

V. IMMUNOLOGICAL SIMILARITIES AND DIFFERENCES BETWEEN EXTRINSIC AND INTRINSIC ATOPIC DERMATITIS

Various immunological parameters have been investigated in peripheral blood cells and in cells from biopsy samples of lesional skin or patch test reactions (Table 5).

A. T Cells

Clinical observations and various studies have shown that T-cells are among the most important cells involved into the pathogenesis of atopic dermatitis (60). The dermal infiltrate consists predominantly of activated CD4+ and CD8+ cells with a CD4+/CD8+ ratio similar to that in peripheral blood (52,61). Aeroallergens, food allergens, and superantigens are involved in the activation of T cells (62,63).

Various immunological differences between intrinsic atopic dermatitis and extrinsic atopic dermatitis have been found in the cytokine pattern of involved T cells as well in peripheral blood as in lesional skin findings. So a differential cytokine pattern in peripheral blood lymphocytes supernatants and skin patients was shown by Kägi et al. in total of 33 patients (48). T-cell activation occurs in both forms, as measurable by expression of soluble IL-2R+ and HLA-DR+ lymphocytes (47). In contrast, 19 patients with extrinsic atopic dermatitis did express elevated levels of IL-4 and IL-5, whereas in 14 patients with intrinsic atopic dermatitis high IL-5 but low IL-4 levels were found. Increased B-cell

Table 5 Various Characteristics of Intrinsic Atopic Dermatitis (IAD) in Comparison with Extrinsic Atopic Dermatitis (EAD)

	IAD	Ref.
Clinical distribution	Similar to EAD	
Onset	Later than EAD	47, 48, 52, 53, 57
Sex	Mild female predominance	47, 48, 52, 53, 57
Frequency	16–45%	
Total serum IgE	<100 kU/L	
Eosinophilia	Mild-moderate	47, 48
Eosinophil survival	No difference from EAD	50
T cells		
Peripheral blood	HLA-DR like in EAD	47, 48, 52, 57
	IL-5 levels = EAD	48
	IL-4 levels < EAD	48
	CD23 + B cells < EAD	47, 52
Derived from lesional skin	IL-5 < EAD	52
	IL-13 < EAD	52
Epidermal dendritic cells	FcεRI/FcεRII expression ratio < 0.5 (>1.5 in EAD)	54

activation by enhanced expression of the CD23 (FcεIgERII) in extrinsic atopic dermatitis has been observed in various studies (47,48,52). In addition, activated skin-homing T cells expressing the selective skin-homing receptor, cutaneous lymphocyte-associated antigen (CLA), induce IgE mainly via IL-13 and prolong eosinophil lifespan, mainly via IL-5 (63,64). Because both IL-4 and IL-13 activate B cells, the decreased expression of the B-cell surface marker CD23 (FcεRII) found in intrinsic atopic dermatitis is possibly a consequence of the lower IL-4/IL-13 levels found there (52). Aside from binding IgE, CD23 seems to be a negative regulator of IgE but may have also a positive regulatory on IgE titers under some conditions (65). Therefore the decreased CD23/FcεRII expression can be as much a secondary effect of decreased IL-4/IL-13 production in intrinsic atopic dermatitis as a primary cause of differences in IgE levels.

In the skin, immunohistological features of eczematous lesions in atopic dermatitis correspond only in the acute stage with a Th2 reponse (with increased IL-4, IL-5, and IL-13) while chronic lesions show preferably a Th1-like pattern with increased levels of IL-12 and IFN-γ (66). Interestingly IFN-γ, a key cytokine involved in the induction of T-cell–mediated apoptosis in eczema, shows no differences between intrinsic and extrinsic atopic dermatitis (67). In contrast, Akdis et al. demonstrated decreased IL-5 and IL-13 production in the dermal cellular infiltrate in intrinsic atopic dermatitis compared to extrinsic atopic dermatitis (52). Thus, T cells isolated from skin biopsies of extrinsic atopic dermatitis induced high IL-13–mediated IgE production in cocultures with normal B cells, whereas intrinsic-type cells did not (63).

In conclusion, in atopic dermatitis activated T cells infiltrate the skin and secrete cytokines. The two types of atopic dermatitis are reflected in these cytokine patterns: extrinsic atopic dermatitis with high IL-5, IL-13, and some IFN-γ and intrinsic atopic dermatitis with low IL-5, IL-13, and also some IFN-γ.

B. Eosinophils, Mast Cells, and Basophils

Eosinophils are the hallmark of the late-stage inflammatory reaction in asthma and other allergic inflammations (68). In asthma and atopic dermatitis eosinophils are recruited differentially to healthy individuals. Apparently prolonged eosinophil apoptosis plays a central role in the pathogenesis of asthma (69). This phenomenon has moreover been shown in atopic dermatitis; however, the role of eosinophils in atopic dermatitis is much less clear (50). Eosinophilic toxic granule proteins as well as eosinophil-attractive chemokines such as eotaxin and its receptor are increased in lesional skin (70,71). Eosinophils are not only effector cells, they also play an active immunoregulatory role; therefore, they may play an important role in the switch from a Th2-cytokine pattern in acute lesions of atopic dermatitis towards a more Th1-like pattern in chronic stage (64,65). Blood eosinophils and eosinophilic cationic protein (ECP) are often elevated in both forms of atopic dermatitis (47,48).

Mast cells and basophils mediate the classical immediate-type hypersensitivity, triggered through allergen-induced cross-linking of specific IgE antibody bound to mast cells through high-affinity receptors. Except acute urticarial reactions, these mechanisms may not be of major importance in the clinical manifestation of atopic dermatitis. In addition, mast cells release a wide range of chemokines and cytokines, which contribute to the recruitment and activation of other cells, in particular eosinophils, and induce local tissue inflammation such as IL-4 and IL-13 (72,73). Differences on a mast cell level are not as expected in atopic dermatitis, since immediate-type allergic reactions are hardly involved. So far investigations comparing mast cells and basophils from the two form of atopic dermatitis have not yet been reported.

C. Antigen-Presenting Cells

The immune response to foreign proteins is strongly dependent on the efficiency and selectivity of antigen uptake by antigen-presenting cells (APC). Therefore, APC play an important role also in asthma and atopic dermatits. Langerhans cells

(LC) and epidermal dendritic cells (EDC) as skin resident cells have been shown to play a crucial role in these diseases. The high-affinity receptor for IgE (FcεRI) has been demonstrated not only on mast cells and basophils, but also on LC and EDC (74,75). An increased expression of the high-affinity receptor for IgE (FcεRI) on epidermal dendritic cells (DC) from nonlesional and lesion skin of atopic dermatitis patients has been found (76). Oppel et al. demonstrated a lower expression of FcεRI on EDC in patients with intrinsic atopic dermatitis compared with extrinsic atopic dermatitis (54). These authors were able to identify 80% of extrinsic atopic dermatitis patients by EDC typing using flow cytometry as they showed an FcεRI/FcεRII expression ratio of >1.5 compared to intrinsic atopic dermatitis with a value of around 0.5 (77,78). It is not yet clear if the lower FcεRI levels found in EDC is a cause or a consequence of lower local or serum IgE. Other cells such as mast cells and basophil FcεRI are upregulated by the serum IgE concentration (75). Independent of the underlying mechanism, these findings make clear the differences in the inflammatory micromilieu between intrinsic and extrinsic atopic dermatitis.

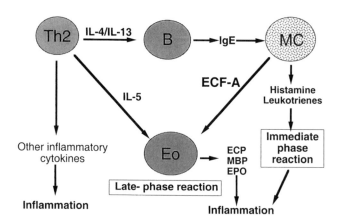

Figure 2 Pathogenetic models in asthma and atopic dermatitis. Role of T-helper 2 cells (Th2) for IgE synthesis in B cells via interleukin 4 (IL-4) and interleukin 13 (IL-13) (extrinsic type of asthma and atopic dermatitis) and of interleukin 5 (IL-5) for activation of eosinophils in both extrinsic and intrinsic asthma and atopic dermatitis. Activation of eosinophils leads to a release of toxic enzymes in the mucosa and in the dermis, which cause chronic tissue inflammation. EA = Extrinsic asthma; EAD = extrinsic atopic dermatitis; IA = intrinsic asthma; IAD = intrinsic atopic dermatitis; B = B cells, MC = mast cells; EO = eosinophils; ECP = eosinophil cationic protein; MBP = major basic protein; EPO = eosinophil peroxides; ECFA = eosinophil chemotactic factor of anaphylaxis. (From Ref. 86.)

VI. CONCLUSIONS

Intrinsic atopic dermatitis is a subtype of atopic dermatitis that fullfills the most commonly used diagnostic criteria, but patients show no elevated total or specific serum IgE and negative immediate-type skin tests. Our conclusions, based on a large experience and a review of the literature, are in contrast to the millenium criteria for the diagnosis of atopic dermatitis formulated by Bos and coworkers (79), who consider the presence of allergen-specific IgE as absolutely mandatory for the diagnosis of atopic dermatitis. The Japanese Dermatological Association Criteria for the diagnosis of atopic dermatitis emphasize that most individuals with atopic dermatitis have an atopic diathesis—defined as having a personal history and overproduction of IgE antibodies (80). However, Uhera has repeatedly shown that there are in Japan atopic dermatitis patients without IgE-mediated hypersensitivity mechanisms (81–83). Other Japanese authors were the first to demonstrate that some atopic dermatitis patients present positive atopy patch tests to aeroallergens without IgE sensitization (84,85). The results of atopy patch tests with aeroallergens and specific IgE (sIgE) could be used to divide atopic dermatitis patients into four distinct subgroups-(1) +APT and −sIgE, (2) +APT and +sIgE, (3) −APT and +sIgE, and (4) −APT and −sIgE. Each subgroup has its own particular clinical morphology, suggesting the heterogeneity of the disease (82,84). The modern immunological findings of a Th2 cell–related activation

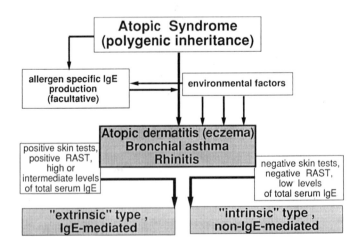

Figure 3 Classification of atopic diseases (atopic dermatitis, bronchial asthma, and rhinitis) in an extrinsic, IgE-mediated and intrinsic, non–IgE-mediated type according to the results of allergy skin and in vitro tests (with or without specific IgE sensitization). (From Ref. 86.)

pattern of cytokine release in both allergic and nonallergic types of bronchial asthma and atopic dermatitis allow a redefinition of the term atopy. This would include the respiratory syndromes of asthma and rhinitis and the atopic skin manifestations, which share a genetic predispostion, a hyperreactivity of the target organ to pharmacological agents (cholinergic hyperreactivity and α-adrenergic hyporesponsiveness) or to irritants, and immunologically a Th2 cell response to allergens (exogenous or endogenous) with a facultative specific IgE production, and eosinophil activation (Fig. 2). So far, the extrinsic and intrinsic types of asthma, rhinitis, and eczema represent an atopic manifestation (Fig. 3) (86).

REFERENCES

1. AF Coca, RA Cooke. On the classification of the phenomena of hypersensitiveness. J Immunol 8:163–182, 1923.
2. C Prausnitz, H Küstner. Studien über die Überempfindlichkeit. Zbl Bakt Parasits Infect I Abt Orig 86:160–169, 1921.
3. AF Coca, EF Grove. Studies in hypersensitiveness. XIII A study of atopic reagins. J Immunol 10:445–464, 1925.
4. F Wise, MB Sulzberger. Footnote on problem of eczema. neurodermatitis and lichenification. In: F Wise, MB Sulzberger, eds. The 1933 Year Book of Dermatology and Syphilogy. Chicago: Year Book Publishers, 1933, pp 38–39.
5. ME Besnier. Première note et observations préliminaires pour servir d' introduction à l' étude des prurigos diathésiques (dermatites multiformes prurigineuses chroniques exacerbantes et paroxystiques, du type du prurigo de Hebra). Ann Derm Syph (Paris) 3:634–648, 1892.
6. L Brocq. Quelques aperçus sur les dermatoses prurigineuses et sur les anciens lichens. Ann Derm Syph (Paris) 3:1100–1117, 1892.
7. M Schwartz. Heredity in bronchial asthma: a clinical and genetic study of 191 asthma probands and 50 probands with baker's asthma. Acta Allergol (Kbh) 5(suppl 2), 1952.
8. UW Schnyder. Neurodermitis—Asthma—Rhinitis. Eine genetisch-allergologische Studie. Int Arch Allergy 178(suppl):1–106, 1960.
9. K Musgrove, JK Morgan. Infantile eczema: a long-term follow-up study. Br J Dermatol 95:365–372, 1967.
10. WC Stiftler. A 21 year follow-up of infantile eczema. J Pediatr 66:166–169, 1965.
11. K Ishizaka, T Ishizaka. Identification of γE antibodies as carrier of reaginic activity. J Immunol 99:1187–1198, 1967.
12. SGO Johansson. Raised levels of a new immunoglobulin (IgND) in asthma. Lancet 2:951–953, 1967.
13. L Juhlin, SGO Johansson, H Bennich, C Högman, N Thyresson. Immunoglobulin E in dermatoses: levels in atopic dermatitis and urticaria. Arch Derm 100:12–16, 1969.

14. M Ogawa, PA Berger, OR McIntyre, WE Clendenning, Hanover NH, Ishizaka K. IgE in atopic dermatitis. Arch Derm 103:575–580, 1971.

15. B Wüthrich, H Storck, P Grob, M Schwarz-Speck. Zur Immunpathologie der Neurodermitis. Arch Derm Forsch 244:327–332, 1972.

16. DR Hoffman, FY Yamamoto, B Geller, Z Haddid Z. Specific IgE antibodies in atopic eczema. J Allergy Clin Imm 55:256–267, 1974.

17. S Öhman, SGO Johansson. Allergen-specific IgE in atopic dermatiitis. Acta Dermat Venerol (Stockh) 54:283–290, 1974.

18. B Wüthrich. Allergen-spezifische IgE im Radio-Allergo-Sorbens-Test bei Neurodermitis. Hautarzt 25:603–605, 1974.

19. WE Clendenning, WE Clack, M Ogawa, K Ishizaka K. Serum IgE studies in atopic dermatitis. J Invest Derm 61:233–236, 1973.

20. B Wüthrich, E Kopper, Chr Virchow. IgE-Bestimmungen bei Neurodermitis und anderen Dermatosen. Hautarzt 24:381–384, 1973.

21. B Wüthrich. Zur Immunpathologie der Neurodermitis constitutionalis. Eine klinisch-immunologische Studie mit besonderer Berücksichtigung der Immunglobuline E und der spezifischen Reagine im zeitlichen Verlauf. Bern: Hans Huber, 1975, pp 92–124.

22. B Wüthrich. Serum IgE in atopic dermatitis. Relationship to severity of cutaneous involvement and course of disease as well as coexistence of atopic respiratory diseases. Clin Allergy 8:241–248, 1978.

23. R Patterson. Laboratory models of reaginic allergy. Prog Allergy 13:332–407, 1969.

24. SL Spector, RS Farr. Atopy reconsidered. Clin Allergy 6:83–90, 1976.

25. FC Lowell. ''Asthma,'' ''rhinitis'' and ''atopy'' reconsidered. N Engl J Med 300:669–670, 1979.

26. HC Williams. Epidemiology of atopic dermatitis: recent advances and future predictions. In: B. Wüthrich, ed. The Atopy Syndrome in the Third Millennium. Basel: S. Karger, 1999, pp 9–17.

27. JM Hanifin, G Rajka. Diagnostic features of atopic dermatitis. Acta Derm Venereol (Stockh) 92 (suppl):44–47, 1980.

28. TL Diepgen, M Fartsch, OP Hornstein. Evaluation and relevance of atopic basic and minor features in patients with atopic dermatitis and in the general population. Acta Derm Venerol (Stockh) 144:50–54, 1989.

29. HC Williams, AC Pembrokle, PGF Burney, H Forsdyke, S Boodoo, RJ Hay. Community validation of the UK Working Party's diagnostic criteria for atopic dermatitis. Br J Dermatol 135:12–17, 1996.

30. F Schultz Larsen, T Diepgen, A Svensonn. Clinical criteria in diagnosing AD. The Lillehammer criteria 1994. In: G. Rajka, ed. Contributions and discussion presented at the 5th International Symposium on Atopic Dermatitis. May 22–25, 1994, Lillehammer, Norway. Acta Derm Venerol (Stockh) 76(suppl. 196):115–119, 1996.

31. A Basex, A Dupré, B Christol. Aspects morphologiques atypiques de l' eczéma atopique. Rev Med 1:62, 1966.

32. MJ Racouchot. Les petits signes cliniques du terrain eczémateux. Bull Soc Dermatol Syphiligr 73:531–535, 1966.

33. P Temime, L Oddoze. La chéilite exfoliatrice et la pulpite digitale craquelée récidi-

vante peuvent être des manifestations atopiques. Bull Soc Dermatol Syphiligr 77: 150–156, 1970.

34. J Herzberg. Wenig bekannte Formen der Neurodermitis. Hautarzt 24:47–51, 1973.

35. B Wüthrich. Minimal forms of atopic eczema. In: T Ruzicka, J Ring, B Przybilla, eds. Handbook of Atopic Eczema. Berlin: Springer, 1991, pp 46–53.

36. B Przybilla. Stigmata of the atopic constitution. In: T Ruzicka, J Ring, B Przybilla, eds. Handbook of Atopic Eczema. Berlin: Springer, 1991, pp 29–45.

37. N Mygind, R Dahl, S Pedersen, K Thestrup-Pedersen. Atopic diseases. Atopic dermatitis, allergic rhinitis and asthma. In: Essential Allergy. 2nd ed. Oxford: Blackwell Science, 1996, p 63.

38. B Wüthrich. Neurodermitis atopica sive constitutionalis. Ein pathogenetisches Modell aus der Sicht des Allergologen. Akt Dermatol 9:1–7, 1983.

39. G Rajka, A Giannetti, B Wüthrich. Atopic dermatitis. In: E Orfanos, R Stadler, H Gollnick, eds. Dermatology in Five Continents. Berlin: Springer, 1988, pp 280–285.

40. B Wüthrich. Atopic dermatitis flare provoked by inhalant allergens. Dermatologica 178:51–53, 1989.

41. ETAC Study Group. Determinants of total and specific IgE in infants with atopic dermatitis. Pediatr Allergy Immunol 8:177–184, 1997.

42. B Wüthrich, A Benz, F Skvaril. IgE and IgG₄ levels in children with atopic dermatitis. Dermatologica 166:229–235, 1983.

43. B Wüthrich, Chr Schindler, TC Medici, J-P Zellweger, PH Leuenberger, SAPAL-DIA-Team. IgE levels, atopy marker and hay fever in relation to age, sex and smoking status in a normal adult Swiss population. Int Arch Allergy Immunol 111:396–402, 1996.

44. DU Kalinke, B. Wüthrich. Clinical and allergologic-immunologic parameters in patients with atopic dermatitis. A prospective study (1989–1997) (abstr). Dermatology 195:191, 1997.

45. ETAC Study Group. Allergic factors associated with the development of asthma and the influence of cetirizine in a double-blind, randomized, placebo-controlled trial: First results of ETAC. Pediatr Allergy Immunol 9:116–124, 1998.

46. B Wüthrich. Clinical aspects, epidemiology, and prognosis of atopic dermatitis. Ann Allergy Asthma Immunol 83:464–470, 1999.

47. C Walker, MK Kägi, P Ingold, P Braun, K Blaser, B Wüthrich. Atopic dermatitis: correlation of peripheral blood T cell activation, eosinophilia and serum factors with clinical severity. Clin Exp Allergy 23:45–153, 1993.

48. MK Kägi, B Wüthrich, E Montano, J Barandun, K Blaser, C Walker. Differential cytokine profiles in peripheral blood lymphocyte supernatants and skin biopsies from patients with different forms of atopic dermatitis, psoriasis and normal individuals. Int Arch Allergy Immunol 103:332–340, 1994.

49. N Cabon, G Ducombs, P Mortureux, M Perromat, A Taieb. Contact allergy to aeroallergens in children with atopic dermatitis: comparison with allergic contact dermatitis. Contact Dermatitis 35:27–32, 1996.

50. B Wedi, U Raap, A Kapp. Significant delay of apoptosis and Fas resistance in eosinophils of subjects with intrinsic and extrinsic type of atopic dermatitis. Int Arch Allergy Immunol 118:234–235, 1999.

51. T Schafer, J Heinrich, M Wjst, H Adam, J Ring, HE Wichmann. Association be-

tween severity of atopic eczema and degree of sensitization to aeroallergens in schoolchildren. J Allergy Clin Immunol 104:1280–1284, 1999.

52. CA Akdis, M Akdis, D Simon, B Dibbert, M Weber, S Gratzl, O Kreyden, R Disch, B Wüthrich, K Blaser, HU Simon. T cells and T cell-derived cytokines as pathogenic factors in the nonallergic form of atopic dermatitis. J Invest Dermatol 113:628–634, 1999.

53. G Fabrizi, A Romano, P Vultaggio, S Bellegrandi, R Paganelli, A Venuti. Heterogeneity of atopic dermatitis defined by the immune response to inhalant and food allergens. Eur J Dermatol 9:380–384, 1999.

54. T Oppel, E Schuller, S Günther, M Moderer, J Haberstok, T Bieber, A Wollenberg. Phenotyping of epidermal dendritic cells allows the differentiation between extrinsic and intrinsic forms of atopic dermatitis. Br J Dermatol 143:1193–1198, 2000.

55. T Schäfer, U. Krämer, D Vieluf, D Abek, H Behrendt, J Ring. The excess of atopic eczema in east Germany is related to the intrinsic type. Br J Dermatol 143:992–998, 2000.

56. M Bradley, I Kockum, C Söderhäll, M Van Hage-Hamsten, H Luthman. Characterization by phenotype of families with atopidermatitis. Acta Derm Venerol (Stockh) 80:106–110, 2000.

57. T Werfel, A Kapp. What do we know about the etiopathology of the intrinsic type of atopic dermatitis? In: B Wüthrich, ed. The Atopy Syndrome in the Third Millennium Curr Probl Dermatol 28:29–36, 1999.

58. M Tengvall Linder, C Johansson, A Zargari, A Bengtsson, I van der Ploeg, I Jones, B Harfast, A Scheynius. Detection of *Pityrosporum orbiculare* reactive T cells from skin and blood in atopic dermatitis and characterization of their cytokine profiles. Clin Exp Allergy 26:1286–1297, 1996.

59. E Jensen-Jarolim, LK Poulsen, H With, M Kieffer, V Ottevanger, P Stahl Skov. Atopic dermatitis of the face, scalp, and neck: type I reaction to the yeast *Pityrosporum ovale*? J Allergy Clin Immunol 89:44–51, 1992.

60. CA Akdis, M Akdis, A Trautmann, K Blaser. Immune regulation in atopic dermatitis. Curr Opin Immunol 12:641–648, 2000.

61. FC van Reijsen, CA Bruijnzeel-Koomen, FS Kalthoff, E Maggi, S Romagnani, JK Westland, GC Mudde. Skin-derived aeroallergen-specific T-cell clones of Th2 phenotype in patients with atopic dermatitis. J Allergy Clin Immunol 90:184–193, 1992

62. KJ Abernathy-Carver, HA Sampson, LJ Picker, DY Leung. Milk-induced eczema is associated with the expansion of T cells expressing cutaneous lymphocyte antigen. J Clin Invest. 95:913–918, 1995.

63. M Akdis, CA Akdis, L Weigl, R Disch, K Blaser. Skin-homing, CLA+ memory T cells are activated in atopic dermatitis and regulate IgE by an IL-13-dominated cytokine pattern: IgG4 counter-regulation by CLA-memory T cells. J Immunol 159:4611–4619, 1997.

64. M Akdis, HU Simon, L Weigl, O Kreyden, K Blaser, CA Akdis. Skin homing (cutaneous lymphocyte-associated antigen-positive) CD8+ T cells respond to superantigen and contribute to eosinophilia and IgE production in atopic dermatitis. J Immunol 163:466–475, 1999.

65. LF Santamaria Babi, LJ Picker, MT Perez Soler, K Drzimalla, P Flohr, K Blaser, C Hauser. Circulating allergen-reactive T cells from patients with atopic dermatitis

and allergic contact dermatitis express the skin-selective homing receptor, the cutaneous lymphocyte-associated antigen. J Exp Med 181:1935–1940, 1995.

66. DB Corry, F Kheradmand. Induction and regulation of the IgE response. Nature 402:B18–23, 1999.

67. Q Hamid, M Boguniewicz, DY Leung. Differential in situ cytokine gene expression in acute versus chronic atopic dermatitis. J Clin Invest 94:870–876, 1994.

68. A Trautmann, M Akdis, D Kleemann, F Altznauer, HU Simon, T Graeve, M Noll, EB Brocker, K Blaser, CA Akdis. T cell-mediated Fas-induced keratinocyte apoptosis plays a key pathogenetic role in eczematous dermatitis. J Clin Invest 106: 25–35, 2000.

69. C Bruijnzeel-Koomen, E Storz, G Menz, P Bruijnzeel. Skin eosinophilia in patients with allergic and nonallergic asthma and atopic dermatitis. J Allergy Clin Immunol 89:52–59, 1992.

70. HU Simon, S Yousefi, C Schranz, A Schapowal, C Bachert, K Blaser. Direct demonstration of delayed eosinophil apoptosis as a mechanism causing tissue eosinophilia. J Immunol 158:3902–3908, 1997.

71. KM Leiferman, SJ Ackerman, HA Sampson, HS Haugen, PY Venencie, GJ Gleich. Dermal deposition of eosinophil-granule major basic protein in atopic dermatitis. Comparison with onchocerciasis. N Engl J Med 313:282–285, 1985.

72. N Yawalkar, M Uguccioni, J Scharer, J Braunwalder, S Karlen, B Dewald, LR Braathen, M Baggiolini. Enhanced expression of eotaxin and CCR3 in atopic dermatitis. J Invest Dermatol 113:43–48, 1999.

73. L Horsmanheimo, IT Harvima, A Jarvikallio, RJ Harvima, A Naukkarinen, M Horsmanheimo. Mast cells are one major source of interleukin-4 in atopic dermatitis. Br J Dermatol 131:348–353, 1994.

74. A Jarvikallio, A Naukkarinen, IT Harvima, ML Aalto, M Horsmanheimo. Quantitative analysis of tryptase- and chymase-containing mast cells in atopic dermatitis and nummular eczema. Br J Dermatol 136:871–877, 1997.

75. T Bieber, B Dannenberg, JC Prinz, EP Rieber, W Stolz, O Braun-Falco, J Ring. Occurrence of IgE-bearing epidermal Langerhans cells in atopic eczema: a study of the time course of the lesions and with regard to the IgE serum level. J Invest Dermatol 93:215–219, 1989.

76. T Bieber. Fc epsilon Rl-expressing antigen-presenting cells: new players in the atopic game. Immunol Today 18:311–313, 1997.

77. D Maurer, S Fiebiger, C Ebner, B Reininger, GF Fischer, S Wichlas, MH Jouvin, M Schmitt-Egenolf, D Kraft, JP Kinet, G Stingl. Peripheral blood dendritic cells express Fc epsilon Rl as a complex composed of Fc epsilon Rl alpha- and Fc epsilon Rl gamma-chains and can use this receptor for IgE-mediated allergen presentation. J Immunol 157:607–616, 1996.

78. A Wollenberg, S Wen, T Bieber. Langerhans cell phenotyping: a new tool for differential diagnosis of inflammatory skin diseases [letter]. Lancet 346:1626–1627, 1995.

79. JD Bos, EJM Leent, JH Sillevis Smitt. The millenium criteria for the diagnosis of atopic dermatitis. Exp Dermatol 7:132–138, 1998.

80. Japanese Dermatological Association Criteria for the diagnosis of atopic dermatitis. J Dermatol 24:opposite to page 561, 1996.

81. M Uehara, S Ofuji. Atopic dermatitis. A discussion of theories concerning its pathogenesis. J Dermatol 7:231–238, 1980.
82. M Uehara. Heterogeneity of serum IgE levels in atopic dermatitis. Acta Derm Venereol (Stockh) 66:404–408, 1986.
83. M Uehara. Family background of respiratory atopy: a factor of serum IgE elevation in atopic dermatitis. Acta Derm Venereol (Stockh) Suppl 144:787–782, 1989.
84. S Imayama, T Hashizume, H Miyahara, T Tanahashi, M Takeishi, Y Kubota, T Koga, Y Hori, H Fukuda. Combination of patch test and IgE for dust mite antigens differentiates 130 patients with atopic dermatitis. J Am Acad Dermatol 27:531–538, 1992.
85. M Tanaka, S Aiba, N Matsumara, H Aoyama, N Tabata, Y Sekita, H Tagami. IgE-mediated hypersensitivity and contact sensitivity to multiple environmental allergens in atopic dermatitis. Arch Dermatol 130:1393–1401, 1994.
86. B Wüthrich. What is atopy? Condition, disease or a syndrome? In: B Wüthrich, ed. The Atopy Syndrome in the Third Millennium. Basel: S. Karger, 1999, pp 1–8.

2
Epidemiology

Carolyn R. Charman and Hywel C. Williams
University Hospital, Nottingham, United Kingdom

I. INTRODUCTION: WHAT IS EPIDEMIOLOGY?

The aim of this chapter is to review the way in which the concepts and methods of epidemiology have been applied to the study of atopic dermatitis to advance our knowledge and understanding of the disease. The science of epidemiology involves the study of the distribution and determinants of disease in specified populations and the application of this study to control of health problems (1). It involves a study of patterns of disease in whole populations in order to allow a broad understanding of etiology and natural history that cannot be gained from the study of individuals alone. The basic principles of epidemiology are to describe the distribution and burden of disease in human populations, to identify etiological factors of the disease, and to provide data essential for the evaluation and planning of services for prevention, control, and treatment of the disease. The findings of such research are not only essential for public health planning, they can contribute greatly to the scientific basis of routine clinical practice and individual patient care.

Epidemiological research can provide a natural foundation for the study of chronic diseases such as atopic dermatitis. In the past much research into atopic dermatitis has been directed around the cellular and immunological mechanisms of the disease. It is only over the last 10 years that epidemiological studies of atopic dermatitis have started to flourish. This recent research has generated important information on disease frequency and provided clues about genetic and environmental risk factors, as well as highlighting associated morbidity and costs to patients and health providers.

This chapter will describe our current knowledge of the distribution and frequency of atopic dermatitis worldwide and review recent advances in our understanding of the natural history of the disease. It is important to note that although research into causes and risk factors for disease forms a key element of epidemiological work,. these are covered in detail in Chapter 6 and will not be discussed here.

In order to ensure that information covered in this chapter is up to date, the authors carried out an electronic literature search of Medline (1966 to August 2000) and Embase (1977 to August 2000), using the key search terms "atopic dermatitis," "atopic eczema," "eczema," "prevalence," "incidence," and "epidemiology." Articles for which an English translation was not available were not considered, which inevitably leads to some degree of bias, although based on the extensive body of literature identified it is hoped that the chapter provides a general overview of past and recent epidemiological research into atopic dermatitis.

II. PREVALENCE AND INCIDENCE

There are many difficulties in providing an overall estimate of atopic dermatitis frequency, as studies have differed greatly in methodology, measuring disease frequency over different time periods, in different age groups, using different techniques of data collection and different diagnostic criteria. The effect of these various factors on the measurement of disease frequency are discussed below.

A. Defining Atopic Dermatitis

Variations in disease definition have made epidemiological studies of atopic dermatitis particularly difficult to interpret and compare. Patients typically present a spectrum of disease distribution, morphology, and severity, along with a variable time course of disease activity. This means that it is not always easy to say whether or not patients definitely have atopic dermatitis at any specified time point, particularly those at the end of the spectrum. Researchers have used a variety of methods to define the presence of disease. Some questionnaire-based surveys have relied on maternal reporting of "eczema" (although the accuracy of parental diagnosis remains unclear), while others have measured those with a history of doctor-diagnosed atopic dermatitis (which may depend on the knowledge and experience of the physician). Other questionnaires have recorded a variety of patient symptoms to establish the diagnosis. Even those studies based on examination by a dermatologist have used various combinations of signs and symptoms to aid diagnosis, reflecting different ideas about what constitutes a typical case of atopic dermatitis.

Although there is no definitive gold standard disease definition, various well-established diagnostic criteria have been developed, both to improve diagnostic accuracy and to aid in the comparison of results from different studies (2,3). These diagnostic criteria are discussed in detail in Chapter 1. The development of Hanifin and Rajka's diagnostic criteria in 1980 (2) represented an important milestone for atopic dermatitis research, but their complexity has limited their use in large-scale epidemiological studies. Furthermore, they were derived largely from experience with the more severe subset of patients attending hospitals, whereas epidemiological studies are often carried out in the community among patients with less severe disease. The UK Working Party's diagnostic criteria developed in 1990 have provided a more simple list of reliable disease criteria based on the original proposal by Hanifin and Rajka (3). The six diagnostic criteria have been independently validated and tested for repeatability (4,5). In order to capture the episodic nature of atopic dermatitis and minimize the effect of possible seasonal variations, the criteria have been developed as a 12-month period prevalence measure.

B. Measuring Disease Frequency

The most common measure of disease frequency in epidemiological research is disease prevalence, defined as the total number of cases in the population under study. Disease prevalence can be measured at any one point in time (point prevalence) or over a defined period, e.g., one year (period prevalence). Prevalence estimates provide useful information about the total *burden* of disease in a population. The majority of epidemiological studies have examined disease prevalence in the community because surveys of disease prevalence in hospital clinics or private practices are subject to referral bias. Prevalence measurements usually involve a cross-sectional study design, and much of the data on atopic dermatitis has arisen from questionnaire surveys in schools. Point prevalence measurements using clinical examination are potentially more accurate but rely on subjects having active eczema at the time of examination. One-year period prevalence measurements are probably the most useful for comparative purposes as they take into account the relapsing and remitting nature of the disease while minimizing the recall bias of lifetime prevalence estimates.

Much harder to obtain are incidence figures that provide information on the number of new cases developing over a period of time (e.g., one year). Incidence data provide a more precise insight into changes in disease frequency over time and minimize the risk of recall bias. However, measuring atopic dermatitis incidence usually requires a cohort study design, and such longitudinal studies are costly and time-consuming to perform. Furthermore, measuring new cases may be difficult because disease chronicity is often quoted as a major diagnostic feature of atopic dermatitis, and it is sometimes difficult to decide whether a child

Table 1 Summary of Studies Measuring Prevalence of Atopic Dermatitis in 1990s

Country (Ref.)	Prevalence (%)	No. in study	Measurements and definitions	Age group	Year
Finland (6)	9.7	1712	12-month period prevalence (questionnaire—symptoms)	15–16 years	1990
Germany (7)	12.9	1273	Point prevalence (dermatologist's examination)	5–7 years	1991
Norway (8)	23.6	551	Lifetime prevalence (questionnaire—symptoms)	7–12 years	1991
UK (9)	14.0	322	Point prevalence (history/examination by trained observer)	1–4 years	1992
Denmark (10)	22.9	437	Lifetime prevalence (questionnaire)	7 years	1992
Germany (10)	13.1	1164	Lifetime prevalence (questionnaire)	7 years	1992
Sweden (10)	15.5	1054	Lifetime prevalence (questionnaire)	7 years	1992
Germany (11)	14.9	2402	Lifetime prevalence (questionnaire—symptoms)	5–14 years	1992
	2.6	2200	Point prevalence (dermatologist's examination)		
Hong Kong (12)	20.1	1062	Lifetime prevalence (questionnaire—symptoms)	11–20 years	1992
Malaysia (12)	7.6	409	Lifetime prevalence (questionnaire—symptoms)		
China (12)	7.2	737	Lifetime prevalence (questionnaire—symptoms)		
Norway (13)	23	424	Point prevalence (dermatologist's examination)	7–12 years	1992
	37	424	Lifetime prevalence (interview)		
UK (14)	10.7	413	Point prevalence (dermatologist's examination)	1 year	1993
	15.5	413	12-month period prevalence (interview—symptoms)		
Turkey (15)	5.0	1334	Lifetime prevalence (questionnaire—doctor diagnosis)	6–14 years	1993
UK (16)	11.7	693	Point prevalence (dermatologist's examination)	3–11 years	1994
Germany (17)	11.3	1511	Point prevalence (dermatologist's examination)	5–6 years	1994
Russia (18)	5.9	3368	Lifetime prevalence (questionnaire about symptoms)	Adults	1994

Turkey (19)	2.2	5412	Lifetime prevalence (questionnaire—doctor diagnosis)	7–12 years	1994
	0.9	5412	12-month period prevalence (questionnaire—doctor diagnosis)		1994
Japan (20)	24	994	Point prevalence (dermatologist's examination)	5–6 years	1994
	19	1240	Point prevalence (dermatologist's examination)	7–9 years	1994
	15	1152	Point prevalence (dermatologist's examination)	10–12 years	1995
	14	1670	Point prevalence (dermatologist's examination)	13–15 years	1995
Japan (21)	14.2	1378	Point prevalence (Japanese Dermatological Association Diagnostic Criteria)	Elementary schools	1995
Norway (22)	19.6	8676	Lifetime prevalence (questionnaire)	7–13 years	1995
	5.2	8676	12-month period prevalence (questionnaire)		1995
UK (23)	2.3	9786	12-month period prevalence (medical records and examination)	All ages	1995
UK (24)	8.5	695	Point prevalence (dermatologist's examination)	3–11 years	1995
	5.9	695	Point prevalence (UK Working Party Diagnostic Criteria)		1995
Japan (20)	11	2159	Point prevalence (dermatologist's examination)	16–18 years	1996
UK (25)	16.5	1523	12-month period prevalence (history/dermatologist's examination)	1–5 years	1996
UK (26)	14.2	260	Point prevalence (dermatologist's examination)	4 years	1996
	12.3	260	UK Working Party Diagnostic Criteria (dermatologist's examination)		1996
Turkey (27)	4.3	738	12-month prevalence (questionnaire—doctor diagnosis)	6–13 years	1997
	6.5	738	Lifetime prevalence (questionnaire—doctor diagnosis)		1997
Australia (28)	16.3	2491	Point prevalence (dermatologist's examination)	4–18 years	1997
	10.8	2491	UK Working Party's Diagnostic Criteria (dermatologist's examination)		1997
Romania (29)	2.4	1114	Point prevalence (dermatologist's examination)	6–12 years	1997
	1.8	1114	UK Working Party Diagnostic Criteria (dermatologist's examination)		1997
USA (30)	17.2	1465	Lifetime prevalence (questionnaire—symptoms)	5–9 years	2000

developing eczematous inflammation for the first time will go on to develop the disease. Rather than describing the number of new cases per year, some studies have reported cumulative incidence, defined as the number of new cases developing since birth over a defined period. However, such studies have often relied on patients' recall of ever having had eczema at a certain age rather than being based on a prospective study design. A commonly used measure is cumulative lifetime incidence, which is synonymous with lifetime prevalence, although the latter term is preferable when data have been collected retrospectively.

III. HOW COMMON IS ATOPIC DERMATITIS?

Taking into account these difficulties, prevalence estimates taken from studies of varying methodology over the last 10 years are shown in Table 1 (6–30). The majority of studies have been carried out in children with lifetime prevalence figures in temperate developed countries ranging from 13 to 37% up until early adolescence. Point prevalence figures are lower, partly reflecting the fluctuating nature of the disease. The few studies of adults have shown lower prevalence rates of 0.2–2% in temperate developed countries such as the United Kingdom (23).

In order to compare the prevalence of atopic dermatitis on a more global scale using standardized methodology, a worldwide cross-sectional survey known as the International Study of Asthma and Allergies in Childhood (ISAAC) has been recently reported (31). Most previous surveys of atopic dermatitis prevalence had been conducted in northern Europe, giving the impression that the disease mainly occurs in developed countries in cooler climates. The ISAAC study comprised a questionnaire survey conducted on random samples of school children aged 6–7 years and 13–14 years from centers in 56 countries throughout the world. Children with a positive response to questions about the presence of an itchy relapsing skin rash in the last 12 months that had affected their skin creases were considered to have atopic dermatitis (Table 2). This study generated complete data for 256,410 children aged 6–7 years in 90 centers and 458,623

Table 2 Questions Relating to Eczema Symptoms Used in International Study of Asthma and Allergies in Childhood (ISAAC), Phase 1

1. Have you (Has your child) ever had an itchy rash that was coming and going for at least 6 months?
2. Have you (Has your child) had this itchy rash at any time in the last 12 months?
3. Has this itchy rash at any time affected any of the following places: the folds of the elbows, behind the knees, in front of the ankles, under the buttocks, or around the neck, ears, or eyes?

children aged 13–14 years in 153 centers. The 12-month period prevalence estimates for the 6 to 7 year age group ranged from under 2% in Iran to over 16% in Japan and Sweden. In the 13- to 14-year age group, disease prevalence ranged from less than 1% in Albania to over 17% in Nigeria (Fig. 1). Many of these variations cannot be completely explained by known risk factors or established hypotheses concerning the disease. Although the results of the ISAAC study still need to be validated with more objective measures such as skin examination (as will occur in Phase 2 of the study), it has provided much-needed basic information about the distribution of the disease and has confirmed that atopic dermatitis is a worldwide problem rather than being a disease confined to northern and western Europe.

IV. DISEASE SEVERITY

Overall prevalence data may include many mild or asymptomatic cases. In public health terms the severity distribution of atopic dermatitis is of greater importance than total prevalence because this is more likely to closely reflect the need for health services. As with the diagnosis of atopic dermatitis, there are numerous methods of measuring disease severity. Epidemiological studies that have included a measurement of disease severity have generally used simple scales such as Rajka and Langeland's scoring system (32) or global severity estimates undertaken by the assessor. Some studies have graded severity according to the percentage of body surface area involved, although this may not provide an accurate reflection of patient morbidity because involvement of small but functionally or cosmetically important sites such as the hands and face can be extremely disabling. More complex measures such as Costa's scoring system (33) and the SCORAD index (34) are generally too complex and time-consuming for large epidemiological studies, although the SCORAD index been used successfully in one large cross-sectional multicenter survey (17).

Overall data from epidemiological studies in many countries has shown that the majority of cases of atopic dermatitis can be managed in primary care, with between 65 and 90% of cases in the community being of mild severity and only 1–2% or less being classified as severe. In a recent survey of Australian school students aged 4–18 years, 86% were classified as minimal to mild on clinical examination (28), and among U.K. preschool children 84% were classified as mild by a dermatologist (25). A recent study of Romanian school children showed that 93% were very mild or mild (29), and in Japanese kindergarten and school children between 81 and 87% were classified as mild depending on age (20). In a further study of Norwegian school children two thirds showed mild and one third moderate symptoms, with less than 0.01% having severe disease confirmed by clinical examination (13). Although data relating disease severity

Charman and Williams

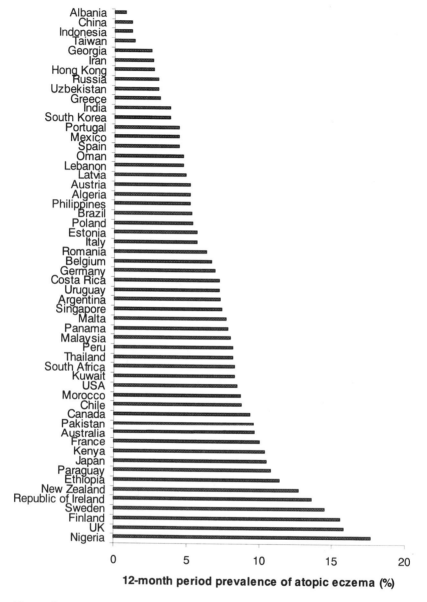

Figure 1 Summary of 12-month period prevalences for atopic dermatitis from the International Study of Asthma and Allergies in Childhood (ISAAC), Phase 1.

to age is sparse, adults with atopic eczema are less likely to be in remission and more likely to have active disease when examined than children (23).

V. MORBIDITY

The physical impact of atopic eczema depends on the severity of the disease and can range from annoying dryness to severely itchy skin with painful cracking, weeping, and secondary infection. Studies suggest that 60–90% of children suffer from sleep disturbance secondary to the severe pruritus usually associated with the disease (35,36). Sleep disturbance and constant scratching may trigger other psychological and social problems, especially in children. Irritability and lack of concentration can lead to detrimental effects on schooling, educational development, and social interactions. Furthermore, the stigmata of a visible skin disease can lead to teasing and bullying (37,38). Higher levels of dependency and clinginess have been found in children attending hospital outpatient clinics for their atopic dermatitis (39). The stress of caring for a child with eczema can have profound effects on all family members, especially for mothers of severely affected children, who have been shown to have higher stress levels than mothers of healthy control children (39).

Compared to other skin diseases atopic dermatitis rates highly on morbidity scores designed to capture the impact of disease on aspects of everyday life (40). In the past much of the emphasis in atopic dermatitis research has been on the measurement of physical signs, although the concept of measuring disease-related disability and quality of life is being increasingly recognized and will be discussed fully in the next chapter.

VI. WHO GETS IT?

A. Age

Atopic dermatitis is predominantly a disease of childhood, as reflected in the prevalence data in Table 1. Prevalence estimates show a continuous reduction with increasing age (20,23). A recent Norwegian study based on review of medical records found a prevalence of atopic dermatitis of 13% in patients under the age of 20 years compared to 2% for those over the age of 20 years (41). In the United Kingdom 2% of adults aged 16–40 years and less than 0.2% of adults over the age of 40 years are affected (23). Adult atopic dermatitis has been relatively ignored in epidemiological research. However, in developed countries adults make up approximately 80% of the population, meaning that up to a third of all subjects with the disease are adults (23). Furthermore, there is evidence that the number of adults presenting to hospital with the disease is increasing in some countries (42).

B. Sex

Although overall no strong relationship with sex has been demonstrated, a slight female preponderance has been demonstrated in some studies (7,8,13,23,28, 30,43), but not in others (11,14,19,41). A small female preponderance was also noted in the ISAAC study with an overall female:male ratio of 1.3:1, being higher in countries with the highest prevalence of atopic dermatitis symptoms. Interestingly in children under the age of 2 years this difference is not observed and the ratio may even be reversed (13,23), suggesting that increased disease chronicity in females may be partly responsible.

C. Ethnicity

Various studies have examined the effect of ethnic group on the prevalence of atopic dermatitis. It is difficult to draw conclusions about ethnic differences in prevalences by examining results from different countries because environmental factors may contribute to any differences seen. Therefore, studies of different ethnic groups in the same environment are particularly helpful. In the United Kingdom atopic dermatitis prevalence is similar in Asian schoolchildren compared to non-Asian schoolchildren (mainly European Caucasian), although Asian patients are three times more likely to be referred to the local dermatology department, perhaps due to less familiarity with the disease (9,14). However, atopic dermatitis is almost twice as common in black Caribbean schoolchildren born in the United Kingdom than their white counterparts (16). Similarly, the disease is more prevalent among Chinese infants born in the United States compared to local Caucasians (44). In Australia the 12-month cumulative incidence of atopic dermatitis is much higher in Chinese babies (44%) compared to Caucasians living under similar environmental conditions (21%) (45). In Norway atopic eczema is more prevalent in schoolchildren of Sami origin compared to Norse white Caucasian schoolchildren (22).

D. Socioeconomic Status

Atopic dermatitis shows a strong relationship to social class, but in contrast to many diseases it is significantly more common in higher social class groups (45–48). The disease is also more frequent in children from smaller families (49) and in those from privately owned properties rather than council rented properties (50). A variety of factors relating to education, lifestyle, type of home furnishing and degree of cross-infection could be responsible for this effect.

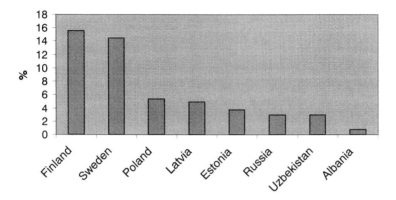

Figure 2   The 12-month period prevalence of atopic dermatitis among 13- to 14-year-old children from northeast Europe participating in the International Study of Asthma and Allergies in Childhood (ISAAC).

The socioeconomic gradient can also be seen on a wider scale, with disease prevalence being generally higher in more affluent countries with a westernized lifestyle and market economy (12,31). A comparison of disease prevalence in northern and eastern Europe (Fig. 2) shows a higher prevalence of atopic dermatitis in industrialized countries such as Scandinavia, compared to the western part of the formally disadvantaged socialist region, e.g., Estonia, Latvia, and Poland, with the lowest frequency in former socialist countries with a lifestyle even more different from that in western Europe, such as Albania.

E.   Other Factors

Atopic dermatitis is significantly more prevalent in those with a personal or family history of atopy. The role of genetic factors and other risk factors in disease expression will be discussed fully in Chapters 5 and 6.

VII.   WHERE DOES IT OCCUR?

A.   International Variation

Describing the geographical occurrence of disease comprises a basic component of epidemiological research and can lead to the identification of many important risk factors. Although the lack of standardized methodology has been a significant obstacle in comparing international data, research suggests large geographical variations in atopic dermatitis prevalence both within and between countries (Table 1). The most comprehensive and standardized comparisons can be made from the ISAAC study, which found a 60-fold variation in prevalence between the 56 countries studied, with 12-month prevalences ranging from 0.3 to 20.5% (31). The study revealed some interesting patterns of disease frequency, such as a band of low prevalence running from China through central Asia to eastern Europe, and low prevalences throughout the former socialist eastern Europe. In contrast, very high prevalences were observed in developed countries such as Scandinavia, the United Kingdom, Japan, Australia, and New Zealand. The study also revealed that atopic dermatitis is a major problem in African cities such as Addis Ababa and Ibadan. Prior to this study there had been few epidemiological studies of atopic dermatitis in developing countries. Some caution must be taken in the interpretation of results in countries such as India and Nigeria where the sensitivity of the ISAAC questionnaire may have been reduced due to the high prevalence of other itchy dermatoses in childhood such as scabies and onchocerciasis. Interestingly the prevalence of eczema diagnosed by a doctor was also high in Nigeria (38.3%) (51). Interpretation of the ISAAC results also needs to take into account cultural factors such as differing thresholds for complaining about skin symptoms or an association of skin disease with stigmata of uncleanliness in some countries, which may have affected responses. Phases 2 and 3 of the ISAAC study will use more detailed questionnaires and objective measures to confirm the differences seen in Phase 1.

Another international study using standardized methodology has also found large variations in atopic dermatitis prevalence between genetically similar secondary school students in three different countries—Malaysia, China, and Hong Kong (Table 1) (12). As with the results of the ISAAC study, both genetic and environmental factors such as climate and air pollution may all contribute to these differences in disease prevalence, and these factors will be discussed further in Chapter 6.

B. Regional Variation

Wide regional variations in atopic dermatitis prevalence have been demonstrated across the United Kingdom, with higher prevalences in the southern and eastern areas of the country after adjustment for confounders such as social class (46,52). Several studies found a higher prevalence of atopic dermatitis in eastern Germany compared to western Germany (53–55). Higher prevalences of atopic dermatitis have also been noted in urban versus rural areas in the United States (30), Southeast Asia (12), Sweden (56), Finland (57), and Germany (7). On a smaller geographical scale the disease has also been associated with water hardness in a recent U.K. study (58). These regional differences highlight the potential role of a variety of environmental exposures that may be amenable to public health manipulation. The role of airborne pollutants, climatic factors, and water quality are all possible risk factors that may contribute to such regional variation.

C. Migrant Studies

The study of disease in migrant groups compared to genetically similar groups in their country of origin allows insight into the role of environmental factors in disease expression. Children from Tokelau who migrated to New Zealand have higher prevalences of atopic dermatitis compared to genetically similar children who remained in Tokelau (59). The risk of atopic dermatitis in Asian migrants is significantly larger for those born in Australia compared to those of the same age who have recently immigrated to Australia (60). There is some evidence that people from less developed countries who move to industrialized countries may become more vulnerable than the local population. For example, IgE levels are significantly higher in migrant Turks residing in Sweden than among similar Swedish residents, with levels declining with increasing periods of residence in the country (61). These studies suggest that environmental factors associated with urbanization and development may be important in the etiology of atopic dermatitis in genetically susceptible individuals. Furthermore, the timing of migration may play a critical role in the expression of the disease.

VIII. TIME TRENDS

A. Seasonal Trends

Many studies have focused attention on the importance of month of birth on subsequent development of atopic dermatitis. These studies have arisen from the hypothesis that exposure to seasonal allergens during the initial few months of life when the immune response is maturing may result in sensitization and subsequent disease. Some studies have suggested that infants born in the autumn have higher prevalences of atopic dermatitis compared to those born in the spring (62). However, other studies have found no significant association with month of birth (63,64).

The effect of seasonality on the expression of established atopic dermatitis has also been studied. Atopic dermatitis characteristically runs a relapsing and remitting course, and point prevalence measurements can be used to compare the prevalence of active disease in different seasons. A recent study in Japan found no significant difference in disease prevalence in school children examined in the spring and autumn, although half of the children showed symptoms in only one season (21). However, a recent questionnaire study of teenagers in Finland found distinct seasonal variation, with atopic dermatitis occurring most commonly in the winter and least commonly in the summer (6). The majority of patients with established eczema report deterioration in winter months and improvement in the summer. The extent to which these changes are related to the effects of centrally heated houses or to the immuno-modulatory effect of sunlight remains to be fully established.

B. Long-Term Trends

Epidemiological research suggests that the prevalence of atopic dermatitis has increased two- to threefold over the last 30–50 years (65,66). It is important to separate out real changes in disease frequency from secular changes in diagnosis or reporting over time. Changes in the acceptability of eczema as a diagnosis or changes in the medical use of the word eczema, along with improved diagnostic methods and higher parental awareness and expectations, may all have exaggerated the trends seen in recent years. However, the increased prevalence has been consistently observed in different studies, suggesting that at least some of the observed changes are due to a true change in disease frequency.

The increasing prevalence of atopic eczema has been reported mainly in developed countries. One of the most widely quoted epidemiological studies supporting an increasing prevalence has been the study of three British cohorts of children born in 1946, 1958, and 1970. The prevalence of a history of eczema determined when the children were aged between 5–7 years increased from 5.1% to 7.3% to 12.2% in children born in the three successive cohorts, respectively, although the results of the three cohorts were drawn from three separate studies using slightly different methodologies (48). A further study of atopic twins in Denmark has shown that the percentage of at-risk individuals who developed atopic dermatitis between 0–7 years rose from 3% for the 1960–64 birth cohort to 10% for the 1970–74 birth cohort (67). Another study from Sweden has shown that the prevalence of atopic dermatitis had increased from 7% to 18% in school children between 1979 and 1991 (68). In Japan there is evidence that the prevalence of atopic dermatitis has doubled in 9- to 12-year-olds and increased five times in 18-year-olds over the last 20 years (20). The increasing disease prevalence reported over the last three to five decades cannot be explained by genetic factors alone because the time span is too short to allow specific genetic selection. It may be that specific environmental changes have led to a shift in the distribution of latent atopic disease, with more genetically predisposed individuals going on to express the disease. Changes in environmental exposure to irritants, decreased exposure to infectious agents, changes in domestic house dust mite levels with increased indoor humidity, carpets, and soft furnishing, and increasing exposure to allergens in childhood and pregnancy have all been investigated as potential contributing factors. These risk factors will be discussed further in later chapters.

IX. NATURAL HISTORY

Much of the data on the natural history of atopic dermatitis has been generated from the hospital setting, with a paucity of long-term follow-up studies of community cases. Summaries of the percentage of cases of atopic dermatitis developing with age are clearly dependent on the age group studied, as surveys of very young children may include many who will later go on to develop the disease. Atopic dermatitis usually begins in infancy when it may be confused with seborrheic dermatitis (69). However, the former usually clears in the first year of life, whereas atopic dermatitis is characterized by a more chronic relapsing and remitting course. The distribution of atopic dermatitis may change early in life, from involvement of the scalp and face to involvement of the neck and flexures between 1 and 2 years of age (70). Age of onset in community cases of atopic eczema may be later than that reported in hospital-based studies. From the available epidemiological data approximately 70% of cases begin before the age of 5 years, suggesting that factors in early life may be crucial in determining disease expression (71). In a recent U.K. study, the disease developed within the first 6 months of life in 47.5% and within the first year of life in 60% of cases (72). The National Child Development Study (NCDS) is a U.K. birth cohort study of children born in March 1958 with cases of atopic eczema based on examination by a medical officer. Of the 870 cases with examined or reported eczema by the age of 16 years, 43% had onset before the age of 1 year and 66% had onset before the age of 7 years (73). In a study of 551 Norwegian children, the onset of eczema occurred before 1 year of age in 25% of children and before 5 years of age in 75% (8). A recent prospective study including a large number of high-risk infants (family history of atopic dermatitis and elevated IgE) showed a lifetime prevalence of 4.8, 8.7, 13, and 18% at 3, 6, 12, and 24 months of age, respectively (74,75).

Because there is currently no cure for atopic dermatitis, epidemiological data on clearance rates can be extremely helpful when it comes to making predictions about patients' long-term prognosis. It is generally agreed that a number of mild to moderate cases clear spontaneously in early life, although good prospective studies are lacking. Given the limitations of comparing research of varying methodology, examination of studies including representative cases (milder community cases as well as hospital patients) suggests clearance rates of approximately 60% by early adolescence (71,76). Data from the National Child Development Study (NCDS) have shown that at the age 11 and 16 years, 65 and 74% of children, respectively, are clear of their disease in terms of examined eczema or a history of eczema in the previous year (73). In a recent study of 260 children in the United Kingdom, of those who had atopic dermatitis at age 1 year, almost 50% no longer had the disease by age 4 years (26). Cessation of atopic dermatitis occurred in 13% before the age of 5 years and 17% before the age of 7 years in a recent interview study of 156 Norwegian children (13). However, it is not always easy to say whether the disease has resolved permanently because atopic eczema is characterized by a relapsing and remitting course, and recurrences in adult life are not uncommon (73,77). Such recurrences often occur on the hands and may be triggered by occupations such as food preparation, housework, or hairdressing. In the hospital setting approximately 10% of patients still suffer from eczema in adult life (78). The strongest and most consistent factors that appear to predict more persistent atopic dermatitis are early onset, severe widespread disease in early infancy, concomitant asthma or hay fever, and a family history of atopic dermatitis (71,76,79).

X. PRIMARY, SECONDARY, AND TERTIARY PREVENTION

One of the major goals of epidemiological research is to identify groups who are at high risk for the disease with the hope of modifying potential risk factors to prevent the disease. In this respect it is important to distinguish between primary, secondary, and tertiary prevention. Primary prevention refers to action taken to prevent the development of the disease in individuals who are free from the disease. Because atopic dermatitis usually begins in the first 5 years of life, there is potential for epidemiological research to identify prenatal or early life factors that may be involved in sensitization and development of the disease. This raises the real possibility of primary prevention, either by altering exposures during pregnancy or by the prevention of sensitization in early infancy. Much interest has been focused on the role of dietary factors, breast-feeding, the timing of introduction of potentially antigenic solid foods, and the reduction of house dust mite levels around the home. Several cohort studies are currently evaluating manipulation of such factors, especially in individuals at a genetically high risk of developing atopic disease. If simple manipulation of these factors can be shown to be important in the development of the disease, this would have huge health implications, but at the present time further research is still needed before primary prevention becomes a reality (80).

Secondary prevention refers to the identification of those who have already developed the disease at an early stage in its natural history, with the implication of intervention measures to reduce the associated morbidity and complications. Epidemiological research can help identify key genetic and environmental factors involved in disease expression, and manipulation of these factors may help to diminish the progression of established atopic dermatitis (81).

Tertiary prevention involves the treatment of established disease, which will be covered in detail in later chapters. A recent systematic review has summarized all the published data available from randomized controlled clinical trials of treatments for atopic dermatitis, covering more than 284 different trials (82). Unfortunately, prospective studies evaluating the effect of common treatments such as topical steroids on long-term disease progression are lacking. Most trials have been of less than 6-week duration, and while they may show beneficial effects in controlling the acute phase of the disease, they do not capture the chronic relapsing course or the long-term effects of treatment such as the number of disease-free periods per year. For many other commonly employed therapies such as emollients and wet wrap bandaging, there are as yet no randomized controlled trials.

XI. FUTURE RESEARCH AGENDA

The epidemiological developments of the last 20 years have provided a strong foundation on which to build our knowledge and understanding of this common and distressing skin condition. These advances have included the development of valid and reliable disease definitions, the production of a worldwide map of the disease in the ISAAC study, and developments in the understanding of the genetic basis of the disease from family and twin studies. As we begin a new millennium there remain a number of unanswered questions, and future research is desperately needed to fill in the gaps of knowledge identified by recent studies. In particular, further investigation is needed into the factors associated with the ''western'' lifestyle that seems so strongly associated with atopic eczema expression. Prospective cohort studies are required to examine how the incidence and natural history of the disease is changing with time. The challenge remains to identify factors that can be easily manipulated at a population level in order to prevent the inexorable increase in disease prevalence.

REFERENCES

1. JM Last. A Dictionary of Epidemiology. 2nd ed. New York: Oxford University Press, 1988.
2. JM Hanifin, G Rajka. Diagnostic features of atopic dermatitis. Acta Derm Venereol (Stockh) Suppl 92:44–47, 1980.
3. HC Williams, PGJ Burney, RJ Hay, CB Archer, MJ Shipley, JJA Hunter, EA Bingham, AY Finlay, AC Pembroke, RAC Graham-Brown, DA Atherton, MS Lewis-Jones, CA Holden, JI Harper, RH Champion, TF Poyner, J Launer, TJ David. The UK Working Party's diagnostic criteria for atopic dermatitis I. Derivation of a minimum set of discriminators for atopic dermatitis. Br J Dermatol 131:383–396, 1994.
4. HC Williams, PGJ Burney, AC Pembroke, RJ Hay. The UK Working Party's diagnostic criteria for atopic dermatitis III: independent hospital validation. Br J Dermatol 131:406–416, 1994.

5. HC Williams, PGJ Burney, D Strachan, RJ Hay. The UK Working Party's diagnostic criteria for atopic dermatitis II: observer variation of clinical diagnosis and signs of atopic dermatitis. Br J Dermatol 131:397–405, 1994.

6. E Varjonen, K Kalimo, K Lammintausta, P Terho. Prevalence of atopic disorders among adolescents in Turku, Finland. Allergy 47:243–248, 1992.

7. T Schäfer, D Vieluf, H Behrendt, U Krämer, J Ring. Atopic eczema and other manifestations of atopy: results of a study in East and West Germany. Allergy 51:532–539, 1996.

8. LK Dotterud, B Kvammen, R Bolle, E Falk. A survey of atopic disease among school children in Sør-Varanger community. Acta Derm Venereol (Stockh) 74:124–128, 1994.

9. RL Neame, J Berth-Jones, JJ Kurinczuk, RAC Graham-Brown. Prevalence of atopic dermatitis in Leicester: a study of methodology and examination of possible ethnic variation. Br J Dermatol 132:772–777, 1995.

10. F Schultz Larsen, T Diepgen, A Svensson. The occurrence of atopic dermatitis in northern Europe: an international questionnaire study. J Am Acad Dermatol 34:760–764, 1996.

11. T Schäfer, J Heinrich, M Wjst, C Krause, H Adam, J Ring, HE Wichmann. Indoor risk factors for atopic eczema in school children from East Germany. Environmental Research Section A 81:151–158, 1999.

12. R Leung, P Ho. Asthma, allergy and atopy in three south-east Asian populations. Thorax 49:1205–1210, 1994.

13. LK Dotterud, B Kvammen, E Lund, E Falk. Prevalence and some clinical aspects of atopic dermatitis in the community of Sør-Varanger. Acta Derm Venereol (Stockh) 75:50–53, 1995.

14. J Berth-Jones, S George, RAC Graham-Brown. Predictors of atopic dermatitis in Leicester children. Br J Dermatol 136:498–501, 1997.

15. GS Kendirli, DU Altinta, N Alparslan, N Akmanlar, Z Yurdakul, B Bolat. Prevalence of childhood allergic diseases in Adana, Southern Turkey. Eur J Epidemiol 14:347–350, 1998.

16. HC Williams, AC Pembroke, H Forsdyke, G Boodoo, RJ Hay, PGJ Burney. London-born black Caribbean children are at increased risk of atopic dermatitis. J Am Acad Dermatol 32:212–217, 1995.

17. T Schäfer, D Dockery, U Krämer, H Behrendt, J Ring. Experiences with the severity scoring of atopic dermatitis in a population of German pre-school children. Br J Dermatol 137:558–562, 1997.

18. LK Dotterud, ES Falk. Atopic disease among adults in northern Russia, an area with heavy air pollution. Acta Derm Venereol 79:448–450, 1999.

19. ZT Selçuk, T Caglar, T Enunlu, T Topal. The prevalence of allergic diseases in primary school children in Edirne, Turkey. Clin Exp Allergy 27:262–269, 1997.

20. H Sugiura, N Umemoto, H Deguchi, Y Murata, K Tanaka, T Sawai, M Omoto, M Uchiyama, T Kiriyama, M Uehara. Prevalence of childhood and adolescent atopic dermatitis in a Japanese population: comparison with the disease frequency examined 20 years ago. Acta Derm Venereol (Stockh) 78:293–294, 1998.

21. Y Kimura, Y Kanazawa, K Kida, R Mita, Y Nishizawa, I Hashimoto. A study of

atopic dermatitis in elementary school children in Hirosaki City, Aomori Prefecture, Japan. Environ Health Prevent Med 3:141–145, 1998.
22. A Selnes, R Bolle, J Holt, E Lund. Atopic diseases in Sami and Norse schoolchildren living in northern Norway. Pediatr Allergy Immunol 10:216–220, 1999.
23. RM Herd, MJ Tidman, RJ Prescott, JAA Hunter. Prevalence of atopic eczema in the community: the Lothian atopic dermatitis study. Br J Dermatol 135:18–19, 1996.
24. HC Williams, PGJ Burney, AC Pembroke, RJ Hay. Validation of the UK diagnostic criteria for atopic dermatitis in a population setting. Br J Dermatol 135:12–17, 1996.
25. RM Emerson, HC Williams, BR Allen. Severity distribution of atopic dermatitis in the community and its relationship to secondary referral. Br J Dermatol 139:73–76, 1998.
26. TO Bleiker, H Shahidullah, E Dutton, RAC Graham-Brown. The prevalence and incidence of atopic dermatitis in a birth cohort: The importance of a family history of atopy. Arch Dermatol 136:274, 2000.
27. AF Kalyoncu, ZT Selçuk, T Enünlü, AU Demir, L Cöplü, AA Sahin, M Artvinli. Prevalence of asthma and allergic diseases in primary school children in Ankara, Turkey: Two cross-sectional studies, five years apart. Pediatr Allergy Immunol 10: 261–265, 1999.
28. M Marks, M Kilkenny, A Plunkett, K Merlin. The prevalence of common skin conditions in Australian school students: 2. Atopic dermatitis. Br J Dermatol 140:468–473, 1999.
29. CM Popescu, R Popescu, H Williams, D Forsea. Community validation of the United Kingdom diagnostic criteria for atopic dermatitis in Romanian schoolchildren. Br J Dermatol 138:436–442, 1998.
30. D Laughter, JA Istvan, SJ Tofte, JM Hanifin. The prevalence of atopic dermatitis in Oregon schoolchildren. J Am Acad Dermatol 43:649–655, 2000.
31. HC Williams, C Robertson, A Stewart, N Aït-Khaled, G Anabwani, R Anderson, I Asher, R Beasley, B Björkstén, M Burr, T Clayton, J Crane, P Ellwood, U Keil, C Lai, J Mallol, F Martinez, E Mitchell, S Montefort, N Pearce, J Shah, B Sibbald, D Strachan, E von Mutius, SK Weiland. Worldwide variations in the prevalence of symptoms of atopic eczema in the international study of asthma and allergies in childhood. J Allergy Clin Immunol 103:125–138, 1999.
32. G Rajka, T Langeland. Grading of the severity of atopic dermatitis. Acta Derm Venereol (Stockh) 144(suppl):13–14, 1989.
33. C Costa, A Rilliet, M Nicolet, JH Saurat. Scoring atopic dermatitis: the simpler the better? Acta Derm Venereol (Stockh) 69:41–45, 1989.
34. European Task Force on Atopic Dermatitis. Severity scoring of atopic dermatitis: the SCORAD index. Dermatology 186:23–31, 1993.
35. V Lawson, MS Lewis-Jones, P Reid et al. Family impact of childhood atopic eczema. Br J Dermatol 133(suppl 45):19, 1995.
36. P Reid, M Lewis-Jones. Sleep difficulties and their management in preschoolers with atopic eczema. Clin Exp Dermatol 20:38–41, 1995.
37. M Fennessy, S Coupland, J Popay, K Naysmith. The epidemiology and experience of atopic eczema during childhood: a discussion paper on the implications of current knowledge for health care, public health policy and research. J Epidemiol Community Health 54:581–589, 2000.

38. S Jowett, T Ryan. Skin disease and handicap: an analysis of the impact of skin conditions. Soc Sci Med 20:425–429, 1985.
39. LR Daud, ME Garralda, TJ David. Psychosocial adjustment in preschool children with atopic eczema. Arch Dis Childhood 69:670–676, 1993.
40. AY Finlay, GK Khan. The Dermatology Life Quality Index. A simple practical measure for routine clinical use. Clin Exp Dermatol 19:210–216, 1994.
41. E Falk. Atopic Diseases in Norwegian Lapps. Acta Derm Venereol (Stockh) Suppl 182:10–14, 1993.
42. K Nishioka. Atopic eczema of the adult type in Japan. Australas J Dermatol 37:S7–S9, 1996.
43. P Saval, G Fuglsang, O Østerballe. Prevalence of atopic disease among Danish school children. Pediatr Allergy Immunol 4:117–122, 1993.
44. RM Worth. Atopic dermatitis among Chinese infants in Honolulu and San Francisco. Hawaii Med J 22:31–34, 1962.
45. A Mar, M Tam, D Jolley, R Marks. The cumulative incidence of atopic dermatitis in the first 12 months among Chinese, Vietnamese, and Caucasian infants born in Melbourne, Australia. J Am Acad Dermatol 40:597–602, 1999.
46. J Golding, TJ Peters. The epidemiology of childhood eczema. Pediatr Perinat Epidemiol 1:67–79, 1987.
47. B Wüthrich. Epidemiology and natural history of atopic dermatitis. Allergy Clin Immunol Int 8(3):77–82, 1996.
48. B Taylor, J Wadsworth, M Wadsworth, C Peckham. Changes in the reported prevalence of childhood eczema since the 1938–45 war. Lancet 2:1255–1257, 1984.
49. DP Strachan. Hay fever, hygiene, and household size. Br Med J 299:1259–1260, 1989.
50. HC Williams, DP Strachan, RJ Hay. Childhood eczema: disease of the advantaged? Br Med J 308:1132–1135, 1994.
51. AG Falade, F Olawuyi, K Osinusi, BO Onadeko. Prevalence and severity of symptoms of asthma, allergic rhino-conjunctivitis and atopic eczema in secondary school children in Ibadan, Nigeria. East African Med J 75(12):695–698, 1998.
52. DP Strachan, J Golding, HR Anderson. Regional variations in wheezing illness in British children: effect of migration during early childhood. J Epidemiol Community Health 44:231–236, 1990.
53. SK Weiland, E von Mutius, T Hirsch, H Duhme, C Fritzsch, B Werner, A Hüsing, M Stender, H Renz, W Leupoid, U Keil. Prevalence of respiratory and atopic disorders among children in the east and west of Germany five years after unification. Eur Respir J 14:862–870, 1999.
54. H Behrendt, U Krämer, R Dolgner et al. Elevated levels of total serum IgE in East German children: atopy, parasites or pollutants? Allergy J 2:31–40, 1993.
55. T Schäfer, J Ring. Epidemiology of allergic diseases. Allergy 52(suppl 38): 14–22, 1997.
56. B Kjellman, R Petterson, B Hyensjö. Allergy among school children in a Swedish country. Allergy 37(suppl 1):5, 1982.
57. I Pösä, M Korppi, M Pietikäinen, K Remes, K Juntunen-Backman. Asthma, allergic rhinitis and atopioc eczema in Finnish children and adolescents. Allergy 46:161–165, 1991.

58. NJ McNally, HC Williams, DR Phillips, M Smallman-Raynor, S Lewis, AJ Venn, J Britton. Water hardness and atopic eczema. Lancet 352:527–553, 1998.

59. DA Waite, EF Eyles, SL Tonkin, et al. Asthma prevalence in Tokelauan children in two environments. Clin Allergy 10:71–75, 1980.

60. R Leung. Asthma, allergy and atopy in south-east Asian immigrants in Australia. Aust NZ J Med 24:255, 1994.

61. AF Kalyoncu, ZT Selcuk, Y Karakoca, et al. Prevalence of childhood asthma and allergic diseases in Ankara, Turkey. Allergy 49:485–488, 1994.

62. T Kusunoki, A Kouichi, M Harazaki, S Korematsu, S Hosoi. Month of birth and prevalence of atopic dermatitis in schoolchildren: Dry skin in early infancy as a possible etiological factor. J Allergy Clin Immunol 103(6):1148–1152, 1999.

63. HR Anderson, PA Bailey, JM Bland. The effect of birth month on asthma, eczema, hayfever, respiratory symptoms, lung function, and hospital admissions for asthma. Int J Epidemiol 10:45–51, 1981.

64. T Schäfer, B Przybilla, J Ring, B Kunz, A Grief, K Überla. Manifestation of atopy is not related to patient's month of birth. Allergy 48:291–294, 1993.

65. F Schultz-Larsen, JM Hanifin. Secular changes in the occurrence of atopic dermatitis. Acta Derm Venereol (Stockholm) Suppl 176:7–12, 1992.

66. HC Williams. Is the prevalence of atopic dermatitis increasing? Clin Exp Derm 17: 385–391, 1992.

67. F Schultz Larson, NV Holm, K Henningsen. Atopic dermatitis. A genetic-epidemiological study in a population-based twin sample. J Am Acad Dermatol 15:487–494, 1986.

68. N Åberg, B Hesselmar, B Åberg, B Eriksson. Increase of asthma, allergic rhinitis and eczema in Swedish schoolchildren between 1979 and 1991. Clin Exp Allergy 25:815–819, 1995.

69. VM Yates, REI Kerr, RM MacKie. Early diagnosis of infantile seborrhoeic dermatitis and atopic dermatitis—clinical features. Br J Dermatol 108:633–638, 1983.

70. T Aoki, T Fukuzumi, J Adachi, K Endo, M Kojima. Re-evaluation of skin lesion distribution in atopic dermatitis. Acta Derm Venereol (Stockh) Suppl 176:19–23, 1992.

71. HC Williams, B Wüthrich. The natural history of atopic dermatitis. In: HC Williams, ed. Atopic Dermatitis: The Epidemiology, Causes and Prevention of Atopic Eczema. Cambridge: Cambridge University Press, 2000, pp 41–59.

72. J Kay, DJ Gawkrodger, MJ Mortimer, AG Jaron. The prevalence of childhood atopic eczema in a general population. J Am Acad Dermatol 30:35–39, 1994.

73. HC Williams & DP Strachan. The natural history of childhood eczema: observations from the 1958 British cohort study. Br J Dermatol 139:834–839, 1998.

74. RL Bergmann, KE Bergmann, S Lau-Schadensdorf, W Luck, A Dannermann, CP Bauer, W Dorsch, J Forster, E Schmidt, J Schultz, U Wahn. Atopic diseases in infancy. The German multicenter atopy study (MAS-90). Pediatr Allergy Immunol 5(suppl 1):19–25, 1994.

75. RL Bergmann, G Edenharter, KE Bergmann et al. Predictability of early atopy by cord blood-IgE and parental history. Clin Exp Allergy 27:752–760, 1997.

76. I Rystedt. Long term follow-up in atopic dermatitis. Acta Dermatol Venereol (Stockh) Suppl 114:117–120, 1986.

77. CFH Vickers. The natural history of atopic eczema. Acta Dermatol Venereol (Stockh) Suppl 92:113–115, 1980.

78. F Scuultz Larsen. The epidemiology of atopic dermatitis. In: ML Burr, ed. Epidemiology of Clinical Allergy. Monogr Allergy. Vol. 31. Basel: Karger, 1993, pp 9–28.

79. K Musgrove, JK Morgan. Infantile eczema. A long-term follow-up study. Br J Dermatol 95:365–372, 1976.

80. A Mar, R Marks. Prevention of atopic dermatitis. In: HC Williams, ed. Atopic Dermatitis: The Epidemiology, Causes and Prevention of Atopic Eczema. Cambridge: Cambridge University Press, 2000, pp 205–218.

81. Anonymous. Allergic factors associated with the development of asthma and the influence of cetirizine in a double-blind, randomised, placebo-controlled trial: first results of ETAC. Early Treatment of the Atopic Child. Pediatr Allergy Immunol 9: 116–124, 1998.

82. C Hoare, A Li Wan Po, HC Williams. Systematic review of treatments for atopic eczema. Health Technology Assessment 2000; 4 (37).

3
Psychoimmunology and Evaluation of Therapeutic Approaches

Uwe Gieler, Volker Niemeier, and Burkhard Brosig
Justus Liebig University Giessen, Giessen, Germany

I. HISTORY

In 1850 a translation was published of the works of Erasmus Wilson (110) on *Diseases of the Skin*, in which, in a chapter on skin neuroses, he attributed "itching, alopecia and leukoderma" to insufficient stimulation of the skin. In another part of the text dealing with the causes of eczema, however, he states that "the primary cause is . . . disorders of the nervous system, like emotions, especially of a depressive nature." And "eczema very commonly acts as a safety valve for the health of the organism and the associated exsudation must be very gradually brought under control. . . ." In this sense, it appears reasonable to consider Erasmus Wilson (1809–1894) as one of the first dermatologists with an understanding of psychosomatics (111).

At the beginning of scientific dermatology in the second half of the nineteenth century, insights into psychosomatic relationships were repeatedly published. Even before Erasmus Wilson published his chapter on "skin neuroses" (111), Hillier (43) expressed the conviction that "nervous excitement may lead to urticaria. Shock is known as a cause of eczema, and fear turns the hair white." We must remember that at that time, nothing was known of parallel studies or of the detailed relationships within the nervous system, the function of which was elucidated only after development of embryology and the horrible revelations presented on brain damage related to injuries during the First World War.

Late in the nineteenth century, Brocq and Jacquet (19) coined the term "neurodermatitis," which they considered to be weakness of the nerves and which has remained unchanged, especially among patients, to the present day.

II. STRESS AND ATOPIC DERMATITIS

Psychological factors seem to be important in atopic dermatitis as significant modulators of the disease. Stress increases atopic dermatitis symptoms depending on the severity of stress.

In a very large population of 1457 patients questioned after the Japanese earthquake in Hanshin in 1995, Kodama et al. (60) showed that 38% of patients with atopic dermatitis in the most severely hit region and 34% in a moderately hit region reported exacerbation, compared to only 7% in a control group without earthquake stress. However, 9 and 5% in the respective earthquake regions and only 1% in the control region reported a marked improvement in atopic dermatitis. In a multiple regression analysis, subjective stress was the best indicator predicting exacerbation compared to genetic and treatment-related factors. The results of this study show that stress apparently has an immunological effect, which can, though to a slighter extent, exert an opposite inflammatory effect.

Similar influencing factors had already been described by Brown and Bettley (20). In a prospective controlled study of children with asthma, it could also be demonstrated that psychosocial stress had the greatest influence in eliciting an asthma attack (91).

The relationship between stress and atopic dermatitis is underlined by studies showing that daily hassles could be associated with symptom severity. Using a diary technique for severity and emotional state, King and Wilson (56) demonstrated a significant positive relationship between interpersonal stress on a given day and skin condition 24 hours later. This study, as well as further time-series analyses (42,64), indicated the influence of daily hassles on the exacerbation of atopic dermatitis.

III. NEUROANATOMY

Atopy-relevant effector cells, such as mast cells and Langerhans cells, form a close anatomical relationship with nerve fibers staining positive for a number of neuroactive substances, for instance substance P, vasoactive peptide, or nerve growth factor (NGF) (101). Regarding this close anatomical relationship of nerve terminals and effector cells in atopic dermatitis, it seems possible that stress-induced stimulation of nerve fibers induces secretion of neuroactive substances. There is a growing number of studies indicating that atopic dermatitis patients show disturbances in the cyclic adenosine monophosphate (cAMP) system, suggesting an altered catecholamine responsiveness. This concept was introduced by Szentivany (102), who reported reduced responsiveness of β-adrenergic receptors in atopic dermatitis patients, and has been confirmed by Niemeier et al. (82).

IV. PSYCHONEUROENDOCRINOLOGY

Functional changes in the hypothalamus–pituitary–adrenal cortex axis are under discussion (4,21). Buske-Kirschbaum et al. (22) compiled an overview of the psychobiological aspects of neurodermatitis and confirmed by means of hypotheses the various endocrine, immunological, and psychophysiological influences on atopic dermatitis.

Pathophysiological studies follow the behavioral approach and address the pathophysiological reactibility of neurodermatitis patients and conditioning as a means of influence. The following are among the parameters used: heart rate, electrical skin resistance, electromyographic activity, and skin temperature under defined stress situations. In addition, psychometric data, such as scores for anxiety and hostility and depressivity, are measured.

Jordan and Whitlock (48,49) compared neurodermatitis patients with a control group of neurological and internal medicine patients with no atopic-type diseases either themselves or in any family member. In the first phase, psychometric data (Cattel Personality Inventory, Esenck Personality Inventory, Buss-Durkee Hostility Inventory, Depression and Anxiety Scales of the Minnesota Multiphasic Personality Inventory) were recorded, and in a second phase the authors examined the scratching reaction and changes in skin resistance in eliciting by both an unconditioned stimulus (itching via electrodes) and a conditioned stimulus (bell tone). The neurodermatitis patients had significantly higher values in the scales Neuroticism (EPI), Anxiety (MMPI), and Suppressed Hostility (BDHI).

No correlation could be demonstrated between emotional alteration (elevated scores for Neuroticism, Anxiety, Hostility) and vasomotor reactivity in the sense of Eysenecks ''autonomic reactivity.''

A study by Faulstich et al. (30) compared 10 neurodermatitis patients with a conception of autonomic reactivity to a control group with regard to measured values of heart rate, electromyography, peripheral vasomotor response, skin temperature, and skin resistance. The patients were subjected to emotional (intelligence test) and physical stress. The neurodermatitis patients reacted remarkably only with elevation of heart rate and of muscle tone under provocation by placing the hand in ice-water (''cold-pressor test''). The neurodermatitis subjects attained significantly high values in the scores for anxiety in the Symptom Checklist 90 (SCL-90R). However, no other connection to pathophysiological data could be made.

In a similar study, Münzel and Schandry (78) compared 18 atopic dermatitis patients with a healthy-skin control group. In this study, heart rate, skin resistance, axial skin temperature, and pulse volume amplitude were also measured under emotional stress in the form of mental arithmetic and social (expressing an opinion on a topic in front of a group). The patients reported their feelings with respect to tension, annoyance, and restlessness using constant scales (0–100) during the breaks.

All physiological parameters of the neurodermatitis patients, as well as the feeling of tension, were significantly higher than in the control group. The skin temperature also increased in the neurodermatitis patients and decreased in the control group. The authors divided the neurodermatitis patient group with respect to subjective malaise due to itching; the values of the subgroup of patients suffering greatly from itching were responsible for the statistical increase in skin temperature in the entire group. The assumption was that there is a relationship between emotional stress and the course of the disease, especially in patients with sustained high levels of activation.

By contrast, Köhler and Weber (61) found absolutely no evidence of a general hyperreactivity in relation to the skin system of neurodermatitis patients in a study of similar design.

These results demonstrate that a general hyperreactivity in neurodermatitis patients can apparently not be assumed.

The influence of serious events in life and of stressors of various degrees on the immune system is known. The autonomic nervous system acts as the connector between feelings and subsequent somatic response. Lymph nodes contain sympathic afferents; adrenergic and cholinergic fibers are found in the thymus, the lymphocytes also have adrenergic and cholinergic receptors (6).

In a study of 75 students in the phase preceding final exams, Kiecolt-Glaser et al. (55) found considerably reduced activity of the natural killer (NK) cells. These cells play a special role in carcinogenesis and virus defense. The study group was subdivided on the basis of psychometric tests (Brief Symptom Inventory, Symptom Checklist 90, Social Readjustment Rating Scale, UCLA Loneliness Scale), which revealed a correlation between loneliness and feeling of distress due to stressors and a reduced NK cell activity. Moreover, the tested students had an elevated serum IgA level. In additional studies with similar conditions and populations (54), reduced interferon levels were found, as was a correlation between the extent of relaxation exercises and the number of T-helper cells. Moreover, Kiecolt-Glaser et al. (55) found evidence of influence by stressors in DNA repair of lymphocytes.

Baker (6) emphasizes that the altered reactivity of defense cells is decisive, rather than the fluctuations in their counts. He also points out the significantly higher incidence of neurodermatitis in depressive patients compared to schizophrenic patients. A large number of studies has demonstrated a reduced T-cell count as well as an increase in eosinophils, B lymphocytes, and serum IgE in neurodermatitis patients (23). Eosinophils and IgE correlate with the degree of skin eruptions in eczema (72). Stone et al. (99) registered a reduction in the IgE levels when the eczema abated in half of the neurodermatitis patients they examined. Wüthrich (112) ascribed a prognostic value to the eosinophil count in eczema therapy.

Kupfer (64) examined the interaction between the severity of skin symptoms, the expression of individual emotions, and the excretion of salivary cortisol and salivary IgA. Aggression, depression, and anxiety were found to be emotions particularly related to skin symptoms.

McGeady und Buckley (72) found a limited cellular defense. They examined 21 neurodermatitis patients by applying intracutan-*Candida-Candida albicans* antigen and streptokinase-streptodornase. A pronounced anergie was found, which correlated with the severity of the eczema. It is a fact that neurodermatitis patients more frequently suffer sometimes generalized viral infections (herpes-, coxsackie-, and other viruses) and bacterial superinfections (17,112).

Ring (88) has delineated the central immunoetiological role of vasoactive mediators such as histamine and ECF-A (eosinophil-chemotactic factor of anaphylaxis) in neurodermatitis patients. He cites the following factors as the decisive influence of this mediator liberation: Increased readiness of the basophiles to excrete histamines, so-called "leaky" mast cells, a β_2-adrenergic control defect among other things at the level of the intracellular cAMP system, increased sensitivity to α-adrenergic and cholinergic stimuli demonstrated in vivo and in vitro, and elevated IgE levels. The histamine effect, besides its effect on the capillary-bronchial system, lies in a limitation of T-suppressor activity with consecutive IgE elevation. Increased sensitivity to histamine was found in nearly all atopics at the T-cell level.

V. STUDIES OF ANXIETY, HOSTILITY, AND DEPRESSION

Developments in research recognize atopic dermatitis as a psychosomatic illness (2,14,59). Psychosomatic causes are considered important eliciting factors. Numerous studies on the personality of the neurodermatitis patient have shown, however, that there is no "specific neurodermaitis personality." According to studies by Pürschel (85), up to 40% of patients themselves cite emotional factors as eliciting neurodermatitis, while Griesemer and Nadelsohn (39) report up to 70%.

Anxiety was studied by Jordan and Whitlock (49) as one partial aspect of the etiological discussion in neurodermatitis patients. The results showed elevated anxiety values among neurodermatitis patients compared to a control group with other types of disease; the MMPI additional scale was used to measure anxiety. Garrie et al. (32) arrived at similar results in their studies. Faulstich et al. (30) performed a pathophysiological study in which elevated anxiety could be demonstrated in neurodermatitis patients.

In a study by Gieler et al. (34) using the HESTIBAR test procedure, the neurodermatitis patients also recorded considerably elevated anxiety values. In this study, cluster analysis showed subgroups, some of which presented extremely high anxiety values and others in which values were in the normal range. It can be assumed that the elevated anxiety values of neurodermatitis patients are not a component of a "neurodermatitis personality," but that they do influence the course of the disease and the patient's coping with the disease.

Suppressed hostility is frequently cited as one characteristic of the supposed "neurodermatitis personality." The study by Jordan and Whitlock (49) using the Bus-Durkey Hostility Inventory Test determined that neurodermatitis patients had elevated values with respect to felt but not outwardly expressed hostility compared to the control group. However, no differences were measured with respect to openly expressed hostility. Other authors, like Borrelli (12), Cleveland and Fischer (24), Fiske and Obermeier (31), Jordan and Whitlock (49), Levy (66), McLaughlin et al. (73), and Ott et al. (84), also reported on studies using projective procedures in which elevated hostility parameters were measured.

Gieler et al. (34) found elevated neuroticism values in their emotionally remarkable subgroup of neurodermatitis patients, already mentioned above. Elevated values toward depressive moods were also remarkable in this group.

It appears as if personal aspects like suppressed hostility and anxiety, as well as depression, are frequently confirmed in neurodermatitis patients in these studies, but these aspects might also be interpreted as a consequence of the disease.

VI. PSYCHOTHERAPY IN ATOPIC DERMATITIS

Suggested therapies in the literature refer mainly to behavioral therapeutic and in-depth psychological forms of therapy. In addition, there are numerous suggestions for combined therapy (for example, with relaxation training, dermatological training) (36). According to the in-depth psychology concept, psychotherapy can be performed with individual patients, with families, or even in groups. The treatment technique does not differ in these groups. The basis of psychoanalytical-psychotherapeutic treatment is the creation of a viable therapeutic relationship via acceptance. On this basis, latent conflicts can be made accessible and conscious during the course of treatment. Correspondingly arising inner resistance and defense processes can be made accessible in order to be dealt with and overcome. This usually results in stabilization of the emotional balance and improved coping with the actual disease episodes. Supportive interventions alternate with revelatory interventions.

In in-depth psychological psychotherapy, special attention is paid to the affects (sadness, rage, etc.) and fantasies that arise during treatment. Making these affects and fantasies conscious should help the patient to obtain better insight into his own world and thus to attain altered coping ability in experiencing his disease.

An analytically oriented psychotherapeutic treatment may be indicated, especially in conjunction with chronic skin diseases, since stable and supportive family relationships appear to considerably improve the coping with disease in chronically ill patients.

VII. BEHAVIORAL THERAPY

Treatment begins initially with behavior analysis, which records certain behaviors that are elicited by certain situations (stimulus constellations or specific stimuli) or promoted by certain situations (controlling stimuli, which precede the problem, and stimuli that follow as a consequence of expressed behavior). In this connection, it is also interesting to note the importance of the patient's person of reference, especially how this person reacts to the patient's problems. From a behavioral-therapeutic point of view, it is important that the patient see the causes of his disorder, i.e., attribute them. At the end of the session, considerations are addressed concerning which therapeutic procedures could be applied. An important treatment procedure is thus based on rational development of new coping strategies in dealing with "stress situations," i.e., the patient is taught to expand his behavioral repertoire (75). In behavioral therapy, behavior analysis always serves targeted therapeutic planning for the individual patient, whereby the controlling momentary stimulus conditions (operant, classical, conditional, and cognitive aspects) in the maintenance of a disease are isolated, which are then further documented in parallel to the individual phases in the course of treatment. Changes in the goal of therapy and the use of new treatment methods may occur during treatment. The active participation of the patient by means of so-called homework or documentation of strategies, which the patient uses or which are suggested by the therapist, is in any case part of treatment. Operant "conditioning" with application of so-called positive rewards plays an important role in the differentiated psychotherapy program of the behavioral therapist. Operant reward models are more effective if certain aspects are taken into account:

1. Self-confidence training or social training seeks to attain improvement in the possibility of realizing one's own wishes and needs in face of the environment. This is made possible by role-playing, training, and social confrontations, taking nonverbal aspects of behavior into account.

2. In learning models in role-playing, the patient observes therapeutically desirable behaviors in other persons and the positive consequences that result from their behavior. Certain characteristics of these persons (sex, age, social attractiveness) may promote or limit this learning model.

3. Many behavior-therapeutic interventions are carried out in complex or chronic behavioral problems that do not immediately offer a chance to attain completely different (desired) behavior within a short time. Various therapeutic steps may lead ultimately to a desired therapy modification (shaping). Parts of behavioral patterns are analyzed and influenced, especially in individual steps. These steps are related to one another and potentiate the patient's willingness to change.

4. In biofeedback the patient cognitively registers physiological parameters, and support in changing these parameters is given a particular direction by means of light and sound signals. Additional techniques are counterconditioning (e.g., in overcoming anxiety), aversion techniques, operant deleting, exposition therapy—especially in phobic states, confrontation with the situation that elicits the fear.

To complete the picture, the behavioral-therapeutic approach in itching should be mentioned (11). In a presentation of the dynamics of the scratch reaction, they reveal the unconscious aspect of this process. Diffuse distress and not the visual or haptic perception of a scratch site precedes the scratching reaction typical of neurodermatitis.

At the start of the scratching phase, the need to scratch increases, only to decrease rapidly again when pain and bleeding have begun. The curve of circadian scratching rate recorded on a large patient collective is a mirror image of the daily activity curve. This makes it apparent that wakefulness and nonwakefulness exert a control function and are one criterion of scratching.

The vicious circle of scratching begins when a frustrating, fear-eliciting stimulus (S) meets an organism (O) with a characteristic behavioral deficit (deficit in recognition, permissiveness, and dealing with one's own emotions). These patients tend, according to the authors' observations, to reject a psychological interpretation of the scratching symptoms. The authors attribute this attitude to the fact that "the organ skin in our culture is the one which most readily permits expression of emotional distress, without being unmasked by the patient or his environment" (11). The tension reduction (C1) appears more spontaneously under reaction (R) in the form of scratching when S meets O than the negative consequences (C2) like pain and exacerbation of the skin condition.

The therapy concept of Böddecker and Böddecker (11) is based on positive reinforcement of not scratching, punishment preceding reward (tension reduction) (e.g., by protocolling before scratching), and withdrawal of reinforcement (e.g., armbands with alarm devices).

VIII. ANALYTICAL AND PSYCHODYNAMIC-ORIENTED SINGLE, FAMILY, AND GROUP THERAPY

At the center of the psychoanalytical treatment method is making the patient aware of unrecognized meanings in respect to his own life situation. This is made without behavioral instructions from the therapist (104). The treatment techniques consist essentially of "elucidation," "confrontation," "interpretation," especially perception of "transfer" and "countertransfer." The individual terms are explained briefly below.

Elucidation proceeds via examination of experience and behavior patterns in dealing with others in the patient's personal environment. Important interaction and experience patterns are to be worked out in connection with the patient's internalized importance.

In confrontation, blocked and denied modes of behavior and experience and their effect on others are made clear, whereby the therapeutic situation is also made clear by using everyday situations.

Interpretations are intended to reveal unrecognized relationships of the experience and behavioral patterns between significant others. Past experiences, such as in childhood, which are blocked and denied are addressed.

The aspect of transfer and countertransfer plays a special role in analytically oriented psychotherapeutic treatment. It is based on the idea that working through emotions and relationship fantasies in connection with behavior represents a particular psychodynamic configuration and is understood as a mutual process of therapist and patient, or as a therapeutic process. Within the therapeutic framework, wishes for independence and the fear of consequences and reaching a compromise between wishes and fears are understood and their defense mechanisms with resultant modes of behavior dissipated. Psychotherapeutic treatment is considered successful when the patient is able to work out more satisfying possibilities in his personal life.

Analytic in-depth psychology–oriented psychotherapeutic group therapy enables a therapeutic relationship constellation in which patients have the possibility of experiencing and working out neuroticizing or pathological relationships within the group, where a multiple transfer resource arises between the group leader and group participants, with the possibility of working out personal conflicts as well as conflicts with one another. Psychotherapeutic treatment procedures are relatively effective for neurodermatitis patients (10).

IX. FAMILY ASPECTS

Some studies take special notice of the family situation of neurodermatitis patients. It appears that the family environment is co-responsible to a high degree for the course of the disease. Essentially, the studies concentrate on the mother-child relationship.

Gieler and Effendy (33) reported on disrupted communication between infants and their environment, elicited by neurodermititis skin disease. In their view, no delineated body image can crystallize because of the early disruption of communication, which leads to impairment in the child's overall emotional development with a tendency to withdrawal to the organ skin. Adult atopic dermatitis patients engaged in a problem discussion with their mothers or with their partners showed less acceptance, less self-disclosure, and more justification than a nonatopic control group (108).

Rechenberger (1993) also sees an altered body image of patients with neurodermatitis as essential. The neurodermatitis patient is incapable of experiencing his skin as a protective, enveloping shell.

Pürschel (85) is of the opinion that a child with skin disease experiences marked limitations in respect to his relationship to his environment, which results in a persistent impairment of contact to that environment.

It was remarkable in the study by Ring et al. (89) that children with neurodermatitis displayed more aggression toward their parents and reported more separation events in their lives to that point. The mothers in these studies were also seen to be rather cool and to show little emotion; they were sparing in their praise of their children, which they limited essentially to performance. Bräutigam et al. (16) are of the opinion that mothers of neurodermitic children feel stressed by the outward appearance of the child with skin disease and from the experience that the child apparently desire physical contact, which they are unable to accept. It is assumed that the distancing posture of the mothers is elicited mostly by the child's disease. By contrast, Pürschel (85) points out that parents react with overprotection toward their skin-diseased child and thus inhibit the child's development.

Generally, the particular stress for the child with neurodermatitis, as well as for the other family members in early-onset and chronic course of the disease, appears to give the skin a special value as an "organ of limitation" in these families and complicated neuroticizing interactions may result.

X. AFFECTIVE AREA AND NEUROTIC SYMPTOMS

According to the study by Kuypers (65), psychosocial factors coupled with emotional conflicts have a marked influence on the onset or exacerbation of neurodermatitis. The tensions caused by certain emotional states and their resolution are accompanied in many cases by a reduction in skin symptoms. The importance of emotions and the experience of related conflicts are variously experienced by neurodermatitis patients. Decisive for elicitation of skin reactions is probably not the conflict itself, but rather the emotional quality ascribed to the conflict.

In a study with 448 neurodermatitis patients, Pürschel (85) found that 57.5% had problems in private areas, with women reporting difficulties more often (76.1%) than men (29%). Stress situations were viewed as a central theme with regard to onset of neurodermatitis episodes. Of the 448 patients, 187 (41%) ascribed the exacerbation to problems at work and especially in interpersonal relationships. The skin reactions in the sense of neurodermatitis were also reported in connection with examinations, engagements, and weddings. Apparently general stress situations are decisive; according to Pürschel (85), the individual tolerance limits are lower than among healthy individuals. Rechardt (86) found that feelings of dependence and hopelessness occurred more often during episodes of the disease but did not occur in an episode-free interval 9 years later. He attributed the emotional disturbances to stress caused by the skin disease. Likewise, according to Bosse (13), neurodermatitis episodes occur in connection with actual conflict situations. These conflict situations are age-related threshold situations, which may lead to a subsequent exacerbation of the skin condition. In children, he typically observed absence or lack of one or both parents, tensions in the parents' marriage or within the family, job situations, change of schools, move, periods of looking for a job, looking for a partner, or examinations. In adults, weddings, interpersonal problems, death, or temporary emotional or physical overload led to recurrent exacerbation of the skin condition.

XI. STRESS IN CONNECTION WITH LIFE EVENTS

King and Wilson (56) examined 50 neurodermatitis patients over a period of 14 days. In a subsequent meta-analysis, the calculated correlation coefficients revealed that the skin condition cross-correlated synchronously with values for anxiety/tension, interpersonal stress, depression, frustration, feelings of aggression, expressed aggression, and suppressed aggression (in that order). The authors showed that stress on the previous day correlated with the actual skin condition, and the actual skin condition led to increased stress and elevated depression values on the following day.

Hospitalized neurodermatitis patients were examined in a pilot study by Hünecke et al. (47). An attempt was made to discover certain events that elicited the episodes. It was found that demonstrable psychosocial events (weekends, visits, discharge) were coupled significantly frequently with disease exacerbation. Schubert (93) was also able to demonstrate a number of cross-correlations between stress events and disease outbreak, as well as between emotional well-being and skin symptoms in a timed series study of 6 neurodermatitis patients. Conversely, it was not possible to predict the skin condition on the subsequent day from the occurrence of stress events or any particular mood.

XII. STATUS OF RESEARCH INTO
THERAPEUTIC EFFECTIVENESS

Research into the effectiveness of psychotherapy in skin diseases, especially neurodermatitis, is still largely in the beginning phase. To date, differential aspects in adult neurodermatitis patients have only limited value with respect to prognostically relevant indication criteria, since the studies thus far refer usually to individual cases or very small numbers of patients. In general, clinical dermatology does not appear to have paid sufficient attention to psychological factors and psychotherapeutic possibilities.

A high level of motivation for therapy is considered prognostically positive (93), while early onset of disease and other additional atopical diseases are viewed as prognostically unfavorable (63).

Another study was performed at the request of the Institute for Social Medicine Epidemiology and Health Systems Research (ISEG Study) to evaluate therapeutic measures in neurodermatitis (10). In cooperation with the Gmünder Ersatzkasse health insurance group, it could be demonstrated that, among other forms of therapy, psychotherapy was rated by the patients as having the most positive long-term effect.

In a meta-analysis (1) various psychotherapeutic procedures were examined with respect to skin condition and subjective well-being. It was found that the psychotherapeutic procedures were clearly more effective than somatic-medical standard measures. The neurodermatitis personality postulated in this study could not be confirmed, but the characteristics of anxiety, depression, and neuroticism were significantly high. A total of 865 subjects were examined: 553 adult neurodermatitis patients and 129 children. The effects of various combined psychotherapeutic interventions were examined. The skin symptoms improved significantly with all measures in the patients receiving psychotherapy. Their medication consumption and scratching frequency were also reduced.

Kaschel (52) studied various methods and developed a training program especially for neurodermatitis patients, taking psychotherapeutic aspects into account. Positive affects were also described by Klein (57) Walsh and Kierland (106), Williams (109), and Thomä (104). Since skin diseases may be caused, according to psychoanalytical theory, by disruptions in early childhood development, other psychological therapy forms, like gestalt therapy or client-centered conversation (defined by Rogers) may be effective. However, no results with respect to neurodermatitis have yet been published.

Neurodermatitis has considerable influence on a patient's quality of life. Satisfaction with life is of central importance in experiencing and coping with disease (5). A number of stresses with corresponding psychosocial consequences make high demands on coping resources (25). It can therefore be assumed that various aspects of the disease will elicit various coping reactions, and they, in turn, may differ from the coping reactions in other stress situations (9). Chronic skin diseases like neurodermatitis may lead to serious limitations in emotional well-being and are frequently coupled with social problems. It can be demonstrated that these stressing effects are underestimated in relation to other chronic diseases. Dermatological diseases like neurodermatitis are particularly likely to be of considerable detriment to self-image and social relationships, since the symptoms are so visible. It happens frequently that persons with skin diseases experience negative social reactions from other persons, starting with ambivalent reserve to distancing and on to open rejection (15). Occasionally, fear of contagion makes social contact more difficult (46). Expectation of rejection and avoidance, for example, in public, leads to a consistent coping strategy of avoidance, which in turn leads to generalization and exacerbation of the symptoms (68).

Itching is one skin symptom of neurodermitis. The intensive need to scratch is a serious limitation of well-being. Since itching can be elicited by external and internal stimuli, like heat, skin dryness, or simply imagining such sensations (100), it is a particularly stressful symptom. Likewise, the itching threshold can be lowered by "stress" (27,37). The scratching impulse to itching stimuli is a reflex that can be inhibited spinal by cortical structures (100). Scratching irritates the pain receptors. For a time, this reduces the sensation of itching, accompanied by a feeling of relief. With a slight delay, the itching threshold is reduced, which brings increased sensation of itching and in turn increased scratching. When the skin is finally bleeding, it hardly itches (77). Pain takes precedence over itching. In this constantly widening vicious circle, new skin damage arises, neurodermatitis becomes chronic with the known symptoms of thickening of the afflicted epidermis and coarsening of the skin structures. It was demonstrated (49) that even slight diffuse tensions or malaise can elicit scratching. According to Bosse and Hünecke (14), helplessness in the face of this vicious circle and guilt feelings of having failed in self-control give rise to additional emotional stress for the patients, which in turn can maintain the itching-scratching cycle. The ever-recurrent sequence of recurrences and freedom from episodes is also often accompanied by feelings of helplessness, of being thrown to the wolves, and by anxious-depressive moods (96). The stress of constant itching is also frequently underestimated. Sleep deficits and reduced ability to concentrate during episodes of the disease are frequent symptoms (44).

Due to disease-related habits like constant scratching or the experienced limitation of attractiveness, the negative effects on communication increase (108). This, in turn, leads to additional unsolved problems in social relationships. The resultant increase in tension and aggression is expressed by more scratching and contributes to further exacerbation of the disease.

XIII. EXPERIENCES WITH ATOPIC ECZEMA
PREVENTION PROGRAMS

In 1951 and 1955 Williams (109) and Shoemaker et al. (94) published their experiences with supportive group therapy, the latter with 25 patients. In some cases improvements of symptoms were noted together with an improvement of emotional responses (e.g., anger), but the size and heterogeneous composition of the groups were on the whole rather disadvantageous.

In the behavior-oriented therapeutic interventions of the studies published so far, it was predominantly attempted to interrupt the itching-scratching cycle (80). This can be activated by (1) reduction of excessive physiological stress reactions, (2) methods concerning the perception of itching, and (3) strategies to avoid scratching. Further therapeutic approaches involve measures aimed at the reduction of negative effects on social behavior by (1) development of behavioral competence for an improved coping with stress and (2) improving the handling of illness-specific psychological stress. Thus, dermatological education constitutes an attempt to enable the patient to become active in a competent manner by acquiring knowledge.

XIV. MEASURES TO INFLUENCE THE
ITCHING-SCRATCHING CYCLE

A. Reduction of Physiological Stress Reactions

There is a wealth of experience concerning the reduction of the physiological excitation level. The following relaxation methods are practiced: autogenic training (AT), EMG-feedback training, cue-controlled relaxation, and the progressive muscle relaxation according to Jacobson.

Horne et al. (45), Kaschel et al. (51), and Niebel (79) were successful in combination therapies with progressive muscle relaxation. The balancing of vegetative and immunological dysfunction as well as improved body perception and an active conviction concerning physical reactions (8), are considered as effective factors in muscle relaxation and autogenic training.

The technique of so-called cue-controlled relaxation, i.e., the flexible deployment of relaxation techniques following an exciting cue (e.g., scratching impulse), has been proven successful by Horne et al. (45), Kaschel et al. (51), and Niebel (79). Another effective method for the reduction of stress, EMG-feedback training, was demonstrated in eight patients (41). The extent to which the ability to relax led to an improvement of her skin state (over 30 months) is, however, unclear, for an improved ability to relax could not be proven (38).

In an EMG-biofeedback study with progressive muscle relaxation, McMenamy et al. (74) were able to achieve a complete remission of symptoms, which persisted in three patients during a 2-year follow-up. Unfortunately, this study, like many others, had no control group without therapy (placebo effect).

Kämmerer (50) and Cole et al. (26) employed AT in combination with other behavioral therapies, e.g., self-observation, self-control following a scratching impulse, and the alteration of stress-evoking basic convictions. Following therapy a significantly improved skin condition was diagnosed. In the study by Cole et al. (26) the problem of the control group was solved by using the patients during the 3-month period before the begin of the therapy as "controls." Unfortunately, the follow-up period amounted to only 1 month. But even in this study (as in many other studies) the problem remains that AT was employed only in combination with other behavioral therapies. Therefore, it is not clear which therapy was responsible for the positive results. In a prospective randomized study of 125 atopic eczema patients treated with different therapies, Stangier et al. (97) showed that AT was unexpectedly effective. Besides the therapy studies (unfortunately executed in combination) investigations with other aims showed positive effects of AT on skin reaction. Through AT the extent of skin reactions to standardized allergy testing could be reduced (103). Ely et al. (28a) found that inflammatory reactions of the skin following allergen contact rose if anxiety and stress were artificially produced by experimental conditions. According to Kämmerer (50) AT can lead to a reduction of affective tension provoking itch and to an improved perception of one's body. In addition, AT can contribute to an alteration of the perception of itching and to a lowering of the elevated psycho-physiological excitation level. The effects of suggestive procedures like hypnosis depend on previous experience, expectations, and, above all, on the inclination of the person to be hypnotized; of great importance is imaginative capability.

For the alteration of the itching perception there are several approaches: Schubert (92) transformed some suggestion techniques of hypnosis studies into an imagination training, and Luthe and Schulz (71) used imagination techniques (imagination of coolness) (see also Refs. 38 and 45). Suggestive techniques like hypnotherapy were used successfully in some studies (58,95,98,105). Hajek et al. (40) reported long-lasting positive effects in the sense of raising of the itching threshold. These results suggest that imaginative methods can be effective because of the relationship between perceptions, (auto-) suggestive reaction expectations, and physiological skin functions in skin diseases.

B. Strategies for Scratching Avoidance

Bar and Kuypers (7) reported their work with children whose scratching behavior was simply ignored, while abstaining from scratching was rewarded. During the 18-month follow-up, the children remained symptom-free. The technique, based on a better perception of an automated procedure and the learning of alternative behavior incompatible with scratching (pinching, muscle tension), has proved a success (76,90).

Melin and coworkers (76) and Noren and Melin (83) compared the effect of behavior-oriented and medical treatment with that of medical treatment (corticosteroids) alone. The interventions carried out with control groups, but unfortunately without long-time follow-up, included several habit-reversal techniques. Following the early perception of the scratch impulse and its accompanying conditions, the patients reacted with two kinds of behavior incompatible with scratching. The marked reduction of scratching and the improvement of symptoms correlated highly, leading to the conclusion that these were the results of scratching-avoidance strategies.

Rosenbaum and Ayllon (90) were able to obtain long-term success (6 months follow-up) with such habit-reversal techniques in four patients. Scratching, eliciting risk situations, and consequences were described in detail by the patients, a signal was installed for the interruption of the time course, then an alternative behavior, e.g., pinching, was learned, and this course sequence practiced repeatedly.

Niebel (79,80) also applied training with specific scratch-control and stress-control techniques (habit-reversal, "scratching-blocks" replacing skin). Similar to the comparison group, which was more directed to coping with stress, a reduction of the scratching frequency and severity of symptoms was observed during the 6-month follow-up ($n = 15$). However, there were no significant differences between the groups, which is not surprising given the minimal therapeutic differences between the groups.

XV. METHODS TO REDUCE NEGATIVE EFFECTS ON SOCIAL RELATIONSHIPS BY ATOPIC ECZEMA PREVENTION PROGRAMS

Development of behavorial competence for improved coping with stress and improved coping with the illness-specific mental stress have received little attention in studies so far. Training for attaining social competence with the aim of improved coping with situations stressing atopic eczema patients was practiced successfully by Kaschel et al. (51) and Niebel (79,80) in combination with relaxation exercises.

Schubert et al (93) found significant differences when comparing a group with unspecific discussion therapy and a behavioral therapy group (reduction of scratching, stress-coping techniques). In five case studies Kaschel et al. (51) noted essentially short-term success concerning the reduction of scratching and medication. Great individual differences were pointed out.

The attempt to improve the control over the disease (self-therapeutic competence) by acquiring knowledge in the framework of dermatological teaching has been neglected in the studies published. However, the various psychotherapeutic approaches have obviously stood the test.

XVI. STATUS OF EMPIRICAL RESEARCH WITH ATOPIC ECZEMA PREVENTION PROGRAMS

The effect of different combined psychotherapeutic interventions was investigated in 12 studies (26,28,40,41,69,70,76,79,80,93,95,107). Melin et al. (76) and Cole et al. (26) studied the effects of medical treatment on skin symptoms. Melin et al (76) compared a hydrocortisone therapy alone with concomitant self-control strategies for the reduction of scratching, and Cole et al.(26) investigated different topical applications including systemic steroids in comparison to a combined psychotherapy. The skin symptoms improved following all the methods, but significantly moreso in patients with psychotherapy. The use of drugs decreased and systemic steroids were no longer used, even at one-month follow-up (76). The paper of Cole et al. (26) had no follow-up.

In four methodically well-controlled studies (28,79,80,93), the effects of different forms of therapy were compared. Dermatological symptoms and scratching frequency were reduced by all the evaluated therapies studies (28,79,80,93) better by combined behavior therapy and scratching control techniques (78,81) and in tendency better by behavior therapy compared with dermatological education and school medical therapy (28). No significant differences were obtained in one study (93). In a further study the scratching frequency declined in one group, while another group yielded better results with regard to itching, skin symptoms, and scratching frequency; in the first group the psychological variables "depressions," "fear of failure," "restrictions through atopic eczema," and "lack of self-assurance and attractiveness" were reduced; dermatological state and itching improved only in individual cases (79,80).

In a subsequent study (80) the psychological variables improved, especially following combined behavioral therapy and least in the control group. The fear tendency was most effectively reduced in the group with relaxation training and the combined behavior therapy group (28). The variable "anxiety" was in one study improved by dermatological teaching and combination therapy, but not significantly. The follow-up after 6 and 12 months showed that psychotherapeutical inverventions had more positive long-term effects on the course of the disease. The skin improved further following all psychological interventions (28). Eleven out of 15 patients in the study of Niebel (80) stopped using cortisone, and the skin remained improved in all groups and the positive effects of the behavior therapy persisted in contrast to those of the dermatological standard therapy (93). The combination of behavioral therapy and education (28) and the combined behavior therapy (80) yielded marginally better results than the other forms of psychotherapy.

There are also studies concerning the effectivity of therapies in children with atopic eczema or their parents. In one study with children (107) a complex dermatological therapy in a rehabilitation clinic was compared with an additional behaviour therapy of 7 hours per week. At the end of the treatment the skin was similarly improved in both atopic eczema groups. Broberg et al. (18) Allen and Harris (3), Köhnlein et al. (62), and Gieler et al. (35) demonstrated that parent education is effective.

In two recent controlled studies it was shown that educational measures were superior to routine therapy. Niebel (81) observed similar effects in two groups, one of which underwent direct training devised to change behavior, while the other was schooled by video tapes. In a randomized study with 204 families, Kehrt et al. (53) showed that the quality of life of the mothers had improved significantly in the invervention groups compared to the control group.

REFERENCES

1. Al Abesie S. Atopische Dermatitis und Psyche. Dissertation des Fachbereichs Human Medizin, Giessen, 2000.
2. Alexander F. Psychosomatische Medizin. Berlin: Verlag De Gruyter, 1971.
3. Allen K, Harris E. Elimination of a child's excessive scratching by the training of the mother in reinforcement procedures. Behav Res Ther 1966; 4:79–84.
4. Arnetz BB, Fjellner B, Eneroth P, Kallner A. Endocrine and dermatological concomitants of mental stress. Acta Derm Venereol (Stockh) 1991; 156:9–12.
5. Augustin M, Zschocke I, Lange S, Seidenglanz K, Amon U. Lebensqualität bei Hauterkrankungen: Vergleich verschiedener Lebensqualitäts-Fragebögen bei Psoriasis und atopischer Dermatitis. Hautarzt 1999; 50:715–722.
6. Baker GHB. Invited Review. Psychological Factors and Immunity. J Psychosom Res 1987; 31:1–10.
7. Bar LHJ, Kuypers BRM. Behaviour therapy in dermatological practice. Br J Dermatol 1973; 88:591–598.
8. Bernstein DA, Borkovec ID. Entspannungstraining. Munich: Pfeiffer, 1978.
9. Beutel M. Bewältigungsprozesse bei chronischen Erkrankungen. Berlin: Springer, 1988.
10. Bitzer EM, Grobe TG, Dorning H. Die Bewertung therapeutischer Maßnahmen bei atopischer Dermatitis und Psoriasis aus der Perspektive der Patienten unter Berücksichtigung komplementär medizinischer Verfahren. ISEG Studie Endbericht, 1997.
11. Böddecker KW, Böddecker M. Verhaltenstherapeutische Ansätze bei der Behandlung des endogenen Ekzems unter besonderer Berücksichtigung des zwanghaften Kratzens. Z Psychosom Med Psychoanal 1976; 21:61–101.

12. Borelli S. Untersuchungen zur Psychosomatik des Neurodermitikers. Hautarzt 1950; 1:250–256.

13. Bosse K. Psychosomatische Gesichtspunkte bei der Betreuung atopischer Ekzematiker. Zeitschr Hautkr 1990; 65:543–545.

14. Bosse K, Hünecke P. Der Juckreiz des endogenen Ekzematikers. Münch Med Wochenschr 1981; 123:1013–1016.

15. Bosse K, Fassheber P, Hünecke P, Teichmann AT, Zauner J. Zur sozialen Situation des Hautkranken als Phänomen interpersoneller Wahrnehmung. Psychosom Med Psychoanal 1976; 21:3–6.1

16. Bräutigam W, Christian P, v Rad M. Psychosomatische Medizin. 5th ed. Stuttgart: Thieme Verlag, 1992.

17. Braun-Falco O, Ring J. Zur Therapie des Atopischen Ekzems. Hautarzt 1984; 35: 447–454.

18. Broberg A, Kalimo K, Lindblad B, Swanbeck G. Parental education in the treatment of childhood atopic eczema. Acta Derm Venereol 1990; 70:495–499.

19. Brocq L, and Jacquet L. Notes pour servir a l'histoire des neurodermatitis. Ann Dermatolo Venerol 1891; 97:193–195.

20. Brown DG, Bettley FR. Psychiatric treatment of eczema: a controlled trial. Br Med J 1971; 2:729–734.

21. Buske-Kirschbaum A, Jobst S, Wustmans A, Kirschbaum C, Rauh W, Hellhammer D. Attenuated free cortisol to psychosocial stress in children with atopic dermatitis. Psychosom Med 1997; 59:419–426.

22. Buske-Kirschbaum A, Geiben A, Hellhammer D. Psychobiological aspects of atopic dermatitis: an overview. Psychother Psychosom 2001; 70:6–16.

23. Byrom NA, Timlin DM. Immune status in atopic eczema. A survey. Br J Derm 1979; 100:491–498.

24. Cleveland SE, Fischer S. Psychological factors in the neurodermatoses. Psychosom Med 1956; 18:209–220.

25. Cohen F, Lazarus R. Coping with the stresses of illnes. In: G Stone, N Adler, F Cohen, eds. Health Psychology. San Francisco: Jossey-Bass, 1979 pp 217–254.

26. Cole WC, Roth HL, Lewis B, Sachs D. Group psychotherapy as an aid in the medical treatment of eczema. J Am Acad Dermatol 1988; 18:286–291.

27. Cormia FE. Experimental histamine pruritus. Influence of physical and psychological factors on threshold reactivity. J Invest dermatol 1952; 19:21–29.

28. Ehlers A, Stangier U, Gieler U. Treatment of atopic dermatitis: a comparison of psychological and dermatological approaches to relapse prevention. J Consult Clin Psychol 1995; 63(4):624–635.

28a. Ely DL, Henry JP. Ethological and physiological theories. In: Kutash IL, Schlesinger LB, et al. (eds.) Handbook on Stress and Anxiety. Jossey-Bass, San Francisco, 1980.

29. Faulstich ME, Williamson DA. An overview of atopic dermatitis. Toward a biobehavioral integration. J Psychosom Res 1985; 29:647–654.

30. Faulstich ME, Williamson DA, Duchmann EG, Conerly LS, Brantley PJ. Psychophysiological analysis of atopic dermatitis. J Psychosom Res 1985; 29:415–417.

31. Fiske CE, Obermayer ME. Personality and emotional factors in chronic disseminated neurodermatitis. Arch Dermatol Syphilol 1954; 70:261–267.

32. Garrie E, Garrie S, Mote T. Anxiety and atopic dermatitis. J Consult Clin Psychol 1974; 42:742–748.

33. Gieler U, Effendy I. Psychosomatische Aspekte in der Dermatologie. Akt Dermatol 1984; 10:103–106.

34. Gieler U, Ehlers A, Höhler T, Burkhard G. Die psychosoziale Situation der Patienten mit endogenem Ekzem. Der Hautarzt 1990; 41:416–423.

35. Gieler U, Köhnlein B, Schauer U, Freiling G, Stangier U. Eltern-Beratung bei Kindern mit atopischer Dermatitis. Hautarzt 1992; 11(43):37–42.

36. Gieler U, Stangier U, Ernst R. Psychosomatische Behandlung im Rahmen der klinischen Therapie von Hautkrankheiten. In: K Bosse, U Gieler, eds. Seelische Faktoren bei Hautkrankheiten. Bern: Huber, 1985, pp 154–160.

37. Graham DT, Wolf S. Pathogenesis of urticaria. JAMA 1950; 143:1396–1402.

38. Gray SG, Lawlis GF. A case study of pruritic eczema treated by relaxation and imagery. Psychol Rep 1982; 51:627–633.

39. Griesemer R, Nadelsohn T. Emotional aspects of cutaneous disease. In: Fitzpatrick T, et al. (eds.) Dermatology in General Medicine. 1979; 1353–1363; New York, McGraw-Hill.

40. Hajek P, Jakoubek B, Radil T. Gradual increase in cutaneous threshold induced by repeated hypnosis of healthy individuals and patients with atopic eczema. Percept Mot Skills 1990; 70(2):549–550.

41. Haynes SN, Wilson CC, Jaffe FG, Britton BV. Biofeedback treatment of atopic dermatitis: controlled case studies of eight cases. Biofeedback Self Reg 1979; 4:195–209.

42. Helmbold P, Gaisbauer G, Kupfer J, Haustein UF. Longitudinal case analysis in atopic dermatitis. Acta Derm Venereol 2000; 80:348–352.

43. Hillier T. Handbook of Skin Disease. London: Walton & Maberly, 1865.

44. Hofmann S, Ehlers A, Stangier U, Gieler U. Zusammenhang von Juckreiz und Kratzverhalten mit Befindlichkeit und Aufmerksamkeit bei Neurodermitis. Unveröff. Vortrag Dtsch. Kolleg. Psychosomatische Medizin, 10.11.1989, Gießen.

45. Horne DJ, White AE, Varigos GA. A preliminary study of psychological therapy in the management of atopic eczema. Br J Med Psychol 1989; 62:241–248.

46. Hornstein O, Brückner G, Graf V. Über die soziale Bewertung von Hautkrankheiten in der Bevölkerung. Hautarzt 1973; 24:230–235.

47. Hünecke P, Bosse K, Finckh H. Krankheitsverlauf und psychosoziale Ereignisse während der stationären Behandlung atopischer Ekzematiker. Pilostudie. Zeitschr Hautkr 1990; 65:428–434.

48. Jordan JM, Whitlock FA. Atopic dermatitis, anxiety and conditioned scratch responses. J Psychosom Res 1974; 18:297–299.

49. Jordan JM, Whitlock FA. Emotions and the skin. The conditioning of scratch responses in the cases of atopic dermatitis. Br J Dermatol 1972; 86:574–585.

50. Kämmerer W. Die psychosomatische Ergänzungstherapie der Neurodermitis-Atopica. Autogenes Training und andere Maßnahmen. Allergologie 1987; 10:536–541.

51. Kaschel R, Miltner H, Egenrieder H, Lischka G. Verhaltenstherapie bei atopischem Ekzem: Ein Trainingsprogramm für ambulante und stationäre Patienten. Aktuel Dermatol 1990; 15:275–280.

52. Kaschel R. Neurodermitis in den Griff bekommen. Heidelberg: Verlag für Medizin, 1990.

53. Kehrt R, von Rüden U, Wenninger K, Wahn U, Staab D. Schulung von 204 Eltern von neurodermitiskranken Kindern. Poster 21. Tagung der Deutschen Gesellschaft für Allergologie und klinische Immunologie, München, 1999.

54. Kiecolt-Glaser JK, Glaser R. Psychological influences on immunity. Psychosom Med 1986; 27:621–624.

55. Kiecolt-Glaser JK, Garner W, Speicher C. Psychosocial modifiers of Immunocompetence in medical students. Psychosom Med 1984; 46:7–14.

56. King RM, Wilson GV. Use of a diary technique to investigate psychosomatic relations in atopic dermatitis. J Psychosom Res 1991; 35:697–706.

57. Klein HS. Psychogenic factors in dermatitis and their treatment by group therapy. Br J Med Psychol 1949; 22:32–45.

58. Kline MV. Neurodermatitis and hypnotherapy: the acceptance of resistance in the treatment of a long-standing neurodermatitis with a sensory imagery techniques. J Clin Exp Hypnosis 1954; 2:313–322.

59. Koblenzer CS, Koblenzer P. Chronic intractable atopic eczema. Its occurrence as a physical sign of impaired parent-child relationships and psychologic developmental arrest: improvement through parent insight and education. Arch Dermatol 1988; 124(11):1673–1677.

60. Kodama A, Horikawa T, Suzuki T, Ajiki W, Takashima T, Harada S, Ichihasha M. Effects of stress on atopic dermatitis: investigations in patients after the great Hanshin earthquake. J Allergy Clin Immunol 1999; 104:173–176.

61. Köhler T, Weber D. Psychophysical reactions of patients with atopic dermatitis. J Psychosom Res 1992; 36:391–394.

62. Köhnlein B, Stangier U, Freiling G, Schauer U, Gieler U. Elternberatung von Neurodermitiskindern. In: U Gieler, U Stangier, E Brähler, eds. Hautkrankheiten in psychologischer Sicht; Jahrbuch für Medizinische Psychologie. Bd 9. Hofgrefe-Verlag, Göttingen, 1993.

63. Korting GW, Laux B, Niemöller M. Das endogene Ekzem. Persistenz und Wandel während der vergangenen Jahrezehnte. Dtsch Ärztebl 1987; 84:224–229.

64. Kupfer J. Psychoimmunologische Verlaufsstudie bei Patientinnen mit atopischer Dermatitis. Dissertation, University of Gießen, Germany, 1994.

65. Kuypers BRM. Atopic dermatitis. Some observations from a psychological viewpoint. Dermatologica 1967; 136:387–394.

66. Levy RJ. The Rorschach pattern of neurodermatitis. Psychosom Med 1952; 14:41–49.

67. Liebermann RP, King LW, DeRisi WJ, McCann M. Personal effectiveness. Research Press Campaign, 1975.

68. Liebowitz MR, Gormann HM, Fyer AJ, Klein AB. Social phobia: review of a neglected anxiety disorder. Arch Gen Psychiatry 1985; 12:729–736.

69. Löwenberg H, Peters M. Psychosomatic dermatology: results of an integrated inpatient treatment approach from the patients perspective. Prax Psychother Psychosom 1992; 37:138–148.

70. Löwenberg H, Peters M. Evaluation of in-patient psychotherapeutic and dermatological treatment in atopic dermatitis. Psychother Psychosom Med Psychol 1994; 44(8):267–272.

71. Luthe W, Schultz JH. Autogenic Therapy. Vol II. Medical Applications. New York: Grune and Stratton, 1969.

72. McGeady SJ, Buckley RH. Depression of cell-mediated immunity in atopic eczema. J Allergy Clin Immunol 1975; 56:393–406.
73. McLaughlin JT, Shoemaker RJ, Guy WB. Personality factors in adult atopic eczema. Arch Dermatol Syphilol 1953; 68:506–516.
74. McMenamy CJ, Katz RC, Gipson M. Treatment of eczema by EMG biofeedback and relaxation training: a multiple baseline analysis. J Behav Ther Exp Psychiatry 1988; 19:221–227.
75. Meichenbaum D. Kognitiv-behavioral Modifikation. New York: Plenum Press, 1977.
76. Melin L, Fredericksen T, Noren P, Swebelius BG. Behavioral treatment of scratching in patients with atopic dermatitis. Br J Dermatol 1986; 115:467–474.
77. Münzel K. Atopische Dermatitis. Ergebnisse und Fragen aus verhaltensmedizinischer Sicht. Verhaltensmodif Verhaltensmed 1988; 9:169–193.
78. Münzel K, Schandry R. Atopisches Ekzem. Pathophysiologische Reaktivität unter standardisierter Belastung. Hautarzt 1990; 41:606–611.
79. Niebel G. Verhaltensmedizinisches Gruppentraining für Patienten mit atopischer Dermatitis in Ergänzung zur dermatologischen Behandlung; Pilotstudie zur Erprobung von Selbsthilfestrategien. Verhaltenmodif Verhaltensmed 1990; 11:24–44.
80. Niebel G. Entwicklung verhaltensorientierter Gruppentrainingsprogramme für AD-Patienten—eine experimentelle Studie. In: Behavior Medicine of Chronical Dermatological Disorders—Interdisciplinary Perspectives on Atopic Dermatitis and Its Treatment. Niebel G, ed. Bern: Huber, 1990:420–525.
81. Niebel G. Direkte versus videovermittelte Elternschulung bei atopischen Ekzem im Kindesalter als Ergänzung fachärztlicher Behandlung. Hautarzt 2000; 51:401–411.
82. Niemeier V, Gieler U, Bärwald C, Kupfer J, Schill WB, Happle R. Decreased density of β-adrenergic receptors on peripheral blood mononuclear cells in patients with atopic dermatitis. Eur J Dermatol 1996; 6:377–380.
83. Noren P, Melin L. The effect of combined topical steroids and habit-reversal treatment in patients with atopic dermatitis. Br J Dermatol 1989; 121:359–366.
84. Ott G, Schönberger A, Langenstein B. Psychologisch-psychosomatische Befunde bei einer Gruppe von Patienten mit endogenem Ekzem. Aktuel Dermatol 1986; 12:209–213.
85. Pürschel W. Neurodermitis und Psyche. Zeitschr Psychosom Med Psychoanal 1976; 22:62–70.
86. Rechardt E. An investigation in the psychosomatic aspects of prurigo Besnier. Monographs of the Psychiatric Clinic Helsinki, University-Central Hospital, Helsinki, 1970.
87. Rechenberger I. Das Körperbild bei Hautkranken. Mat Psychoanal Anal Orientierten Psychother 1993; 9:31–34.
88. Ring J. Atopic dermatitis. A disease of general vasoactive mediator dysregulation. Int Arch Allergy Appl Immunol 1979; 59:233–239.
89. Ring J, Palos E, Zimmermann F. Psychosomatische Aspekte der Eltern-Kind-Beziehung bei atopischem Ekzem im Kindesalter. Erziehungsstil, Familiensituation im Zeichentest und strukturierten Interview. Hautarzt 1986; 1/37:560–567.
90. Rosenbaum MS, Ayllon T. The behavioral treatment of neurodermitis through habit reversal. Behav Res Ther 1981; 19:313–318.

91. Sandberg S, et al. The role of acute and chronic stress in asthma attacks in children. Lancet 2000; 356:982–987.

92. Schubert HJ. Psychosoziale Faktoren bei Hauterkrankungen. Göttingen: Vandenhoek & Ruprecht, 1988.

93. Schubert HJ. Evaluation of effects of psychosocial interventions in the treatment of atopic eczema. In: Psychosoziale Faktoren bei Hauterkrankungen. Verlag für Medizinische Psychologie. Göttingen: Vandenhoeck & Ruprecht, 1989:158–215.

94. Shoemaker RJ, Guy WB, McLaughlin JT. The usefulness of group therapy in the treatment of atopic eczema. Penn Med J 1955; 58:603–609.

95. Sokel B, Christie D, Kent A, Lansdown R, Atherton D, Glover M, Knibbs J. A comparison of hypnotherapy and biofeedback in the treatment of childhood atopic eczema. Contemp Hypnosis 1993; 10:145–154.

96. Stangier U, Kirn U, Ehlers A. Ein ambulantes psychologisches Gruppenprogramm bei Neurodermitis. Prakis der klinischen verhaltens medizin und rehabilitation 1993; 6:103–113.

97. Stangier U, Gieler U, Ehlers A. Autogenes Training bei Neurodermitis. Z Allgemeinmed 1992; 68:392–400.

98. Stewart AC, Thomas SE. Hypnotherapy as a treatment for atopic dermatitis in adults and children. Br J Dermatol 1995; 132(5):778–783.

99. Stone SP, Gleich GJ, Muller SA. Atopic dermatitis and IgE. Arch Dermatol 1976; 112:1254–1255.

100. Stüttgen G. Physiologie und Pathophysiologie des Juckreizes. Münch Med Wochenschr 1981; 123:987–991.

101. Sugiura H, Maeda T, Uehara M. Mast cell invasion of peripheral nerve in skin lesions of atopic dermatitis. Acta Derm Venereol 1992; 90:613–622.

102. Szentivany A. The beta adrenergic theory of the atopic abnormality in bronchial asthma. J Allergy 1968; 42:201–232.

103. Teshima I. Psychosomatic aspects of skin diseases from the standpoint of immunology. Psychother Psychosom 1982; 37:165–175.

104. Thomä H. Über die Unspezifität psychosomatischer Erkrankungen am Beispiel einer Neurodermitis mit zwanzigjähriger Katamnese. Psyche 1980; 7:589–624.

105. Twerski AJ, Naar R. Hypnotherapy in a case of refractory dermatitis. Am J Clin Hypnosis 1974; 16:202–205.

106. Walsh MN, Kierland RR. Psychotherapy in the treatment of neurodermatitis. Proc Mayo Clin 1947; 22:578–583.

107. Warschburger P. Psychologie der atopischen Dermatitis im Kindes-und Jugendalter. Munich: Quintessenz MMV Medizin Verlag GmbH, 1996.

108. Wenninger K, Ehlers A, Gieler U. Kommunikation von Neurodermitis-Patienten mit ihrer Bezugsperson. Eine empirische Analyse. Z Klin Psychol 1991; 20:251–264.

109. Williams D. Management of atopic dermatitis in children; control of the maternal rejection factor. Arch Dermatol Syphilol 1951; 63:545–556.

110. Wilson E. Die Krankheiten der Haut; aus dem Englischen übersetzt von Dr. Schröder. Leipzig: Verlag von Christian Ernst Kollmann, 1850.

111. Wilson E. Diseases of the Skin London: Churchill, 1867.

112. Wüthrich B. Immunologische Befunde bei endogenem Ekzem. In: Dermatologie in Praxis und Klinik. Vol. 2. Stuttgart: Thieme, 1980.

4

Socioeconomic Impact of Atopic Dermatitis

Candace S. Lapidus and Philip E. Kerr
Brown Medical School, Providence, Rhode Island

I. INTRODUCTION

Atopic dermatitis (AD) is one of the most commonly diagnosed skin disorders worldwide. It is a chronic disease that affects 5–20% of infants and children (1). A recent study by Hanifin and coworkers (2) examined the prevalence of AD in Oregon schoolchildren less than 9 years of age. Their prevalence estimates ranged between 6.8% and 17.2%. Approximately two thirds of those afflicted with AD are under the age of 16 (3), with most cases beginning before age 5 (4). AD has been shown to have a lifetime prevalence of 30% or higher in certain geographic areas (5–7). We are in the midst of a worldwide epidemic of AD, with the prevalence of this important skin disorder increasing significantly over the past 30–40 years (4,8).

Despite the frequency and natural history of AD, it is often viewed by society and the medical community as a minor dermatological condition. Dermatologists, pediatricians, and other practitioners who care for patients with AD recognize the hardship caused by the disease not only to the patient, but also to the family and society. Atopic dermatitis can have a major effect on the patient's quality of life, disrupting family and social relationships, and interfering with work, school, and recreational activities. Given its frequency, it is not surprising that the treatment of AD is accompanied by significant costs. These costs are borne not only by health insurance carriers and patients for prescriptions and physician consultations, but also by families and society for time lost from work and school for treatment and resulting restrictions in employment opportunities.

II. PSYCHOSOCIAL IMPACT OF ATOPIC DERMATITIS

A. Impact on Quality of Life

As previously stated, AD is particularly common in children under 5 years of age. The effects of a chronic, symptomatic disease at such a young age may certainly be expected to have an impact on the overall well-being of a child. In these formative years, the disease often interferes with the child's important emotional and social development. A study by Daud et al. (9) in England directly assessed psychosocial adjustment in children affected by atopic dermatitis (average age approximately 3 years). The parents completed questionnaires and were interviewed, and the children were placed in stressful situations to evaluate their reactions. The scores on the behavioral questionnaire indicated that while the majority of children with AD were well adjusted psychologically, about a third had scores above morbidity levels. This rate was meaningfully higher than in controls or samples from the general population. In fact, the proportion of children with major disturbance was similar to those seen in other severe chronic illnesses in childhood. In comparison to the control groups, children with AD demonstrated significantly more clinginess, dependency, and fearfulness. They were considered poorly adaptable and were twice as likely to have problems with sleep. The presence of these behavioral problems was directly correlated with the severity of the atopic dermatitis.

Children with AD did not exhibit significantly greater incidence of other behavioral disturbances, such as mood changes, eating problems, or difficult relationships with siblings and peers. Importantly, children with AD did not display the more ominous behavioral signs of hyperactivity, attention seeking, disobedience, or aggressiveness. Overall development was equal between subjects and controls in this study, with 85% of both groups scoring within the normal range on the Denver Developmental Screening Test. Therefore, these young children had relatively mild behavioral problems, and the presence of these problems was linked to the severity of the eczema. This led the authors to conclude that the psychosocial disturbance in most children with AD is closely related to the their physical condition and is not likely to be severe or permanent in the majority of cases.

Atopic dermatitis may lower self-image, self-esteem, and confidence in older children just as they are beginning a stage of social interaction (9). This point was illustrated in a study by Lewis-Jones and Finlay (10), in which the authors applied the Children's Dermatology Life Quality Index (Table 1) to 233 school-aged dermatology outpatients in England. The study revealed several important findings regarding patients in this age group. Of the dermatoses that commonly affect children, only scabies was shown to have a greater impact on quality of life than AD. Atopic dermatitis scored higher than other inflammatory disorders such as psoriasis as well as infectious diseases such as viral warts and mol-

Table 1 The Children's Dermatology Life Quality Index Questionnaire

1. Over the last week, how itchy, "scratchy," sore, or painful has your skin been?
2. Over the last week, how embarrassed or self-conscious, upset or sad have you been because of your skin?
3. Over the last week, how much has your skin affected your friendships?
4. Over the last week, how much have you changed or worn different or special clothes/shoes because of your skin?
5. Over the last week, how much has your skin trouble affected going out, playing, or doing hobbies?
6. Over the last week, how much have you avoided swimming or other sports because of your skin trouble?
7. Last week, was it school time or holiday time?
   a. If school time: Over the last week, how much did your skin affect your schoolwork?
   b. If holiday time: How much over the last week has your skin problem interfered with your enjoyment of the holiday?
8. Over the last week, how much trouble have you had because of your skin with other people calling you names, teasing, bullying, asking questions, or avoiding you?
9. Over the last week, how much has your sleep been affected by your skin problem?
10. Over the last week, how much of a problem has the treatment for your skin been?

Source: Ref. 10.

luscum contagiosum. Atopic dermatitis even scored higher than such highly visible diseases as acne and alopecia, which might be expected to have a substantially greater impact on the quality of life of patients in this age group. Interestingly, skin diseases in general were not considered by the children to have impacted friendships despite a high percentage of patients reporting feelings of embarrassment, self-consciousness, or sadness due to their skin. Not surprisingly, symptoms such as pruritus, soreness, or pain appeared to have the greatest impact on quality of life. Other ways in which skin diseases impacted quality of life included the following: restrictions in sporting activities, disruption of sleep, and problems with continuity of treatment.

Atopic dermatitis can have an equally detrimental impact on the quality of life of adults. This was demonstrated initially by Finlay and Khan (11), who developed and used the Dermatology Life Quality Index (DLQI) (Table 2) on a group of adult dermatology outpatients. Using this questionnaire, in which a higher score theoretically corresponds to greater impact on quality of life, the authors found that patients with AD were the highest scoring group when com-

Table 2   The Dermatology Life Quality Index Questionnaire

1. Over the last week, how itchy, sore, painful or stinging has your skin been?
2. Over the last week, how embarrassed or self-conscious have you been because of your skin?
3. Over the last week, how much has your skin interfered with you going shopping or looking after your home or garden?
4. Over the last week, how much has your skin influenced the clothes you wear?
5. Over the last week, how much has your skin affected your social or leisure activities?
6. Over the last week, how much has your skin made it difficult for you to do any sport?
7. Over the last week, has your skin prevented you from working or studying? If 'No,' over the last week how much has your skin been a problem at work or studying?
8. Over the last week, how much has your skin created any problems with your partner or any of your close friends or relatives?
9. Over the last week, how much has your skin caused any sexual difficulties?
10. Over the last week, how much of a problem has the treatment for your skin been, for example, by making your home messy, or by taking up time?

Source: Ref. 11.

pared to patients with other common skin diseases. These patients exhibited Index scores higher than patients with psoriasis, acne, basal cell carcinomas, or viral warts. The DLQI has been used in a number of other studies, and the deleterious affect AD has on quality of life has been consistently demonstrated (12,13).

Atopic dermatitis has also been associated with increased anxiety. A recent study by Linnet and Jemec (12) demonstrated a higher level of anxiety in adult patients with AD compared to controls. The AD was shown to have a significant affect on their quality of life. Interestingly, the degree of anxiety in the AD patients was not dependent upon the severity of disease. Anxiety related directly to the extent the disease interfered with social, recreational, and sexual activities. The study found these activities to be relatively independent of disease severity. The severity of AD seemed to primarily affect symptoms, self-image, and daily activities. Therefore, the quality of life of patients with AD seemed to relate relatively independently to both disease severity and anxiety. In order to best improve quality of life, the authors emphasized the need to treat not only the dermatological manifestations of AD, but the psychological aspects as well.

Since atopic dermatitis is a disease with numerous predisposing and precipitating factors (14), it follows that certain occupations may contribute to the signs and symptoms of AD. Examples include flare-ups in veterinarians, farmers, groomers, and other animal workers who develop allergic reactions and hand eczema in patients with occupational or domestic exposure to irritants. In their review of the occupational aspects of AD, Coenraads and Diepgen (15) reported that occupational irritants could precipitate atopic dermatitis, especially hand eczema. The authors observe that the risk of hand eczema in the general population is at least doubled simply by having a history of AD, and exposure to occupational irritants multiplies this risk by a factor of two or more. Patients with AD may be forced to change occupations, observe special precautions at their workplace, or avoid certain jobs altogether. It is unclear, however, to what extent this occurs.

B. Impact on the Family and Society

Given the substantial impact atopic dermatitis can have on the quality of life of patients afflicted with this disorder, it is not surprising that having a child with AD can markedly disrupt family function. A study by Su et al. in Australia (16) examined the degree to which a child's atopic dermatitis impacted the family. In this cross-sectional study of the families of 48 children with AD, parents were asked to agree or disagree with statements pertaining to the affect this chronic illness has had on the family. Examples of statements provided to parents include: (1) My child's eczema is causing financial problems for the family; (2) People in the neighborhood treat us differently because of my child's eczema; and (3) Nobody understands the burden I carry. Other statements in the survey examined the positive effects the child's eczema may have had on the parents, for example: Learning to manage my child's eczema has made me feel better about myself. To get an idea of how AD compared to other chronic childhood diseases, a control population was formed of children with insulin-dependent diabetes mellitus (IDDM) from a nearby hospital clinic. Overall, AD had a *greater* impact on the family than did diabetes. When AD was categorized according to severity, those groups with moderate and severe eczema had significantly higher impact scores. Despite the significant burden one might expect IDDM to place on the families of affected children, even mild AD had a similar impact as did diabetes on the family.

In a study by Lawson et al. (17) in England, intensive interviews with 34 families of children with AD were conducted. With the information gathered, a questionnaire (Table 3) was synthesized and results were collected from 56 families. The findings from this study revealed the many different ways in which having a child with AD can impact the family. The authors reported that most parents of children with AD described psychological pressures including feelings of guilt, exhaustion, frustration, resentment, and helplessness. Family lifestyle was similarly affected, with many parents stating that they did not lead a "normal" family life, including restrictions in choices of foods, pets, and household products and location of family vacations. Having a child with AD requires a

Table 3   The Dermatitis Family Impact Questionnaire

1. Over the last week, how much effect has your child having eczema had on housework, e.g., washing, cleaning?
2. Over the last week, how much effect has your child having eczema had on food preparation and feeding?
3. Over the last week, how much effect has your child having eczema had on the sleep of others in the family?
4. Over the last week, how much effect has your child having eczema had on family leisure activities, e.g., swimming?
5. Over the last week, how much effect has your child having eczema had on time spent on shopping for the family?
6. Over the last week, how much effect has your child having eczema had on your expenditure, e.g., costs related to treatment, clothes, etc.?
7. Over the last week, how much effect has your child having eczema had on causing tiredness or exhaustion in your career(s)?
8. Over the last week, how much effect has your child having eczema had on causing emotional distress such as depression, frustration or guilt in your career(s)?
9. Over the last week, how much effect has your child having eczema had on relationships between the main caregiver and partner or between the main caregiver and other children in the family?
10. Over the last week, how much effect has helping with your child's treatment had on the main caregiver's life?

Source: Ref. 17.

substantial commitment of treatment time on the part of the whole family. In one study (16) the mean daily time spent by the parents for treatment of the child was 2–3 hours, excluding time spent in preventing children from scratching. The mean hours of sleep lost by parents was 1–2; the same was true for the affected child. Lawson and coworkers (17) noted that approximately two thirds of children reported sleep problems. The authors reported that nighttime scratching led to delays in settling the child down to sleep and increased rates of nighttime reawakening. Both of these may be expected to contribute to frustration and exhaustion in the parents. Of note, approximately two thirds of siblings also reported lost sleep. In addition to the time required to perform treatments, supervision is also necessary to avoid trigger factors, such as food, pets, woolen clothes, and certain soaps. Overall, this caused the parents to describe a sense of increased burden due to the extra time and effort required to care for the child (9,17).

In the study by Daud et al. (9), most mothers reported that their child's atopic dermatitis had a detrimental effect on family life. Compared to controls, the study found that significantly more mothers of children with AD described the child as being generally difficult to handle. The mothers in the AD group reported feeling more distressed, tired, and "fed up." It is not surprising, then, that when the authors directly investigated maternal psychosocial stress, large differences were noted in the overall stress levels reported, with significantly more mothers in the AD group describing themselves as highly stressed. The mothers, not coincidentally, also reported being less active and involved socially, with few if any friends, and had difficulty finding babysitters. They reported that their friends were uncomfortable or frightened by the responsibility of babysitting for a child with AD. The mothers were also less frequently employed outside the home. It is apparent from these reports that parental social functioning can be markedly impaired due to stress and the practical demands of caring for their child's eczema. These findings were confirmed in the study by Lawson et al. (17), in which parents described having difficulty leaving the house to enjoy entertainment or hobbies due to fatigue and the inability to find responsible babysitters. Athletic activities, especially swimming, were similarly restricted. The child was still considered an important and valued member of the family despite the added stress and strain the disease caused. In fact, when mothers were specifically asked, there was no difference in the child's level of acceptance in the family, and there was no difference in the level of warmth expressed by mothers about their child (9).

Given the added stress, fatigue, and lack of social support, it is not surprising that parenting skills can also be adversely affected by having a child with a burdensome condition such as atopic dermatitis. In the study by Daud et al. (9), two thirds of mothers indicated that their child's AD had a substantial effect on their parenting. Their study revealed differences in the quality of parenting between the mothers of children with atopic dermatitis versus controls, although the overall care provided was evaluated as adequate in most cases from both groups. The area of parenting in which mothers of children with AD reported feeling ineffective was discipline. Fewer mothers regarded their disciplining of the child to be adequate. Though mothers of children with AD were similar to those in the control group in their use of various (appropriate) techniques to discipline their child, they more commonly "gave in" in the end. Two factors may contribute to a parent's capitulation instead of discipline. The first is their empathy for a sick child—60% of the mothers reported feeling sorry for the child. Second, mothers likely "give in" to avoid conflict with the child. Conflict may cause distress, followed by an episode of scratching and a subsequent deterioration of their condition. The authors concluded that this might contribute to increased behavioral difficulties in the children, since "giving in" reduced their opportunities to learn to cope with the frustration, fears, and separation anxieties that are common in young children.

The association of having a child with a chronic medical condition such as atopic dermatitis and reduced parental employment is notable. At least two studies (9,16) indicated a negative impact on the employment status of one or both of the parents. In the first of the two studies (9), the authors did not ascertain the reason for the discrepancy in rates of employment. Although the children's medical condition may have prevented the mothers from achieving gainful employment outside the home, the difference may have been due to the higher socioeconomic status of the AD group compared to controls. The study by Su et al. (14) specifically indicated that mothers of children with moderate or severe AD were often forced to reduce, cease, or not initiate employment due to their child's eczema. Furthermore, the job status of some fathers may be negatively impacted by time taken off work to take the child to medical appointments. Lack of gainful employment by either parent may increase the financial stress in less economically advantaged homes. If the family's primary caregiver, often the mother, preferred to work outside the home, having a child with AD may deprive her of that opportunity. There are certainly advantages to having the mother (or father) stay home with the child full time, especially in terms of maintaining continuity of care and establishing a strong parent-child bond in the face of chronic illness. Nonetheless, a satisfying career may help to reduce the stress of having a child with a significant medical illness by developing in the caregiving parent a sense of confidence and accomplishment. This may then translate into a stronger ability to care for the child's eczema. A parent with outside employment may also develop more relationships with other adults, which would expand the realm of her or his social support system.

The added burden of caring for an atopic child can affect spousal and other familial relationships. In the study by Lawson and coworkers (17), subjects reported that caring for a child with AD often had a detrimental effect on familial interpersonal relationships. Reasons cited included tiredness from sleep loss and overprotectiveness by the caregiver, which could lead to feelings of jealousy in the partner and siblings. Furthermore, sibling rivalry may develop. Although uncommon, having a child with AD has been reported as a contributing factor to significant marital problems (16,17). It is reasonable to expect that these issues may contribute to dysfunctional family relationships, and such families have been shown to exhibit poor treatment compliance and, therefore, inadequate control of symptoms (18).

Psychosocial issues associated with AD extend beyond the home. Delayed academic achievement may result from school missed for hospitalizations or physician consultations, sedation from medications, sleep deprivation, and distractions from physical discomfort. Acceptance by peers and teachers may be affected by the appearance of the child and concerns about infectivity, especially if the AD affects exposed skin. As noted above, the atopic child's participation in sports may be limited. These problems can lead to environmental, social, and emotional deprivations, which can negatively affect the course of the disease. Children who have AD may be an even greater challenge for low-income families. Approximately 10% of the families in one study (17) felt that the added financial costs of treating AD adversely affected their family life. In a slightly smaller percentage of families the financial impact was considered severe.

As mentioned earlier, dysfunctional families frequently have problems following treatment regimens, which may contribute to poor control of the AD in the child. Single females head 50% of families below the poverty level in the United States. These caregivers have fewer personal, social, and economic resources to devote to the care of a child who has a chronic illness. Poverty has been shown to be associated with ill health and poor access to care. Starfield (19) describes the poor access to care by low-income families and their noncompliance with treatment regimens. Alternative ways of providing care might be of particular value in this population.

A study by Lapidus et al. (20) in a large urban setting in the United States found that a large fraction of the cost of care for children with AD in this setting was for emergency department visits. The majority of patients seen in the emergency department for AD were government-insured low-income patients, and they were also the more severe cases. The authors concluded that low-income families with atopics are at high risk and need alternative ways to provide treatment for their disease. The literature indicates that the emergency department is an inappropriate setting in which to treat chronic non–life-threatening conditions (21), including atopic dermatitis. The use of the emergency department for treatment of AD is neither desirable nor optimal for the child, hospital, or society. Given the high prevalence of atopic dermatitis (especially in urban centers), its associated morbidity, its costs, and the pressing need to cut health care expenditures, attention must be focused on improving the organization of treatment for AD.

III. FINANCIAL IMPACT OF ATOPIC DERMATITIS

The economic aspects of atopic dermatitis have received little attention over the years. However, since the practice of medicine is becoming increasingly constrained by financial considerations, some understanding of the economic impact different diseases have on the system's limited resources is now necessary, particularly for the most common diseases such as AD (16). Analysis of the cost borne by a community for a given disease must include not only the direct costs incurred by health insurance carriers, government, and patients for such items as office consultations, hospitalization, and prescriptions, but also the indirect costs to patients, their families, and society for lost work or school time and restrictions in employment opportunities (Table 4). Over the past several years, studies outlining the financial burden of atopic dermatitis were conducted in the United States (20), United Kingdom (22), and Australia (16).

Table 4   Financial Impact of Atopic Dermatitis

Direct costs incurred by health insurance carriers and the government
Hospitalizations
Emergency department visits
Office visits to health care professionals
Prescription medications
Direct costs incurred by patients and their families
Payments or co-payments for the above
Over-the-counter treatments
Appropriate clothing and bed linens and their laundering
Changes to the patient's environment, such as new carpets and air filters
Special diet considerations
Transportation to and from appointments
Indirect costs incurred by patients, their families, and society
Lost work and school due to illness, clinic visits, or hospitalization
Time required to administer treatments
Restrictions in employment opportunities

A.   Financial Impact in the United States

Lapidus and coworkers (20) used national data sets to estimate the expense of care for children with AD in the United States. The authors totaled the estimated national costs (in 1990 dollars) for hospitalizations ($49 million), office visits ($107 million), emergency department visits ($87 million), and outpatient prescriptions ($121 million) for an annual total cost of pediatric AD care of $364 million. Despite this high figure, it is considered a conservative estimate of the total direct amount spent annually on atopic dermatitis because it did not include the amount spent on the following:

1.   Adults with atopic dermatitis
2.   Hospitalizations at children's hospitals (the study was only able to gather national data from general, nonfederal, short-term hospitals)
3.   Ambulatory visits at health maintenance organizations or hospital-based practices
4.   Cases in which atopic dermatitis was the secondary diagnosis

This estimation did not include the direct cost incurred by patients or their families for such items as over-the-counter treatments, appropriate clothing/bedding, new carpets or air filters, or co-payments for office visits or prescriptions. This figure also does not include the indirect costs such as lost work or restrictions in employment options for the patients' caregivers.

    The authors also used institution-specific data to examine the service use and expense of care for children with AD at a large urban U.S. children's hospital.

These data revealed that 63% of outpatient visits for AD occurred in the emergency department setting, 40% of which were graded as mild in severity. It was also noted that 60% of emergency department visits for atopic dermatitis occurred during regular clinic hours. In 1990–1991, the projected annual reimbursement for atopic dermatitis in this hospital alone was approximately $410,000.

The authors suggested one way to reduce the cost of care is through utilizing home visits by trained medical personnel. These visits would serve the following purposes: demonstrate proper use of medication, deliver vital education to families, and encourage compliance with follow-up appointments. The home visits would likely increase compliance with medical instructions and may reduce parental absence from work through better control of the disease. The authors anticipated a considerable direct cost saving if establishing this continuity of care resulted in significant reduction in emergency department visits and hospital admissions. Another solution to reduce the financial burden created by emergency department management of atopic dermatitis (estimated annual cost of $87 million) is to shift daytime visits to dermatology practice settings. Using this strategy in the above-mentioned children's hospital, the authors projected a cost savings of 35%. Given the pressing need to cut health care expenditures, attention must be focused on improving the organization of treatment of common chronic diseases such as AD.

B. Financial Impact in the United Kingdom

A study by Herd et al. (22) in Scotland estimated that the total annual expenditure for atopic dermatitis in the United Kingdom was £465 million. This included a total annual personal cost to patients of £297 million, a cost to the national health service of £125 million, and a cost to society of £43 million due to lost working days. To arrive at these figures the authors extrapolated the results from a detailed study of 155 patients with AD from a semi-rural community of approximately 10,000 people. The authors noted that these figures likely underestimate the actual expenditure for the following reasons:

1. The prevalence of AD in Scotland is less than in the rest of the United Kingdom.
2. The general practitioners in the study group were low prescribers.
3. None of the patients in the study population required hospital treatment during the study.
4. Travel costs were minimized since all patients lived within walking distance of the health center.
5. The time spent by parents caring for their child's AD, with its consequent cost to society, was not included.

Based on this study, the annual per capita cost of treating atopic dermatitis in the United Kingdom was calculated at £7.38. In comparing this figure to other common diseases, Herd and coworkers noted that the amount spent on AD was significantly more than the annual per capita amount spent on benign prostatic hypertrophy, was similar to that of venous ulceration, and was approximately half the amount spent on strokes. This is surprising since venous ulceration is considered to be an expensive disease to treat, and the treatment of strokes usually requires prolonged hospitalization. While there are certain limitations to this type of study, which extrapolates to the entire U.K. population the data derived from a community of approximately 10,000 people, it does give some estimation of the startling amount spent on the treatment of this disease.

It is important to note that when the cost to society for lost working days was excluded, a full 70% of the total estimated expenditure of £422 million is borne by the patients and their families. The single most costly element of treating AD in the study group was prescription medication. Interestingly, the next most costly item was new clothing/bedding and extra laundry expenses that were necessary because of the patient's skin condition. Each patient in the study group also spent an average of £31 annually for over-the-counter preparations. In total, the average amount spent by patients and their families in the study group was £153 per year. Remembering that none of these patients had disease severe enough to require hospital treatment, it is clear that AD can exact a substantial financial toll on patients and their families.

C. Financial Impact in Australia

In the study by Su and coworkers in Australia (16), the authors also examined the cost of managing AD that was borne by the family. The annual personal financial cost of managing mild, moderate, and severe AD was Aus$330, 818, and 1,255, respectively, which included medication, dressings, diet, and other management strategies. Predictably, the largest direct costs were for medications and dressings. The authors compared these figures to similar expenditures by families of children with asthma and found that treating AD was substantially more expensive. Even for a child with asthma requiring hospitalization in the past year, the annual costs to the family were similar to those associated with moderate or severe AD. They also demonstrated that the direct financial cost to the family of a child with AD was similar to those reported for children with diabetes. This helps support the conclusion that AD is a significant financial burden for patients, families, and health care systems worldwide.

IV. SUMMARY

Atopic dermatitis is a common and important skin condition that most often arises in infants and children and can persist into adulthood. It can have a tremendous impact on quality of life by affecting psychosocial adjustment in children, creating embarrassment, disrupting sporting activities in older children, and interfering with employment opportunities in adults. Having a child with AD can have a substantial impact on family function. Parents describe feelings of guilt, exhaustion, frustration, and helplessness. Atopic dermatitis disrupts sleep not only in patients but also in parents and family members. Having a child with AD can affect the social functioning of the parents and can cause parents to miss work or avoid outside employment altogether. Parenting skills can also be affected, as can spousal and other familial relationships. All of these challenges become even greater in low-income families, who often have minimal social support mechanisms.

The costs are high for the treatment of AD, not only for health insurance carriers and the government, but also for patients and society. The allocation of limited resources to manage AD, one of the most common diseases, requires an analysis of the therapeutic cost-effectiveness of each treatment modality. Such an analysis ensures that evidence-based decisions can be made when considering the various treatment options available. An evidence-based approach may also be used to examine the means with which care is delivered and to develop and test innovative methods of organizing treatment. A resourceful attitude would be particularly helpful for examining novel ways to manage chronic diseases such as AD in low-income families.

The importance of effective treatment and control of AD to patients, their families, and society is clear. There is a profound need for enhanced and expanded efficacy and cost research, followed by wise and thoughtful changes in public policy, to minimize its future socioeconomic toll.

REFERENCES

1. H Williams, C Robertson, A Stewart, N Aït-Khaled, G Anabwani, R Anderson, I Asher, R Beasley, B Björkstén, M Burr, T Clayton, J Crane, P Ellwood, U Keil, C Lai, J Mallol, F Martinez, E Mitchell, S Montefort, N Pearce, J Shah, B Sibbald, D Strachan, E von Mutius, S Weiland. Worldwide variations in the prevalence of symptoms of atopic eczema in the international study of asthma and allergies in childhood. J Allergy Clin Immunol 103:125–138, 1999.
2. D Laughter, JA Istvan, SJ Tofte, JM Hanifin. The prevalence of atopic dermatitis in Oregon schoolchildren. J Am Acad Dermatol 43:649–655, 2000.
3. RM Herd, MJ Tidman, RJ Prescott, JA Hunter. Prevalence of atopic eczema in the community: the Lothian Atopic Dermatitis study. Br J Dermatol 135(1):18–19, 1996.
4. HC Williams. Epidemiology of atopic dermatitis: recent advances and future predictions. In: B Wüthrich, ed. The Atopy Syndrome in the Third Millennium. Basel: Karger, 1999, pp 9–17.

5. JK Peat, RH van den Berg, WF Green, CM Mellis, SR Leeder, AJ Woolcock. Changing prevalence of asthma in Australian children. Br Med J 308:1591–1596, 1994.
6. N Åberg, B Hesselmar, B Åberg, B Eriksson. Increase of asthma, allergic rhinitis and eczema in Swedish schoolchildren between 1979 and 1991. Clin Exp Allergy 25(9):815–819, 1995.
7. LK Dotterud, B Kvammen, E Lund, ES Falk. Prevalence and some clinical aspects of atopic dermatitis in the community of Sørvaranger. Acta Derm Venereol 75(1): 50–53, 1995.
8. F Schultz Larsen. Epidemiology and socioeconomic impact of allergic skin diseases. In: DYM Leung, MW Greaves, eds. Allergic Skin Disease: A Multidisciplinary Approach. New York: Marcel Dekker, 2000, pp 1–19.
9. LR Daud, ME Garralda, TJ David. Psychosocial adjustment in preschool children with atopic eczema. Arch Dis Child 69:670–676, 1993.
10. MS Lewis-Jones, AY Finlay. The Children's Dermatology Life Quality Index (CDLQI): initial validation and practical use. Br J Dermatol 132:942–949, 1995.
11. AY Finlay, GK Khan. Dermatology Life Quality Index (DLQI)—a simple practical measure for routine clinical use. Clin Exp Dermatol 19(3):210–216, 1994.
12. J Linnet, GBE Jemec. An assessment of anxiety and dermatology life quality in patients with atopic dermatitis. Br J Dermatol 140:268–272, 1999.
13. L Lundberg, M Johannesson, M Silverdahl, C Hermansson, M Lindberg. Quality of life, health-state utilities and willingness to pay in patients with psoriasis and atopic eczema. Br J Dermatol 141:1067–1075, 1999.
14. CS Lapidus, PJ Honig. Atopic dermatitis. Pediatr Rev 15(8):327–332, 1994.
15. PJ Coenraads, TL Diepgen. Occupational aspects of atopic dermatitis. In: HC Williams, Ed. Atopic Dermatitis: The Epidemiology, Causes, and Prevention of Atopic Eczema. Cambridge: Cambridge University Press, 2000, pp 60–68.
16. JC Su, AS Kemp, GA Varigos, TM Nolan. Atopic eczema: its impact on the family and financial cost. Arch Dis Child 76:159–162, 1997.
17. V Lawson, MS Lewis-Jones, AY Finlay, P Reid, RG Owens. The family impact of childhood atopic dermatitis: the Dermatitis Family Impact questionnaire. Br J Dermatol 138:107–113, 1998.
18. AM La Greca. Adherence to prescribed medical regimens. In: DK Routh, ed. Handbook of Pediatric Psychology. New York: Guilford Publications, 1988.
19. B Starfield. Social factors in child health. In: M Green, RJ Haggerty, eds. Ambulatory Pediatrics. Philadelphia: WB Saunders, 1990, pp 30–36.
20. CS Lapidus, DF Schwarz, PJ Honig. Atopic dermatitis in children: Who cares? Who pays? J Am Acad Dermatol 28(5):699–703, 1993.
21. JA Witkowski. Compliance: the dermatologic patient. Int J Dermatol 27:608–611, 1988.
22. RM Herd, MJ Tidman, RJ Prescott, JAA Hunter. The cost of atopic eczema. Br J Dermatol 135:20–23, 1996.

5

Genetics of Atopic Dermatitis

Kate Elliott and Susan Forrest
Murdoch Childrens Research Institute, Melbourne, Australia

I. INTRODUCTION

Atopic dermatitis is a member of a growing class of diseases referred to as common complex diseases. This reflects the frequency of the disease in the general population and the number of genes likely to cause disease. Early genetic studies focused on single gene disorders in which only one genetic locus was found to be responsible for a particular disease phenotype, even though the mutation in each family could differ. The complexity with atopic dermatitis arises because genetic factors and the environment interact to determine disease susceptibility. Therefore, the challenging task exists to actually identify these various factors and understand how they interact.

The importance of accurate phenotype definition for the study of complex traits cannot be emphasized strongly enough. It is crucial for the replication of others findings or indeed to facilitate pooling of results into a meta-analysis. It is essential that comparable criteria are used by different research groups. Ideally, one clinician should be responsible for coding all phenotypes, but often this is not possible.

Asthma and atopy in general have been the focus of many genetic studies using total serum IgE as a phenotypic marker. The benefits of studying atopic dermatitis in particular to find atopy loci seem to have been overlooked by a number of researchers in this field. The diagnosis is consistent between clinicians, and well-established scoring systems such as the SCORAD are used to ascertain the severity of disease (1). This is certainly not the case with asthma and atopy in general, thus atopic dermatitis is a better defined clinical phenotype. In our genetic study of atopic dermatitis, we purposely chose an early-onset severely affected cohort (2). With this tight phenotypic group we maximized the chance that the same set of genes were involved.

II. EVIDENCE FOR GENETIC INFLUENCES ON ATOPIC DERMATITIS

In order to ascertain what proportion of the dermatitis phenotype is attributable to a genetic component, traditional genetic studies are undertaken. The two most common are family studies and twin studies.

A. Family Studies: Increased Risk to First-Degree Relatives

The early studies to determine whether or not atopy has a genetic component involved ascertaining the prevalence of allergic disease in first-degree relatives of atopic individuals (3). Not surprisingly, the prevalence was higher in relatives of affected individuals than in relatives of unaffected individuals (Fig. 1). A prospective study of several hundred newborns over a 5-year period gave more convincing evidence that atopic dermatitis and other forms of atopy were passed from parent to child (4). Fifty-one percent of children with a family history of atopy compared to 19% of children with no family history of atopy developed symptoms of allergic disease within the first 5 years of life. In particular, Dold

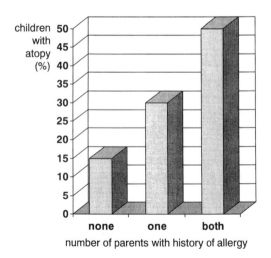

Figure 1   Family history and risk of allergy. (Adapted from Ref. 129.)

et al. (5) found that children of parents with atopic dermatitis are more likely to develop atopic dermatitis than children of asthmatic parents or those with allergic rhinitis. This could be interpreted as the genetic component manifesting itself in a tissue-specific manner, suggesting that genes specific for atopic dermatitis might exist.

B. Twin Studies

Twin studies provide additional evidence for a genetic contribution. In such studies, the frequency of the trait of interest is assessed in pairs of monozygous (MZ) and dizygous (DZ) twins. The difference in concordance rates between MZ and DZ twins gives an indication of the heritability of the disorder. Initially, measurements of quantitative traits such as skin prick test results and total serum IgE levels have indicated a twofold higher correlation between MZ twins when compared to DZ twins (6) (Fig. 2). In a genetic epidemiological study in a population-based twin sample, Schultz-Larsen (7) showed that the concordance rate for MZ twins was 0.72 and for dizygotic twins 0.23. This study therefore showed that genetic factors have a far greater influence on the atopic dermatitis phenotype than was previously believed.

Multigeneration family studies as well as twin studies have indicated that there is a strong genetic component to atopic dermatitis. No clear mode of inheritance can be identified, indicating that it is a complex trait, with multiple gene interactions and environmental influences. From studying population frequencies and sibling recurrence risks for atopy, it has been hypothesized that at least two

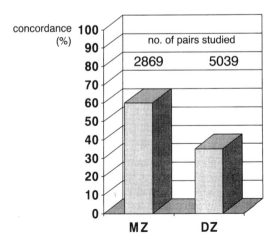

Figure 2 Concordance for atopic disease in twins. (Adapted from Ref. 129.)

disease susceptibility genes exist that segregate independently and interact with each other (8).

III. GENETIC STUDIES

Once convincing arguments were put forward in the literature for a strong genetic component, researchers in the field of atopic dermatitis embarked on the challenging task of gene identification. This task has been greatly slowed by the genetic complexity of atopic dermatitis, asthma, and atopy in general.

A. Candidate Genes Versus Whole Genome Scan

In order to find these genes, two major approaches can be utilized. One method for the localization of the candidate region is a genome-wide scan whereby genetic markers spaced at intervals between 5 and 10 cM across the genome are analyzed. A whole genome scan does not presuppose the involvement of any particular locus. An alternative approach is candidate gene analysis. Depending on the knowledge of the underlying biology of the trait, it is sometimes possible to predict genes that might be involved in particular diseases. The gene that encodes mast cell chymase, for example, is a logical candidate as this protein is part of the pathway for developing atopic dermatitis.

Two types of genetic markers can be used in linkage and association analyses. Microsatellites are simple repeat sequences, most often dinucleotide or tetranucleotide repeats, which occur randomly throughout the genome and have on average 5–10 different alleles at each locus. Single nucleotide polymorphisms, on the other hand, are biallelic and therefore less informative as fewer individuals are heterozygous for the marker. However, they are found more often in the genome both within and near genes and are more likely to have functional consequences.

B. Linkage Analysis

The aim of genetic linkage studies is to determine the position of the predisposing gene(s) for the phenotype under study relative to marker loci that have known chromosomal localizations. The localization step relies on the principle of linkage where two genetic markers that cosegregate when transmitted in pedigrees are said to be linked. When the gene has been roughly positioned, fine mapping studies using a denser array of polymorphic markers and positional cloning followed by detailed sequence analysis identify the predisposing gene.

Genetic markers that are polymorphic between individuals are used for linkage analysis. Linkage is determined by the recombination fraction theta (θ)

between two markers in the genome, which in turn is determined by the distance between the two markers (9). The recombination fraction is $\theta = 0.5$ for loci that assort independently or are located on different chromosomes, and ranges from 0 to 0.5 for linked loci.

The probability of genetic linkage is determined by the maximum likelihood method or the LOD score. The LOD score is the ratio between the probability of linkage at a certain θ and the probability of no linkage ($\theta = 0.5$) (9). The LOD score is calculated with different values of θ to determine the distance between the marker and the trait under study where the LOD score is maximal. For single gene disorders, a LOD score of 3 is required to establish linkage with statistical significance and a value of -2 is regarded to be statistically significant for exclusion (9). The value of 3 for linkage is only valid for the study of single gene disorders and should be adjusted for more complex disorders in which multiple genes are involved (10).

Different sample-collection strategies, such as extended pedigrees and affected sib pairs, have been used in genome-wide scans. Extended pedigrees will have the most power to detect linkage as they contain a large number of meiotic events that assist with gene localization. When large pedigrees are unavailable, identification of simple kinships of sibpairs, preferably with parents and/or triads (the affected individual plus parents), are preferred to just collecting unrelated affected individuals, as the latter only allows for association and linkage disequilibrium studies (11).

C. Specifying a Model or Model-Free Analysis

Linkage analysis can be accomplished with the aid of a variety of programs that perform the statistical calculations, such as Genehunter (12). Two different methods are utilized to calculate linkage, parametric and nonparametric, and both essentially rely on testing for a deviation in the frequency of alleles or haplotypes that segregate with the disease. Parametric methods are based on specifying a model for the disease inheritance. The parameters to be chosen include disease gene frequency, mode of inheritance, and penetrance. However, with complex traits it is often the case that these are estimates at best and are very sensitive to misspecification of the genetic model. Thus, most researchers use model-free, nonparametric methods and analyze multiple marker results at once.

D. Association Analysis

Association studies compare allele frequencies of polymorphic variants in candidate genes between a case group of unrelated affected people and a control group of unrelated unaffected people. No mode of inheritance needs to be specified. Alleles are said to be associated if they are present at a higher frequency in the case group, and the significance of the finding is measured using the chi-square test. It is important to note that in different populations, different alleles at the locus might be associated with disease. If positive associations are detected between an allele and the disease of interest, they are said to be in linkage disequilibrium.

However, association results can be positive for a number of different reasons, apart from linkage disequilibrium, which may help explain the number of inconsistent results when comparing findings between laboratories. The allele under study could actually be the causal factor such that having that allele predisposes the individual to developing the disease. Second, the apparent association may be due to population stratification/admixture where the disease and the associated allele happen, by virtue of population ancestry, to be more frequent in a subset. Unidentified population stratification can result in differences in allele frequency between unrelated affecteds, unrelated controls, or both. The choice of control group is therefore vital to ensure that results of association studies are meaningful, and Terwilliger and Goring advise selection of appropriate controls (11).

E. Transmission Disequilibrium Tests

Methods have been developed to overcome the problems of false-positive association results. The transmission disequilibrium test confirms whether a marker allele is associated with a disease (13). Samples are collected from both the parents as well as the affected offspring. This then means that simple triads (mother, father and affected child) can be used as a genetic resource rather than having to find affected sib pairs, which is a far more arduous task. Parents are tested for heterozygosity at the associated allele. The test determines whether the ''associated'' allele is transmitted to the affected offspring more than expected by chance (50%). If multiple affected sibs happen to be available, corrections can be invoked to allow inclusion of this extra data in the analysis (14).

F. Recommendations

The recent completion of the first draft of the human genome has meant that many more microsatellite genetic markers as well as SNPs are now available all over the genome. The preferred approach for complex traits with our current knowledge base is linkage disequilibrium studies. Functional polymorphisms in coding regions (see NCBI's dbSNP database at http://www.ncbi.nlm.nih.gov/SNP/) are the variants of first choice to search for linkage disequilibrium (LD) between marker and disease. It needs to be noted that there is not an exact inverse linear relationship between strength of LD and distance from the causative allele. LD varies over chromosomal regions (15), thus posing additional challenges to the development of efficient mapping strategies to identify predisposing genes for complex traits.

Terwilliger and Goring (11) in a recent article recommend three approaches for collecting the sample set that maximizes the number of informative meioses:

1. Selecting idiosyncratic forms of the disease that may reflect a particular defect in one gene, thereby reducing the locus or allelic heterogeneity
2. Selecting a very small homogenous population, which increases the possibility that many of the disease risk factors are either absent or fixed in the population, thus reducing the locus heterogeneity
3. Finding large pedigrees with the disease phenotype present in many individuals and generations, presumably enriching for genetic components

IV. SUMMARY OF THE ATOPY PATHWAY

The atopic pathway has been studied extensively, and many of the molecules involved in allergic responses have been identified. This makes the task of the geneticist easier since it gives an array of candidate genes to choose from either when searching for genes beneath a linked region or when looking for variants within molecules that might be associated with atopic diseases. Figure 3 is a

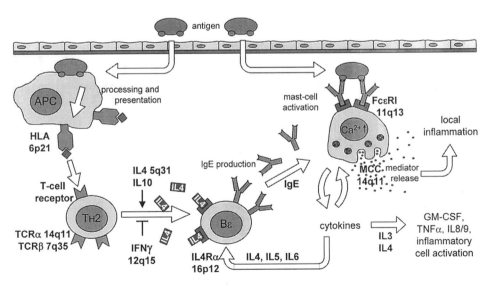

Figure 3 IgE hyperproduction and effector mechanisms in atopy. See Sec. IV for a description of the atopic pathway. (Adapted from Ref. 129.)

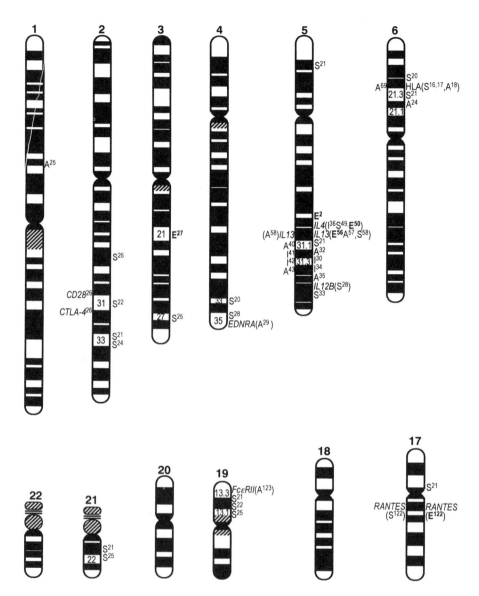

Figure 4   A representation of the current linkages and associations reported with atopy, asthma, and eczema. A = Atopy; S = asthma; I = IgE levels; E = eczema or atopic dermatitis (shown in bold). Positive reports are shown on the right of the chromosomes, negative reports are shown on the left. The corresponding references are superscripted.

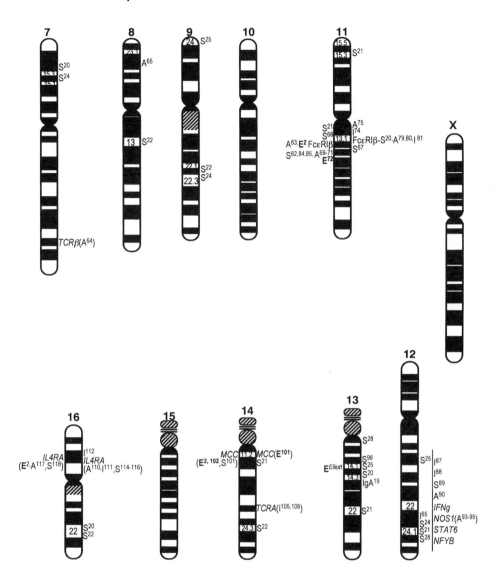

schematic diagram of the atopy pathway. Antigens enter via the skin (eczema) or lungs (asthma) and are taken up by antigen-presenting cells, processed, and presented to T cells via the MHC molecules encoded by the MHC genes on chromosome 6p21. The T-cell receptor is encoded by the α subunit gene on chromosome 14q11 and the β subunit gene on chromosome 7q35.

The T_H2 cells signal to the B cells via a cocktail of cytokines to upregulate the production of IgE (IL4, IL5, IL13—chromosome 5q31) or suppress the production of IgE (INFγ—chromosome 12q14). The IgE then binds to the Fcε receptors (FcεRI encoded on chromosome 11q13) on mast cells, thus sensitizing them. When an allergen then reaches the sensitized mast cell it cross-links with the surface bound IgE and triggers a reaction that leads to the release of histamine and proteases such as mast cell chymase encoded on chromosome 14q11. Theoretically mutations that upregulate, downregulate, or alter the function of the genes encoding these molecules could have an effect on the susceptibility of an individual to atopy. A number of these genes have already been studied with respect to atopic susceptibility, and the results in many cases have been contradictory, underlining the complexity of atopy genetics.

V.   ATOPY GENES AND LOCI

Since the very first reports of linkage of atopy to HLA in the mid-1970s (16–18) atopic dermatitis, asthma, and elevated serum IgE have been linked to almost every chromosome. An illustration of this complexity can be seen by looking at the results of genome scans of cohorts of patients with atopy and asthma phenotypes (19–24). These scans reveal multiple peaks, only a few of which are duplicated between different studies. There are relatively few studies of the genetics of atopic eczema specifically. Therefore, we will also be describing loci that have been linked and associated with asthma and atopy in general, since it is predictable that a large proportion of asthma and general atopy genes will also play a role in eczema susceptibility. Figure 4 illustrates the reported linkages and associations of atopy, asthma, and atopic dermatitis with different chromosomal locations and is intended to give a pictorial summary of the current knowledge of atopy genetics.

A.   Chromosome 1

Chromosome 1 has been linked to susceptibility to atopy by Ober et al. in a genome wide screen of Hutterites (25). Using a second-generation genome screen they reconfirmed this linkage at D1S239 (22), but this region has not been reported as an atopy susceptibility locus in any other studies.

B. Chromosome 2

Four genome scans have linked chromosome 2 to atopic phenotypes; two studies linked chromosome 2q33 in Hispanics (21) and a German and Swedish cohort (24) and two generations of genome scans of Hutterites linked 2q22 and 2q31 (22,25). Within the 2q22-33 region the CD28 and CTLA-4 genes are both good candidates for asthma and atopy since their encoded proteins have been shown to be involved as an important costimulatory signal in the regulation of allergic inflammation and T_H2 cytokine production. However, no association was found between polymorphisms in these genes and asthma or atopy phenotypes (26).

C. Chromosome 3

Interestingly, until 2000 no region on chromosome 3 had been convincingly implicated in atopy. Lee et al. ascertained 199 families, each with at least two affected offspring with moderate to severe eczema with the age of onset under 2 years (27). They performed a genome-wide linkage study that revealed highly significant evidence for linkage on chromosome 3q21. Two type I membrane proteins, CD80 and CD86, are located within this region. These two proteins interact with CD28, which has been implicated in T-cell activation.

D. Chromosome 4

Chromosome 4q35 has been linked to asthma in two genome scans in Australians (20) and Japanese (28), but no other linkages have been reported. However, an association has been observed between a variant of the endothelin-1 receptor type A (EDNRA) gene at 4q35 and atopic asthma (29). Endothelin-1 is a 21-amino-acid peptide that has various roles in the pathophysiology of asthma, and therefore genes encoding endothelin-1 and its receptors are candidates for atopy genes.

E. Chromosome 5 (Interleukin Cluster)

The genetic location that has attracted the greatest interest after the major histocompatibility complex (MHC) with respect to disposition to allergic diseases is 5q23-31. Chromosome 5 has been repeatedly associated with or linked to asthma, atopy, and atopic eczema in a large number of studies (2,21,30–36). Most reports have linked 5q23-31, and within this region is a cluster of cytokine genes (37–39). However, there have also been some reports refuting these findings (40–43).

1. Interleukin 4 (IL4)

IL4 plays an important role in IgE synthesis by activating the pre-T-helper cells that trigger isotype switching from IgM/IgG to IgE in B cells by promoting T_H2

cell development (44). This has led to its emergence as the most studied gene in terms of its linkage or association with atopic disease. To date, three polymorphisms have been identified in the IL4 gene: −590C/T in the promoter (45), −34C/T in the 5′ untranslated region (46), and a dinucleotide repeat, IL4-R1, in intron 2 (47).

In 1994, in a study of IL4 and the surrounding region, linkage was found between IL4 (IL4-R1) and elevated serum IgE (30). The majority of studies since then have focused on association of the single nucleotide polymorphisms with atopic disease. In 1996 the group of Cookson found weak association of the −590C/T allele with asthma and atopy in Australians (48). Further study of the −590C/T polymorphism together with the IL4-R1 dinucleotide repeat suggested that these polymorphisms were linked to serum IgE levels, but no evidence could be found to suggest that the −590C/T polymorphism contributed to disease (36). Two studies in the Japanese population have linked this polymorphism to asthma (49,50), and reporter gene transfection studies have suggested that the −590T allele is associated with increased promoter activity (51). The recently discovered −34C/T polymorphism (46) was also tested together with the −590C/T polymorphism for association with atopic eczema. Even though there was no evidence for association, when separated into haplotypes, the −590C/−34C haplotype was weakly associated, suggesting that it was either mildly causative or in linkage disequilibrium with a causative allele (130).

2. Interleukin 13 (IL13)

IL13 shares several biological profiles with IL4 (52,53), including IgE production, MHC class II expression and binding to receptors containing the IL4RI subunit (54). The IL13 gene is tandemly positioned very close to the IL4 gene and comprises many similarities in terms of its structure and functional sequence elements (55). Seven polymorphisms have been identified within the IL13 gene. One of these, Gln110Arg has been associated with atopic dermatitis in a German cohort (56), elevated serum IgE in three Caucasian populations (57), and asthma, but not serum IgE, in British and Japanese populations (58).

3. CD14 Antigen

CD14 is found on the surface of monocytes and macrophages and may play a role in regulating IgE. The −159C/T promoter polymorphism has been associated with serum CD14 levels and elevated IgE (59,60). A genome scan of Hutterites also found association of this promoter polymorphism with asthma, but only when it was preferentially transmitted with the 185-base-pair allele of the adjacent D5S642 marker, suggesting that these alleles are in linkage disequilibrium with a nearby susceptibility locus (22).

4. Interleukin 12B (IL12B)

IL12 is a key cytokine in the induction of T_H1-type immune responses, and a reduced capacity to produce this cytokine could lead to aberrant T_H2-type responses in atopic patients (61). It is comprised of p35 (IL12A) and p40 (IL12B) subunits located on chromosomes 3 and 5q31-33 (62). Studies have detected linkage to bronchial hyperresponsiveness in a Danish population (32) and weak linkage to asthma in the Hutterites (25). A recent genome scan of mite-sensitive asthmatic Japanese detected significant linkage at 5q31. Fine mapping of this region localized the linkage peak to markers close to the IL12B gene (28).

F. Chromosome 6—Major Histocompatibility Complex

In the mid-1970s, the first reports of genetic susceptibility to asthma and atopy were reported as linkages with particular HLA haplotypes (16–18). The first serious studies of the segregation of atopy within multigeneration families began in the early 1980s and this coincided with a flood of interest in the products of the major histocompatibility complex. The MHC class II genes became the first "candidate" genes to be analyzed for association with atopy and have been repeatedly implicated since then. Dozens of studies investigated the role of MHC genes in predisposition to atopy with respect multiple atopic phenotypes and multiple-defined allergens. One study analyzing 100 individuals with a positive or negative family history of atopy associated the HLA-DR4 and DR7 alleles with susceptibility for atopic disease (63). A number of genome scans have also linked MHC to asthma (20,21,24).

G. Chromosome 7

Two genome scans have detected linkage to asthma on chromosome 7 at 7p15-21 in Australians (20) and 7p15 in Swedish and Germans (24), but there are no known candidate genes in this region. However, a study of Japanese asthmatics reported linkage to markers flanking the T-cell receptor β gene at 7q33 (64).

H. Chromosome 8

Two linkages have been reported on chromosome 8, to asthma at 8q13 (22), and to mite-specific IgE responses at chromosome 8p23-21 (65). Although there are no obvious candidates on chromosome 8, it is interesting to note that 8p23-21 shares synteny with the major atopic dermatitis locus in the NOA mouse model (66).

I. Chromosome 9

Three genome scans have detected linkage to chromosome 9: two to 9q22 in Hutterite (22) and German and Swedish asthmatics (24) and one to two separate chromosome 9 peaks in the first-generation screen of asthmatic Hutterites (25). Again there is a lack of candidate genes on chromosome 9.

J. Chromosome 11

Like chromosome 5q, follow-up studies of the initial reports of linkage to chromosome 11 have either confirmed or failed to confirm the initial findings. In 1989 the laboratory of Cookson were the first to report linkage to 11q to IgE levels with the observation of maternal transmission (67). Studies by many others failed to replicate these findings (68–72), and since this early phase of studies the field has been split as to whether or not real linkage exists between 11q and atopy.

In 1993 the high-affinity IgE receptor (FcεRI) was then mapped to 11q13 (73). This is obviously a strong candidate gene for atopy since it encodes the receptor for IgE on mast cells. Two Japanese groups then reported linkages to D11S97 adjacent to FcεRI and to a dinucleotide repeat within intron 5 of the gene (74,75). To add further controversy, 11q13 was reported as being linked to bronchial hyperresponsiveness in the absence of atopy (76). Several polymorphisms have now been identified in the FcεRI gene, including the Leu181Ile (77) and Gly237Glu (78) coding variants and the 1109C/T promoter polymorphism. Again Cookson and his collaborators plus others (79–81) have published reports of positive associations of these polymorphisms with atopic markers, but many investigators have failed to replicate these findings (2,82–85). The issue of true linkage of the FcεRI gene to atopic disease remains contentious and factors such as population differences (74) and phenotypic heterogeneity (76) will undoubtedly make a significant contribution to these discrepancies.

K. Chromosome 12

The initial demonstrations of genetic linkage of asthma and atopy to chromosome 12 (86,87) have been confirmed by several genome-wide screens (21,24,25,65). The region showing the most convincing and reproducible linkage is 12q22-24, which has been linked to asthma in Caucasians and Hispanics (21) and Japanese (28). Four other studies have concentrated on fine mapping the 12q region against (a) total serum IgE and asthma in Afro-Carribean and Caucasian populations (87), (b) asthma and total serum IgE in Germans (88), (c) asthma in a U.K. cohort (89), and (d) asthma and atopy in subjects from Barbados (90). All of these studies detected linkage in a region spanning approximately 30 centimorgans from 12q13-24.

This region contains a number of strong candidate genes, including interferon-gamma (IFNγ), which inhibits IL4-induced class switching to IgE production in B lymphocytes (91). The exons and 5'-flanking region were screened for polymorphisms, but no variants could be found to test association of the IFNγ gene with asthma (92). Also present in this region is the gene encoding neuronal nitric oxide synthase (NOS1), which is known to have a role in bronchomotor control in animals. Although this gene is clearly not a candidate for atopic eczema, polymorphisms have been associated with asthma (93–95). Signal transducer and activator of transcription 6 (STAT6), which is essential for IL4 signaling and T_H2 development (96,97), and the β subunit of nuclear transcription factor Y (NFYB), which binds to the promoter of HLA genes, are also good candidates found in this interval. However, to date no genetic studies have been undertaken to test the association with atopic disease.

L.   Chromosome 13

The majority of genome scans for asthma loci have detected linkage to chromosome 13 (20–22,25,28). However linkage has only reproducibly been detected at 13q14 (20,25). Interestingly, this region was also detected in a genome scan for loci influencing IgA levels (19). A linkage and association study of atopic asthma to markers on chromosome 13 in the Japanese population confirmed linkage to 13q14 and additionally found association of asthma with the D13S153 marker (98). However, when this marker was tested for linkage to atopic eczema in Australians, a highly negative linkage score was obtained, indicating that this region could be excluded as an eczema locus (K. Elliott et al., unpublished). This suggests that 13q14 may harbor an asthma-specific gene, but there are no obvious candidates.

M.   Chromosome 14

Only two genome screens (21,22) have detected linkage of asthma with chromosome 14 at different locations, making it an unconvincing candidate for atopy loci. However, this has not deterred other researchers from conducting linkage and association studies on candidate genes harbored within chromosome 14.

1.   Mast Cell Chymase

Mast cell chymase (MCC) is a chymotrypsin-like serine protease secreted by skin mast cells and has proinflammatory properties (99). The MCC gene is located within the Cathepsin/granzyme gene cluster (100). In 1996 Mao et al. identified a *Bst*XI polymorphism in the MCC gene and found association with eczema, but not with asthma or hayfever in the Japanese population (101). However, two other studies have failed to find association of atopic eczema and MCC in Japanese and Caucasian populations (2,102). In a second study by Mao et al., the same polymorphism was found to be associated with eczematous Japanese children with lower IgE levels (103). This suggests that MCC may play an important role in inflammatory skin disease, but not atopy.

2. T-Cell Receptor Alpha (TCRA)

The T-cell receptor recognizes antigenic peptide fragments presented by MHC, which initiates T-cell activation and cytokine release with subsequent recruitment of inflammatory cells. The α subunit of the T-cell receptor is encoded by the TCRA gene located on 14q23 (104). Linkage to specific IgE reactions was detected to a microsatellite marker within the TCRA gene in U.K. and Australian families (105). This result was supported by linkage of total serum IgE levels to markers within and flanking the TCRA gene, and one of the flanking markers showed evidence of association (106).

N. Chromosome 16

Linkage to chromosome 16 has been detected in three genome scans for atopy and asthma loci. 16q23 was detected in two scans for serum IgE in an Australian population (20) and asthma in a second-generation screen of Hutterites (22), but there are no candidate genes in this region. The first screen of Hutterites by Ober et al. found linkage to a different locus at 16p12, which is where the interleukin-4 receptor alpha (IL4RA) gene is located (107).

IL4RA constitutes a subunit of the respective receptors for IL4 and IL13, the T_H2 cytokines whose function overlaps and include mediating isotype switching to IgE (108,109). Thirteen polymorphisms have been identified in the coding region of the IL4RA gene, 7 of which result in amino acid substitutions (110–112). Associations between atopic phenotypes and IL4RA polymorphisms, ile50 and arg551, were reported in two case-control studies (110,113). After a linkage study (112), Kruse et al. (111) reported significant associations between the pro478 and arg551 alleles and low IgE levels and further demonstrated that these two variants act synergistically to influence signal-transduction pathways via the IL4RA gene. Additional evidence of association of the arg551 allele with asthma severity supports this (114–116). However, two studies have failed to replicate the finding of association of IL4RA polymorphisms with atopic eczema in Caucasians (2) and atopy and asthma in Japanese (117,118).

O. Chromosome 17 (RANTES)

Two genome scans have linked asthma to chromosome 17 in African Americans and Hutterites (21,25). Located on chromosome 17 is the gene encoding

RANTES or small inducible cytokine A5 (SCYA5). This is one of a family of C-C chemokines, which play a crucial role in the pathogenesis of allergic inflammation (119–121). Given the linkage and potential role for the RANTES gene in atopy, Nickel et al. (122) screened the promoter for polymorphisms. A single polymorphism was identified at base pair −401 and results in a new consensus binding site for the GATA transcription factor family. In vitro transfection studies demonstrated that the difference conferred an eightfold increase in promoter activity. Association studies indicated that this polymorphism contributed to the development of atopic dermatitis but not asthma in African and Caucasian study populations (122).

P. Chromosome 19

Linkage to chromosome 19 has been detected by three genome scans to asthma traits in Hutterites (22,25) and Caucasians (21), all at the same interval, 19p13, where there are no obvious candidate genes. Further along the chromosome is the gene encoding the low-affinity IgE receptor (FcεRII), but a study of this gene and 10cM of the surrounding chromosome in Finnish and Catalonian families suggested that it was only weakly associated with atopic disease (123).

Q. Chromosome 21

Two genome scans have detected linkage to atopy phenotypes at chromosome 21q21-22 in Hutterites and Hispanics (21,25). However, there are no association studies of candidate genes in this region.

VI. GENETICS OF ANIMAL MODELS

A. Inbred Mouse Strains

1. NOA Mouse

The NOA mouse model is a strain that develops spontaneous ulcerative skin lesions similar to atopic dermatitis, associated with an accumulation of mast cells and significantly increased serum IgE (124). Natori et al. carried out an experiment to map the genes responsible for the eczema by backcrossing the mice to five different wild-type strains (125). They carried out a genome-wide scan of the offspring and scored for the eczema phenotype. Their results indicated the presence of a single major atopic dermatitis locus on chromosome 14 in a region that shares synteny with human chromosomes 8p32-23 and 13q14.3-22 (Fig. 5). There has been only one report of linkage to human 8p32-23 and mite-specific IgE responses (65), and reports of linkage of atopic phenotypes to 13q14.3-22

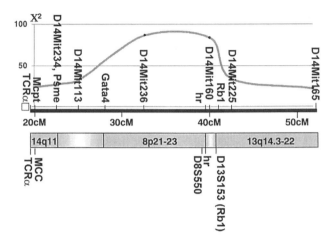

Figure 5 Map of human synteny on mouse chromosome 14, showing the approximate boundaries of the syntenies. Aligned with the left-hand side of the picture is a curve of the chi-squared values along this region of mouse chromosome 14 showing the linkage to atopic dermatitis in the NOA mouse.

have been contradictory (98). There are no obvious atopy genes identified in the chromosome 13 interval, but interestingly it does harbor the *hairless* gene. Although Natori et al. found no molecular differences in the *hr* gene, it is still difficult to reconcile the coincidence that the major atopy locus lies within the vicinity of the *hairless* gene when this strain has a pronounced *hairless* phenotype.

In a further study the same group tried isolating genes responsible for the atopic dermatitis in NOA mice by looking at the differential expression of genes in the spleens of NOA mice compared with controls. The platelet factor 4 (PF4) gene was identified as being significantly more highly expressed in NOA mice compared to controls (125). PF4 encodes a heparin-binding protein and belongs to the CXC motif chemokine molecules. However, the gene does not map to the chromosome 14 peak identified in their genome scan and the human gene is located on chromosome 4q25, a region that has not been reported as linked to any atopic disorders.

2. Other Studies

To study the genetics of atopy, Daser et al. developed a mouse model that provides the general phenotype of atopy—the early response characteristic of IgE-dependent eczema and the diagnostic test of atopy, the skin-prick test. Using a

skin-prick test against birch pollen extract they could classify A/J and C57BL/
6 (B6) inbred mouse strains, respectively, as high and low responders. The F1
hybrids were found to be high responders with incomplete penetrance. Backcrossing F1 mice to the low-responder B6 strain yielded three classes of responders:
high, intermediate, and low. A genome-wide scan of the backcross progeny dis-
closed suggestive linkage to chromosome 6 close to the locus of the IL-5 receptor
α chain. The human IL5 receptor gene is located on chromosome 3p24, and this
region has not been previously linked to atopic disorders.

The Biozzi BP2 mouse shows features of asthma when sensitized and subsequently challenged with ovalbumin. Zhang et al. set out to map the genes influencing the asthma phenotype by backcrossing the mice to BALBc mice and carrying out a genome-wide scan (126). Five loci were identified that were linked
to the asthma phenotype. Four of these had previously been identified as linked at
asthma in syntenic human regions: chromosome 9 (syntenic with human 11q23—
IL10R), chromosome 10 (syntenic with human 12q22-24—IFNγ), chromosome
11 (syntenic with human 5q31—IL4 cluster), and chromosome 17 (syntenic with
human 6p21—MHC and TNF).

B. Transgenic Mice

1. CNS1, a Coordinate Regulator of IL4, IL5, and IL13 Expression

The group of Loots et al. have identified a long-range regulatory element coordinately controlling the expression of the IL4, IL5, and IL13 genes (127). Using
computational methods, one megabase of orthologous human and mouse sequences covering the region of the IL4, IL5, and IL13 genes was searched for
conserved elements and a total of 90 extragenic conserved sequences were identified. Fifteen of these were found to be conserved across other mammals including
cows, pigs, dogs, and cats. The largest of these extragenic regions, termed CNS1
(*c*onserved *n*oncoding *s*equence) is 401 base pairs lying between the IL4 and
IL13 genes (Fig. 6).

Loots et al. chose this element for functional study using transgenic mice
bearing a 450kb YAC encompassing CNS1 and 9 genes including IL4, IL5, and
IL13. A comparison was made of T_H2 cells in mice with the same human
transgene insertions, with or without CNS1. They found a decrease in human
IL4 and IL13 production due to a decrease in T_H2 cells expressing these cytokines
and an overall decrease in human IL5 production in mice bearing transgenes
with the CNS1 element removed. Besides providing important insights into the
mechanism of control of the IL4 cluster, this finding clearly demonstrates the
importance of the elements as a potential source of variation predisposing to
complex diseases.

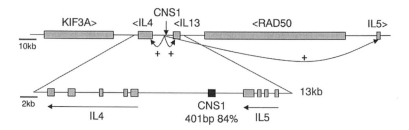

Figure 6   The relationship between CNS1 and the IL4, IL5, and IL13 genes on chromosome 5q31.

2.   IL4 Transgenic Mice

By fusing the IL4 gene to a immunoglobulin enhancer/promoter construct, Tepper et al. demonstrated that deregulation of the IL4 gene in vivo can induce a complex inflammatory reaction resembling that observed in human allergic disease (128). Overexpression of IL4 results in a marked increase in serum IgE levels and the appearance of an inflammatory eye lesion with characteristic histopathalogical features seen in allergic reactions.

VII.   CONCLUSION

In summary, no one gene can be implicated as the gene responsible for the development of atopic dermatitis. However, a clearer picture of the most likely candidate genes or regions is emerging from complementary studies in humans and mice. The MHC complex has certainly been implicated as well as the cluster of interleukins on human chromosome 5. One of the major outcomes of a better understanding of the contribution of genetics to the overall phenotype is the possibility of developing improved therapeutics for atopic dermatitis. Topical administration of therapeutic molecules such as antisense RNAs, which have the capability of knock out or significantly reduce the function of key genes, may be the goal for the future for this increasing common disorder.

ACKNOWLEDGMENTS

Dr. David Hill is thanked for his clinical expertise and Professor Bob Williamson for his support of this manuscript. This work is supported by the Murdoch Childrens Research Institute and the Cooperative Research Centre for the Discovery of Genes for Common Human Diseases. The CRC is established and supported by the Australian Governments Cooperative Research Centres Program.

REFERENCES

1. Severity scoring of atopic dermatitis: the SCORAD index. Consensus Report of the European Task Force on Atopic Dermatitis. Dermatology 1993; 186(1):23–31.
2. Forrest S, Dunn K, Elliott K, Fitzpatrick E, Fullerton J, McCarthy M, Brown J, Hill D, Williamson R. Identifying genes predisposing to atopic eczema. J Allergy Clin Immunol 1999; 104(5):1066–1070.
3. Ono SJ. Molecular genetics of allergic diseases. Annu Rev Immunol 2000; 18:347–366.
4. Luoma R, Koivikko A, Viander M. Development of asthma, allergic rhinitis and atopic dermatitis by the age of five years. A prospective study of 543 newborns. Allergy 1983; 38(5):339–346.
5. Dold S, Wjst M, von Mutius E, Reitmeir P, Stiepel E. Genetic risk for asthma, allergic rhinitis, and atopic dermatitis. Arch Dis Child 1992; 67(8):1018–1022.
6. Hopp RJ, Bewtra AK, Watt GD, Nair NM, Townley RG. Genetic analysis of allergic disease in twins. J Allergy Clin Immunol 1984; 73(2):265–270.
7. Schultz-Larsen F. Atopic dermatitis: a genetic-epidemiologic study in a population-based twin sample. J Am Acad Dermatol 1993; 28(5 Pt 1):719–723.
8. Xu J, Levitt RC, Panhuysen CI, Postma DS, Taylor EW, Amelung PJ, Holroyd KJ, Bleecker ER, Meyers DA. Evidence for two unlinked loci regulating total serum IgE levels. Am J Hum Genet 1995; 57(2):425–430.
9. Ott J. Analysis of Human Genetic Linkage. Revised ed. Baltimore: The Johns Hopkins University Press, 1991.
10. Lander E, Kruglyak L. Genetic dissection of complex traits: guidelines for interpreting and reporting linkage results [see comments]. Nat Genet 1995; 11(3):241–247.
11. Terwilliger JD, Goring HH. Gene mapping in the 20th and 21st centuries: statistical methods, data analysis, and experimental design. Hum Biol 2000; 72(1):63–132.
12. Kruglyak L, Daly MJ, Reeve-Daly MP, Lander ES. Parametric and nonparametric linkage analysis: a unified multipoint approach. Am J Hum Genet 1996; 58(6):1347–1363.
13. Spielman RS, McGinnis RE, Ewens WJ. Transmission test for linkage disequilibrium: the insulin gene region and insulin-dependent diabetes mellitus (IDDM). Am J Hum Genet 1993; 52(3):506–516.
14. Martin ER, Kaplan NL, Weir BS. Tests for linkage and association in nuclear families. Am J Hum Genet 1997; 61(2):439–448.
15. Moffatt MF, Traherne JA, Abecasis GR, Cookson WO. Single nucleotide polymorphism and linkage disequilibrium within the TCR alpha/delta locus. Hum Mol Genet 2000; 9(7):1011–1019.
16. Wagatsuma Y, Yakura H, Nakayama E, Wakisaka A, Aizawa M. Inheritance of asthma in families and its linkage to HLA haplotypes. Acta Allergol 1976; 31(6):455–462.

17. Brostoff J, Mowbray JF, Kapoor A, Hollowell SJ, Rudolf M, Saunders KB. 80% of patients with intrinsic asthma are homozygous for HLA W6. Is intrinsic asthma a recessive disease? Lancet 1976; 2(7991):872–873.

18. Geerts SJ, Pottgens H, Limburg M, van Rood JJ. Letter: Predisposition for atopy or allergy linked to HL-A. Lancet 1975; 1(7904):461.

19. Wiltshire S, Bhattacharyya S, Faux JA, Leaves NI, Daniels SE, Moffatt MF, James A, Musk AW, Cookson WO. A genome scan for loci influencing total serum immunoglobulin levels: possible linkage of IgA to the chromosome 13 atopy locus. Hum Mol Genet 1998; 7(1):27–31.

20. Daniels SE, Bhattacharyya S, James A, Leaves NI, Young A, Hill MR, Faux JA, Ryan GF, le Souef PN, Lathrop GM, Musk AW, Cookson WO. A genome-wide search for quantitative trait loci underlying asthma. Nature 1996; 383(6597):247–250.

21. A genome-wide search for asthma susceptibility loci in ethnically diverse populations. The Collaborative Study on the Genetics of Asthma (CSGA). Nat Genet 1997; 15(4):389–392.

22. Ober C, Tsalenko A, Parry R, Cox NJ. A Second-Generation Genomewide Screen for Asthma-Susceptibility Alleles in a Founder Population. Am J Hum Genet 2000; 67(5):1154–1162.

23. Malerba G, Trabetti E, Patuzzo C, Lauciello MC, Galavotti R, Pescollderungg L, Boner AL, Pignatti PF. Candidate genes and a genome-wide search in Italian families with atopic asthmatic children. Clin Exp Allergy 1999; 29(suppl 4):27–30.

24. Wjst M, Fischer G, Immervoll T, Jung M, Saar K, Rueschendorf F, Reis A, Ulbrecht M, Gomolka M, Weiss EH, Jaeger L, Nickel R, Richter K, Kjellman NI, Griese M, von Berg A, Gappa M, Riedel F, Boehle M, van Koningsbruggen S, Schoberth P, Szczepanski R, Dorsch W, Silbermann M, Wichmann HE, et al. A genome-wide search for linkage to asthma. German Asthma Genetics Group. Genomics 1999; 58(1):1–8.

25. Ober C, Cox NJ, Abney M, Di Rienzo A, Lander ES, Changyaleket B, Gidley H, Kurtz B, Lee J, Nance M, Pettersson A, Prescott J, Richardson A, Schlenker E, Summerhill E, Willadsen S, Parry R. Genome-wide search for asthma susceptibility loci in a founder population. The Collaborative Study on the Genetics of Asthma. Hum Mol Genet 1998; 7(9):1393–1398.

26. Heinzmann A, Plesnar C, Kuehr J, Forster J, Deichmann KA. Common polymorphisms in the CTLA-4 and CD28 genes at 2q33 are not associated with asthma or atopy. Eur J Immunogenet 2000; 27(2):57–61.

27. Lee YA, Wahn U, Kehrt R, Tarani L, Businco L, Gustafsson D, Andersson F, Oranje AP, Wolkertstorfer A, Berg A, Hoffmann U, Kuster W, Wienker T, Ruschendorf F, Reis A. A major susceptibility locus for atopic dermatitis maps to chromosome 3q21. Nat Genet 2000; 26(4):470–473.

28. Yokouchi Y, Nukaga Y, Shibasaki M, Noguchi E, Kimura K, Ito S, Nishihara M, Yamakawa-Kobayashi K, Takeda K, Imoto N, Ichikawa K, Matsui A, Hamaguchi H, Arinami T. Significant evidence for linkage of mite-sensitive childhood asthma to chromosome 5q31-q33 near the interleukin 12 B locus by a genome-wide search in Japanese families. Genomics 2000; 66(2):152–160.

29. Mao XQ, Gao PS, Roberts MH, Enomoto T, Kawai M, Sasaki S, Shaldon SR,

Coull P, Dake Y, Adra CN, Hagihara A, Shirakawa T, Hopkin JM. Variants of endothelin-1 and its receptors in atopic asthma. Biochem Biophys Res Commun 1999; 262(1):259–262.

30. Marsh DG, Neely JD, Breazeale DR, Ghosh B, Freidhoff LR, Ehrlich-Kautzky E, Schou C, Krishnaswamy G, Beaty TH. Linkage analysis of IL4 and other chromosome 5q31.1 markers and total serum immunoglobulin E concentrations. Science 1994; 264(5162):1152–1156.

31. Meyers DA, Postma DS, Panhuysen CI, Xu J, Amelung PJ, Levitt RC, Bleecker ER. Evidence for a locus regulating total serum IgE levels mapping to chromosome 5. Genomics 1994; 23(2):464–470.

32. Postma DS, Bleecker ER, Amelung PJ, Holroyd KJ, Xu J, Panhuysen CI, Meyers DA, Levitt RC. Genetic susceptibility to asthma—bronchial hyperresponsiveness coinherited with a major gene for atopy. N Engl J Med 1995; 333(14):894–900.

33. Levitt RC, Holroyd KJ. Fine-structure mapping of genes providing susceptibility to asthma on chromosome 5q31-q33. Clin Exp Allergy 1995; 25(suppl 2):119–123.

34. Ulbrecht M, Eisenhut T, Bonisch J, Kruse R, Wjst M, Heinrich J, Wichmann HE, Weiss EH, Albert ED. High serum IgE concentrations: association with HLA-DR and markers on chromosome 5q31 and chromosome 11q13. J Allergy Clin Immunol 1997; 99(6 Pt 1):828–836.

35. Palmer LJ, Daniels SE, Rye PJ, Gibson NA, Tay GK, Cookson WO, Goldblatt J, Burton PR, LeSouef PN. Linkage of chromosome 5q and 11q gene markers to asthma-associated quantitative traits in Australian children. Am J Respir Crit Care Med 1998; 158(6):1825–1830.

36. Dizier MH, Sandford A, Walley A, Philippi A, Cookson W, Demenais F. Indication of linkage of serum IgE levels to the interleukin-4 gene and exclusion of the contribution of the (−590 C to T) interleukin-4 promoter polymorphism to IgE variation. Genet Epidemiol 1999; 16(1):84–94.

37. Huebner K, Nagarajan L, Besa E, Angert E, Lange BJ, Cannizzaro LA, van den Berghe H, Santoli D, Finan J, Croce CM, et al. Order of genes on human chromosome 5q with respect to 5q interstitial deletions. Am J Hum Genet 1990; 46(1): 26–36.

38. Warrington JA, Hall LV, Hinton LM, Miller JN, Wasmuth JJ, Lovett M. Radiation hybrid map of 13 loci on the long arm of chromosome 5 [published erratum appears in Genomics 1992; 14(3):832]. Genomics 1991; 11(3):701–708.

39. Warrington JA, Wasmuth JJ. A contiguous high-resolution radiation hybrid map of 44 loci from the distal portion of the long arm of human chromosome 5. Genome Res 1996; 6(7):628–632.

40. Kamitani A, Wong ZY, Dickson P, van Herwerden L, Raven J, Forbes AB, Abramson MJ, Walters EH, Harrap SB. Absence of genetic linkage of chromosome 5q31 with asthma and atopy in the general population. Thorax 1997; 52(9):816–817.

41. Laitinen T, Kauppi P, Ignatius J, Ruotsalainen T, Daly MJ, Kaariainen H, Kruglyak L, Laitinen H, de la Chapelle A, Lander ES, Laitinen LA, Kere J. Genetic control of serum IgE levels and asthma: linkage and linkage disequilibrium studies in an isolated population. Hum Mol Genet 1997; 6(12):2069–2076.

42. Blumenthal MN, Wang Z, Weber JL, Rich SS. Absence of linkage between 5q

markers and serum IgE levels in four large atopic families. Clin Exp Allergy 1996; 26(8):892–896.

43. Mansur AH, Christie G, Turner A, Bishop DT, Markham AF, Helms P, Morrison JF. Lack of linkage between chromosome 5q23–33 markers and IgE/bronchial hyperreactivity in 67 Scottish families. Clin Exp Allergy 2000; 30(7):954–961.

44. Vercelli D, Geha RS. Regulation of IgE synthesis: from the membrane to the genes. Springer Semin Immunopathol 1993; 15(1):5–16.

45. Borish L, Mascali JJ, Klinnert M, Leppert M, Rosenwasser LJ. SSC polymorphisms in interleukin genes [published erratum appears in Hum Mol Genet 1995; 4(5): 974]. Hum Mol Genet 1994; 3(9):1710.

46. Takabayashi A, Ihara K, Sasaki Y, Kusuhara K, Nishima S, Hara T. Novel polymorphism in the 5′-untranslated region of the interleukin-4 gene. J Hum Genet 1999; 44(5):352–353.

47. Mout R, Willemze R, Landegent JE. Repeat polymorphisms in the interleukin-4 gene (IL4). Nucleic Acids Res 1991; 19(13):3763.

48. Walley AJ, Cookson WO. Investigation of an interleukin-4 promoter polymorphism for associations with asthma and atopy. J Med Genet 1996; 33(8):689–692.

49. Noguchi E, Shibasaki M, Arinami T, Takeda K, Yokouchi Y, Kawashima T, Yanagi H, Matsui A, Hamaguchi H. Association of asthma and the interleukin-4 promoter gene in Japanese. Clin Exp Allergy 1998; 28(4):449–453.

50. Kawashima T, Noguchi E, Arinami T, Yamakawa-Kobayashi K, Nakagawa H, Otsuka F, Hamaguchi H. Linkage and association of an interleukin 4 gene polymorphism with atopic dermatitis in Japanese families. J Med Genet 1998; 35(6): 502–504.

51. Rosenwasser LJ. Promoter polymorphism in the candidate genes, IL-4, IL-9, TGF-beta l, for atopy and asthma. Int Arch Allergy Immunol 1999; 118(2–4):268–270.

52. Shirakawa I, Deichmann KA, Izuhara I, Mao I, Adra CN, Hopkin JM. Atopy and asthma: genetic variants of IL-4 and IL-13 signalling. Immunol Today 2000; 21(2): 60–64.

53. Izuhara K, Shirakawa T. Signal transduction via the interleukin-4 receptor and its correlation with atopy. Int J Mol Med 1999; 3(1):3–10.

54. Murata T, Taguchi J, Puri RK. Interleukin-13 receptor alpha' but not alpha chain: a functional component of interleukin-4 receptors. Blood 1998; 91(10):3884–3891.

55. Smirnov DV, Smirnova MG, Korobko VG, Frolova EI. Tandem arrangement of human genes for interleukin-4 and interleukin-13: resemblance in their organization. Gene 1995; 155(2):277–281.

56. Liu X, Nickel R, Beyer K, Wahn U, Ehrlich E, Freidhoff LR, Bjorksten B, Beaty TH, Huang SK. An IL13 coding region variant is associated with a high total serum IgE level and atopic dermatitis in the German multicenter atopy study (MAS-90). J Allergy Clin Immunol 2000; 106(1 Pt 1):167–170.

57. Graves PE, Kabesch M, Halonen M, Holberg CJ, Baldini M, Fritzsch C, Weiland SK, Erickson RP, von Mutius E, Martinez FD. A cluster of seven tightly linked polymorphisms in the IL-13 gene is associated with total serum IgE levels in three populations of white children. J Allergy Clin Immunol 2000; 105(3):506–513.

58. Heinzmann A, Mao XQ, Akaiwa M, Kreomer RT, Gao PS, Ohshima K, Umeshita

R, Abe Y, Braun S, Yamashita T, Roberts MH, Sugimoto R, Arima K, Arinobu Y, Yu B, Kruse S, Enomoto T, Dake Y, Kawai M, Shimazu S, Sasaki S, Adra CN, Kitaichi M, Inoue H, Yamauchi K, Tomichi N, Kurimoto F, Hamasaki N, Hopkin JM, Izuhara K, Shirakawa T, Deichmann KA. Genetic variants of IL-13 signalling and human asthma and atopy. Hum Mol Genet 2000; 9(4):549–559.

59.	Gao PS, Mao XQ, Baldini M, Roberts MH, Adra CN, Shirakawa T, Holt PG, Martinez FD, Hopkin JM. Serum total IgE levels and CD14 on chromosome 5q31 [letter]. Clin Genet 1999; 56(2):164–165.

60.	Baldini M, Lohman IC, Halonen M, Erickson RP, Holt PG, Martinez FD. A Polymorphism* in the 5′ flanking region of the CD14 gene is associated with circulating soluble CD14 levels and with total serum immunoglobulin E. Am J Respir Cell Mol Biol 1999; 20(5):976–983.

61.	van der Pouw Kraan TC, Boeije LC, de Groot ER, Stapel SO, Snijders A, Kapsenberg ML, van der Zee JS, Aarden LA. Reduced production of IL-12 and IL-12-dependent IFN-gamma release in patients with allergic asthma. J Immunol 1997; 158(11):5560–5565.

62.	Sieburth D, Jabs EW, Warrington JA, Li X, Lasota J, LaForgia S, Kelleher K, Huebner K, Wasmuth JJ, Wolf SF. Assignment of genes encoding a unique cytokine (IL12) composed of two unrelated subunits to chromosomes 3 and 5. Genomics 1992; 14(1):59–62.

63.	Aron Y, Desmazes-Dufeu N, Matran R, Polla BS, Dusser D, Lockhart A, Swierczewski E. Evidence of a strong, positive association between atopy and the HLA class II alleles DR4 and DR7. Clin Exp Allergy 1996; 26(7):821–828.

64.	Noguchi E, Shibasaki M, Arinami T, Takeda K, Kobayashi K, Matsui A, Hamaguchi H. Evidence for linkage between the development of asthma in childhood and the T-cell receptor beta chain gene in Japanese. Genomics 1998; 47(1):121–124.

65.	Hizawa N, Freidhoff LR, Chiu YF, Ehrlich E, Luehr CA, Anderson JL, Duffy DL, Dunston GM, Weber JL, Huang SK, Barnes KC, Marsh DG, Beaty TH. Genetic regulation of Dermatophagoides pteronyssinus-specific IgE responsiveness: a genome-wide multipoint linkage analysis in families recruited through 2 asthmatic sibs. Collaborative Study on the Genetics of Asthma (CSGA). J Allergy Clin Immunol 1998; 102(3):436–442.

66.	Natori K, Tamari M, Watanabe O, Onouchi Y, Shiomoto Y, Kubo S, Nakamura Y. Mapping of a gene responsible for dermatitis in NOA (Naruto Research Institute Otsuka Atrichia) mice, an animal model of allergic dermatitis. J Hum Genet 1999; 44(6):372–376.

67.	Cookson WO, Sharp PA, Faux JA, Hopkin JM. Linkage between immunoglobulin E responses underlying asthma and rhinitis and chromosome 11q. Lancet 1989; 1(8650):1292–1295.

68.	Lympany P, Welsh K, MacCochrane G, Kemeny DM, Lee TH. Genetic analysis using DNA polymorphism of the linkage between chromosome 11q13 and atopy and bronchial hyperresponsiveness to methacholine. J Allergy Clin Immunol 1992; 89(2):619–628.

69.	Amelung PJ, Panhuysen CI, Postma DS, Levitt RC, Koeter GH, Francomano CA, Bleecker ER, Meyers DA. Atopy and bronchial hyperresponsiveness: exclusion of linkage to markers on chromosomes 11q and 6p. Clin Exp Allergy 1992; 22(12): 1077–1084.

70. Hizawa N, Yamaguchi E, Ohe M, Itoh A, Furuya K, Ohnuma N, Kawakami Y. Lack of linkage between atopy and locus 11q13. Clin Exp Allergy 1992; 22(12): 1065–1069.

71. Lympany P, Welsh KI, Cochrane GM, Kemeny DM, Lee TH. Genetic analysis of the linkage between chromosome 11q and atopy. Clin Exp Allergy 1992; 22(12): 1085–1092.

72. Coleman R, Trembath RC, Harper JI. Chromosome 11q13 and atopy underlying atopic eczema. Lancet 1993; 341(8853):1121–1122.

73. Sandford AJ, Shirakawa T, Moffatt MF, Daniels SE, Ra C, Faux JA, Young RP, Nakamura Y, Lathrop GM, Cookson WO, et al. Localisation of atopy and beta subunit of high-affinity IgE receptor (Fc epsilon RI) on chromosome 11q [see comments]. Lancet 1993; 341(8841):332–334.

74. Hizawa N, Yamaguchi E, Furuya K, Ohnuma N, Kodama N, Kojima J, Ohe M, Kawakami Y. Association between high serum total IgE levels and D11S97 on chromosome 11q13 in Japanese subjects. J Med Genet 1995; 32(5):363–369.

75. Shirakawa T, Hashimoto T, Furuyama J, Takeshita T, Morimoto K. Linkage between severe atopy and chromosome 11q13 in Japanese families. Clin Genet 1994; 46(3):228–232.

76. van Herwerden L, Harrap SB, Wong ZY, Abramson MJ, Kutin JJ, Forbes AB, Raven J, Lanigan A, Walters EH. Linkage of high-affinity IgE receptor gene with bronchial hyperreactivity, even in absence of atopy. Lancet 1995; 346(8985):1262–1265.

77. Shirakawa T, Li A, Dubowitz M, Dekker JW, Shaw AE, Faux JA, Ra C, Cookson WO, Hopkin JM. Association between atopy and variants of the beta subunit of the high-affinity immunoglobulin E receptor [see comments]. Nat Genet 1994; 7(2): 125–129.

78. Shirakawa T, Mao XQ, Sasaki S, Enomoto T, Kawai M, Morimoto K, Hopkin J. Association between atopic asthma and a coding variant of Fc epsilon RI beta in a Japanese population [published erratum appears in Hum Mol Genet 1996; 5(12): 2068]. Hum Mol Genet 1996; 5(8):1129–1130.

79. Hill MR, James AL, Faux JA, Ryan G, Hopkin JM, le Souef P, Musk AW, Cookson WO. Fc epsilon RI-beta polymorphism and risk of atopy in a general population sample [see comments] [published erratum appears in Br Med J 1995; 311(7014): 1196]. Br Med J 1995; 311(7008):776–779.

80. Mao XO, Shirakawa T, Sasaki S, Enomoto T, Morimoto K, Hopkin JM. Maternal inheritance of atopy at the Fc epsilon RI beta locus in Japanese sibs. Hum Hered 1997; 47(3):178–180.

81. Palmer LJ, Pare PD, Faux JA, Moffatt MF, Daniels SE, LeSouef PN, Bremner PR, Mockford E, Gracey M, Spargo R, Musk AW, Cookson WO. Fc epsilon R1-beta polymorphism and total serum IgE levels in endemically parasitized Australian aborigines. Am J Hum Genet 1997; 61(1):182–188.

82. Martinati LC, Trabetti E, Casartelli A, Boner AL, Pignatti PF. Affected sib-pair and mutation analyses of the high affinity IgE receptor beta chain locus in Italian

families with atopic asthmatic children. Am J Respir Crit Care Med 1996; 153(5): 1682–1685.

83. Wong ZY, Tsonis D, van Herwerden L, Raven J, Forbes A, Abramson MJ, Walters EH, Harrap SB. Linkage analysis of bronchial hyperreactivity and atopy with chromosome 11q13. Electrophoresis 1997; 18(9):1641–1645.

84. Amelung PJ, Postma DS, Xu J, Meyers DA, Bleecker ER. Exclusion of chromosome 11q and the FcepsilonRI-beta gene as aetiological factors in allergy and asthma in a population of Dutch asthmatic families [see comments]. Clin Exp Allergy 1998; 28(4):397–403.

85. Simon Thomas N, Wilkinson J, Lonjou C, Morton NE, Holgate ST. Linkage analysis of markers on chromosome 11q13 with asthma and atopy in a United Kingdom population. Am J Respir Crit Care Med 2000; 162(4):1268–1272.

86. Wilkinson J, Thomas NS, Lio P, Holgate ST, Morton NE. Evidence for linkage for atopy and asthma to markers on chromosome 12q. Eur Respir J 1996; 9(suppl 23):435s.

87. Barnes KC, Neely JD, Duffy DL, Freidhoff LR, Breazeale DR, Schou C, Naidu RP, Levett PN, Renault B, Kucherlapati R, Iozzino S, Ehrlich E, Beaty TH, Marsh DG. Linkage of asthma and total serum IgE concentration to markers on chromosome 12q: evidence from Afro-Caribbean and Caucasian populations. Genomics 1996; 37(1):41–50.

88. Nickel R, Wahn U, Hizawa N, Maestri N, Duffy DL, Barnes KC, Beyer K, Forster J, Bergmann R, Zepp F, Wahn V, Marsh DG. Evidence for linkage of chromosome 12q15-q24.1 markers to high total serum IgE concentrations in children of the German Multicenter Allergy Study. Genomics 1997; 46(1):159–162.

89. Wilkinson J, Grimley S, Collins A, Thomas NS, Holgate ST, Morton N. Linkage of asthma to markers on chromosome 12 in a sample of 240 families using quantitative phenotype scores. Genomics 1998; 53(3):251–259.

90. Barnes KC, Freidhoff LR, Nickel R, Chiu YF, Juo SH, Hizawa N, Naidu RP, Ehrlich E, Duffy DL, Schou C, Levett PN, Marsh DG, Beaty TH. Dense mapping of chromosome 12q13.12-q23.3 and linkage to asthma and atopy. J Allergy Clin Immunol 1999; 104(2 Pt 1):485–491.

91. Pene J, Chretien I, Rousset F, Briere F, Bonnefoy JY, de Vries JE. Modulation of IL-4-induced human IgE production in vitro by IFN-gamma and IL-5: the role of soluble CD23 (s-CD23). J Cell Biochem 1989; 39(3):253–264.

92. Hayden C, Pereira E, Rye P, Palmer L, Gibson N, Palenque M, Hagel I, Lynch N, Goldblatt J, Lesouef P. Mutation screening of interferon-gamma (IFNgamma) as a candidate gene for asthma. Clin Exp Allergy 1997; 27(12):1412–1416.

93. Grasemann H, Yandava CN, Drazen JM. Neuronal NO synthase (NOS1) is a major candidate gene for asthma. Clin Exp Allergy 1999; 29(suppl 4):39–41.

94. Gao PS, Kawada H, Kasamatsu T, Mao XQ, Roberts MH, Miyamoto Y, Yoshimura M, Saitoh Y, Yasue H, Nakao K, Adra CN, Kun JF, Moro-oka S, Inoko H, Ho LP, Shirakawa T, Hopkin JM. Variants of NOS1, NOS2, and NOS3 genes in asthmatics. Biochem Biophys Res Commun 2000; 267(3):761–763.

95. Grasemann H, Yandava CN, Storm van's Gravesande K, Deykin A, Pillari A, Ma J, Sonna LA, Lilly C, Stampfer MJ, Israel E, Silverman EK, Drazen JM. A neuronal

NO synthase (NOS1) gene polymorphism is associated with asthma. Biochem Biophys Res Commun 2000; 272(2):391–394.

96. Hou J, Schindler U, Henzel WJ, Ho TC, Brasseur M, McKnight SL. An interleukin-4-induced transcription factor: IL-4. Stat. Science 1994; 265(5179):1701–1706.

97. Takeda K, Tanaka T, Shi W, Matsumoto M, Minami M, Kashiwamura S, Nakanishi K, Yoshida N, Kishimoto T, Akira S. Essential role of Stat6 in IL-4 signalling. Nature 1996; 380(6575):627–630.

98. Kimura K, Noguchi E, Shibasaki M, Arinami T, Yokouchi Y, Takeda K, Yamakawa-Kobayashi K, Matsui A, Hamaguchi H. Linkage and association of atopic asthma to markers on chromosome 13 in the Japanese population. Hum Mol Genet 1999; 8(8):1487–1490.

99. Caughey GH, Zerweck EH, Vanderslice P. Structure, chromosomal assignment, and deduced amino acid sequence of a human gene for mast cell chymase. J Biol Chem 1991; 266(20):12956–12963.

100. Caughey GH, Schaumberg TH, Zerweck EH, Butterfield JH, Hanson RD, Silverman GA, Ley TJ. The human mast cell chymase gene (CMA1): mapping to the cathepsin G/granzyme gene cluster and lineage-restricted expression. Genomics 1993; 15(3):614–620.

101. Mao XQ, Shirakawa T, Yoshikawa T, Yoshikawa K, Kawai M, Sasaki S, Enomoto T, Hashimoto T, Furuyama J, Hopkin JM, Morimoto K. Association between genetic variants of mast-cell chymase and eczema [see comments] [published erratum appears in Lancet 1997; 349(9044):64]. Lancet 1996; 348(9027):581–583.

102. Kawashima T, Noguchi E, Arinami T, Kobayashi K, Otsuka F, Hamaguchi H. No evidence for an association between a variant of the mast cell chymase gene and atopic dermatitis based on case-control and haplotype- relative-risk analyses. Hum Hered 1998; 48(5):271–274.

103. Mao XQ, Shirakawa T, Enomoto T, Shimazu S, Dake Y, Kitano H, Hagihara A, Hopkin JM. Association between variants of mast cell chymase gene and serum IgE levels in eczema [published erratum appears in Hum Hered 1998; 48(2):91]. Hum Hered 1998; 48(1):38–41.

104. Croce CM, Isobe M, Palumbo A, Puck J, Ming J, Tweardy D, Erikson J, Davis M, Rovera G. Gene for alpha-chain of human T-cell receptor: location on chromosome 14 region involved in T-cell neoplasms. Science 1985; 227(4690):1044–1047.

105. Moffatt MF, Hill MR, Cornelis F, Schou C, Faux JA, Young RP, James AL, Ryan G, le Souef P, Musk AW, et al. Genetic linkage of T-cell receptor alpha/delta complex to specific IgE responses. Lancet 1994; 343(8913):1597–1600.

106. Mansur AH, Bishop DT, Markham AF, Morton NE, Holgate ST, Morrison JF. Suggestive evidence for genetic linkage between IgE phenotypes and chromosome 14q markers. Am J Respir Crit Care Med 1999; 159(6):1796–1802.

107. Pritchard MA, Baker E, Whitmore SA, Sutherland GR, Idzerda RL, Park LS, Cosman D, Jenkins NA, Gilbert DJ, Copeland NG, et al. The interleukin-4 receptor gene (IL4R) maps to 16p11.2-16p12.1 in human and to the distal region of mouse chromosome 7. Genomics. 1991; 10(3):801–806.

108. Barner M, Mohrs M, Brombacher F, Kopf M. Differences between IL-4R alpha-

deficient and IL-4-deficient mice reveal a role for IL-13 in the regulation of Th2 responses. Curr Biol 1998; 8(11):669–672.

109. Aman MJ, Tayebi N, Obiri NI, Puri RK, Modi WS, Leonard WJ. cDNA cloning and characterization of the human interleukin 13 receptor alpha chain. J Biol Chem 1996; 271(46):29265–29270.

110. Hershey GK, Friedrich MF, Esswein LA, Thomas ML, Chatila TA. The association of atopy with a gain-of-function mutation in the alpha subunit of the interleukin-4 receptor [see comments]. N Engl J Med 1997; 337(24):1720–1725.

111. Kruse S, Japha T, Tedner M, Sparholt SH, Forster J, Kuehr J, Deichmann KA. The polymorphisms S503P and Q576R in the interleukin-4 receptor alpha gene are associated with atopy and influence the signal transduction. Immunology 1999; 96(3):365–371.

112. Deichmann K, Bardutzky J, Forster J, Heinzmann A, Kuehr J. Common polymorphisms in the coding part of the IL4-receptor gene. Biochem Biophys Res Commun 1997; 231(3):696–697.

113. Mitsuyasu H, Izuhara K, Mao XQ, Gao PS, Arinobu Y, Enomoto T, Kawai M, Sasaki S, Dake Y, Hamasaki N, Shirakawa T, Hopkin JM. Ile50Val variant of IL4R alpha upregulates IgE synthesis and associates with atopic asthma [letter]. Nat Genet 1998; 19(2):119–120.

114. Rosa-Rosa L, Zimmermann N, Bernstein JA, Rothenberg ME, Khurana Hershey GK. The R576 IL-4 receptor alpha allele correlates with asthma severity. J Allergy Clin Immunol 1999; 104(5):1008–1014.

115. Sandford AJ, Chagani T, Zhu S, Weir TD, Bai TR, Spinelli JJ, Fitzgerald JM, Behbehani NA, Tan WC, Pare PD. Polymorphisms in the IL4, IL4RA, and FCERIB genes and asthma severity. J Allergy Clin Immunol 2000; 106(1 Pt 1):135–140.

116. Takabayashi A, Ihara K, Sasaki Y, Suzuki Y, Nishima S, Izuhara K, Hamasaki N, Hara T. Childhood atopic asthma: positive association with a polymorphism of IL-4 receptor alpha gene but not with that of IL-4 promoter or Fc epsilon receptor I beta gene. Exp Clin Immunogenet 2000; 17(2):63–70.

117. Noguchi E, Shibasaki M, Arinami T, Takeda K, Yokouchi Y, Kobayashi K, Imoto N, Nakahara S, Matsui A, Hamaguchi H. No association between atopy/asthma and the ILe50Val polymorphism of IL-4 receptor. Am J Respir Crit Care Med 1999; 160(1):342–345.

118. Noguchi E, Shibasaki M, Arinami T, Takeda K, Yokouchi Y, Kobayashi K, Imoto N, Nakahara S, Matsui A, Hamaguchi H. Lack of association of atopy/asthma and the interleukin-4 receptor alpha gene in Japanese. Clin Exp Allergy 1999; 29(2):228–233.

119. Leung DY. Atopic dermatitis: the skin as a window into the pathogenesis of chronic allergic diseases. J Allergy Clin Immunol 1995; 96(3):302–318; quiz 319.

120. Bousquet J, Chanez P, Lacoste JY, Barneon G, Ghavanian N, Enander I, Venge P, Ahlstedt S, Simony-Lafontaine J, Godard P, et al. Eosinophilic inflammation in asthma [see comments]. N Engl J Med 1990; 323(15):1033–1039.

121. Alam R. Chemokines in allergic inflammation. J Allergy Clin Immunol 1997; 99(3):273–277.

122. Nickel RG, Casolaro V, Wahn U, Beyer K, Barnes KC, Plunkett BS, Freidhoff

LR, Sengler C, Plitt JR, Schleimer RP, Caraballo L, Naidu RP, Levett PN, Beaty TH, Huang SK. Atopic dermatitis is associated with a functional mutation in the promoter of the C-C chemokine RANTES. J Immunol 2000; 164(3):1612–1616.

123. Laitinen T, Ollikainen V, Lazaro C, Kauppi P, de Cid R, Anto JM, Estivill X, Lokki H, Mannila H, Laitinen LA, Kere J. Association study of the chromosomal region containing the FCER2 gene suggests it has a regulatory role in atopic disorders. Am J Respir Crit Care Med 2000; 161(3 Pt 1):700–706.

124. Kondo T, Shiomoto Y, Kondo T, Kubo S. The NOA mouse: a new hair deficient mutant (a possible animal model of allergic dermatitis). Mouse Genome 1997; 95: 609–700.

125. Watanabe O, Natori K, Tamari M, Shiomoto Y, Kubo S, Nakamura Y. Significantly elevated expression of PF4 (platelet factor 4) and eotaxin in the NOA mouse, a model for atopic dermatitis. J Hum Genet 1999; 44(3):173–176.

126. Zhang Y, Lefort J, Kearsey V, Lapa e Silva JR, Cookson WO, Vargaftig BB. A genome-wide screen for asthma-associated quantitative trait loci in a mouse model of allergic asthma. Hum Mol Genet 1999; 8(4):601–605.

127. Loots GG, Locksley RM, Blankespoor CM, Wang ZE, Miller W, Rubin EM, Frazer KA. Identification of a coordinate regulator of interleukins 4, 13, and 5 by cross-species sequence comparisons. Science 2000; 288(5463):136–140.

128. Tepper RI, Levinson DA, Stanger BZ, Campos-Torres J, Abbas AK, Leder P. IL-4 induces allergic-like inflammatory disease and alters T cell development in transgenic mice. Cell 1990; 62(3):457–467.

129. Roitt I, Brostoff J, Male D. Immunology. 5th ed. St. Louis: Mosby International Ltd., 1998.

130. Elliot K, Fitzpatrick E, Hill D, Brown J, Adams S, Chee P, Stewart G, Fulcher D, Tang M, Kemp A, King E, Varigos G, Bahlo M, Forrest S. The −590C/T and −34C/T interleukin-4 promoter polymorphisms are not associated with atopic eczema in childhood. J Allergy Clin Immunol 2001; 108(2):285–287.

6
Risk Factors for Atopic Dermatitis

Erika von Mutius
University Children's Hospital, Munich, Germany

I. INTRODUCTION

Atopic eczema is a common health problem for children and adolescents through-out the world. The International Study of Asthma and Allergies in Childhood (ISAAC) has shown that symptoms of atopic eczema exhibit wide variations in prevalence both within and between countries inhabited by similar ethnic groups, suggesting that environmental factors may be critical in determining disease expression. Epidemiology offers the methodological framework to answer questions relating to potential environmental and genetic determinants of atopic dermatitis. Yet it is only during the last 10 years that research into the epidemiology of atopic dermatitis has started in earnest. In many of these studies striking differences in the distribution and risk factor profile of atopic eczema as compared to asthma and hay fever have become apparent. For example, the striking differences in the prevalence of hay fever, atopy, and asthma seen between eastern and western Europe are not found for atopic dermatitis (1,2). Children exposed to farming environments early in life have strikingly low prevalences of asthma, hay fever, and atopy, yet the prevalence of atopic eczema is unaffected by early childhood farming exposures (3–5). Therefore, it seems likely that risk factors determining the development of atopic dermatitis may differ significantly from those affecting the incidence of asthma and hay fever.

  In the following sections I have therefore restricted the discussion to studies focusing on atopic dermatitis and have excluded reports relating to "atopic ill-nesses" without specification of the different atopic conditions. Because subjects with atopic eczema share certain characteristics with individuals affected by asthma and hay fever, such as elevated IgE production and a deviated immune response, this restriction may have been too tight. Yet it seems likely that atopic dermatitis is a multifactorial syndrome, and the many components of the disease may be even harder to identify if too loose criteria are applied.

As with other chronic conditions, several limitations of population-based studies must be borne in mind when interpreting the findings. First, the definition of atopic eczema varies from study to study, and validations of questionnaire-based estimates have been few. Skin examinations by trained field workers, which can add an objective parameter to questionnaire-based data, do reflect a point prevalence of skin symptoms at the time of examination and can therefore only in limited ways corroborate estimates of lifetime prevalences assessed by questions inquiring about a doctor's diagnosis of eczema ever. Second, assessment of potential determinants in cross-sectional surveys relate to the prevalence of the condition, i.e., the incidence and persistence of the disease. It is therefore often difficult to disentangle aggravating from causal factors in such cross-sectional studies. There are only few prospective surveys aiming at identifying environmental exposures prior to the onset of clinical manifestations of atopic dermatitis.

Third, atopic dermatitis often occurs concomitantly with asthma and hay fever in the same subject, but most studies have not taken into account potential confounding by the presence of two or three atopic conditions in which case no unambiguous association between outcome and exposure exists. Finally, it seems reasonable to suggest that different phenotypic manifestations of atopic dermatitis develop during childhood and adult years. For example, it has been shown that on a population level only 42% of all children with atopic eczema produce IgE antibodies to inhalant and food allergens as assessed by skin prick tests (1). It thus seems likely that different risk factors will be associated with different phenotypes of the disease and that, in addition, different gene-by-environment interactions may occur in subjects with different phenotypic expressions of the condition. Unfortunately, the epidemiology of atopic dermatitis has just commenced, and more detailed information about such potential interactions is still missing.

The following chapter will discuss findings from epidemiological surveys relating the prevalence of atopic dermatitis to environmental risk factors such as migration, socioeconomic conditions, family size, nursing and infant feeding, as well as exposure to environmental pollutants.

II. MIGRANT STUDIES

Migrant studies make comparisons between the morbidity experience of migrant groups and that of their current country of residence and/or their country of origin. Migrant studies can help resolve whether spatial differences in the frequency of disease are attributable to environmental factors in the regions studied or to different genetic compositions of the population.

In children migrating from the Pacific Islands of Tokelau to New Zealand, a large increase in the prevalence of atopic eczema as compared to children of similar ethnic groups in their country of origin were documented in 1980 (6). Asian children born in Australia have been shown to be at higher risk of atopic eczema than those who have recently immigrated (7), which may point towards the importance of environmental factors in the country of residence.

III. SOCIOECONOMIC STATUS

The National Child Development Study in the United Kingdom gathered detailed information on over 98% of babies born in England, Wales, and Scotland during the week of March 3–9, 1958 (8). These infants were followed up at the ages of 7, 11, and 16 years ($n = 8279$). When the children were aged 7, parents were asked by health visitors using a structured questionnaire whether their child had had eczematous rashes during the first year of life or at any time after the first year. When the children were aged 11 and 16, parents were asked whether they had had eczematous rashes in the past 12 months. In addition, skin examinations by experienced school medical officers were recorded at the ages of 7, 11, and 16. Social class was assessed using the registrar general's classification according to the father's occupation when the children were 7 years of age. The prevalence of reported eczema was 1.5–2 times higher in upper social classes I and II than in classes IV and V at each follow-up point. The social class trend was strongest when the children were aged 7 and under. Prevalences for examined eczema showed similar social class gradients to those for reported eczema at all ages in the follow-up study, with a roughly twofold difference in prevalence between the two highest and two lowest social classes. The results retained significance after adjusting for potential confounding factors (8).

The 1970 British birth cohort comprised all children born in England, Scotland, and Wales in one week of April 1970 and follow-up surveys at birth, 5, 10, and 16 years of age (9). As in the 1958 cohort, social advantage was a risk factor for eczema at age 16 years. Similar results were obtained in the Swiss Study on Childhood Allergy and Respiratory Symptoms with Respect to Air Pollution, Climate and Pollen (SCARPOL) conducted as a cross-sectional survey in several areas in Switzerland in 1992/93 among school-aged children (10). The lifetime prevalence of atopic dermatitis was assessed via questionnaires inquiring about itching skin disease persisting for at least 6 months and eczema in typical locations ever. The SCARPOL findings confirmed the British results showing the highest prevalence in social class I (15.9%) as compared to the lowest prevalence in social class V (9.6%, $p = 0.006$ for trend).

The increase in the prevalence of atopic dermatitis in British adolescents aged 16 years over a time period of 12 years (1974–1986) was, however, not

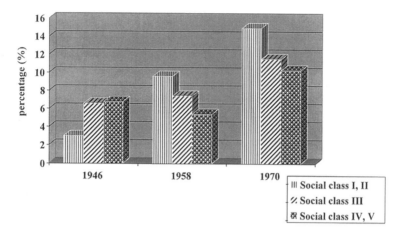

Figure 1   Relationship between social class and atopic eczema in three national cohorts in the United Kingdom. (From Ref. 13.)

attributable to changes in social class over time (11). Likewise, no clear relation was found between social class and atopic dermatitis among adult parents participating in a large German Multicentre Birth Cohort Study (12), suggesting that factors associated with social class may affect certain phenotypes of atopic dermatitis more prevalent in younger children.

An interesting report from 1984 suggests that the relationship between atopic dermatitis and social class may have changed over time (Fig. 1). Rates of reported childhood eczema between the ages of 4 and 7 years were studied in three national British cohorts of children born in 1946, 1958, and 1970 (13). Social classes I and II children born in 1946 were less likely to be reported as having eczema, compared with children from lower social classes, whereas children born into higher social classes in 1958 and 1970 had higher rates. These findings may reflect secular changes in factors associated with higher socioeconomic status in previous years.

IV. FAMILY SIZE

There is conflicting evidence with respect to the role of birth order in the development of atopic dermatitis. A number of reports have documented inverse associations between family size and the occurrence of childhood atopic dermatitis. In a large prospective birth cohort study in Denmark, parity was strongly inversely related to a specialist diagnosis of atopic dermatitis at a mean age of around 6 years [adjusted OR = 0.26 (95% CI: 0.10–0.73) comparing four siblings to one sibling] (14). Likewise, the prevalence of parental-reported atopic dermatitis was found to be inversely related to family size after adjusting for potential confounders using data from the National Child Development Study in the United Kingdom and the 1970 British birth cohort (9,15). In a large Finnish birth cohort study over 8000 infants were followed up to the age of 7 years. Again, parity was significantly inversely related to the prevalence of parental-reported allergic eczema after adjusting for potential confounding factors (16).

Such inverse associations were, however, not seen in all studies. An Australian cross-sectional survey investigating school children 7 years of age found only a nonsignificant trend towards lower prevalences of parental-reported atopic dermatitis in this population [23.3% in children without siblings as compared to 19.5% in children with at least 5 siblings (OR = 0.80; 95% CI: 0.49–1.31)] (17). Likewise, in a recent prospective birth cohort study from the United Kingdom, atopic dermatitis at age 2 years defined either as doctor-diagnosed eczema, as visible dermatitis, or as maternally reported eczema showed a nonsignificant inverse association with the number of older siblings [adjusted OR = 0.86 (95% CI: 0.36–2.06) when comparing no sibling to at least 3 older siblings] (18). Furthermore, in young adults no relationship between birth order and the prevalence of atopic dermatitis was seen (19,20). None of these studies specified the phenotypic presentation of atopic eczema, e.g., as intrinsic or extrinsic, which may account for the apparent discrepancies since it is mainly atopic sensitization and hay fever that so far have shown the strongest and most consistent inverse associations with family size (21).

Several hypotheses have been put forward to explain the sibling effect. It seems very unlikely that the age of the mother is the underlying causal factor, since in most reports the sibling effect was still seen after adjusting for the age of the mother at birth of her child. Furthermore, the age of the mother has been investigated in several surveys, but no significant association between maternal age and the prevalence of atopic eczema was found (14,16,20).

David Strachan, who first described the phenomenon in 1989 (15), proposed that "infection in early childhood, transmitted by unhygienic contact with older siblings, or acquired prenatally from a mother infected by contact with her older children" may prevent the development of allergic diseases. Recent studies relating surrogate markers of an increased burden of infections such as daycare attendance and number of rhinitis episodes early in life, as well as a positive serology for hepatitis A to a decreased risk of atopy and asthma (21), seem to support this notion. However, no convincing evidence exists at present to suggest that infections early in life are similarly protective for the development of atopic dermatitis.

The strong inverse relation between sibship size and the expression of atopy in families may, however, also be attributable to other mechanisms. The number of older siblings might be a surrogate measure for multiple pregnancies in which feto-maternal immune responses may change with each pregnancy. If this notion were correct, then not only the number of older siblings but also the number of pregnancies, including miscarriages, should be related to the occurrence of atopic diseases in the offspring. No data are at present available to test this hypothesis.

V. NURSING AND INFANT FEEDING

Conflicting evidence exists with respect to the role of breastfeeding in the development of childhood atopic dermatitis. The three early British birth cohorts of children born in 1946, 1958, and 1970 show interesting results (13). In the later cohorts of children born in 1958 and 1970, there was a positive association between eczema and breastfeeding. The longer the child was breastfed, the more likely he or she was to be reported as having eczema, whereas no such relationship was found in the 1946 cohort. This discrepancy may point towards changing factors over time which are carried over to the infant through the breast milk, suggesting that the nursing of an infant may have different effects depending on the maternal environment and status. Thus, beneficial effects of breastfeeding as recently reported from a large Breastfeeding Intervention Trial (PROBIT) in Belarus (22), which showed a 50% reduction in risk of developing atopic eczema in the first year of life, may not be applicable to other populations. In fact, several studies have shown either no effect of breastfeeding (14,18) or an increased risk of developing atopic dermatitis with prolonged breastfeeding (23).

A significant proportion of children with atopic dermatitis are sensitized to food allergens, mostly cows' milk, egg, nuts, and wheat. In this subgroup of children with food allergy, which manifests as atopic dermatitis early in life, the introduction of certain foods into the infant's diet after weaning may be associated with an increased risk of developing food allergy and concomitantly atopic eczema. There are few prospective studies investigating the role of nutrition for the development of food allergy and atopic dermatitis in the general population. In a New Zealand birth cohort following over 1200 infants up to the age of 10 years, the exposure to a diverse solid food diet during the first 4 months produced risks of eczema in early childhood about 1.6 times those of children who were not introduced to solid food by age 4 months (24). These associations remained significant after adjusting for potential confounding factors. Similar relationships were seen between early infant diet and risks of chronic and recurrent eczema up to the age of 10 years (25). Recurrent or chronic eczema was defined by the following criteria: (1) the child had attended a family doctor on at least 3 occasions for eczema; (2) the condition had lasted for a period of at least 3 consecutive years; (3) the child was receiving regular medication for eczema. Another, smaller prospective study following roughly 450 infants up to age 2 years concluded that there was an increase in the incidence of eczema in the infants who received solids at 8–12 weeks of age but that the effect was weaker than previously reported (26).

Several subsequent intervention studies in high-risk populations combining lactation dietary restriction and delayed solid feeding have shown transient reductions in the incidence of atopic eczema in the first 12–18 months of life, as will be discussed in more detail later in this book. These findings suggest that for certain subtypes of atopic dermatitis in children at high risk, most likely those phenotypes related to sensitization to cows' milk may be triggered or incited by feeding of cows' milk and solids early in life. Since the effect is only transient and does not abolish risks completely, the role of infant feeding for the development of childhood atopic eczema in the general population must be interpreted with caution.

VI. ENVIRONMENTAL POLLUTANTS

Unlike hay fever and asthma, which have been shown to occur less frequently in highly polluted areas in eastern Germany (2,27,28), the prevalence of atopic dermatitis either assessed via parental reports or as visible flexural dermatitis was found to be higher in eastern Germany (1,2). Interestingly, the excess of atopic dermatitis in eastern Germany as assessed by an experienced senior dermatologist was attributable to the intrinsic phenotype, i.e., to eczematous children without atopic sensitization to common allergens in skin prick tests (1). In subsequent investigations in these polluted areas of eastern Germany (Zerbst, Bitterfeld, and Hettstedt), the body burden of arsenic and heavy metals was measured, but no relationship to the prevalence of atopic dermatitis in the school-aged children was found (29). However, the overall prevalence of atopic eczema was slightly higher in industrial areas as compared to control areas in eastern Germany, but this difference did not reach statistical significance (2.9% vs. 1.6%).

Indoor heating with a gas heater with an exhaust pipe connection to the wall was furthermore found to be associated with an increased risk of eczema in east German children (OR = 8.22; 95% CI: 2.44–27.66), whereas a central heating system was associated with a decreased risk (OR = 0.30; 95% CI: 0.10–0.90) (29). The same authors had previously reported in a comparative survey of east and west German preschool-aged (5–7 year old) children that the prevalence of eczema as assessed by physical examination was associated with indoor use of gas without hood (adjusted OR = 1.68; 95% CI: 1.11–2.56) and distance of homes from a busy road (<50 m adjusted OR = 1.71; 95% CI: 1.07–2.73) (30). Similar questions inquiring about self-reported increased traffic exposure on busy roads did not, however, find any association with the prevalence of atopic eczema in one west German study (31), and inconsistent results in Malta (32).

Subsequent extensive exposure studies in eastern Germany (Dresden), using a 1 km grid to assess personal exposure at home and school addresses of study children, were furthermore unable to reproduce these findings when investigating parental reports and skin examinations for atopic eczema in school-aged children (33). Thus, more comprehensive studies including objective assessment of visible dermatitis and comprehensive pollution exposure assessment are needed before any firm conclusions can be drawn.

Environmental tobacco smoke exposure has been related to the prevalence of atopic eczema in German 5- to 6-year-old preschool children (34). In this survey 12.6% of the mothers reported that they had smoked during pregnancy and/or lactation. Of the children exposed to maternal smoking, 33.8% had reported atopic dermatitis as compared to 18.1% of unexposed children. This difference amounts to a roughly twofold increased risk of atopic eczema in children exposed to environmental tobacco smoke early in life (adjusted OR = 2.30; 95% CI: 1.32–3.12). Other studies failed to confirm these results (29,32,35), which may either reflect differences in the timing of the exposure (prenatal or infant versus childhood exposure) or confounding by concomitant manifestations of asthma and wheezy bronchitis, which have consistently been shown to be related to maternal smoking. Interestingly, no consistent relationship between environmental tobacco smoke exposure and atopic sensitization was found, again pointing towards potential confounding between wheeze and atopic eczema in studies reporting positive associations between the prevalence of atopic dermatitis and maternal smoking.

Besides pollution, other environmental factors may be relevant, such as domestic water supply. Water hardness is believed to be important in the development of eczema, and water-softening units are recommended by manufacturers and by some physicians for the management of eczema. To test this hypothesis, an ecological study of the relation between domestic water hardness and the prevalence of eczema among Nottinghamshire school children was conducted (36). Questionnaire details of 1-year and lifetime prevalence of eczema were obtained from parents of over 7500 school children. Geographical information systems were used to link the geographical distribution of eczema in the study area to four categories of domestic water-hardness data. Among the primary school children aged 4–16 years, a significant relation between the prevalence of atopic eczema and water hardness, both before and after adjustment for potential confounding factors, was found (Fig. 2). The 1-year period prevalence was 17.3% in the highest water-hardness category and 12.0% in the lowest category (adjusted OR = 1.54; 95% CI: 1.19–1.99). The effect on recent eczema symptoms was stronger than on lifetime prevalence, which may indicate that water hardness acts more on existing dermatitis by exacerbating the disorder or prolonging its duration rather than as a cause of new cases. Eczema prevalence trends in the second-

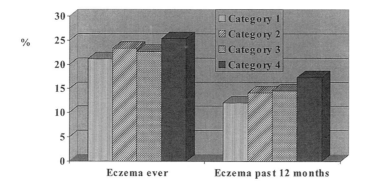

Figure 2 Water hardness categories and prevalence of atopic eczema among primary school children in the United Kingdom. (From Ref. 36.)

ary school population of children aged 11–16 years were furthermore not significant, pointing to age-specific effects of exposure.

VII. CONCLUSIONS

Very little is known about determinants of atopic dermatitis among children, adolescents, and adults. The worldwide variation in prevalence both within and between countries inhabited by similar ethnic groups suggests that environmental factors may be critical in determining disease expression. Likewise, the findings of migrant studies, though scarce for atopic eczema, point towards the importance of environmental risk factors for the expression of the disease. From the findings referred to in this chapter it seems likely that factors associated with recent advantaged lifestyle may in part determine the inception of atopic dermatitis. Whether family size contributes to this effect is unknown, but higher parity has been reported in a number of studies to be inversely related to atopic dermatitis. The strength of the effect is, however, much weaker than for atopic sensitization and hay fever, which may be due to a significant proportion of subjects with atopic eczema belonging to the intrinsic phenotype, i.e., atopic eczema without atopic sensitization as assessed by skin prick tests or serum IgE antibodies. Conversely, the atopic eczema related to food allergy early in life may represent a subgroup of children in whom nutritional aspects of infant feeding may play a role, particularly the introduction of solid foods. Finally, some aspects of the environment may play a role in either aggravating atopic eczema, as in the case of water hardness, or in inciting new cases of intrinsic atopic eczema, as seen in polluted areas of eastern Germany. Overall, the epidemiological findings relating to atopic dermatitis are still few and need replenishment. Not only should environmental exposures be assessed more rigorously, but attention must be paid in future studies to potential gene-environment interactions, since an atopic family history is still one of the main and consistent risk factors for the development of the disease.

REFERENCES

1. Schäfer T, Krämer U, Vieluf D, Abeck D, Behrendt H, Ring J. The excess of atopic eczema in east Germany is related to the intrinsic type. Br J Dermatol 2000; 143: 992–998.
2. Weiland S, von Mutius E, TH, Duhme H, Fritzsch C, Werner B, et al. Prevalence of respiratory and atopic disorders among children in the east and west Germany five years after unification. Eur Respir J 1999; 14:862–870.
3. Braun-Fahrländer C, Gassner M, Grize L, Neu U, Sennhauser F, Varonier H, et al. Prevalence of hay fever and allergic sensitization in farmer's children and their peers living in the same rural community. SCARPOL team. Swiss Study on Childhood Allergy and Respiratory Symptoms with Respect to Air Pollution. Clin Exp Allergy 1999; 29:28–34.
4. Riedler J, Eder W, Oberfeld G, Schreuer M. Austrian children living on a farm have less hay fever, asthma and allergic sensitization. Clin Exp Allergy 2000; 30:194–200.
5. von Ehrenstein O, von Mutius E, Illi S, Hachmeister A, von Kries R. Reduced risk of hay fever and asthma among children of farmers. Clin Exp Allergy 2000; 30: 187–193.
6. Waite D, Eyles E, Tonkin S, O'Donnell T. Asthma prevalence in Tokelauan children in two environments. Clin Allergy 1980; 10:71–75.
7. Leung R. Asthma, allergy and atopy in south-east Asian immigrants in Australia. Austr New Zeal J Med 1994; 24:255–257.
8. Williams H, Strachan D, Hay R. Childhood eczema: disease of the advantaged? Br Med J 1994; 308:1132–1135.
9. Lewis S, Britton J. Consistent effects of high socioeconomic status and low birth order, and the modifying effect of maternal smoking on the risk of allergic disease during childhood. Respir Med 1998; 92:1237–1244.
10. Wuethrich B. Clinical aspects, epidemiology, and prognosis of atopic dermatitis. Ann Allergy Asthma Immunol 1999; 83:464–470.
11. Butland B, Strachan D, Lewis S, Bynner J, Butler N, Britton J. Investigation into the increase in hay fever and eczema at age 16 observed between the 1958 and 1970 British birth cohorts. Br Med J 1997; 315:717–721.
12. Bergmann R, Edenharter G, Bergmann K, Lau S, Wahn U, and the Multicenter Allergy Study Research Group. Socioeconomic status is a risk factor for allergy in parents but not in their children. Clin Exp Allergy 2000; 30:1740–1745.
13. Taylor B, Wadsworth J, Wadsworth M, Peckham C. Changes in the reported prevalence of childhood eczema since the 1939–45 war. Lancet 1984; 1255–1257.

14. Olesen A, Ellingsen A, Olesen H, Juul S, Thestrup-Pedersen K. Atopic dermatitis and birth factors: historical follow up by record linkage. Br Med J 1997; 314:1003–1008.

15. Strachan D. Hay fever, hygiene, and household size. Br Med J 1989; 299:1259–1260.

16. Xu B, Järvelin MJP. Prenatal factors and occurrence of rhinitis and eczema among offspring. Allergy 1999; 54:829–836.

17. Ponsonby A, Couper D, Dwyer T, Carmichael A. Cross sectional study of the relation between sibling number and asthma, hay fever, and eczema. Arch Dis Child 1998; 79:328–333.

18. Harris J, Cullinan P, Williams H, Mills P, Moffat S, White C, et al. Environmental associations with eczema in early life. Br J Dermatol 2001; 144:795–802.

19. Jarvis D, Chinn S, Luczynska C, Burney P. The association of family size with atopy and atopic disease. Clin Exp Allergy 1997; 27:240–245.

20. Steffensen F, Sörensen H, Gillman M, Rothman K, Sabroe S, Fischer P, et al. Low birth weight and preterm delivery as risk factors for asthma and atopic dermatitis in young adult males. Epidemiology 2000; 11:185–188.

21. von Mutius E. The environmental predictors of allergic diseases. JACI 2000; 105:9–19.

22. Kramer M, Chalmers B, Hodnett E, Sevkovskaya Z, Dzikovich I, Shapiro S, et al. Promotion of Breastfeeding Intervention Trial (PROBIT). A randomized trial in the Republic of Belarus. JAMA 2001; 285:413–420.

23. Taylor B, Wadsworth J, Golding J, Butler N. Breast feeding, eczema, asthma, and hay fever. J Epidemiol Com Health 1983; 37:95–99.

24. Fergusson D, Horwood L. Early solid food diet and eczema in childhood: a 10-year longitudional study. Pediatr Allergy Immunol 1994; 5:44–47.

25. Fergusson D, Horwood J, Shannon F. Early solid feeding and recurrent childhood eczema: a 10-year longitudinal study. Pediatrics 1990; 86:541–546.

26. Forsyth J, Ogston S, Clark A, Florey C, Howie P. Relation between early introduction of solid food to infants and their weight and illnesses during the first two years of life. Br Med J 1993; 306:1572–1576.

27. von Mutius E, Fritzsch C, Weiland S, Roell G, Magnussen H. Prevalence of asthma and allergic disorders among children in united Germany: a descriptive comparison. Br Med J 1992; 305:1395–1399.

28. von Mutius E, Martinez F, Fritzsch C, Nicolai T, Reitmeir P, Thiemann H. Prevalence of asthma and atopy in two areas of west and east Germany. Am J Respir Crit Care Med 1994; 149:358–364.

29. Schäfer T, Heinrich J, Wjst M, Krause C, Adam H, Ring J, et al. Indoor risk factors for atopic eczema in school children from east Germany. Environ Research Sect A 1999; 81:151–158.

30. Schafer T, Vieluf D, Behrendt H, Kramer U, Ring J. Atopic eczema and other manifestations of atopy: results of a study in east and west Germany. Allergy 1996; 51:532–539.

31. Weiland S, Mundt K, Ruckmann A, Keil U. Self-reported wheezing and allergic rhinitis in children and traffic density on street of residence. Ann Epidemiol 1994; 4:243–247.

32. Montefort S, Lenicker H, Caruna S, Agius Muscat H. Asthma, rhinitis and eczema in Maltese 13–15 year-old schoolchildren—prevalence, severity and associated factors (ISAAC). Clin Exp Allergy 1998; 28:1089–1099.

33. Hirsch T, Weiland S, von Mutius E, Safeca A, Gräfe H, Csaplovics E, et al. Inner city air pollution and respiratory health and atopy in children. Eur Respir J 1999; 14:669–677.

34. Schäfer T, Dirschedl P, Kunz B, Ring J, Überla K. Maternal smoking during pregnancy and lactation increases the risk for atopic eczema in the offspring. J Am Acad Dermatol 1997; 36:550–556.

35. Arshad S, Stevens M, Hide D. Te effect of genetic and environmental factors on the prevalence of allergic disorders at the age of two years. Clin Exp Allergy 1993; 23:504–511.

36. McNally N, Williams H, Phillips D, Smallman-Raynor M, Lewis S, Venn A, et al. Atopic eczema and domestic water hardness. Lancet 1998; 352:527–531.

7
Epidermal Barrier in Atopic Dermatitis

Ehrhardt Proksch
University of Kiel, Kiel, Germany

Peter M. Elias
University of California, San Francisco, California

I. INTRODUCTION

The epidermal permeability barrier resides in the stratum corneum (SC), a hetero-geneous, two-compartment tissue. Whereas the cells (corneocytes) of the SC are lipid-depleted, they are embedded in a continuous, lipid-enriched extracellular matrix organized into characteristic, multilamellar membrane unit structures, which mediate barrier function (22). The formation of the permeability barrier is the goal of epidermal proliferation and differentiation, processes that begin in the basal layer. The quantitatively most important cell type of the epidermis, the keratinocyte, derives from stem cells, and en route to the SC it synthesizes spe-cific basal (K5 and K14) and suprabasal (K1 and K10) keratins, as well as corni-fied envelope (CE)–associated proteins (20). The CE begins to form with the deposition and cross-linking of involucrin and envoplakin on the intracellular surface of the plasma membrane in the upper spinous and granular cell layers of the epidermis. The process begins at or near desmosomal sites, followed by the subjacent addition of elafin, small prolin-rich proteins, and loricrin. With cornifi-cation, the phospholipid-enriched plasma membrane disappears, followed by the formation of a ceramide-containing membrane bilayer (see below), which is cova-lently attached to involucrin, envoplakin, and periplakin moieties on the extracel-lular surface of the CE by ω-hydroxyester bonds (57).

The lipid synthesis required for barrier function occurs in keratinocytes within all nucleated cell layers of the epidermis. Newly synthesized lipids then are delivered to and stored within epidermal lamellar bodies (Odland bodies, keratinosomes). Lamellar body formation is first visible ultrastructurally at the level of the spinous layer and continues throughout the granular layer. In the outermost granular layer the contents of lamellar bodies are secreted into the intercellular domains at the stratum granulosum/SC interface. Lamellar bodies contain mainly cholesterol, phospholipids, and glucosylceramides, as well as hydrolytic enzymes, which also are delivered to the SC interstices, where they convert the newly secreted phospholipids, glucosylceramides, and sphingomyelins to free fatty acids and ceramides. These biochemical transformations, which may be regulated by the stratum corneum pH gradient (60,61), provoke sequential changes in membrane structure, leading to the formation of lamellar membrane unit membranes. This type of membrane organization is required for life in a terrestrial environment. In addition to lamellar body–derived lipid hydrolytic enzymes, a variety of proteases, required for desquamation, are delivered to the SC interstices by lamellar body secretion present as well.

SC lipids comprise approximately equimolar quantities of ceramides, cholesterol, and free fatty acids, as well as lesser amounts of other nonpolar lipids and cholesterol sulfate (91a). Of the three key lipids, ceramides comprise a family of at least seven subfractions (89,91a), which account for up to 50% of SC lipids by weight. Not only because of the preponderance, but also because of their amphiphilic structure and extremely long-chain, constituent N-acyl fatty acids, ceramides are presumed to be critical for barrier function. Studies with different inhibitors of ceramide formation (41,42,47) demonstrate a broad requirement for the ceramide family in barrier function. However, the function and the requirement for specific species within the ceramide family are still incompletely understood. Substantial indirect evidence points to the importance of the most nonpolar species, ceramides 1 and 4, which contain linoleic acid ω-esterified to an unusually long-chain, N-acyl fatty acid (C → 30; acyl-ceramide) for permeability barrier function (89). The ω-hydroxyceramides in the ceramide family are generated by a cytochrome P450–dependent process (7). In essential fatty acid deficiency, oleate substitutes for linoleate as the predominant ω-esterified species in basal ceramides 1 and 4 (107) in association with a profound barrier abnormality (21). Moreover, only when acylceramides are added to model lipid mixtures of cholesterol, free fatty acids, and non-ω-esterified ceramides do membrane structures form that resemble those present in SC extracellular domains (10). In addition to their putative role in extracellular lamellar membrane organization, a portion of the ω-hydroxyceramides is linked to the external surface of the CE, where they are attached covalently to involucrin and other constituent cornified envelope peptides (57,97,108), apparently through the action of keratinocyte transglutaminase 1 (77). The resulting monolayer of ω-hydroxyceramides forms the corneocyte-bound lipid envelope (CLE) (108). Although the cornified CE itself possesses no intrinsic water barrier properties, the CLE may be important for either normal deposition of the extracellular lamellae (scaffold function) and/or for intercorneocyte cohesion.

The epidermis is a highly active site of lipid synthesis, which is largely autonomous from the influence of circulating lipids, but regulatable by alterations in barrier status (24,29). Injury to the skin resulting in perturbations of the permeability barrier, regardless of type, provokes a recovery response that leads to a normalization of barrier function within hours to days, depending on species, age, and severity of the initial insult (24,29). Barrier recovery results from restoration of sufficient extracellular lipids to the SC interstices (32), with the organization of newly delivered lipid into lamellar membrane unit structures (68). Restoration of lipids to the SC is driven by a metabolic response limited to the epidermis underlying the site of acute injury. The initial response is secretion of a substantial pool of preformed lamellar bodies from the outer granular cells by 30 minutes (68), followed by an increase in cholesterol and fatty acid synthesis over the next 30 minutes to 4 hours (31) and increased ceramide synthesis in 6–9 hours. The increase in formation of these lipids, in turn, is regulated by (1) increased activities of key enzymes in each of their synthetic pathways, (2) an tecedent increases in mRNA levels for the same enzymes, (3) changes in the phosphorylation (activation) state of at least one key enzyme, HMG CoA reductase), and (4) putative role for sterol regulatory element binding proteins (SREBPs) as regulators of both epidermal cholesterol and fatty acid synthesis.

The delivery of ceramides results not only from the synthetic pathway, regulated by serine palmitoyl transferase, but also from hydrolysis of glucosylceramides and sphingomyelins by the enzymes β-glucosecerebrosidase and acid sphingomyelinase respectively. An increase in the activity and mRNAs of β-glucosecerebrosidase occurs somewhat later, i.e., not until 6–9 hours after acute disruption (43). As noted above, ceramides also are derived from the hydrolysis of sphingomyelins during a step regulated by the enzyme acid sphingomyelinase. Acid sphingomyelinase activity increases more quickly after acute barrier disruption, i.e., by 1 hour after treatment, which suggests the importance of this enzyme in the generation of ceramides for early permeability barrier repair (47,91). Uchida et al. found that epidermal sphingomyelins of different structures are precursors for two of the seven SC ceramides, i.e., ceramides 2 and 5, but other ceramide species, including the ω-hydroxyceramide species, do not derive from sphingomyelin (101).

In addition to enhanced lipid synthesis, epidermal DNA synthesis increases by about 16 hours after acute barrier disruption in mouse skin (84). Accordingly, acute as well as chronic barrier disruption results in the induction of the hyperproliferation-associated keratins K6 and K16, as well as the inflammation-associated K17. Also, the expression of suprabasal keratins, K1 and K10, increase in a delayed fashion after acute barrier disruption, while expression of the CE protein involucrin, which normally is restricted to the granular and upper spinous layers, extends to the lower spinous layers after acute barrier disruption. In contrast, loricrin expression remains unchanged. These results suggest that lipid, DNA, keratin, and involucrin synthesis are regulated coordinately in response to epidermal permeability barrier requirements (20).

Integrity of the permeability barrier also regulates epidermal Langerhans cell density. Experimental barrier disruption in mouse skin by treatment with either acetone, sodium dodecylsulfate solution (SDS), or tape stripping increases Langerhans cell density (85). The increase in epidermal Langerhans cell density is accompanied, in turn, by an enhanced propensity for allergic contact dermatitis (85,86). Immunofluorescence staining of epidermal sheets, as well as flow cytometric analyses, showed that subpopulations of Langerhans cells expressed the major histocompatibility complex class II antigens, CD54 and CD86, at levels higher than in control. Therefore, barrier compromise leads not only to increased permeability of allergens through the SC, but also to altered immune functions of epidermal dendritic cells that can potentiate T-cell activation. Such overregulation of immune reactivity, coupled with barrier repair, may be critical to the restriction of penetration of environmental noxious agents into epidermis (78).

II. SIGNALS OF BARRIER HOMEOSTASIS

The fact that external perturbations initiate homeostatic (repair) responses in underlying layers of the epidermis implies that signaling mechanisms are operative. The epidermis generates a plethora of candidate signaling molecules, and several potential candidates (e.g., neuropeptides, nitric oxide, polar lipids) have not yet been studied. However, it is clear that changes in the concentration of selected ions, particularly Ca^{2+} and K^+, are important for barrier recovery after acute disruption. These ions regulate lamellar body secretion from the outermost granular cell by a mechanism that involves both voltage-sensitive calcium channels and calmodulin. A steep ionic gradient exists across the nucleated layers of the epidermis, with the highest concentrations in the outer granular layer (60). In the presence of an unperturbed barrier, the extracellular Ca^{2+} gradient restricts lamellar body secretion, while loss of the gradient coincident with barrier disruption accelerates lamellar body secretion (53,61). The inhibitory effects of Ca^{2+} and other ions on barrier homeostasis may explain the increased incidence of dermatitis in geographic areas where ''hard water'' provides the principle water supply (62).

Ionic mechanisms probably do not, however, regulate synthetic events proximal to the outer granular layers. Therefore, we next examined cytokines and growth factors, known to be produced in abundance by keratinocytes (30,74), as potential autocrine regulators of barrier homeostasis. Indeed, both the mRNA and protein levels of several cytokines and growth factors increase after acute barrier perturbations, although the kinetics of these changes differed (111). TNF and GM-CSF are among the first cytokines that increase at an mRNA level, followed by both IL-1α/β and IL-1ra. Furthermore, IL-1α (but not TNF) is also released from a large preformed pool in the outer epidermis (112). The localization of these cytokines within the epidermis under basal conditions is consistent with the role of one or more of these substances as a homeostatic regulator, i.e., IL-1α, IL-1ra, amphiregulin, and TNF are concentrated in the outer nucleated layers.

We explored the TNF and IL-1 signal transduction pathways in permeability barrier repair. We showed that topical application of either TNF or IL-1 enhances barrier repair after acute perturbations of hairless mouse skin. Moreover, in TNF p55 receptor–deficient mice, cutaneous barrier repair was delayed in comparison to either wild-type or TNF p75 receptor–deficient animals. After barrier disruption in hairless and wild-type, but not in TNF-p55–deficient mice, the activities of acid and neutral sphingomyelinase, downstream targets of the TNF p55 receptor, are significantly enhanced. Stimulation of acid sphingomyelinase activity is accompanied by both a decrease in sphingomyelin content and an increase in ceramide levels. Furthermore, reduction of epidermal acid sphingomyelinase activity by the inhibitor imipramine results in a delay in permeability barrier repair after SC injury (47). The WD-40 repeat protein FAN binds to a distinct domain of the TNF-p55 receptor and signals the activation of neutral sphingomyelinase. In FAN-deficient mice we found delayed kinetics of recovery after cutaneous barrier disruption, further suggesting a physiological role of TNF/FAN in epidermal barrier repair. Also, epidermal proliferation after tape stripping is reduced in FAN-deficient animals, suggesting a role for neutral sphingomyelinase-generated ceramides in the regulation of the proliferative response to barrier disruption (51). Together, these results suggest that the TNF p55 receptor signaling pathway contributes to permeability barrier homeostasis through sphingomyelinase-mediated generation of ceramides (47).

Finally, these cytokines are likely to serve not only as homeostatic signals, but also as pathogenic signals. For example, repeated barrier disruption (''subacute model'') leads to epidermal hyperplasia and inflammation, accompanied by increased IL-1α and TNF expression (17). Together, these alterations can be presumed to mirror increases in barrier-initiated cytokine generation (cytokine cascade) that occurs in skin diseases, such as atopic dermatitis and psoriasis, which, it should be noted, are inevitably characterized by abnormal barrier function.

III. BARRIER FUNCTION IN ATOPIC DERMATITIS

The existence of a defect in skin permeability barrier function in atopic dermatitis (AD) is well accepted, but the epidermal abnormality generally is viewed as a downstream consequence of the inflammatory phenotype (11). Several studies have shown a two- to fivefold increase in basal transepidermal water loss (TEWL) over clinically uninvolved skin in AD. The extent of the barrier abnormality appears to correlate with the state of dermatitis—acute, subacute, and chronic—as well as the degree of inflammation in lesional skin (94,95). Moreover, barrier function in clinically uninvolved skin of normal appearance or dry noneczematous skin of patients with dermatitis elsewhere shows a from 30–50% up to a twofold increase in TEWL (3,28,94,104). Conversely, TEWL levels and the SC water content in normal-appearing skin of completely healed patients (free from symptoms of AD for more than 5 years) are not different from normal controls (60). As noted above, active dermatitis is associated with a further disturbance in skin barrier function (four- to eightfold increase) (1), as well as enhanced percutaneous absorption of small molecules, such as hydrocortisone, theophylline, and dimethylsulfoxide (1,114). Together, these studies suggest that skin barrier function in AD undergoes fluctuations according to the phase of the disease, supporting the hypothesis that the presence of active eczema provokes impaired barrier function in uninvolved skin, even at sites far from active lesions (95).

It is also well accepted that patients with a history of AD have an increased tendency for certain other dermatoses. Tupker et al. showed that patients with a history of AD had lower preexposure TEWL levels, but higher TEWL measurements following irritant exposure than groups with a history of either allergic contact dermatitis alone or unaffected controls. Moreover, clinically dry skin was more susceptible to irritants than normal-appearing skin (100). Hanifan's patients also showed a significantly greater irritant response to sodium dodecylsulfate both in atopic subjects with no skin disease and in subjects with inactive AD (76). They hypothesized that abnormal, intrinsic hyperreactivity to inflammatory cells in atopic individuals predisposes to a lower threshold of responsiveness to irritants (76). Conti et al. (13) examined skin reactivity in patients with a history of respiratory atopy, but no AD. Tests were performed first in winter and repeated in spring when patients showed respiratory symptoms from seasonal allergic rhinitis. A parallel group of 15 subjects with AD served as the control population. After a standard sodium dodecyl sulfate challenge, AD patients showed a greater extent of skin barrier damage and inflammation than did patients with seasonal allergic rhinitis. Together, these findings suggest that subjects with seasonal allergic rhinitis without atopic dermatitis have normal epidermal barrier function and normal skin reactivity during both the inactive and the active phases of their disease. Further, inflammatory mediators, presumably released by mucous membranes during active allergic rhinitis, do not appear to influence skin barrier function adversely (13,14).

Surprisingly, Gfesser et al. (35) described that the early phase of epidermal barrier regeneration after experimental disruption by tape stripping is faster in patients with AD than in normals. The authors speculated (and we would agree) that repair mechanisms are permanently activated, because of the persistent, mild disturbance in barrier function in patients with AD. Yet, despite accelerated repair kinetics, normal barrier function is never completely achieved (35). The same authors described a disturbance of epidermal barrier function in patch test reactions in AD (36). Positive patch test reactions to aeroallergens were only observed in AD patients, and these bore macroscopic and microscopic resemblance to lesional AD skin. After patch test to grass pollen, birch pollen, cat dander, and house dust mite, the patients developed positive skin reactions and showed a high two- to fourfold increase in TEWL in the patch test area. After patch test reactions to common type IV (contact) allergens (nickel sulfate, potassium dichromate, thiuram-mix, and paraphenylenediamine), only a twofold increase in transepidermal water loss levels occurred. The authors concluded that as a consequence of aeroallergen-induced alterations in barrier function, aeroallergens can penetrate the skin more easily, inducing a vicious circle that perpetuates eczematous lesions (35).

IV. EPIDERMAL LIPIDS

Changes in SC lipid content have long been regarded as the cause of the disturbed permeability barrier function in atopic skin, and numerous studies have addressed this hypothesis. Skin surface lipids from the forearm repeatedly are significantly lower in AD than in either normal controls or in patients with ichthyosis vulgaris (6,46), suggesting a decrease in total SC lipids. Mustakallio et al. (75) characterized and quantitated the epidermal lipids in AD by thin-layer chromatography. Full-thickness epidermal sheets were obtained by the suction blister method during the winter months from the volar aspect of nonlichenified forearm skin of 12 patients with Besnier's prurigo (chronic, lichenified AD). Compared with normal controls of the same age, atopic epidermis displayed a decrease in the contents of total lipids, phospholipids and sterol esters, as well as an increase in free fatty acids and sterols (75). It is likely that the decrease in phospholipids actually reflected a decrease in sphingolipid content; specifically sphingomyelin, based upon more recent work (see below). The phospholipid and fatty acid content of lesional vs. lesion-free epidermis was also determined by Schäfer and Kragballe (90). They found an increased activity of phospholipase A_2 and an incomplete transformation of phospholipids into other lipid classes in AD (90).

More recently, special attention has focused on the role of ceramides in the barrier abnormality in AD. When SC lipids of untreated noninflamed plantar skin of patients with AD vs. 10 healthy age-matched controls were examined by sequential high-performance thin-layer chromatography, significant decrease in the ceramide fraction, expressed as a percentage of total lipids, was found in the AD patients (64). Moreover, a decrease in ceramides was also found in SC from back skin and in toenails from patients with AD (66). A marked reduction in the amount of ceramides was also found in lesional forearm SC in AD by Imokawa et al. (45). Interestingly, nonlesional SC from affected patients also exhibited a similar, significant decrease in ceramides. Among the six ceramide subfractions, ceramide 1 was most significantly reduced in both lesional and nonlesional skin. However, ceramides 2, 3, 4 plus 5, and 6 were also reduced significantly in both lesional and nonlesional SC (45). Likewise, a reduced content of ceramide 1 in the SC of clinically dry skin, with no signs of eczema, was found in AD by Yamamoto et al. (113). It is noteworthy that the relative amount of all other SC lipid classes in AD, including squalene, cholesterol esters, triglycerides, free fatty acids, cholesterol, cholesterol sulfate, and phospholipids, did not differ significantly from controls (113). Furthermore, a reduced content of total ceramides and ceramide 1 was also found in the SC of atopic dry skin by Matsumoto et al. (59). Whereas the content of ceramide 2, 3, 4 plus 5, and 6 was also reduced, it did not reach statistical significance (58). Di Nardo et al. (18) correlated SC ceramide content with barrier function in AD. First, they found significantly lower levels of ceramide 1 and 3 and higher levels of cholesterol in AD vs. control subjects. Second, they found that the decrease in ceramide 3 correlated significantly with the barrier impairment (18). Finally, Bleck et al. (9) found two monohydroxylated and monounsaturated ceramide subfractions of different chain length, containing either C_{16} or C_{18} or C_{22}, C_{24}, C_{26} α-hydroxy fatty acids in nonlesional skin of AD by MALDI-TOF mass spectrometry. In contrast, only a single peak occurred in the SC ceramides from senile xerosis, psoriasis, and seborrheic dermatitis (9).

As described above, skin ceramides derive both from the newly synthesized compound, serine palmitoyl transferase, and from hydrolysis of both glucosylceramides (by β-glucocerebrosidase) and sphingomyelin (by acidic sphingomyelinase) (42,43,47). The rates of ceramide synthesis and the activity of the rate-limiting enzyme, serine palmitoyl transferase, in the epidermis of AD has not yet been determined, because of both the invasive nature of such studies and the sample size needed for such experiments. In contrast, it has been easier to examine hydrolytic enzymes, because their levels peak in the SC. Jin et al. (48) examined β-glucocerebrosidase and ceramidase activities in the SC of AD and age-related dry skin. Since they found differences in neither β-glucocerebrosidase nor ceramidase activities in uninvolved SC of AD, the decrease of ceramides in AD could not be attributed to enhanced ceramide degradation (48). Likewise, the presence of unchanged β-glucocerebrosidase in SC from noneczematous dry skin of AD was confirmed by Redoules et al. (88). Of five enzymatic activities examined by these authors, AD displayed significantly reduced trypsin activity, increased acid phosphatase activity, and no changes in either secretory phospholipase A_2 or chymotryptic protease activities were seen (88).

Prosaposin is a large precursor protein that is proteolytically cleaved to form a family of sphingolipid activator proteins, which stimulate enzymatic hydrolysis of sphingolipids, including glucosylceramides and sphingomyelin. It has been shown that prosaposin is required for normal epidermal barrier formation and function (19). Decreased levels of prosaposin were found in atopic epidermis by ELISA, using a polyclonal antibody to saposin D, suggesting that reduced activation of β-glucocerebrosidase and acid sphingomyelinase in AD could be due to decreased prosaposin levels in AD (15).

As noted above, sphingomyelinase was shown recently to be important for the generation of ceramides during permeability barrier repair of the skin (47,91). The epidermis contains two sphingomyelinase isoenzymes, an acidic sphingomyelinase, which is localized in epidermal lamellar bodies and which generates ceramides for the extracellular lipid bilayers of the SC, as well as a neutral sphingomyelinase, which is important for cell signaling during permeability barrier repair (51). The localization and amount of acid sphingomyelinase was measured in lesional skin of AD by Kusuda et al. (52). The authors generated a polyclonal antibody and found immunostaining extending from the upper spinous cell layers to the upper SC. Moreover, total amounts of enzyme protein, measured by quantitative immunoblot analysis, was slightly increased in lesional vs. non-lesional SC from AD patients (52). Although these results suggest that acidic sphingomyelinase activity is minimalized in AD, direct assays of enzyme activity have not yet been performed. Likewise, the activity of the neutral sphingomyelinase has not yet been determined in AD.

An alternative explanation for reduced Cer in AD was explored by Murata et al. (73). They found that the AD epidermis contains a novel enzyme, glucosylceramide/sphingomyelin deacylase, which cleaves the *N*-acyl linkage of both sphingomyelins and glucosylceramides. Moreover, they found that sphingomyelin hydrolysis is extremely elevated in the SC of both uninvolved and involved skin in AD (a five- and eightfold increase in sphingomyelin deacylase activity in uninvolved and involved skin, respectively). Moreover, the increase in sphingomyelin hydrolysis in AD again was not related to changes in acid sphingomyelinase activity, which increased only slightly (not significant). Sphingomyelin deacylase releases free fatty acids and sphingosyl-phosphorycholine, rather than ceramides, generating additional classes of lipid signalling agents that could participate in the pathophysiology of AD. These findings suggest that sphingomyelin metabolism is altered in AD, resulting in decreased levels of ceramides, providing a possible basis for the barrier abnormality in AD (37,73).

An alternative explanation for the decrease in ceramide content in AD was provided recently by Ohnishi et al. (81). These authors collected bacteria from the skin surface of eczematous and the normal-appearing skin of AD, erythematous skin lesions of psoriasis, and normal control skin. After selective bacterial culture, they assayed ceramidase and sphingomyelinase activities and found that more ceramidase was secreted from the bacterial flora of both lesional and the nonlesional skin of AD than from either lesional psoriasis or normal subjects.

In contrast, sphingomyelinase activity was secreted at similar levels by bacteria obtained from AD, psoriasis, and controls. The authors suggest, therefore, that the skin of patients with AD is colonized by ceramidase-secreting bacteria, and that these microorganisms contribute to the ceramide deficiency in the SC of AD (81). Finally, a disturbed extruding mechanism of lamellar bodies in the dry, non-eczematous skin of AD was described by Fartasch et al. (28), who suggested that this mechanism could account, at least partly, for the SC lipid abnormalities found in AD. Thus, comprehensive studies on lipid metabolism in AD suggest that a decrease in ceramides is the cause of the impaired permeability barrier in AD.

Epidermal differentiation is of great importance for the integrity of the permeability barrier. As noted above, barrier disruption induces K6, K16, and K17 keratin expression, as well as suprabasal expression of K10, while expression of basal keratins K5 and K14 is reduced. Moreover, expression of the CE protein involucrin changes, while, in contrast, loricrin expression remains unchanged (20). Accordingly, reduced expression of involucrin, cystatin A, and filaggrin has been found in lesional skin of AD, while filaggrin expression is also decreased in nonlesional skin of AD (93). Filaggrin expression has been related to SC hydration (92), which is known to be reduced in atopic dry skin. Although involucrin serves as substrate for the covalent attachment of ceramides to the CE (58), the levels of covalently bound ceramides in AD have not yet been determined. This relationship could be interest, since there appears to be a relationship between the content of covalently bound ceramides and TEWL levels (63).

V. ESSENTIAL FATTY ACID METABOLISM IN ATOPIC ECZEMA

Research from the 1930s to the 1950s established that a deficit of n-6 essential fatty acids (EFAs) leads to an inflammatory skin condition in both animals and humans. Later, an essential fatty acid–deficient (EFAD) diet was shown to induce extremely scaly, red skin and an up to 10-fold increase in transepidermal water loss rates in mice (27,69,87). The progressive increase in transepidermal water loss levels correlated with membrane structural alterations (21), explained by replacement of linoleate by oleate in both epidermal ceramides and glucosylceramides (69). The signs of EFAD in animals can be reversed by either systemic or topical administration of n-6 essential fatty acids like linoleic acid, γ-linolenic acid, or columbinic acid (87). Although there is evidence for a low blood EFA concentration in AD, there is no deficit of linoleic acid. Whereas linoleic acid concentrations tend to be elevated in blood, skin, and adipose tissue of patients with AD, levels of downstream metabolites of linoleic acid are substantially reduced (44). These observations suggested that conversion of linoleic acid to γ-linolenic acid (GLA) might be impaired in AD (66,44). Although several studies have assessed the efficacy of systemic or topical n-6 essential fatty acids in AD, the results have been conflicting. In most of the studies, however, administration of γ-linolenic acid appeared to improve the clinical severity (71). However, the largest placebo-controlled trials of either n-6 or n-3 fatty acids supplementation in AD found no consistent benefit. Berth-Jones et al. (8) treated 123 patients with AD with evening primrose oil (n-6) fatty acids, fish oil (n-3) fatty acid, or placebo for 16 weeks. No effects of essential acid supplementation by n-6 or by n-3 fatty acids were found (8). Henz et al. (38) performed a double-blind, multicenter analysis of the efficacy of borage oil (>23% γ-linolenic acid) in 160 patients with AD. Patients took either 500 mg of borage oil-containing capsules or a bland lipid placebo over a 24-week period. Although several clinical symptoms improved in comparison to placebo, the overall response to borage oil did not attain statistical significance. Significant differences in favor of borage oil were, however, observed in a subgroup of AD patients. Moreover, γ-linolenic acid levels increased in borage oil–treated patients only, and serum IgE levels tended to decrease, suggesting that a subgroup of AD patients might benefit from this treatment (38). The mechanisms of action of γ-linolenic acid are only understood in part. γ-Linolenic acid could either influence epidermal barrier function, modulate eicosanoid metabolism, and/or modulate cell signaling (11a). Although a reduced content of linoleic acid in ceramide 1 has been reported in AD (115), whether topically or systematically applied n-6 fatty acids normalize linolenic or γ-linolenic acid content of ceramide 1 is not known. However, preliminary data from Michelsen et al. showed that oral treatment with n-6 fatty acids did not change ceramide content or composition significantly (Michelsen et al., poster at the German Dermatology Meeting, 1995). A different mechanism for the fatty acids has been forwarded recently: linoleic acid and other unsaturated free fatty acids are potent, naturally occurring activators of PPARα. PPARα ligands promote epidermal differentiation in vivo, and topically applications of PPARα activators restore tissue homeostasis in hyperplastic models that bear some resemblance to AD (49,50). Prior studies on EFAs in the treatment of AD should be reevaluated in the light of their status as potential PPARα activators.

VI. BARRIER REPAIR STRATEGIES IN ATOPIC DERMATITIS

Most treatment strategies for AD, such as corticosteroids, tacrolimus, and cyclosporine, are aimed primarily at the immunogenic abnormalities in AD. These approaches generally result in an improvement repair of barrier function that parallels the clinical response. Similarly, treatment with UV light reduces the content of inflammatory cells and also improves barrier function in AD. A commonly employed therapeutic strategy in AD is the use of topically applied cremes and ointments aimed at increasing SC hydration. Creams and ointments contain lipids or lipid-like substances, such as hydrocarbons (petrolatum), long-chain alcohols, free fatty acids, cholesterol esters, and triglycerides. The effects of topical treatment with ointments in AD has been examined in several studies. Aalto-Korte (1) evaluated parallel changes in skin barrier function, assessed as TEWL and percutaneous absorption of hydrocortisone, during treatment of AD. Aalto-Korte found a rapid improvement in skin barrier function during treatment and that TEWL changes reflect decreased systemic absorption of topical hydrocortisone (1).

However, the described effect could be related to either the emollient or co-applied hydrocortisone. Therefore, the effect of moisturizing creams on barrier function in AD is still controversial. Improvement in skin barrier function in patients with AD after treatment (54) as well as unchanged water barrier function (98) has been described. Because it has been shown that lipid composition in AD is reduced, topical applied lipids and hydrocarbons may interfere with the SC permeability barrier. It has been shown that hydrocarbons (petrolatum) enhanced permeability barrier repair after artificial disruption by intercalating into the extracellular lamellar membranes of the SC (36). In contrast, a physiological mixture containing free fatty acid, cholesterol, and ceramides penetrate a disrupted SC, reaching the nucleated epidermal cell layers, followed by uptake into keratinocytes, and release into nascent lamellar bilayers in the SC interstices (55). This strategy recently was applied to the therapy of stubborn-to-recalcitrant childhood AD (12). A phase I trial of ceramide-dominant barrier repair moisturizer in childhood AD significantly reduced severity scoring of AD, normalized TEWL rates, and improved SC integrity in children with recalcitrant AD. TEWL levels declined significantly at both 3 and 6 weeks in involved skin vs. pretreatment measurements and almost normalized in adjacent, uninvolved skin by 6 weeks. In contrast, hydration improved more slowly. Finally, electron microscopy of tape-stripped SC showed significant replenishment of lamellar membrane bilayers in SC treated with the ceramide-dominant mixture (12). Further controlled studies are needed to validate this approach in the therapy of AD.

VII. RELATIONSHIP OF EPIDERMAL BARRIER DYSFUNCTION TO THE PATHOGENESIS OF ATOPIC DERMATITIS

Ogawa and Yoshiike (80) published an interesting account of the pathogenesis of AD. They speculated that the broad clinical spectrum of AD cannot be explained simply by allergy or immunological abnormalities, suggesting instead a primary role for barrier dysfunction in disease pathogenesis. They consider immunological abnormalities and mucocutaneous barrier dysfunction as two major but linked manifestations of atopy or AD. Besides the skin, barrier dysfunction may be operative in the mucous membranes of the nose, the lung, and the gut leading to rhinitis, asthma bronchiale, or type 1 allergy. A mucocutaneous barrier defect would readily allow penetration of multiple antigens or haptens. Repeated encounters with allergens would induce not only tolerance, but also nonspecific hypersensitivity leading to enhancement of the allergic inflammation. Furthermore, an allergic inflammation stemming from the immunological abnormalities would further degrade barrier function. This sequence would result in a "vicious circle," which could be the most important contributor to the pathogenesis of AD and probably of other atopic diseases, as well. The increased frequency of positive patch tests to house dust mite antigens in patients with AD suggests enhanced percutaneous absorption of macromolecules, indirectly supporting this hypothesis (2,70). Deteriorated mucosal barrier function is another important issue: following ingestion of egg or milk, greater amounts of protein antigen appear in the circulation of subjects with AD than in controls (82). Possible explanations for such a phenomenon include either increased intestinal permeability or maldigestion. Increased permeability of the gut wall has been reported in AD (83,102) but is still considered controversial (5,82).

Ogawa and Yoshiike (80) admit that most observers consider the barrier defect to result from the underlying inflammation. It is difficult to determine whether barrier dysfunction is a primary initiator or only a secondary event that participates in the vicious circle. Even in the normal-appearing skin of atopics, injuries sustained by scratching lead to eczematous dermatitis and enhanced penetration of allergens. Therefore, among allergy, immunological abnormalities, and barrier dysfunction/biochemical abnormalities, we are unable to confirm which is the initiator of AD. However, the recent increase in incidence of AD is also explained by barrier dysfunction: alterations of life-styles, such as excessive use of soaps or shampoos, and residuals of detergents or rinses in clothes, appear to enhance skin barrier dysfunction and irritability of skin (25,26,33). Environmental antigens, i.e., house dust mites and pollens, are increasingly available to penetrate the skin due to air conditioning, poor ventilation, and changes in levels of hygiene (4). Finally, too early feeding of animal proteins to babies also could allow more opportunities for antigen penetrations through intestinal barriers (82).

Mar et al. (56) observed that some patients never accommodate to either occupational or topical irritants and that many of these individuals are in fact atopics. For example, a large proportion of Asians from south Asia are atopics, but their disease may be masked by the high ambient humidity of parts of the Pacific Rim (16,56). Conversely, these subclinical atopics often develop cutaneous symptoms when they are geographically displaced to cool, temperate locations. Since atopics display abnormal barrier function, even in clinically uninvolved skin (95), it can be assumed that a barrier-initiated cytokine cascade is always operative. Taieb (99) speculated that some common genetic polymorphism, causing a functional impairment of the epidermal barrier in the first month of age, could increase the probability of being sensitized to allergens and especially to "atopens." At least two genetic epidermal disorders associated with an increased prevalence of AD could be considered as good candidates. Ichthyosis vulgaris is an autosomal dominant disorder linked to defective filaggrin expression in the epidermis. This condition occurs in association with about 4% of AD cases. However, the distinction of this phenotype from AD alone can be blurred because of the overlapping phenotypes, so that the true rate of association is unclear. The known maternal effect of the inheritance of AD might be associated with a predisposing gene on the X chromosome. X-linked hypohydrotic ectodermal displasia is associated with a very high frequency with mild atopic dermatitis and asthma (96). Also, Wiskott-Aldrich syndrome, an X-linked disorder (affecting only boys), according to its standard clinical definition, involves immunodeficiency, low blood platelet levels, and eczema. Eczema closely resembles atopic dermatitis and is prone to eczema herpeticum. Wiskott-Aldrich patients have relatively intact immune systems. Their immune cells attack certain antigens but no others, suggesting a possible defect in antigen presentation or processing (79,96).

Some years ago Williams (109) stated that we should look to the environment to explain atopic eczema. One possible explanation for the threefold increase in the prevalence of eczema over the past 30 years could be that changes in the indoor climate as a result of central heating and better insulation have increased children's exposure to allergens such as house dust mite. It has been

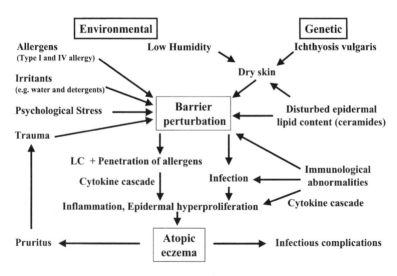

Figure 1 Relationship of epidermal barrier dysfunction to the pathogenesis of atopic dermatitis.

shown that reduction of indoor humidity reduces house mite content (4). It is feasible also that exposure to low-grade irritance and atmospheric indoor pollution makes children vulnerable to sensitization (109) (Fig. 1).

REFERENCES

1. Aalto-Korte K. Improvement of skin barrier function during treatment of atopic dermatitis. J Am Acad Dermatol 33:969–972, 1995.
2. Adinoff AD, Tellez P, Clark RA. Atopic dermatitis and aeroallergen contact sensitivity. J Allergy Clin Immunol 81:736–742, 1988.
3. Agner T. Noninvasive measuring methods for the investigation of irritant patch test reactions. A study of patients with hand eczema, atopic dermatitis and controls. Acta Derm Venereol Suppl (Stockh) 173:1–26, 1992.
4. Arlian LG, Neal JS, Morgan MS, Vyszenski-Moher DL, Rapp CM, Alexander AK. Reducing relative humidity is a practical way to control dust mites and their allergens in homes in temperate climates. J Allergy Clin Immunol 107:99–104, 2001.
5. Barba A, Schena D, Andreaus MC, Faccini G, Pasini F, Brocco G, Cavallini G, Scuro LA, Chieregato GC. Intestinal permeability in patients with atopic eczema. Br J Dermatol 120:71–75, 1989.
6. Barth J, Gatti S, Jatzke M. Skin surface lipids in atopic eczema and ichthyosis. Chron Derm 10:609–612, 1989.
7. Behne M, Uchida Y, Seki T, de Montellano PO, Elias PM, Holleran WM. Omega-hydroxyceramides are required for corneocyte lipid envelope (CLE) formation and normal epidermal permeability barrier function. J Invest Dermatol 114:185–192, 2000.
8. Berth-Jones J, Graham-Brown RA. Placebo-controlled trial of essential fatty acid supplementation in atopic dermatitis. Lancet 342:564, 1993.
9. Bleck O, Abeck D, Ring J, Hoppe U, Vietzke JP, Wolber R, Brandt O, Schreiner V. Two ceramide subfractions detectable in Cer(AS) position by HPTLC in skin surface lipids of non-lesional skin of atopic eczema. J Invest Dermatol 113:894–900, 1999.
10. Bouwstra JA, Gooris GS, Dubbelaar FE, Weerheim AM, Ijzerman AP, Ponec M. Role of ceramide 1 in the molecular organization of the stratum corneum lipids. J Lipid Res 39:186–196, 1998.
11. Bos JD, Kapsenberg ML, Smitt JH. Pathogenesis of atopic eczema. Lancet 343:1338–1341, 1994.
11a. Burton JL. Dietary fatty acids and inflammatory skin disease. Lancet 1(8628):27–31, 1989.
12. Chamlin SL, Frieden IJ, Fowler A, Williams M, Kao J. Ceramide-dominant barrier repair moisturizer in childhood dermatitis. Submitted.
13. Conti A, Di Nardo A, Seidenari S. No alteration of biophysical parameters in the skin of subjects with respiratory atopy. Dermatology 192:317–320, 1996.
14. Conti A, Seidenari S. No increased skin reactivity in subjects with allergic rhinitis during the active phase of the disease. Acta Derm Venereol 80:192–195, 2000.

15. Cui CY, Kusuda S, Seguchi T, Takahashi M, Aisu K, Tezuka T. Decreased level of prosaposin in atopic skin. J Invest Dermatol 109:319–323, 1997.

16. Denda M, Sato J, Masuda Y, Tsuchiya T, Koyama J, Kuramoto M, Elias PM, Feingold KR. Exposure to a dry environment enhances epidermal permeability barrier function. J Invest Dermatol 111:858–863, 1998.

17. Denda M, Wood LC, Emami S, Calhoun C, Brown BE, Elias PM, Feingold KR. The epidermal hyperplasia associated with repeated barrier disruption by acetone treatment or tape stripping cannot be attributed to increased water loss. Arch Dermatol Res 288:230–238, 1996.

18. Di Nardo A, Wertz P, Giannetti A, Seidenari S. Ceramide and cholesterol composition of the skin of patients with atopic dermatitis. Acta Derm Venereol 78:27–30, 1998.

19. Doering T, Holleran WM, Potratz A, Vielhaber G, Elias PM, Suzuki K, Sandhoff. Sphingolipid activator proteins are required for epidermal permeability barrier formation. J Biol Chem 274:11038–11045, 1999.

20. Ekanayake-Mudiyanselage S, Aschauer H, Schmook FP, Jensen JM, Meingassner JG, Proksch E. Expression of epidermal keratins and the cornified envelope protein involucrin is influenced by permeability barrier disruption. J Invest Dermatol 111: 517–523, 1998.

21. Elias PM, Brown BE. The mammalian cutaneous permeability barrier: defective barrier function is essential fatty acid deficiency correlates with abnormal intercellular lipid deposition. Lab Invest 39:574–583, 1978.

22. Elias PM, Menon GK. Structural and lipid biochemical correlates of the epidermal permeability barrier. Adv Lipid Res 24:1–26, 1991.

23. Elias PM. Stratum corneum architecture, metabolic activity, and interactivity with subjacent cell layers. Exp Dermatol 5:191–201, 1996.

24. Elias PM, Ansel JC, Woods LC, Feingold KR. Signalling networks in barrier homeostasis: the mystery widens. Arch Dermatol 132:1505–1506, 1996.

25. Elias PM, Wood LC, Feingold KR. Relationship of the epidermal permeability barrier to irritant contact dermatitis. In: Beltrani V, ed. Immunology and Allergy Clinics of North America. Vol. 17. Contact Dermatitis: Irritant and Allergic. Philadelphia: Saunders, 1997, pp 417–430.

26. Elias PM, Wood LC, Feingold KR. Epidermal pathogenesis of inflammatory dermatoses. Am J Contact Derm 10:119–126, 1999.

27. Elias PM, Brown BEJ. The mammalian cutaneous permeability barrier: defective barrier function in essential fatty acid deficiency correlates with abnormal intercellular lipid deposition. Lab Invest 39:574–583, 1978.

28. Fartasch M, Diepgen TL. The barrier function in atopic dry skin. Disturbance of membrane-coating granule exocytosis and formation of epidermal lipids? Acta Derm Venereol Suppl (Stockh) 176:26–31, 1992.

29. Feingold KR. The regulation and role of epidermal lipid synthesis. Adv Lipid Res 24:57–82, 1991.

30. Feliciani C, Gupta AK, Sauder DN. Keratinocytes and cytokine/growth factors. Crit Rev Oral Biol Med 7:300–318, 1996.

31. Grubauer G, Feingold KR, Elias PM. The relationship of epidermal lipogenesis to cutaneous barrier function. J Lipid Res 28:746–752, 1987.

32. Grubauer G, Elias PM, Feingold KR. Transepidermal water loss: the signal for recovery of barrier structure and function. J Lipid Res 30:323–334, 1989.

33. Garg A, Chren M-M, Sands LP, Matsui MS, Marenus KD, Feingold KR, Elias PM. Psychological stress perturbs epidermal permeability barrier homeostasis: implications for the pathogenesis and treatment of stress-associated skin disorders. Arch Dermatol 137:53–59, 2001.

34. Gfesser M, Abeck D, Riigemer J, Schreiner V, Stab F, Disch R, Ring J. The early phase of epidermal barrier regeneration is faster in patients with atopic eczema. Dermatology 195:332–336, 1997.

35. Gfesser M, Rakoski J, Ring J. The disturbance of epidermal barrier function in atopy patch test reactions in atopic eczema. Br J Dermatol 135:560–565, 1996.

36. Ghadially R, Halkier-Sorensen L, Elias PM. Effects of petrolatum on stratum corneum structure and function. J Am Acad Dermatol 26:387–396, 1992.

37. Hara J, Higuchi K, Okamoto R, Kawashima M, Imokawa G. High-expression of sphingomyelin deacylase is an important determinant of ceramide deficiency leading to barrier disruption in atopic dermatitis. J Invest Dermatol 115:406–413, 2000.

38. Henz BM, Jablonska S, van de Kerkhof PC, Stingl G, Blaszczyk M, Vandervalk PG, Veenhuizen R, Muggli R, Raederstorff D. Double-blind, multicentre analysis of the efficacy of borage oil in patients with atopic eczema. Br J Dermatol 140(4): 685–688, 1999.

39. Higuchi K, Hara J, Okamoto R, Kawashima M, Imokawa G. The skin of atopic dermatitis patients contains a novel enzyme, glucosylceramide sphingomyelin deacylase, which cleaves the N-acyl linkage of sphingomyelin and glucosylceramide. Biochem J 350:747–756, 2000.

40. Holleran WM, Man MQ, Gao WN, Menon GK, Elias PM, Feingold KR. Sphingolipids are required for mammalian epidermal barrier function. Inhibition of sphingolipid synthesis delays barrier recovery after acute perturbation. J Clin Invest 88: 1338–1345, 1991.

41. Holleran WM, Takagi Y, Menon GK, Legler G, Feingold KR, Elias PM. Processing of epidermal glucosylceramides is required for optimal mammalian cutaneous permeability barrier function. J Clin Invest 91:1656–1664, 1993.

42. Holleran WM, Takagi Y, Menon GK, Jackson SM, Lee JM, Feingold KR, Elias PM. Permeability barrier requirements regulate epidermal beta-glucocerebrosidase. J Lipid Res 35:905–912, 1994.

43. Holleran WM, Gao WN, Feingold KR, Elias PM. Localization of epidermal sphingolipid synthesis and serine palmitoyl transferase activity: alterations imposed by permeability barrier requirements. Arch Dermatol Res 287:254–258, 1995.

44. Horrobin DF. Essential fatty acid metabolism and its modification in atopic eczema. Am J Clin Nutr 71:367S–372S, 2000.

45. Imokawa G, Abe A, Jin Y, Higaki Y, Kawashima M, Hidano A. Decreased level of ceramides in stratum corneum of atopic dermatitis: an etiologic factor in atopic dry skin? J Invest Dermatol 96:523–526, 1991.

46. Jakobza D, Reichmann G, Langnick W, Langnick A, Schulze P. [Surface skin lipids

in atopic dermatitis (author's transl)] [article in German]. Dermatol Monatsschr 167:26–29, 1981.

47. Jensen JM, Schutze S, Forl M, Kronke M, Proksch E. Roles for tumor necrosis factor receptor p55 and sphingomyelinase in repairing the cutaneous permeability barrier. J Clin Invest 104:1761–1770, 1999.

48. Jin K, Higaki Y, Takagi Y, Higuchi K, Yada Y, Kawashima M, Imokawa G. Analysis of beta-glucocerebrosidase and ceramidase activities in atopic and aged dry skin. Acta Derm Venereol 74:337–340, 1994.

49. Komuves LG, Hanley K, Man MQ, Elias PM, Williams ML, Feingold KR. Keratinocyte differentiation in hyperproliferative epidermis: topical application of PPARalpha activators restores tissue homeostasis. J Invest Dermatol 115:361–367, 2000.

50. Komuves LG, Hanley K, Lefebvre AM, Man MQ, Ng DC, Bikle DD, Williams ML, Elias PM, Auwerx J, Feingold KR. Stimulation of PPARalpha promotes epidermal keratinocyte differentiation in vivo. J Invest Dermatol 115:353–360, 2000.

51. Kreder D, Krut O, Adam-Klages S, Wiegmann K, Scherer G, Plitz T, Jensen JM, Proksch E, Steinmann J, Pfeffer K, Kronke M. Impaired neutral sphingomyelinase activation and cutaneous barrier repair in FAN-deficient mice. EMBO J 18:2472–2479, 1999.

52. Kusuda S, Cui CY, Takahashi M, Tezuka T. Localization of sphingomyelinase in lesional skin of atopic dermatitis patients. J Invest Dermatol 111:733–738, 1998.

53. Lee SH, Elias PM, Proksch E, Menon GK, Mao-Qiang M, Feingold KR. Calcium and potassium are important regulators of barrier homeostasis in murine epidermis. J Clin Invest 89:530–538, 1992.

54. Loden M, Andersson AC, Lindberg M Improvement in skin barrier function in patients with atopic dermatitis after treatment with a moisturizing cream (Canoderm). Br J Dermatol 140:264–267, 1999.

55. Mao-Qiang M, Brown BE, Wu-Pong S, Feingold KR, Elias PM. Exogenous nonphysiologic vs. physiologic lipids. Divergent mechanisms for correction of permeability barrier dysfunction. Arch Dermatol 131:809–816, 1995.

56. Mar A, Tarn M, Jolley D, Marks R. The cumulative incidence of atopic dermatitis in the first 12 months among Chinese, Vietnamese, and Caucasian infants born in Melbourne, Australia. J Am Acad Dermatol 40:597–602, 1999.

57. Marekov LN, Steinert PM. Ceramides are bound to structural proteins of the human foreskin epidermal cornified cell envelope. J Biol Chem 273:17763–17770, 1998.

58. Matsumoto M, Sugiura H, Uehara M. Skin barrier function in patients with completely healed atopic dermatitis. J Dermatol Sci 23:178–182, 2000.

59. Matsumoto Y, Hamashima H, Masuda K, Shiojima K, Sasatsu M, Arai T. The antibacterial activity of plaunotol against Staphylococcus aureus isolated from the skin of patients with atopic dermatitis. Microbios 96:149–155, 1998.

60. Mauro T, Bench G, Sidderas-Haddad E, Feingold K, Elias P, Cullander C. Acute barrier perturbation abolishes the Ca2+ and K+ gradients in murine epidermis: quantitative measurement using PIXE. J Invest Dermatol 111:1198–1201, 1998.

61. Mauro T, Holleran WM, Grayson S, Gao WN, Mao-Qiang M, Kriehuber E, Behne, Feingold KR, Elias PM. Barrier recovery is impeded at neutral pH, independent of ionic effects: implications for extracellular lipid processing. Arch Dermatol Res 290:215–222, 1998.

62. McNally NJ, Williams HC, Phillips DR, Smallman-Rayanor M, Lems S, Venn A, Britton J. Atopic eczema and domestic water hardness. Lancet 352:527–531, 1998.
63. Meguro S, Arai Y, Masukawa Y, Uie K, Tokimitsu I. Relationship between covalently bound ceramides and transepidermal water loss (TEWL). Arch Dermatol Res 292:463–468, 2000.
64. Melnik B, Hollmann J, Plewig G. Decreased stratum corneum ceramides in atopic individuals—a pathobiochemical factor in xerosis? Br J Dermatol 119:547–549, 1988.
65. Melnik BC, Hollmann J, Erler E, Verhoeven B, Plewig G. Microanalytical screening of all major stratum corneum lipids by sequential high-performance thin-layer chromatography. J Invest Dermatol 92:231–234, 1989.
66. Melnik BC, Plewig G. Is the origin of atopy linked to deficient conversion of omega-6-fatty acids to prostaglandin E1? J Am Acad Dermatol 21:557–563, 1989.
67. Menon GK, Grayson S, Elias PM. Cytochemical and biochemical localization of lipase and sphingomyelinase activity in mammalian epidermis. J Invest Dermatol 86:591–597, 1986.
68. Menon GK, Feingold KR, Elias PM. Lamellar body secretory response to barrier disruption. J Invest Dermatol 98:279–289, 1992.
69. Melton JL, Wertz PW, Swartzendruber DC, Downing DT. Effects of essential fatty acid deficiency on epidermal O-acylsphingolipids and transepidermal water loss in young pigs. Biochim Biophys Acta 921:191–197, 1987.
70. Mitchell EB, Crow J, Chapman MD, Jouhal SS, Pope FM, Platts-Mills T. Basophils in allergen-induced patch test sites in atopic dermatitis. Lancet. 16:127–130, 1982.
71. Morse PF, Horrobin DF, Manku MS, Stewart JC, Allen R, Littlewood S, Wright S, Burton J, Gould DJ, Holt PJ, et al. Meta-analysis of placebo-controlled studies of the efficacy of Epogam in the treatment of atopic eczema. Relationship between plasma essential fatty acid changes and clinical response. Br J Dermatol 121:75–90, 1989.
72. Motta S, Monti M, Sesana S, Caputo R, Carelli S, Ghidoni R. Ceramide composition of the psoriatic scale. Biochim Biophys Acta 1182:147–151, 1993.
73. Murata Y, Ogata J, Higaki Y, Kawashima M, Yada Y, Higuchi K, Tsuchiya T, Kawainami S, Imokawa G. Abnormal expression of sphingomyelin acylase in atopic dermatitis: an etiologic factor for ceramide deficiency? J Invest Dermatol 106:1242–1249, 1996.
74. Murphy JE, Robert C, Kupper TS. Interleukin-1 and cutaneous inflammation: a crucial link between innate and acquired immunity. J Invest Dermatol 114:602–608, 2000.
75. Mustakallio KK, Kiistala U, Piha HJ, Nieminen E. Epidermal lipids in Besnier's prurigo (atopic eczema). Ann Med Exp Biol Fenn 45:323–325, 1967.
76. Nassif A, Chan SC, Storrs FJ, Hanifin JM. Abnormal skin irritancy in atopic dermatitis and in atopy without dermatitis. Arch Dermatol 130:1402–1407, 1994.
77. Nemes Z, Marekov LN, Steinert PM. Involucrin cross-linking by transglutaminase 1. Binding to membranes directs residue specificity. J Biol Chem 274:11013–11021, 1999.
78. Nishijima T, Tokura Y, Imokawa G, Seo N, Furukawa F, Takigawa M. Altered

permeability and disordered cutaneous immunoregulatory function in mice with acute barrier disruption. J Invest Dermatol 109:175–182, 1997.

79. Ochs HD. The Wiskott-Aldrich syndrome. Clin Rev Allergy Immunol 20:61–86, 2001.

80. Ogawa H, Yoshiike TJ. A speculative view of atopic dermatitis: barrier dysfunction in pathogenesis. Dermatol Sci 5:197–204, 1993.

81. Ohnishi Y, Okino N, Ito M, Imayama S. Ceramidase activity in bacterial skin flora as a possible cause of ceramide deficiency in atopic dermatitis. Clin Diagn Lab Immunol 6:101–104, 1999.

82. Pagnelli R, Atherton DJ, Levinski RI: Differences between normal and milk allergic subjects in their immune response after milk ingestion. Arch Dis Child 58:201–206, 1983.

83. Pike MG, Heddle RJ, Boulton P, Turner MW, Atherton DJ: Increased intestinal permeability in atopic eczema. J Invest Dermatol 86:101–104, 1986.

84. Proksch E, Feingold KR, Mao-Quiang M, Elias PM. Barrier function regulates epidermal DNA-synthesis. J Clin Invest 87:1668–1673, 1991.

85. Proksch E, Brasch J, Sterry W. Integrity of the permeability barrier regulates epidermal Langerhans cell density. Br J Dermatol 134:630–638, 1996.

86. Proksch E, Brasch J. Influence of epidermal permeability barrier disruption and Langerhans' cell density on allergic contact dermatitis. Acta Derm Venereol 77:102–104, 1997.

87. Proksch E, Feingold KR, Elias PM. Epidermal HMG CoA reductase activity in essential fatty acid deficiency: barrier requirements rather than eicosanoid generation regulate cholesterol synthesis. J Invest Dermatol 99:216–220, 1992.

88. Redoules D, Tarroux R, Assalit MF, Peri JJ. Characterisation and assay of five enzymatic activities in the stratum corneum using tape-strippings. Skin Pharmacol Appl Skin Physiol 12:182–192, 1999.

89. Robson KJ, Stewart ME, Michelsen S, Lazo ND, Downing DT. 6-Hydroxy-4-sphingenine in human epidermal ceramides. J Lipid Res 35:2060–2068, 1994.

90. Schafer L, Kragballe K. Abnormalities in epidermal lipid metabolism in 11 patients with atopic dermatitis. J Invest Dermatol 96:10–15, 1991.

91. Schmuth M, Man MQ, Weber F, Gao W, Feingold KR, Fritsch P, Elias PM, Holleran WM. Permeability barrier disorder in Niemann-Pick disease: sphingomyelin-ceramide processing required for normal barrier homeostasis. J Invest Dermatol 115:459–466, 2000.

91a. Schurer NY, Plewig G, Elias PM. Seratum corneum lipid function. Dermatologica 183:77–94, 1991.

92. Scott IR, Harding CR. Filaggrin breakdown to water binding compounds during development of the rat stratum corneum is controlled by the water activity of the environment. Dev Biol 115:84–92, 1986.

93. Seguchi T, Cui CY, Kusuda S, Takahashi M, Aisu K, Tezuka T. Decreased expression of filaggrin in atopic skin. Arch Dermatol Res 288:442–446, 1996.

94. Seidenari S, Giusti G. Objective assessment of the skin of children affected by atopic dermatitis: a study of pH, capacitance and TEWL in eczematous and clinically uninvolved skin. Acta Derm Venereol 75:429–433, 1995.

95. Shahidullah M, Raffle EJ, Rimmer AR, Frain-Bell W. Transepidermal water loss in patients with dermatitis. Br J Dermatol 81:722–730, 1969.

96. Spitz JL. Genodermatosis. Baltimore: Williams and Wilkins, 1996, pp 214–215.

97. Swartzendruber DC, Wertz PW, Madison KC, Downing DT. Evidence that the corneocyte has a chemically bound lipid envelope. J Invest Dermatol 88:709–713, 1987.

98. Tabata N, O'Goshi K, Zhen YX, Kligman AM, Tagami H. Biophysical assessment of persistent effects of moisturizers after their daily applications: evaluation of corneotherapy. Dermatology 200:308–313, 2000.

99. Taieb A. Hypothesis: from barrier dysfunction to atopic disorders. Contact Dermatitis 41:177–180, 1999.

100. Tupker RA, Pinnagoda J, Coenraads PJ, Nater JP. Susceptibility to irritants: role of barrier function, skin dryness and history of atopic dermatitis. Br J Dermatol 123:199–205, 1990.

101. Uchida Y, Hara M, Nishio H, Sidransky E, Inoue S, Otsuka F, Suzuki A, Elias PM, Holleran WM, Hamanaka S. Epidermal sphingomyelins are precursors for selected stratum corneum ceramides. J Lipid Res 41:2071–2082, 2000.

102. Ukabam SO, Mann RJ, Cooper BT. Small intestinal permeability to sugars in patients with atopic eczema. Br J Dermatol 110:649–652, 1984.

103. Vanselow NA, Yamate M, Adams MS, Callies Q. The increased prevalence of allergic disease in anhidrotic congenital ectodermal dysplasia. J Allergy 45:302–309, 1970.

104. Werner Y, Lindberg M. Transepidermal water loss in dry and clinically normal skin in patients with atopic dermatitis. Acta Derm Venereol 65:102–105, 1985.

105. Wertz PW, Cho ES, Downing DT. Effect of essential fatty acid deficiency on the epidermal sphingolipids of the rat. Biochim Biophys Acta 753:350–355, 1983.

106. Wertz PW, Downing DT. Covalent attachment of omega-hydroxyacid derivatives to epidermal macromolecules: a preliminary characterization. Biochem Biophys Res Commun 137:992–997, 1986.

107. Wertz PW, Swartzendruber DC, Abraham W, Madison KC, Downing DT. Essential fatty acids and epidermal integrity. Arch Dermatol 123:1381–1384, 1987.

108. Wertz PW, Swartzendruber DC, Kitko DJ, Madison KC, Downing DT. The role of the corneocyte lipid envelopes in cohesion of the stratum corneum. J Invest Dermatol 93:169–172, 1989.

109. Williams HC, Forsdyke H, Boodoo G, Hay RJ, Burney PG. A protocol for recording the sign of flexural dermatitis in children. Br J Dermatol 133:941–949, 1995.

110. Williams HC. Atopic eczema. Br Med J 311:1241–1242, 1995.

111. Wood LC, Jackson SM, Elias PM, Grunfeld C, Feingold KR. Cutaneous barrier perturbation stimulates cytokine production in the epidermis of mice. J Clin Invest 90:482–487, 1992.

112. Wood LC, Elias PM, Calhoun C, Tsai J-C, Grunfeld C, Feingold KR. Barrier disruption stimulates interleukin-1 alpha expression and release from a preformed pool in murine epidermis. J Invest Dermatol 106:397–403, 1996.

113. Yamamoto A, Serizawa S, Ito M, Sato Y. Stratum corneum lipid abnormalities in atopic dermatitis. Arch Dermatol Res 283:219–223, 1991.

114. Yoshiike T, Aikawa Y, Sindhvananda J, Suto H, Nishimura K, Kawamoto T, Ogawa H. Skin barrier defect in atopic dermatitis: increased permeability of the stratum corneum using dimethyl sulfoxide and theophylline. J Dermatol Sci 5:92–96, 1993.

8

Mechanisms of Allergic Skin Inflammation

Mübeccel Akdis, Axel Trautmann, Kurt Blaser, and Cezmi A. Akdis
Swiss Institute of Allergy and Asthma Research (SIAF), Davos, Switzerland

I. INTRODUCTION

Recent investigations have greatly increased our understanding of immunological mechanisms involved in the pathogenesis of atopic dermatitis (AD) (Fig. 1). The mononuclear cellular infiltrate in lesional skin of AD is mainly constituted of $CD4^+$ T cells and to a lesser extent $CD8^+$ T cells. T cells are activated by aeroallergens, food antigens, autoantigens and bacterial superantigens in AD. They are under the influence of skin-related chemokine network and they show skin-selective homing. Epidermal Langerhans cells and dermal dendritic cells are able to activate allergen-specific T cells through allergen-specific IgE-antibodies bound to Fc receptors for IgE (FcεRI and FcεRII). This leads to continuous stimulation of T cells in the skin. T cells play important roles in AD with induction of hyper IgE, eosinophil survival. In addition activated T cells induce keratinocyte apoptosis as a key pathogenetic event in the formation of eczema. To mediate these effector functions after skin-specific homing, activated T cells show continuous survival in the skin. Apoptosis of activated T cells (activation-induced cell death) is prevented by cytokines and extracellular matrix components in the eczematous skin.

II. T-CELL ACTIVATION IN ATOPIC DERMATITIS

A. Mechanisms of $CD4^+$ and $CD8^+$ T-Cell Activation

T cells constitute a large population of cellular infiltrate in atopic dermatitis, and a dysregulated, cytokine-mediated immune response appears to be an important

145

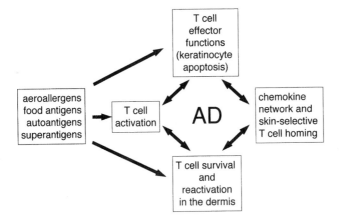

Figure 1 Mechanisms of T cell mediated allergic inflammation in atopic dermatitis. T cells are activated by aeroallergens, food antigens, autoantigens and bacterial superantigens. They are under the influence of skin related chemokine network and they show skin-selective homing. In the skin they show increased survival and they are continuously stimulated. Activated T cells induce keratinocyte apoptosis as a key pathogenetic event in the formation of eczema.

pathogenetic factor. Numerous studies pointed to the role of activated CD4$^+$ T cells in atopic dermatitis and other allergic inflammatory diseases (1). Systemic activation of T cells in AD is supported by the observation that these patients possess increased numbers of activated cutaneous lymphocyte-associated antigen (CLA)–bearing T cells in the circulation and increased levels of serum L-selectin, a marker for leukocyte activation correlating with AD disease severity (2–4). Dermal cellular infiltrate in AD mainly consists of CD4$^+$ and CD8$^+$ T cells with a CD4/CD8 ratio similar to peripheral blood levels (5,6). In recent studies, CD8$^+$CLA$^+$ T cells were demonstrated to be as potent as CD4$^+$CLA$^+$ T cells in induction of IgE and inhibition of eosinophil survival (5,6).

A number of pathogenetic mechanisms leading to T-cell activation in AD including aeroallergens, food allergens, and superantigens have been emphasized. The role of aeroallergens in T-cell activation in AD has been extensively studied (7,8). Aeroallergens can induce both immediate-type and delayed-type responses in the skin (8). The frequency of aeroallergen-specific T cells was investigated in AD lesions, and they were found to be less than 1% in nonchallenged AD lesions (9). Besides, such allergen-specific T cells can be detected in the skin of atopic patients after allergen administration without any signs of AD lesions (10). The contribution of food allergens in the exacerbation of AD by T-cell activation has also been demonstrated (11). Normally allergen-specific T-cell responses in food and aeroallergen allergy are confined to CD4$^+$ T cells. This, however, may not explain the activation and recruitment of CD8$^+$ T cells in AD skin lesions. It is known that bacterial superantigens can interact with certain Vβ elements of the TCR leading to activation, expansion, anergy, or deletion of T cells. It is evident from mouse studies that superantigen response of T cells is not restricted to CD4$^+$ T cells. CD8$^+$ T cells (12) and even CD4$^-$ CD8$^-$ T cells can respond to superantigenic stimuli (13). This may explain the existence and activation of CD8$^+$ T cells in eczema lesions and their contribution to IgE production and eosinophil survival and development, chronicity, and exacerbation of AD (5,6).

Another widely supported view is that dermal dendritic cells and epidermal Langerhans cells display an abnormal hyperstimulatory function for T cells, in addition to IL-12 and IL-18 production. IgE FcϵRI and FcϵRII (CD23) are upregulated in CD1a-positive cells in AD. CD1a is a marker of dermal dendritic cells and Langerhans cells (14). Their role in IgE-facilitated antigen presentation and T-cell activation will be discussed below.

B. Role of Superantigens in T-Cell Activation in Atopic Dermatitis

From a number of studies it can be concluded that bacterial superantigens contribute to the pathogenesis and exacerbation of AD. Staphylococcal superantigens were isolated from AD skin (15). Superantigen patch test elicits skin inflammation in AD patients (16) and in human severe combined immunodeficiency mouse model (17). In addition, specific IgE antibodies to bacterial superantigens exist in AD (18). It was also demonstrated that CD8$^+$ T cells isolated from skin or CLA$^+$CD8$^+$ T cells isolated from peripheral blood efficiently proliferate by superantigenic stimulation (5). Furthermore, purified CD4$^+$ or CD8$^+$ T cells cultured from skin biopsies secrete high IL-5 and IL-13 by staphyloccocal enterotoxin B (SEB) stimulation (5). Induction of CLA expression by superantigens may play an important role in the pathogenesis of AD, which is associated with superantigen-producing staphylococci (19). Staphylococcal superantigens secreted at the skin surface may penetrate the inflamed skin and stimulate epidermal macrophages or Langerhans cells to produce IL-1, TNF, and IL-12. Superantigen-stimulated Langerhans cells may migrate to skin-associated lymph nodes and serve as APC. They can upregulate the expression of CLA by IL-12 production (19,20) and alter the functional profile of virgin T cells. Moreover, superantigens presented by keratinocytes, Langerhans cells, and macrophages can stimulate T cells in the skin. This second round of stimulation is able to induce CLA expression (21). Local production of IL-1 and TNF may induce E-selectin on vascular endothelium, allowing an initial migration of CLA$^+$ memory/effector cells (22).

C. Cytokine Profile of Activated T Cells in AD

Elevated IgE levels and eosinophilia in AD suggest increased expression of Th2-type cytokines (23). The majority of allergen-specific T cells derived from skin lesions that have been provoked in AD patients by epicutaneous allergen application or peripheral blood skin homing T cells produce predominantly Th2 cytokines such as IL-4, IL-5, and IL-13 (2,3,5,24). Previously, such polarized Th2 cytokine pattern was regarded as a specific feature reflecting immune dysregulation in AD. However, current studies demonstrate that IFN-γ predominates over IL-4 in chronic skin lesions and older patch test reactions in AD, whereas IL-5 and IL-13 still remain at high levels (6,9,25,26). A number of factors may be involved in increased IFN-γ in older skin lesions. IL-12 produced by Langerhans cells, eosinophils, and keratinocytes appears to be a predominant mediator for the induction of IFN-γ in T cells after homing to skin (20,27,28). Furthermore, IL-18 produced in the microenvironment of skin may act in parallel to IL-12 (29). Characterization of the cells in the afferent skin–derived lymph from healthy individuals demonstrated the dominance of a type 1 cytokine profile with IFN-γ in T cells and IL-12 in dendritic cells (30). Such studies performed in AD patients may further help to understand the immune regulation mechanisms. Another widely supported view is that dermal dendritic cells and epidermal Langerhans cells display an abnormal hyperstimulatory functions for T cells in addition to their IL-12 and IL-18 production. IgE FcϵRI and FcϵRII (CD23) are upregulated in CD1a-positive cells in AD (14).

D. The Role of IgE-Facilitated Antigen Presentation in T-Cell Activation in Atopic Dermatitis

The immune response to foreign proteins strongly depends on the efficiency and selectivity of antigen uptake by antigen-presenting cells (APC). Kehry and Yamashita have shown that IgE bound to CD23 on mouse B cells may be used to focus antigen to T cells (31). This finding initialized the understanding of focused antigen presentation via IgE receptors. Previously, the high-affinity receptor for IgE was believed to be present on mast cells and basophils. This was followed by the recent demonstration of IgE RI and Langerhans cells, eosinophils, and epidermal cells (14,32,33). Low-affinity IgE receptor (CD23) has a widespread cellular distribution (34). Both types of IgE Fc receptors are thought to play a role in IgE-mediated antigen presentation (35–38). This mechanism operates selectively at low doses of allergens, and the presentation of extremely low doses of allergen to CD4$^+$ T lymphocytes is greatly enhanced by IgE-facilitated antigen presentation (38,39). Blocking IgG antibodies in IgG-containing serum fractions induced by specific immunotherapy (SIT) of birch pollen allergy inhibits the IgE-facilitated antigen presentation at very low allergen concentrations (39). Accordingly, IgE acts as an immunoglobulin specialized in antigen capture or antigen focusing. Especially in extrinsic type of atopic dermatitis, the presence of high levels of specific IgE in serum and CD23 on APC (activated B cells) (6), together with FcεRI expressing APC (Langerhans cells in the skin) (14), may strongly contribute to the overstimulation of the allergen-specific immune responses.

Capture of antigens via surface IgE and signal transduction through IgE cytoplasmic chain were shown as crucial events in specific IgE responses (40). Clinical trials with a neutralizing nonanaphylactogenic anti-IgE mAb treatment have demonstrated an inhibition in bronchial late phase responses and decreased the number of eosinophils in sputum of allergic asthma patients (41). Correspondingly, the production of IL-4 and IL-5 and lung eosinophilia in house dust mite–sensitized mice is inhibited by anti-CD23 or anti-IgE mAb treatment (42). Moreover, studies performed using anti-CD23 mAb and CD23-deficient mice suggest that IgE-mediated antigen presentation play a major role in Th2 cytokine production and lung eosinophilia (42). The recent development of humanized anti-IgE antibodies may also offer the possibility of reduced IgE-facilitated antigen presentation (43). However, elimination of IgE may not be adequate in individuals with persisting T-cell–mediated inflammation, because in animal models of AD, allergic inflammation of the skin was elicited to the same extent in wild-type and IgE knockout mice (44).

III. SKIN-SELECTIVE T-CELL HOMING IN ATOPIC DERMATITIS

Skin represents a functionally distinct immune compartment, and location of the allergic/inflammatory disease in the skin is determined by tissue compartmentalization of the immune response. This is controlled by the expression of chemokines and chemokine receptors, the expression of skin-selective homing ligand, and the route of allergen/superantigen sensitization. The great majority of T cells homing to the skin is of the CD45RO$^+$ memory/effector phenotype and express the selective skin homing receptor, CLA (45). The CLA epitope is characterized by specific binding to the monoclonal antibody HECA-452 (45). CLA binds to its vascular counter receptor, E-selectin (CD62E), which is expressed on inflamed superficial dermal postcapillary venules and endothelial cells (46). CLA$^+$ CD45RO$^+$ T cells migrate across activated endothelium using CLA/E-selectin, VLA-4/VCAM-1, and LFA-1/ICAM-1 interactions (47). In addition, CLA is expressed by the malignant T cells of chronic-phase cutaneous T-cell lymphoma (mycosis fungoides and Sezary syndrome), but not by non–skin-associated T-cell lymphomas (45). In both AD and contact dermatitis, T cells specific to skin-related allergens are confined to the CLA$^+$ T-cell population (3). The CLA$^+$ memory/effector cells demonstrate typical features of in vivo activation in AD (2). Freshly isolated, unstimulated CLA^+ T cells show significantly higher levels of CD25 (IL-2 receptor-α chain), CD40-ligand, and HLA-DR expression. Additional evidence for in vivo activation of CLA^+ T cells appears from the spontaneous proliferation immediately after purification without further activation. CLA^+ T cells contain and spontaneously release high amounts of preformed IL-5 and IL-13 but only very little IL-4 and IFN-γ in their cytoplasm as demonstrated by intracellular cytokine staining immediately after purification (2,5). Moreover, CLA^+ memory/effector T cells induce IgE production by B cells and enhance eosinophil survival by inhibiting eosinophil apoptosis in AD (2,5). In contrast, the CLA^- population represents a resting memory T-cell fraction, induces rather IgG in B cells, and does not show any effect on eosinophil survival and apoptosis (2,5).

The CLA epitope consist of a sialyl-Lewis x carbohydrate and corresponds to a posttranslational modification of the P-selectin glycoprotein ligand 1 (PSGL-1) (48). The generation of CLA on T cells undergoing naive to memory transition in skin-draining lymph nodes requires $\alpha(1,3)$-fucosyltransferase (FucT-VII) activity (48,49). Thus, CLA expression predominantly reflects the regulated activity of the glycosyltransferase, FucT-VII (48,49). Recent studies in mice suggest that adaptively transferred Th1 cells are preferentially recruited to cutaneous DTH reactions compared with Th2 cells (50). In addition in vitro differentiated Th1 but not Th2 cells have been shown to bind E-selectin, and expression of functional selectin ligands is upregulated by IL-12 and inhibited by IL-4 by opposite effects on FucT-VII gene expression in mice (21,51,52). We have demonstrated that the skin-selective homing ligand expression is regulated by the same mechanisms in both $CD4^+$ and $CD8^+$ T cells (53). The CLA molecule was expressed on Th1 cells during the differentiation process (21,51–53). More importantly, CLA can be induced on Th2 cells by T-cell stimulation with bacterial superantigen and/or IL-12 challenge (53). These Th2 cells demonstrate the same cytokine profile as the T cells found in skin biopsies and in peripheral blood of atopic dermatitis patients. They show high IFN-γ, IL-5, and IL-13 production with very little or no IL-4 production (6,24,54,55). By IL-12 stimulation, CLA could be expressed on the surface of bee venom phospholipase A2-specific Th1, Th2, Th0, and T regulatory 1 clones, representing non–skin-related antigen-specific T cells (53). In addition, CLA could be reinduced on T cells that had lost CLA expression upon resting (53). Apparently, skin-selective homing is not restricted to functional and phenotypic T-cell subsets. IL-12 and/or superantigen responsiveness, such as certain T-cell receptor variable β chain expression or IL-12Rβ expression, act as factors that control CLA expression on T cells.

IV. CHEMOKINE NETWORK IN THE SKIN

Mechanisms that control infiltration of inflammatory cells into AD skin have been intensely investigated. Recently, cutaneous T-cell–attracting chemokine

CTACK/CCL27 and its receptor CRP-2/CCR10 were demonstrated to play a role in preferential attraction of CLA$^+$ T cells to the skin (56,57). CTACK is predominantly expressed in the skin and selectively attracts a tissue-specific sub-population of memory lymphocytes. It is also reported as ALP in mouse. The terms "Eskine" and "ILC" were also used for the same chemokine (56), designated as CCL27 in the new systematic chemokine nomenclature. CTACK is constitutively expressed in mouse skin, suggesting that other mechanisms of chemoattraction during flares of AD must exist. In a mouse model of AD, the Th2-selective chemokine, the thymus and activation-regulated chemokine (TARC), is selectively induced by mechanical injury. NC/Nga mice spontaneously develop atopic dermatitis-like lesions, and TARC is highly expressed in the basal epidermis with lesions, whereas it is not expressed in the skin without lesions (58). Similarly, the expression of macrophage-derived chemokine (MDC) was increased severalfold in the mouse skin with atopic dermatitis–like lesions (58).

Eotaxin is a CC chemokine and a potent activator of human eosinophils, basophils, and Th2 cells via the chemokine receptor CCR3. Immunohistological staining and mRNA of eotaxin and its receptor CCR3 have been found significantly increased in lesional skin from AD but not in nonatopic controls. No significant difference in the expression of MCP-3, MIP-1α, and interleukin-8 has been observed between skin samples from AD patients and nonatopic controls (59).

IL-16 is a cytokine with selective chemotactic activity for CD4$^+$ T cells. An in situ hybridization study for IL-16 mRNA has demonstrated positive signals for IL-16 both in the basal layer of epidermis and in the dermis of AD skin samples (60). In addition, the numbers of epidermal and dermal IL-16 mRNA$^+$ cells were found significantly increased in acute in comparison to chronic AD skin lesions (60). Furthermore, the same study demonstrated that upregulation of IL-16 mRNA expression in acute AD was associated with increased numbers of CD4$^+$ cells. These results suggest that IL-16 may play a role in initiation of skin inflammation (60).

Transendothelial migration of skin-homing T cells was studied by Santamaria Babi et al. They used a bilayer vascular construct consisting of a fibroblast matrix underneath an activated endothelial cell monolayer (47,61). Transmigration studies through IL-1β– and TNF-α–activated endothelium demonstrated that IL-8 and IL-8 receptor B were selectively involved in the enhanced transendothelial migration of CLA$^+$ T cells (61). Together these studies on chemokine network for skin homing T cells demonstrate a complex system of different chemokines and chemokine receptors during different disease stages and for different T-cell subsets. The involvement of epidermal keratinocytes in the skin-homing process by releasing chemotactic substances requires further investigation. Similarly, the role of dendritic or Langerhans cells in the generation of a chemokine network in the skin is not yet clearly elucidated.

V. EFFECTOR MECHANISMS IN ATOPIC DERMATITIS

A. The Role of IL-5 and IL-13 in Atopic Dermatitis

Although most patients with AD show high concentrations of total and allergen-specific IgE in blood and skin, some of them express normal IgE levels and show no allergen-specific IgE antibodies. The diagnostic criteria of AD by Hanifin and Rajka (62) can be fulfilled also in the absence of elevated total IgE and specific IgE to food or environmental allergens. This suggests that elevated IgE levels and IgE sensitization are not prerequisites in the pathogenesis of the disease. The subgroup of AD patients with normal IgE levels and without specific IgE sensitization has been termed the nonallergic form of AD (NAD), nonatopic eczema, non-AD or intrinsic-type AD (6,63). Recent data suggest that T cells are likely involved in the pathogenesis of AD and NAD. CD4$^+$ and CD8$^+$ subsets of skin-infiltrating T cells as well as skin-homing CLA$^+$ T cells from peripheral blood responded equally to superantigen, SEB, and produce IL-2, IL-5, IL-13, and IFN-γ in both forms of the disease (5,6). Interestingly, skin T cells from AD patients express higher IL-5 and IL-13 levels compared to NAD patients. Thus, T cells isolated from skin biopsies of AD, but not from NAD, induced high IgE production in cocultures with normal B cells that is mediated by IL-13. In addition, B-cell activation with high CD23 expression is observed in the peripheral blood of AD, but not NAD patients (6). These findings suggest a lack of IL-13–induced B cell activation and consequent IgE production in nonatopic eczema, although high numbers of T cells are present in lesional skin of both types (6). More importantly, IL-4 and IL-13 neutralization in B-cell cocultures with peripheral blood CLA$^+$ skin-homing T cells or skin-infiltrating T cells demonstrated that IL-13 represents the major cytokine for induction of hyper-IgE production in AD (2,5,6).

Cytokine determinations from peripheral blood CLA$^+$ T cells and skin biopsies of AD patients show increased IL-5 expression (5,6,24). Accordingly, supernatants from CLA$^+$ T cells of both CD4$^+$ and CD8$^+$ subsets extend the life span of freshly purified eosinophils in vitro, whereas supernatants of CLA$^-$ T cells do not influence eosinophil survival. Neutralization of cytokines demonstrated the predominant role of CLA$^+$ T-cell IL-5 in prolonged eosinophil survival in AD (5).

B. Dysregulated Apoptosis Is a Key Pathogenetic Factor in AD

1. Dysregulated T-Cell Apoptosis in AD

Although the death of certain cells can lead to functional deficiencies, prolonged survival of some effector cells can cause tissue injury and play a role in the pathogenesis of disease (64). Cell death by apoptosis is a tightly regulated process that enables removal of unnecessary, aged, or damaged cells. During apoptosis a complex death program is initiated that ultimately leads to phagocytosis of the apoptotic cell. One way to induce apoptosis is by triggering a family of transmembrane proteins called death receptors, of which Fas (CD95) may be the most important (65).

To ensure self-tolerance and downregulation of an immune response, the elimination of T cells takes place in the periphery and involves induction of apoptosis (66). During the development of the immune response, T cells are stimulated by antigens presented by antigen-presenting cells that leads to T-cell activation and clonal expansion. Some of the activated T cells die by activation-induced T-cell death (AICD) under certain conditions (67). AICD is thought to play an important role in maintaining homeostasis of the immune response and prevention of excessive immune reactivity. Activated T cells can kill themselves (suicide) and other cells in the environment in a fratricidal way (68–70).

Differences in control of life span was observed between peripheral blood CLA$^+$ T cells and T cells infiltrating the eczema lesions. In peripheral blood of AD patients both CD4$^+$ and CD8$^+$ subsets of CLA$^+$CD45RO$^+$ T cells expressed upregulated Fas and Fas ligand and underwent spontaneous activation-induced cell death (AICD). CLA$^-$CD45RO$^+$ T cells are in a resting state, do not express Fas and Fas ligand, and are resistant to anti-Fas mAb-induced apoptosis (71). In contrast, T cells infiltrating the skin of AD patients expressed both Fas and Fas ligand; however, they showed no signs of apoptosis. Apoptosis of CLA$^+$ CD45RO$^+$ T cells is inhibited by IL-2, IL-4, and IL-15 as cytokines; fibronectin, tenascin, laminin, and collagen IV as extracellular matrix proteins (ECM); and transferrin demonstrating a multifactorial survival of skin infiltrating T cells in the tissue (71). Together, these results demonstrate the control of in vivo activated skin-homing T-cell numbers in peripheral blood with increased apoptosis; in contrast, T-cell apoptosis is prevented by cytokines and extracellular matrix components in the eczematous skin.

Inflammatory cells reside in a protein network in the tissues, the extracellular matrix (ECM), which exerts a profound control over them. The effects of ECM are primarily mediated by integrins, a family of cell surface receptors that attach cells to the matrix and mediate mechanical and chemical signals from it. Many ECM signals converge on cell cycle regulation, directing cells to live or die, to proliferate or to differentiate. Integrins can recognize several ECM proteins; conversely, individual ECM proteins can bind to several integrins (72). Most recent studies have concentrated on signaling pathways activated by integrins in adherent cells. Adherent cells must be anchored to an appropriate ECM to survive (73). During inflammation, leukocytes migrate into the affected tissue interacting with extracellular matrix proteins. Cell adhesion to the ECM has been implicated in protection from apoptosis in anchorage-dependent cell types. Apparently, integrin signaling by ECM represents an important survival signal in T cells, although they do not require anchorage in the tissues. Integrins activate various protein tyrosine kinases, including focal adhesion kinase (FAK), Src family kinases, Abl, a serine threonine kinase, and integrin-linked kinase (74,75). In AD skin T cells express both Fas and Fas ligand, but they are resistant to apoptosis. FAK appears to play a major role in conveying survival signals from the ECM (76). Because FAK binds to phosphatidylinositol, 3(Pl3)-kinase and the protective effect against apoptosis may be the result of Pl3-kinase–mediated activation of protein kinase B (77).

In addition to ECM proteins, IL-2, IL-4, and IL-15 also prevent T-cell apoptosis (71). The common γc-chain is an essential signaling component shared by Il-2, IL-4, and IL-15 receptors as well as all other known T-cell growth factor receptors. Interleukin-15 shares many biological activities with IL-2 and signals through the IL-2 receptor beta and gamma chains (78). However IL-15 and IL-12 differ in their controls of expression and secretion, their range of target cells, and their functional activities. IL-2 induces or inhibits T-cell apoptosis in vitro depending on T-cell activation, whereas IL-15 inhibits cytokine deprivation–induced apoptosis in activated T cells (65). Furthermore, blocking the γc-chain in mice inhibits T-cell proliferation and induces T-cell apoptosis, which induces stable allograft survival (79).

2. Dysregulated Keratinocyte Apoptosis in Atopic Dermatitis

The histological hallmark of eczematous disorders is characterized by a marked keratinocyte pathology. Spongiosis in the epidermis is identified by impairment or loss of cohesion between KC and the influx of fluid from dermis, sometimes progressing to vesicle formation. A recent study by Trautmann et al. delineated activated skin-infiltrating T-cell–induced epidermal keratinocyte apoptosis as a key pathogenic event in eczematous disorders (80). IFN-γ released from activated T cells upregulates Fas (CD95) on keratinocytes, which renders them susceptible to apoptosis. When the Fas number on keratinocytes reaches a threshold of approximately 40.000 Fas molecules per keratinocyte, the cells become susceptible to apoptosis. Keratinocytes exhibit a relatively low threshold for IFN-γ–induced Fas expression (0.1–1 ng/mL). This requirement is substantially achieved by low IFN-γ–secreting T cells that also produce high amounts of IL-5 and IL-13 and thereby contribute to eosinophilia and IgE production (80). The lethal hit is delivered to keratinocytes by Fas ligand expressed on the surface of T cells that invade the epidermis and soluble Fas ligand released from T cells. In these studies, the involvement of cytokines other than IFN-γ was eliminated by experiments with different cytokines and anti-cytokine neutralizing antibodies. In addition, apoptosis pathways other than the Fas pathway were ruled out by blocking T-cell–induced keratinocyte apoptosis with caspase inhibitors and soluble Fas-Fc protein. Keratinocyte apoptosis was demonstrated in situ in lesional eczematous skin and patch test lesions of both atopic dermatitis and allergic contact dermatitis. Exposure of normal human skin and cultured skin equivalents to activated T cells demonstrated that keratinocyte apoptosis caused by skin infiltrating T cells represent a key event in the pathogenesis of eczematous dermatitis (80).

Although allergic contact dermatitis and drug-induced skin rashes are not related to atopic dermatitis, the mechanism of epidermal injury should be mentioned because of histopathological similarities. An exaggerated T-cell response to small molecular weight haptens plays a role in allergic contact dermatitis. Traidl et al. demonstrated that keratinocytes could be the target of multiple hapten-specific cytotoxic T-cell responses, which play a role in epidermal injury during allergic contact dermatitis (81). They found that both nickel-reactive CD4[+] and CD8[+] T cells were exclusively cytotoxic against resting keratinocytes and that IFN-γ treatment rendered keratinocytes susceptible to Th1 cytotoxicity. In addition, both Fas and perforin pathways play a role in keratinocyte killing (81). T-cell–mediated cytotoxicity against keratinocytes has also been studied in sulfamethoxazol-induced skin reactions (82). Sulfamethoxazol-specific CD4[+] and CD8[+] T cells expressed high perforin, and IFN-γ–pretreated keratinocytes were predominantly killed by CD4[+] T cells (82).

These studies demonstrate that both CD4[+] and CD8[+] T cells may play a role in keratinocyte injury according to their activation status. A direct contact of T cell with keratinocyte is not always required, and soluble Fas ligand released from activated T cells can also induce keratinocyte apoptosis if keratinocytes are susceptible to apoptosis. IFN-γ appears to be a decisive cytokine to render keratinocytes susceptible to apoptosis (80–82). Recent mice studies also provide evidence for the role of IFN-γ in eczema formation. IFN-γ knockout mice show significantly decreased allergic eczema formation (44), and transgenic mice expressing IFN-γ in the epidermis spontaneously developed eczema (83).

VI. CONCLUSION

Activation and skin-selective homing of peripheral blood T cells and effector functions in the skin represent sequential immunological events in the pathogenesis of atopic dermatitis (Fig. 2). The CLA molecule represents a homing receptor involved in selective migration of memory/effector T cells to the skin. CLA is expressed on Th1 cells during the differentiation process and can be induced on Th2 cells by stimulation with bacterial superantigen and/or IL-12. Both CD4[+] and CD8[+] T cells bearing CLA represent activated memory/effector T-cell subsets in peripheral blood of AD patients. They induce IgE mainly by IL-13 and prolong eosinophil life span mainly by IL-5. A chemokine network involving T cells, dendritic cells, and keratinocytes control infiltration of inflammatory cells

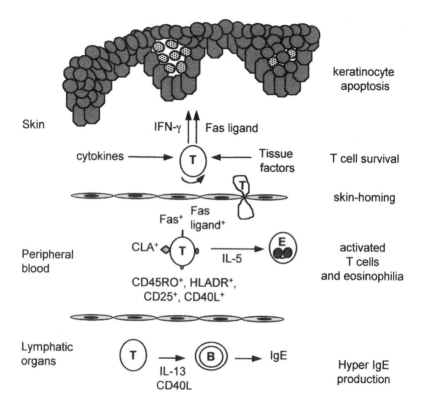

Figure 2 Immune effector mechanisms in atopic dermatitis. T cells infiltrating the skin are CD45RO⁺ and use CLA and other receptors to recognize and cross the endothelium. In the peripheral blood of AD patients, both CD4⁺ and CD8⁺ subsets of CLA+ CD45RO+ T cells are in an activated state (CD25⁺, CD40L⁺, HLADR⁺). They express Fas and Fas ligand and undergo activation-induced apoptosis. In contrast, T cells infiltrating the skin of AD patients-despite expressing both Fas and Fas ligand-do not show any apoptosis, because they are protected from apoptosis by cytokines and ECM proteins. These T cells secrete IFN-γ, which upregulates Fas on keratinocytes and render them susceptible to apoptosis in the skin. Keratinocyte apoptosis is induced by Fas ligand expressed on the surface of activated T cells or released to microenvironment. Both CD4⁺ and CD8⁺ T cells isolated from skin or CLA⁺ CD45RO⁺ T cells from peripheral blood secrete high levels of IL-5 and IL-13 and therefore are capable of prolonging eosinophil life span and inducing IgE production.

into AD skin. Dysregulated apoptosis in skin-infiltrating T cells and epidermal keratinocytes contributes to the elicitation and progress of atopic dermatitis. Activation-induced T-cell apoptosis plays a role in the control of circulating skin-homing memory/effector T-cell numbers in peripheral blood. In contrast, T-cell apoptosis is prevented by cytokines and extracellular matrix components in the eczematous skin to form dermal T-cell infiltrates and mediate effector functions. These activated T cells induce keratinocyte apoptosis via the Fas-dependent pathway representing a key pathogenetic factor in the formation of eczematous lesions. In this context, future studies for treatment of AD should be directed to T cells by inhibition of various modes of activation, inhibition of skin homing, and inhibition of certain cytokines/chemokines that play a role in the pathogenesis. The knowledge of the molecular basis of dysregulated apoptosis is pivotal in understanding the pathology in AD and may lead to more focused therapeutic applications in the future.

ACKNOWLEDGMENTS

The work of the authors is supported by the Swiss National Foundation (32.65661.01). Axel Trautmann is a recipient of a fellowship from the Deutsche Forschungsgemeinschaft (TR460/1.1).

REFERENCES

1. CA Akdis, M Akdis, A Trautmann, K Blaser. Immune regulation in atopic dermatitis. Current Opin Immunol 12:641–646, 2000.
2. M Akdis, CA Akdis, L Weigl, R Disch, K Blaser. Skin-homing, CLA$^+$ memory T cells are activated in atopic dermatitis and regulate IgE by an IL-13-dominated cytokine pattern. IgG4 counter-regulation by CLA$^-$ memory T cells. J Immunol 159: 4611–4619, 1997.
3. LF Santamaria Babi, LJ Picker, MT Perez Soler, K Drzimalla, P Flohr, K Blaser, C Hauser. Circulating allergen-reactive T cells from patients with atopic dermatitis and allergic contact dermatitis express the skin-selective homing receptor, the cutaneous lymphocyte-associated antigen. J Exp Med 181:1935–1940, 1995.
4. Y Shimada, S Sato, M Hasegawa, TF Tedder, K Takehara. Elevated serum L-selectin levels and abnormal regulation of L-selection expression on leukocytes in atopic dermatitis: soluble L-selectin levels indicate disease severity. J Allergy Clin Immunol 104:163–168, 1999.
5. M Akdis, H-U Simon, L Weigl, O Kreyden, K Blaser, CA Akdis. Skin homing (cutaneous lymphocyte-associated antigen-positive) CD8$^+$ T cells respond to superantigen and contribute to eosinophilia and IgE production in atopic dermatitis. J Immunol 163:466–475, 1999.

6. CA Akdis, M Akdis, D Simon, B Dibbert, M Weber, S Gratzl, O Kreyden, R Disch, B Wüthrich, K Blaser, H-U Simon. T cells and T cell-derived cytokines as pathogenic factors in the nonallergic form of atopic dermatitis. J Invest Dermatol 113: 628–634, 1999.

7. FC Van Reijsen, CAFM Bruijnzeel-Komen, FS Kalthoff, E Maggi, S Romagnani, JKT Westland, GC Mudde. Skin-derived aero-allergen specific T cell clones of Th2 phenotype in patients with atopic dermatitis. J Allergy Clin Immunol 90:184–193, 1992.

8. VA Varney, QA Hamid, M Gaga, S Ying, M Jacobson, AJ Frew, AB Kay, SR Durham. Influence of grass pollen immunotherapy on cellular infiltration and cytokine mRNA expression during allergen-induced late-phase cutaneous responses. J Clin Invest 92:644–651, 1993.

9. T Werfel, A Morita, M Grewe, H Renz, U Wahn, J Krutmann, A Kapp. Allergen-specificity of skin-infiltrating T-cells is not restricted to a type 2 cytokine pattern in chronic skin lesions of atopic dermatitis. J Invest Dermatol 107:871–876, 1996.

10. AJ Frew, AB Kay. The relationship between infiltrating CD4+ lymphocytes, activated eosinophils, and the magnitude of the allergen-induced late phase cutaneous reactions in man. J Immunol 141:4158–4164, 1988.

11. KJ Abernathy-Carver, HA Sampson, LJ Picker, DYM Leung. Milk-induced eczema is associated with the expansion of T cells expressing cutaneous lymphocyte antigen. J Clin Invest 95:913–918, 1995.

12. EY Denkers, P Caspar, A Sher. Toxoplasma gondii possesses a superantigen activity that selectively expands murine T cell receptor V β 5-bearing CD8+ lymphocytes. J Exp Med 180:985–994, 1994.

13. MC Chou, SC Lee, YS Lin, HY Lei. V β 8+ CD4− CD8− subpopulation induced by staphylococcal enterotoxin B. Immunol Let 55:85–91, 1997.

14. DA Schmitt, T Bieber, JP Cazenave, D Hanau. Fc receptors of human Langerhans cells. J Invest Dermatol 94:15S–21S, 1990.

15. JE Leyden, RR Marpies, AM Kligman. *Staphylococcus aureus* in the lesions of atopic dermatitis. Br J Dermatol 90:525–530, 1974.

16. P Strange, L Skov, S Lisby, PL Nielsen, O Baadsgaard. Staphylococcal enterotoxin B applied on intact normal and intact atopic skin induces dermatitis. Arch Dermatol 132:27–33, 1996.

17. U Herz, N Schnoy, S Borelli, L Weigl, U Käsbohrer, A Daser, U Wahn, R Köttgen, H Renz. A hu-SCID mouse model for allergic immune responses: bacterial superantigen enhances skin inflammation and supresses IgE production. J Invest Dermatol 110:224–231, 1998.

18. DYM Leung, R Harbeck, P Bina, JM Hanifin, RF Reiser, HA Sampson. Presence of IgE antibodies to staphylococcal exotoxins in the skin of patients with atopic dermatitis: evidence for a new group of allergens. J Clin Invest 92:1374–1380, 1993.

19. DYM Leung, M Gately, A Trumble, B Ferguson-Darnell, PM Schlievert, LJ Picker. Bacterial superantigens induce T cell expression of the skin-selective homing receptor, the cutaneous lymphocyte-associated antigen, via stimulation of interleukin 12 production. J Exp Med 181:747–753, 1995.

20. K Kang, M Kubin, KD Cooper, SR Lessin, G Trinchieri, AH Rook. IL-12 synthesis by human Langerhans cells. J Immunol 156:1402–1407, 1996.

21. Y-C Lim, L Henault, AJ Wagers, GS Kansas, FW Luscinskas, AH Lichtman. Expression of functional selectin ligands on Th cells is differentially regulated by IL-12 and IL-4. J Immunol 162:3193–3201, 1999.

22. DYM Leung, RS Cotran, JS Pober. Expression of an endothelial leukocyte adhesion molecule (ELAM-1) in elicited late phase allergic skin reactions. J Clin Invest 87: 1805–1810, 1991.

23. DYM Leung. Atopic dermatitis: new insights and opportunities for therapeutic intervention. J Allergy Clin Immunol 105:860–876, 2000.

24. Q Hamid, M Boguniewicz, DYM Leung. Differential in situ cytokine gene expression in acute versus chronic atopic dermatitis. J Clin Invest 94:870–876, 1994.

25. M Grewe, CAFM Bruijnzeel-Koomen, E Schöpf, T Thepen, AG Langeveld-Wildschut, T Ruzicka, J Krutmann. A role for Th1 and Th2 cells in the immunopathogenesis of atopic dermatitis. Immunol Today 19:359–361, 1998.

26. T Thepen, EG Langeveld-Wildschut, IC Bihari, DF van Wichen, FC Van Reijsen, GC Mudde, CAFM Bruijnzeel-Koomen. Biphasic response against aeroallergen in atopic dermatitis showing a switch from an initial Th2 response to a Th1 response in situ: an immunochemical study. J Allergy Clin Immunol 97:828–837, 1996.

27. M Grewe, W Czech, A Morita, T Werfel, M Klammer, A Kapp, T Ruzicka, E Schöpf, J Krutmann. Human eosinophils produce biologically active IL-12: implications for control of T cell responses. J Immunol 161:415–420, 1998.

28. G Müller, J Saloga, T Germann, I Bellinghausen, M Mohamadzadeh, J Knop, AH Enk. Identification and induction of human keratinoctye-derived IL-12. J Clin Invest 94:1799–1805, 1994.

29. S Stoll, H Jonuleit, E Schmitt, G Müller, H Yamauchi, M Kurimoto, J Knop, AH Enk. Production of functional IL-18 by different subtypes of murine and human dendritic cells (DC): DC-derived IL-18 enhances IL-12-dependent Th1 development. Eur J Immunol 28:3231–3239, 1998.

30. N Yawalkar, RE Hunger, WJ Pichler, LR Braathen, CU Brand. Human afferent lymph from normal skin contains an increased number of mainly memory/effector CD4$^+$ T cells expressing activation, adhesion and co-stimulatory molecules. Eur J Immunol 30:491–497, 2000.

31. MR Kehry, LC Yamashita. Low-affinity IgE receptor (CD23) function on mouse B cells: role in IgE-dependent antigen focusing. Proc Natl Acad Sci USA 86:7556–7560, 1989.

32. G Stigl, D Maurer. IgE-mediated allergen presentation via Fc epsilon RI on antigen-presenting cells. Int Arch Allergy Immunol 113:24–29, 1997.

33. J-P Kinet. Atopic allergy and other hypersensitivities. Curr Opin Immunol 11:603–605, 1999.

34. D Maurer, G Stigl. Immunoglobulin E-binding structures on antigen-presenting cells present in skin and blood. J Invest Dermatol 104:707–710, 1995.

35. FL Van der Heijden, RJJ van Neerven, M van Katwijk, JD Bos, ML Kapsenberg. Serum IgE-facilitated allergen presentation in allergic disease. J Immunol 150:3643–3647, 1993.

36. D Maurer, C Ebner, B Reininger, E Fiebiger, D Kraft, JP Kinet, G Stingl. The high affinity IgE receptor (FceRI) mediates IgE-dependent allergen presentation. J Immunol 154:6285–6289, 1995.

37. U Pirron, T Schlunck, JC Prinz, EP Rieber. IgE-dependent antigen focusing by human B lymphocytes is mediated by the low-affinity receptor for IgE. Eur J Immunol 20:1547–1551, 1990.

38. LF Santamaria, R Bheekha, FC Van Reijsen, MT Perez Soler, M Suter, CAFM Bruijnzeel-Koomen, GC Mudde. Antigen focusing by specific monomeric immunoglobulin E bound to CD23 on Epstein-Barr virus-transformed B cells. Human Immunol 37:23–30, 1993.

39. RJJ van Neerven, T Wikborg, G Lund, B Jacobsen, A Brinch-Nielsen, J Arnved, H Ipsen. Blocking antibodies induced by specific allergy vaccination prevent the activation of CD4+ T cells by inhibiting serum IgE- facilitated allergen presentation. J Immunol 163:2944–2952, 1999.

40. G Achatz, L Nitschke, MC Lamers. Effect of transmembrane and cytoplasmic domains of IgE on the IgE response. Science 276:409–411, 1977.

41. JV Fahy, HE Fleming, HH Wong, JT Liu, JQ Su, J Reinmann, RB Fick, HA Boushey. The effect of an anti-IgE monoclonal antibody on the early- and late-phase responses to allergen inhalation in asthmatic subjects. Am J Respir Crit Care Med 155:1828–1833, 1997.

42. AJ Coyle, K Wagner, C Bertrand, S Tsuyuki, J Bews, C Heusser. Central role of immunoglobulin-E in the induction of lung eosinophil infiltration and T helper 2 cell cytokine production: inhibition by a non-anaphylactogenic anti-IgE antibody. J Exp Med 183:1303–1308, 1996.

43. C Heusser, P Jardieu. Therapeutic potential of anti-IgE antibodies. Curr Opin Immunol 9:805–814, 1997.

44. JM Spergel, E Mizoguchi, H Oettgen, AK Bhan, RS Geha. Roles of Th1 and Th2 cytokines in a murine model of allergic dermatitis. J Clin Invest 103:1103–1111, 1999.

45. LJ Picker, SA Michie, LS Rott, EC Butcher. A Unique phenotype of skin associated lymphocytes in humans: preferential expression of the HECA-452 epitope by benign and malignant T-cells at cutaneous sites. Am J Pathol 136:1053–1061, 1990.

46. LJ Picker, TK Kishimoto, CW Smith, RA Warnock, EC Butcher. ELAM-1 is an adhesion molecule for skin homing T cells. Nature 349:796–799, 1991.

47. LF Santamaria Babi, R Moser, MT Perez Soler, LJ Picker, K Blaser, C Hauser. The migration of skin- homing T cells across cytokine-activated human endothelial cell layers involves interaction of the cutaneous lymphocyte-associated antigen (CLA), the very late antigen-4 (VLA-4) and the lymphocyte function-associated antigen-1 (LFA-1). J Immunol 154:1543–1550, 1995.

48. RC Fuhlbrigge, JD Kieffer, D Armerding, TS Kupper. Cutaneous lymphocyte antigen is a specialized form of PSGL-1 expressed on skin homing T cells. Nature 389:978–981, 1997.

49. RN Knibbs. The fucosyltransferase FucT-VII regulates E-selectin ligand synthesis in human T cells. J Cell Biol 133:445–456, 1996.

50. F Austrup, D Vestweber, ELöhning Borges, M, R Bräuer, U Herz, H Renz, R Hallmann, A Scheffold, A Radbruch, A Hamann. P- and E-selectin mediate recruitment of T helper 1 but not of T helper 2 cells into inflamed tissues. Nature 385:81–84, 1997.

51. AJ Wagers, CM Waters, LM Stoolman, GS Kansas. Interleukin 12 and interleukin 4 control T cell adhesion to endothelial selectins through opposite effects on $\alpha 1, 3$-fucosyltransferase VII gene expression. J Exp Med 188:2225–2231, 1998.

52. JM Blander, I Visintin, CA Janeway Jr., R Medzhitov. α(1,3)-Fucosyltrasferase VII and α(2,3)-sialyltransferase IV are up-regulated in activated CD4 T cells and maintained after their differentiation into Th1 and migration into inflammatory sites. J Immunol 163:3746–3752, 1999.

53. M Akdis, S Klunker, M Schliz, K Blaser, CA Akdis. Expression of cutaneous lymphocyte-associated antigen on human CD4$^+$ and CD8$^+$ Th2 cells. Eur J Immunol 30:3533–3541, 2000.

54. J Grewe, K Gyufko, K Schöpf, J Krutmann. Lesional expression of interferon-γ in atopic eczema. Lancet 343:25–26, 1994.

55. Q Hamid, T Naseer, EM Minshall, YL Song, M Boguniewicz, DYM Leung. In vivo expression of IL-12 and IL-13 in atopic dermatitis. J Allergy Clin Immunol 98:225–231, 1996.

56. J Morales, B Horney, AP Vicari, S Hudak, E Oldham, J Hedrick, R Orosco, NG Copeland, NA Jenkins, L McEvoy, A Zlotnik. CTACK, a skin-associated chemokine that preferentially attracts skin-homing memory T cells. Proc Natl Acad Sci USA 96:14470–14475, 1999.

57. B Horney, W Wang, H Soto, ME Buchanan, A Wiesenborn, D Catron, A Müller, TK McClanahan, M-C Dieu-Nosjean, R Orozco, T Ruzicka, P Lehmann, E Oldham, A Zlotnik. The orphan chemokine receptor G protein-coupled receptor-2 (CRP-2,CCR10) binds the skin-associated chemokine CCL27 (CTACK/ALP/ILC). J Immunol 164:3465–3470, 2000.

58. C Vestergaard, H Yoneyama, M Murai, K Nakamura, K Tamaki, Y Terashima, T Imai, O Yoshie, T Irimura, H Mizutani, K Matsushima. Overproduction of Th2-specific chemokines in NC/Nga mice exhibiting atopic dermatitis-like lesions. J Clin Invest 104:1097–1105, 1999.

59. N Yawalkar, M Uguccioni, J Schärer, J Braunwalder, S Karlen, B Dewald, LR Braathen, M Baggiolini. Enhanced expression of eotaxin and CCR3 in atopic dermatitis. J Invest Dermatol 113:43–48, 1999.

60. S Laberge, O Ghaffar, M Boguniewicz, A Luster, QA Hamid. Association of increased CD4$^+$ T cell infiltration with increased IL-16 gene expression in atopic dermatitis. J Allergy Clin Immunol 102:645–650, 1998.

61. LF Santamaria Babi, B Moser, MT Perez Soler, R Moser, P Loetscher, B Villiger, K Blaser, C Hauser. The interleukin-8 receptor B and CXC chemokines can mediate transendothelial migration of human skin homing T cells. Eur J Immunol 26:2056–2061, 1996.

62. JM Hanifin, G Rajka. Diagnostic features of atopic dermatitis. Acta Derm Venerol 92:44–47, 1980.

63. B Wüthrich. Serum IgE in atopic dermatitis. Clin Allergy 8:241–248, 1978.

64. H-U Simon, K Blaser. Inhibition of programmed eosinophil death: A key pathogenic event for eosinophilia. Immunol Today 16:53–55, 1995.

65. C Scaffidi, S Kirchhof, PH Krammer, ME Peter. Apoptosis signaling in lymphocytes. Curr Opin Immunol 11:277–285, 1999.

66. CB Thompson. Apoptosis in the pathogenesis and treatment of disease. Science 267:1456–1462, 1995.

67. DR Green, DW Scott. Activation-induced apoptosis in lymphocytes. Curr Opin Immunol 6:476–487, 1994.

68. J Dhein, H Walczak, C Bäumler, KM Debatin, PH Krammer. Autocrine T-cell suicide mediated by APO-1(Fas/CD95). Nature 373:438–441, 1995.
69. T Brunner, RJ Mogil, D LaFace, N Jin Yoo, A Mahboubi, F Echeverri, SJ Martin, WR Force, DH Lynch, CF Ware, DR Green. Cell-autonomous Fas (CD95)/Fas-ligand interaction mediates activation-induced apoptosis in T-cell hybridomas. Nature 373:441–444, 1995.
70. J Shyr-Te, DJ Panka, H Cui, R Ettinger, M El-Khatib, DH Sherr, BZ Stanger, A Marshak-Rothstein. Fas (CD95)/FasL interactions required for programmed cell death after T-cell activation. Nature 373:444–448, 1995.
71. M Akdis, A Trautmann, K Blaser, CA Akdis. Life span of skin homing T cells in atopic dermatitis: survival in skin, activation induced apoptosis in peripheral blood. J Allergy Clin Immunol 105:167, 2000.
72. E Rouslahti, MD Pierschbacher. New perspectives in cell adhesion: RDG and integrins. Science 238:491–497, 1987.
73. EA Clöark, SJ Brugge. Integrins and signal transduction pathways: the road taken. Science 268:233–238, 1995.
74. KK Wary, F Mainiero, SJ Isakoff, EE Marcantonio, FG Giancotti. The adaptor protein Shc couples a class of integrins to the control of cell cycle progression. Cell 87:733–743, 1996.
75. GE Hanningan, C Leung-Hagesteijn, L Fitz-Gibbon, MG Coppolino, G Radeva, J Filmus, JC Bell, S Dedhar. Regulation of cell adhesion and anchorage-dependent growth by a new β1-integrin-linked protein kinase. Nature 379:91–96, 1996.
76. SM Frisch, K Vuori, E Rouslahti, PY Chan-Hui. Control of adhesion-dependent cell survival by focal adhesion kinase. J Cell Biol 134:793–799, 1996.
77. A Khwaja, P Rodriguez-Viciana, S Wennstrom, P Warne, J Downward. Matrix adhesion and Ras transformation both activate a phosphoinositide 3-OH kinase and protein kinase B/Akt cellular survival pathway. EMBO J 16:2783–2793, 1997.
78. JG Giri, S Kumaki, M Ahdieh, DJ Friend, A Loomis, K Shanebeck, R Dubose, D Cosman, LS Park, DM Anderson. Identification and cloning of a novel IL-15 binding protein that is structurally related to the α chain of the IL-2 receptor. EMBO J 14: 3654–3663, 1995.
79. WC Li, A Ima, Y Li, XX Zheng, TR Malek, TB Strom. Blocking the common g-chain of cytokine receptors induces T cell apoptosis and long term islet allograft survival. J Immunol 164:1193–1199, 2000.
80. A Trautmann, M Akdis, D Kleeman, F Altznauer, H-U Simon, T Graeve, M Noll, K Blaser, CA Akdis. T cell-mediated Fas-induced keratinocyte apoptosis plays a key pathogenetic role in eczematous dermatitis. J Clin Invest 106:25–35, 2000.
81. C Traidl, S Sebastiani, C Albanesi, HF Merk, P Puddu, G Girolomoni, A Cavani. Disparate cytotoxic activity of nickel-specific CD8[+] and CD4[+] T cell subsets against keratinocytes. J Immunol 165:3058–3064, 2000.
82. B Schnyder, K Frutig, D Mauri-Hellweg, A Limat, N Yawalkar, WJ Pichler. T-cell mediated cytotoxicity against keratinocytes in sulfamethoxazol-induced skin reactions. Clin Exp Allergy 28:1412–1417, 1998.
83. JM Carroll, T Crompton, JP Seery, FM Watt. Transgenic mice expressing IFN-γ in the epidermis have eczema, hair hypopigmentation and hair loss. J Invest Dermatol 108:412–422, 1997.

9
Animal Models of Atopic Dermatitis

Udo Herz, Ulrike Raap, and Harald Renz
Philipps University Marburg, Marburg, Germany

I. INTRODUCTION

Atopic dermatitis (AD) is a chronically relapsing inflammatory skin condition, exhibiting a variety of unique features (Table 1) (1,2). Over the last few decades, great advancement has been achieved in revealing the inflammatory components of the disease. By histology, acute lesions are characterized by disease: nonspecific acanthosis, para- and hyperkerathoses, and spongiosis (3). Macroscopically, the lesions are characterized by pruritic erythematous excoreated papules. Chronic inflammatory lesions are defined by the presence of lichenification and dry and fybrotic papules.

Lesions are present on characteristic anatomical sites. Childhood AD usually involves the scalp, cheeks, and extensor surfaces of the extremities. In older patients, AD lesions are most commonly localized in the antecubital and popliteal flexoral areas.

Many cellular components of the immune system exhibit striking abnormalities in phenotype and function depending on disease activity. Immunohistological analysis of AD lesions reveal the presence of a mononuclear cell infiltrate predominantly consisting of activated macrophages and CD4+ T cells expressing HLA-DR and CD45 RO (4–6). Although morphologically intact eosinophils are present only in small numbers, eosinophil-derived major basic protein and eosinophil cationic protein in the dermis are deposited (7,8). These data suggest an important role for eosinophils in this condition. Cutaneous mast cells are increased in numbers and show marked degranulation reflecting activation of these cells. Extensive elevation of serum IgE is present in about 80% of all AD patients (9). Since regulation of IgE production and several important aspects of the biol-

Table 1 Key Features of Atopic Dermatitis

Skin inflammation
   Acute (pruritic, erythematous, excoriated papules)
   Chronic (lichenification, dry and fribrotic papules)
   Acanthosis, para-hyperkerathosis, spongiosis
Pruritus (itching-scratching cycle)
Cutaneous hyperreactivity
Elevated IgE ($\sim$80%)
Eosinophilia
Systemic immunological dysbalance
   Acute/early $\rightarrow$ Th2 $\uparrow$
   Chronic/late $\rightarrow$ Tho/Th1 $\uparrow$
Genetic predisposition

ogy of eosinophils are under close control of T cells, these cells have been the focus of many research groups (10). A profound systemic and local immunological dysbalance in T-cell activities has been, indeed, demonstrated in AD. The status of T-cell deregulation has been analyzed in several biological compartments, including peripheral blood, acute and chronic "spontaneous" lesions, lesions induced by epicutaneous allergen application ("atopy patch test"), and nonlesional skin.

Irrespective of the compartment studied, a decreased number and/or function in CD8 T cells has been found, pointing to an important role of CD4+ T cells in the immunopathogenesis of the disease (11). During acute exacerbations and in early phase responses, elicited after epicutaneous allergen exposure, a marked upregulation of T-helper (Th2) T-cell functions has been detected on the transcriptional as well as translational level. Enhanced production and expression of IL-4, IL-5, and IL-13 have been uniformly demonstrated by many groups (12,13). In contrast, chronic lesions and allergic late phase responses following epicutaneous allergen exposure are characterized by a shift in the cytokine profile towards upregulated IL-5 and IFN-γ production, reflecting a Th0 and Th1 phenotype of these T cells (14). These qualitative and quantitative changes in T-cell biology are accompanied by chronic macrophage activation with increased secretion of GM-CSF, PGE2, and IL-10 (15,16). Increased expression of the low-affinity IgE receptor CD23 has been described on mononuclear cells (17).

A further hallmark of the disease is the presence of pruritus and cutaneous hyperreactivity. AD patients have a lower itch threshold than non-AD patients. Furthermore, histamine levels are increased in both involved and uninvolved AD skin (18,19). There are also more mast cells in lesional skin, and an increased releasability of histamine from blood basophils of patients with AD has been also found (20). Increased levels of substance P, a neuropeptide that induces mast cell degranulation, have been detected in AD skin (21). These data point to a neuroimmunological axis of dysregulation in atopic dermatitis, but the underlying molecular mechanisms have not yet been extensively studied.

Family studies, sib-pair analysis, and linkage analysis suggest a genetic predisposition for AD similar to other clinical manifestations of the atopic syndrome. Although it is quite clear that multiple genes as opposed to single genes contribute to AD manifestation, the genetic nature of AD is far from being understood.

Different trigger factors may contribute to acute exacerbation and chronicity of AD. Especially in childhood AD, food allergies are known to cause exacerbations (22). In susceptible individuals, intestinal food antigen uptake can cause acute and chronic worsening of the condition (23). Although the clinical phenomenon is well known, the pathogenetic mechanism of how intestinal food uptake and processing causes dermal inflammatory responses is still unknown. Aeroallergens are also able to elicit atopic reactions on the skin (24). In this regard, the recently developed atopy patch test represents an excellent model to study the effect of epidermally applied allergens on elicitation of atopic reactions (25). AD patients show a markedly increased rate of chronic colonization with microbial organisms, including *Staphylococus aureus*, particularly of exotoxin-producing strains (26). They act in a bidirectional fashion via their superantigenic activity as well as conventional allergens with anti-superantigen–specific IgE production (27,28). Bacterial, viral, and fungal superinfections are well-known risk factors causing acute and severe disease exacerbation (29,30). Stress factors have been determined to cause worsening of the disease in susceptible patients (31,32). Certain climate conditions can cause improvement and/or worsening of the disease. The most important trigger factors are summarized in Table 2. It is important to emphasize that not all of the above-mentioned factors act in the same patient,

Table 2 Trigger Factors of Atopic Dermatitis

Food allergens
(Epicutaneous) aeroallergens
Chronic microbial colonization
S. aureus (exotoxin pos.)
Microbial (super)infection
S. aureus
Herpes simplex
Stress (eu-, dysstress)
Climate conditions

Table 3 Advantages of Animal
Model Systems

Controlled environmental conditions
  Feeding
  Housing
  Day-night rhythm
  Social behavior
  Stress
  Climate
Genetic background and manipulation
Age dependency
Tissue accessibility
Therapeutic manipulation

but that each patient exhibits a unique spectrum of trigger factors influencing the condition.

Although there has been advancement in the understanding of key pathogenetic aspects in atopic dermatitis, several problems still remain to be solved: the current approach of treatment is determined purely symptomatically. A therapeutic concept targeting the cause of the disease still awaits development. Reliable biochemical markers for disease activity are unavailable. Successful strategies for primary prevention of AD have not yet been developed. The individual risk for development of AD cannot be reliably estimated, either pre- or postnatally.

A major reason for these deficiencies is the complex nature of the condition. One approach to better understanding this complexity and multidimensional dysregulation between the immune, endocrine, and nervous systems is the development of suitable animal model systems. Theoretically, such models have a number of advantages, including control of environmental conditions, known genetic background and possibility of genetic manipulations, accessibility of tissues for further molecular studies, and exploration of experimental therapeutic strategies (Table 3). Over the years, a variety of animal model systems have been developed in several species, which mirror at least certain aspects of the disease. Advantages and disadvantages of these models will be discussed in the following chapter. Here we will discuss the key features of the condition currently being modeled in animal systems and what conclusions can be drawn from these results.

II. MURINE MODEL SYSTEMS

The mouse is particularly suitable to study the genetic and molecular nature of immune functions. This species has been extensively used to elicit Th2-dependent

Table 4 MHL Class II and Strain Dependence of Allergic Immune Responses in Mice

Allergen	BALB/c H-2^d	DBA/2 H-2^d	C57 BL/6 H-2^b	A/J H-2^a	SJL/J H-2^s
Ovalbumin	↑	↑	↔	↑	↓
Birch pollen (Bet v)	↑		↓	↑	
House dust mite (Der p)	↑[a]	↓	↑	↓	
Ragweed (Amb a)	↑				
Grass pollen (Phl p)	↑				
Cat (Fel d)	↑				

[a] for BHR: ↓. ↑ High responder; ↓ low responder; ↔ intermediate responder.

IgE and IgG1 responses against a variety of environmental allergens. In contrast to the human immune system, both IgE and IgG1 antibodies elicit immediate hypersensitivity reactions in the mouse. The qualitative and quantitative extend of such responses is dependent on the genetic background. Th2 and/or IgE/IgG1 high- and low-responder strains have been identified. Table 4 summarizes the data from our own laboratory. The BALB/c strain sticks out as an almost universal high-responder mouse for development of Th2 responses. These mice also have elevated baseline IgE antibody levels as compared to other strains. The development of allergen-specific Th2 immune responses also depends on the expression of MHC class II molecules and the expression pattern of the T-cell receptor phenotype. Although these molecular components determine to a large extend the development of specific T-cell responses, other genetic constituents have to be taken in account as playing a critical role in the development of Th2 immunity. In most strains, however, the genetic nature of susceptibility or resistance still remains to be defined.

A.   Per- and Epicutaneous Sensitization

The stratum corneum normally provides a cutaneous permeability barrier against environmental allergens or irritants. Extracellular lipid domains seem to play a critical role in mediating such resistance. In AD patients there is a significant deficiency of ceramides, a major constituent of intercellular lipids in the stratum corneum in both lesional and nonlesional skin (33). AD skin is characterized clinically by cutaneous reactions resulting from barrier-disrupted skin, with the skin being highly susceptible to antigen penetration. Therefore, the question arises whether skin-penetrating antigens are able to elicit a Th2-dominated immune response.

Table 5 Epidermal and Epicutaneous Sensitization in BALB/c and C57BL/6 Mice

Strain	Manipulation	Allergen	Effect
BALB/c wt	Shaving and tape-stripping (8×)	House dust mite	Th2 in regional LN IgE, IgG1 ↑
BALB/c wt C57BL/6 wt	Shaving and 7-day occlusion (3×) plus airway allergen challenge	OVA	Cutaneous inflammation with CD3, mo, eosinophils IgE, IgG1 ↑ AHR airway eosinophils
BALB/c IL-4−/−	Shaving and 7-day occlusion (3×) plus airway allergen challenge	OVA	Similar cutaneous inflammation but eos↓, and T cells↑
BALB/c IFN-γ−/−	Shaving and 7-day occlusion (3×) plus airway allergen challenge	OVA	Reduced dermal thickening
C57BL/6 IL-5−/−	Shaving and 7-day occlusion (3×) plus airway allergen challenge	OVA	Decreased epidermal and dermal thickening No eosinophils

This has been recently investigated utilizing mouse models. In one such model (34), BALB/c mice were barrier-disrupted by repeated application of adhesive cellophane tape to shaved abdominal skin (Table 5). Such manipulations indeed disrupt cutaneous barrier function, as demonstrated by increased transepidermal water loss. The tape-stripping procedure removed most of the stratum corneum but apparently left the living epidermal tissue intact.

Topical application of house dust mite allergens induce mRNA expression for IL-4, but not for IL-2 or IFN-γ in the local draining lymph nodes. In parallel, IgE and IgG1, but not IgG2a, were upregulated after sensitization. When sensitized mice were challenged with the same allergen at a distant site, infiltration of the dermis with eosinophils has been found. These data indicate that high molecular weight proteins can penetrate barrier-disrupted skin and elicit a Th2-dominant cytokine profile in regional lymph nodes.

An extended protocol of epicutaneous sensitization has been employed by another group (35). BALB/c mice were sensitized to ovalbumin applied to a sterile patch on shaved skin. The patch was in place for a 1-week period, and this procedure was repeated three times after 2-week intervals. The effects were compared to mice "conventionally" sensitized by intraperitoneal injection of ovalbumin together with Al(OH)$_3$. Epicutaneous sensitization, but not intraperitoneal immunization to ovalbumin elicited a significant elevation of total serum IgE levels. The IgE and IgG1 antibody response was more pronounced following the epicutaneous sensitization protocol. Epicutaneous sensitization resulted in macroscopically and microscopically skin lesions. This response was characterized by thickening and inflammation of the dermis and epidermis and by infiltration of the dermal layer with neutrophils, eosinophils, mast cells, and mononuclear cells including CD3+ and CD4+ lymphocytes. Furthermore, in epicutaneously sensitized mice, a single airway allergen challenge by aerosolization of ovalbumin-induced eosinophilia in bronchoalveolar lavage (BAL) fluid and airway hyperresponsiveness to intravenous methacholine as assessed by measurement of pulmonary dynamic compliance.

More recently, the investigators extended their initial observation by utilizing gene-targeted mice of both BALB/c and C57BL/6 background (36). BALB/c IL-4−/− mice display similar dermal and epidermal inflammatory responses but had a drastic reduction in eosinophils and a significant increase in infiltrating T cells. These findings were associated with a reduction in eotaxin mRNA and an increase in mRNA for T-cell chemokines makrophage inflammatory protein-2 (MIP-2), MIP-1 β, and RANTES. In C57BL/6 wild-type animals, this model operates similarly as in BALB/c wild-type mice. However, OVA-sensitized skin from C57BL/6 IL-5−/− mice had no detectable eosinophils and exhibited decreased epidermal and dermal thickening as compared to a wild type. Furthermore, when IFN-γ−/− mice of the BALB/c background were exposed to this protocol, the skin was characterized by reduced dermal thickening. The authors concluded that both Th2 and Th1 cytokines play important roles in inflammation and hypertrophy of the skin in this model.

B. The NC/Nga Mouse

NC mice originated from Japanese fancy mice (Nishiki-Nezumi) and were established as an inbred strain in 1955. The NC/Nga strain has been reported to have some biological characteristics similar to the DBA/2 strain, such as high susceptibility to x-ray irradiation and high susceptibility to anaphylactic shock by ovalbumin. Some Japanese researchers noticed development of spontaneous dermatitis (Table 6) just before or after weaning, but its cause and pathogenesis are still unclear (37–39).

When NC/Nga mice were kept under specific pathogen-free (SPF) condition, they remained healthy. Only conventionally housed NC/Nga mice showed AD-likely clinical symptoms, together with other atopic symptoms such as allergic conjunctivitis. The eliciting factor of the dermatitis is not known, but when BALB/c mice were kept under conventional conditions with the NC/Nga mice,

Table 6 Characteristics of the NC/Nga Mouse

Natural history	Starting after weaning, progressive development of lesions from week 8 on only under conventional housing conditions, not under SPF conditions
Clinical signs	Dry skin and scaling, itching, erythema, edema, superficial erosion
Preferential location	Face, nose, dorsal neck, skin
Histology	Hyperkerathosis, acanthosis, paracerathosis
Dermal inflammation	T cells, mast cells, eosinophils, IL-4, and IFN-$\gamma\uparrow$
Antibodies	IgE $\uparrow\uparrow$

they did not develop lesions, indicating that a genetic factor in addition to an environmental factor is responsible for the development of the disease.

Clinical signs and symptoms seen in conventional NC/Nga mice begin with itching, erythema, and hemorrhage followed by edema, superficial erosion deep excoriation, scaling, and rhinus of the skin and retarded growth. Clinical symptoms begin at 8 weeks of age with dryness of the skin and worsen continuously until 17 weeks of age.

The lesions appear on the face, nose, neck, and dorsal skin and disseminate progressively to other regions of the body. The histology of nodular lesions is characterized by hypercarathosis, arcanthosis, and paraceranthosis, all of which resemble lichinification observed in human AD patients (39,40).

In the dermis, an inflammatory cellular response appears with lymphocytes, eosinophils, and mast cells. The latter appear with mild degranulation. Numerous eosinophils with slight or mild degranulation were observed by week 8. IFN-γ and IL-4 are expressed by mast cells and lymphocytes in skin lesions. This cytokine profile is in concordance with the description of chonic AD lesions in which the profile of expressed cytokines changes to a Th0/Th1 pattern.

The level of IgE in the serum gradually increases to very high levels and peaks at the age of 16–18 weeks. This enhanced IgE production has been attributed to an increased sensitivity of the B cells to CD40 lesion and IL-4. The specificity of the IgE antibodies are still unknown. B cells of the NC/Nga mouse with dermatitis lesions show constitutive tyrosin phosphorylation of JAK3, a feature suggested to result in IgE hyperproduction in patients with AD. Treatment of lesions with tacrolimus (FK506) suppresses skin infiltration by CD4 T cells, mast cells, and eosinophils and also suppresses IL-4, IL-5, and IgE production in these mice. Steroid ointment has been found to have only marginal effects (41–43).

Therefore, the NC/Nga mouse exhibits many features of human atopic dermatitis (44). Since these animals develop AD-like lesions only under conventional housing conditions and not when they are housed under SPF conditions, this model system may be particularly useful to assess the contribution of genetic and environmental factors. It can be expected that the identification of environmental factors contributing to the onset and progression of the disease will provide further insight into the nature of human AD.

C. The NAO Mouse

The Naruto Research Institute Otsuka Atrichia (NAO) mouse was originally described in 1997 by Kondo at al. (45). The NAO mouse represents a new hair-deficient mutant of C57BL/6 background. The NAO mouse develops ulcerative skin lesions associated with a remarkable histology that features large numbers of mast cells and eosinophils in and around the lesions. Furthermore, the mouse exhibits significantly elevated serum IgE levels. Also, these animals demonstrate a unique scratching behavior, closely resembling the manifestation of human atopic dermatitis.

To investigate genetic contributors to the pathological process of dermatitis in this model, differentially expressed genes were investigated by means of a differential display technique (46). One gene isolated by this approach appeared to be the murine homolog of human and rat PF4 genes (47,48). PF4 belongs to the family of chemokines that contain a CXC motive. It is produced in megakaryocytes and packaged into α granules for release when platelets are activated. PF4 binds strongly to heparin and neutralizes heparin-like molecules in the serum and on the surface of endothelial cells (49–51). Interestingly, in patients with atopic dermatitis eosinophils show an elevated migratory response towards PF4. Therefore, it was proposed that PF4 may be a molecule that induces eosinophils towards the ulcerative skin lesions in this model. Such lesions develop in about 30% of NAO mice by 10 weeks of age and in 90% by week 20.

D. Immunization of BALB/c Mice with *Shistosoma japonicum*–Derived Glutathione-S-transferase Antigen

When BALB/c mice were immunized with recombinant glutathione-S-tranferase (GST) by intraperitoneal injection with Al(OH)$_3$ followed by boostering 21 days later, these animals develop characteristic skin lesions. Skin pathology was characterized by an inflammatory infiltrate of mononuclear cells and eosinophils in the dermis and mild spongiosis in the epidermis. Numerous IgE-bearing cells were also detected in the dermis. Eosinophilia was detected in peripheral blood. These skin lesions were noted between 2 and 3 weeks after immunization. Macroscopically, hair became sparse and skin erythmatous. These changes were associated by markedly elevated antigen-specific IgE responses.

Immunization of C57BL/6 mice and (BALB/c × C57BL/6) F$_1$ hybrids resulted in development of low and intermediate IgE responses, respectively.

Furthermore, skin lesions were absent in both groups of mice. Although these data suggest a possible linkage between the development of IgE responses and skin lesions, a formal proof of a cause-and-effect relationship still awaits experimental confirmation (52).

GST acts as target molecule, detoxifying enzyme. It binds to hematin and inhibits the formation of large hematin crystals, which could block the evacuation of a parasite gut. GST from house dust mite and cockroaches have been identified as important allergens for humans as well. Their cDNA sequences share up to 40% sequence homology with that of GSP of *Shistosoma japonicum* (53–55). This sequence homology makes it possible that GST from house dust mites and cockroaches could induce similar allergic immune responses, which are accompanied by an allergic disease as shown in this model. This may provide an explanation for the unexpected finding of skin lesions in systemically immunized mice, which has so far not been demonstrated in other models.

E. The Humanized SCID Model

Several of the above-described animal models assess the capacity to elicit cutaneous inflammation via dermal sensitization or antigen challenges. This concept has been further explored by Herz at al. (56), who transferred atopic PBMC into SCID mice. These animals are immunologically severely impaired due to recombinase defect resulting in developmental block of T and B lymphocytes. Therefore, SCID mice cannot reject xenotransplants and, thus, serve as an excellent model system to study human lymphocyte functions under in vivo conditions. When PBMC are transferred from atopic patients sensitized to house dust mite, human antigen specific T- and B-cell responses develop following antigen challenges.

This model was then employed to assess the contribution of epidermally administered superantigens and house dust mite allergens to the development of cutaneous inflammation. Repeated epidermal administration of superantigens [*Staphylococus aureus* enterotoxin B (SEB)] resulted in acute inflammatory responses in the epidermis paralleled by mild dermal influx of human T lymphocytes. A similar but weak inflammatory response was also observed when house dust mite antigen was repeatedly administered to the skin. In this case, the response was characterized by a preferential lymphocyte influx into the dermis. However, when both superantigens and house dust mite allergen were simultaneously applied to the skin, a marked and profound inflammatory response was detected in both epidermis and dermis. The histological features of this inflammatory response were similar as observed in atopic dermatitis patients.

This model provides initial evidence for the synergistic effect of epidermal exposure to allergens and superantigens. House dust mites are ubiquitous allergens of the indoor environment, and more than 50% of children with AD are colonized with toxin-producing *S. aureus* strains. Therefore, this model mimics the situation of antigen and allergen exposure in many AD patients.

III. THE DOG AS AN EXPERIMENTAL MODEL FOR TYPE I HYPERSENSITIVITY AND ATOPIC DERMATITIS

Domestic animals such as dogs, cats, and horses spontaneously develop type I hypersensitivity responses mediated by immunoglobulin E (IgE). In dogs this phenotype is associated with elevated total IgE serum antibody titers and production of allergen-specific IgE antibodies directed against a variety of ubiquitous allergens such as pollen or house dust mites. In addition, dogs develop allergic phenotypes such as atopic dermatitis, rhinitis, and conjunctivitis and, less frequently, asthma.

A. Dogs as a Model for Genetics of Allergy

The level of total serum IgE in healthy dogs seems to be mainly influenced by the genetic background, whereas age and sex were not identified as significant cofactors (57,58). Experimental sensitization by injection of allergen adsorbed to $Al(OH)_3$ in dogs revealed that the capacity to produce high levels of IgE against a variety of allergens, as a characteristic feature of the atopic state, segregates on a genetic basis (59). As in rodents, high and low IgE responder strains were identified, but long-term production of high levels of IgE against various allergens requires repeated exposure to allergens early in life. If the first allergenic contact occurs within the first few weeks of life, dogs will develop strong IgE responses against the allergen (60). The IgE level will remain high as long as contact with the allergen occurs at least every other month. If no early contact with allergen occurs, IgE production will remain low or undetectable for about 3–4 months after birth, and subsequent allergen exposure will result in brief bursts of allergen-specific IgE in high responder animals, which will subside 2–3 months later.

Genetic analysis of IgE responses after allergen sensitization early in life revealed a dominant trait of the atopic phenotype. This mode of inheritants contradicts the experience in humans. Genetic studies in humans suggest a recessive trait and the involvement of multiple genes.

B. Dogs as a Model for Food Allergy

Development of atopic dermatitis in childhood is often associated with clinical manifestation of food allergy. Dogs sensitized to food allergens by serial injection of food extracts absorbed to $Al(OH)_3$ develop positive skin test reactions after intradermal injection of the respective food allergen, as indicated by a wheal-

and-flare reaction (61). These reactions were accompanied by the production of high levels of allergen-specific IgE. Food allergy in dogs is predominantly associated with dermatological manifestations and/or gastrointestinal symptoms. Sensitized dogs develop mucosal changes including swelling and erythema, some petechiae, and in some cases generalized gastric erythema and hyperperistalsis after injection of allergenic food extracts into the gastric mucosa (62,63). Examination of biopsy specimens from early phase responses revealed edema and infiltration with inflammatory cells. Examination of late phase responses revealed increased eosinophil and mononuclear cell infiltration similar to those observed in humans.

C. Naturally Occurring Atopic Dermatitis–Like Phenotype in Dogs

For decades, a chronically relapsing pruritic dermatitis of young adult dogs that is heritable in some breeds has been termed canine AD (64). Dog breeds commonly reported to be predisposed to AD include the German shepherd, Irish setter, poodle, terrier breeds (Scottish terrier, West Highland white terrier, wire haired fox terrier, Cairn terrier, and Boston terrier), Lasa apso, Dalmatian, and miniature schnauzer (65–67).

Canine AD shares many characteristics with its counterpart in humans, such as the presence of a heritable background, early age of onset, a history of seasonal or nonseasonal and chronical pruritus, recurrent and chronic inflammatory dermatitis with morphology of skin lesions typically located at the flexor and extensor sites of extremities, concurrent pyodermas, high number of skin-colonizing bacteria (68), immediate-type skin test reactivity, reaginic antibodies directed toward environmental allergens, and the occurrence of immunosuppression restricted to the skin (69). Moreover, common clinical signs in canine AD include face scratching and/or foot licking and chewing. Consequently, diagnostic criteria for human AD (1) were adopted for use in dogs with major and minor criteria (70,71) (Table 7).

Reported allergens involved in the pathogenesis of canine atopy include house dust mites, plants, arthropods, epithelia, foods, and molds (72–74). Indeed, depending on season, climate, and/or geographic region, clinically important allergens vary. For example in Japan, Japanese cedar pollen is known to be a common and important seasonal allergen in dogs as well as in the human counterparts (75).

Diagnostic methods identifying clinically important allergens in canine atopy are the intradermal skin test (IDST) and allergen-specific IgE testing in the serum (76,77). As in AD humans, serum concentrations of allergen-specific IgE and IgG are increased in AD canines (78).

To date, the most reliable method for the diagnosis of food allergies is the response to restricted dietary trials and provocation test (73). IDST and antigen-specific IgE tests are not considered to be reliable diagnositc tools for identifying clinically relevant food allergies in dogs (79).

Table 7 Diagnostic Criteria for Atopy in Dogs

Major criteria	Minor criteria
Pruritus	Onset before 3 years of age
Facial and/or digital involvement	Facial erythema and cheilitis
Chronic or chronically relapsing dermatitis	Bilateral conjunctivitis
	Superficial staphylococcal pyoderma
Family history and/or breed predisposition	Hyperhidrosis
Lichenification of the flexor surface of the tarsal joint and/or extensor surface of the carpal joint	Immediate skin test reactivity to airborne allergens
	Increased allergen-specific IgG concentrations
	Increased allergen-specific IgE concentrations

Source: Ref. 71.

In addition, atopic dogs show increased concentrations of secretory IgA on their skin in comparison to normal dogs (80). This is in contrast to IgA serum concentrations, which do not differ between atopic and normal dogs. High concentrations of allergen-specific secretory IgA on the skin might be increased in a similar manner as that of IgE. Because of recurrent pyodermas and higher numbers of bacteria, such as *Staphylococcus intermedius*, IgA may also be directed against staphylococcal antigens.

In atopic dogs, eosinophils are not a common histopathological finding in the skin and are not considered of diagnostic relevance (81,82), although one study reports elevated numbers of eosinophils in the skin of canine AD (83).

In lesional skin of canine AD higher numbers of skin-infiltrating CD4+ and CD8+ T cells had been observed with a predominance of CD4+ T cells in the epidermis in comparison with skin of healthy dogs. In nonlesional atopic skin an infiltration with both CD4+ and CD8+ T cells, but without a predominance of CD4+ T cells, was shown compared with the number of skin-infiltrating lymphocytes in healthy skin of nonatopic dogs (84). This is also in accordance with reports on human AD (4).

In a recent study a type 2 cytokine profile with increased m-RNA for the type 2 cytokines IL-4 and IL-5 was detected in lesional and nonlesional skin of atopic dogs (85). On the other hand, IFN-γ m-RNA was amplified in a small number of both atopic and nonatopic canine skin extracts. In contrast to recent studies of human AD, IL-10 transcripts were not amplified from any canine AD skin samples studied. Taken together, a "polarized" type 2 cytokine profile can exist in the skin of atopic dogs, supporting the relevance of canine AD as a model for a human disease.

IV. ATOPIC DERMATITIS IN OTHER ANIMAL MODELS

Epidemiological and immunological studies on horses in Israel reported that 158 of 723 horses suffered from sweet itch lesions. The results of this study indicated that the likelihood of a horse acquiring sweet itch decreased with increasing altitude, but no definite association with rainfall zones was evident. In the population surveyed, stallions were more sensitive than mares and pale horses appeared to be less sensitive than dark ones (86).

Another model of naturally occurring atopic dermatitis has been shown in Finnish reindeer herders. Skin tests consisting of prick and patch test reactivity on 211 randomly selected reindeer herders, 36 of them with past or present atopic dermatitis, showed positive reactions to at least one allergen such as cat, cow epithelium, dog, horse, and reindeer epithelium, house dust mite, birch pollen, meadow grass pollen, and mugwort pollen. These findings suggest that the prevalence of immediate-type and contact allergies and skin diseases is roughly the same as that in other Finns (87).

Feline atopic dermatitis is characterized by cutaneous exanthema as a consequence of exaggerated eczematous reactions to topical and systemic allergens. In a recent study it was shown that MHC class II+ epidermal dendritic cells were CD1a+ in normal feline skin and significantly increased in numbers in the epidermis and dermis of lesional skin, providing the first correlative documentation for CD1a expression by feline dendritic cells containing Birbeck granules (88). In addition, significantly higher numbers of T cells could be observed in lesional skin of domestic short-haired cats with allergic dermatitis as compared to the skin of healthy control animals. A predominant increase of CD4+ T cells and CD4+/ CD8+ ratio was found in lesional skin of 10 cats with allergic dermatitis. Moreover, increase in CD4+ T cells in nonlesional skin of cats with allergic dermatitis compared to the skin of healthy cats is similar to the human counterpart (89).

REFERENCES

1. Hanifin JM, Rajka G. Diagnostic features of atopic dermatitis. Acta Derm Venerol 1980; 92:44–47.
2. Leung DY, Soter NA. Cellular and immunologic mechanisms in atopic dermatitis. J Am Acad Dermatol 2001; 44:S1–S12.
3. Mihm MC, Soter NA, Dvorak HF, Austen KF. The structure of normal skin and the morphology of atopic eczema. J Invest Dermatol 1976; 67:305–312.

4. Leung DY, Bhan AK, Schneeberger EE, Geha RS. Characterization of the mononuclear cell infiltrate in atopic dermatitis using monoclonal antibodies. J Allergy Clin Immunol 1983; 71:47–56.
5. Bos JD, Hagenaars C, Das PK, Krieg SR, Voorn WJ, Kapsenberg ML. Predominance of "memory" T cells (CD4+, CDw29+) over "naive" T cells (CD4+, CD45R+) in both normal and diseased human skin. Arch Dermatol Res 1989; 281:24–30.
6. Beyer K, Niggemann B, Nasert S, Renz H, Wahn U. Severe allergic reactions to foods are predicted by increases of CD4+CD45RO+ T cells and loss of L-selectin expression. J Allergy Clin Immunol 1997; 99:522–529.
7. Leiferman KM, Ackerman SJ, Sampson HA, Haugen HS, Venencie PY, Gleich GJ. Dermal deposition of eosinophil-granule major basic protein in atopic dermatitis. Comparison with onchocerciasis. N Engl J Med 1985; 313:282–285.
8. Omoto M, Gu LH, Sugiura H, Uehara M. Heterogeneity of dermal deposition of eosinophil granule major basic protein in acute lesions of atopic dermatitis. Arch Dermatol Res 2000; 292:51–54.
9. Wuthrich B. Serum IgE in atopic dermatitis: relationship to severity of cutaneous involvement and course of disease as well as coexistence of atopic respiratory diseases. Clin Allergy 1978; 8:241–248.
10. Herz U, Bunikowski R, Renz H. Role of T cells in atopic dermatitis. New aspects on the dynamics of cytokine production and the contribution of bacterial superantigens. Int Arch Allergy Immunol 1998; 115:179–190.
11. McCoy JP, Hanley-Yanez K, McCaslin D, Tharp MD. Detection of decreased cytotoxic effector CD8+ T lymphocytes in atopic dermatitis by flow cytometry. J Allergy Clin Immunol 1992; 90:688–690.
12. Chan SC, Brown MA, Willcox TM, Li SH, Stevens SR, Tara D, Hanifin JM. Abnormal IL-4 gene expression by atopic dermatitis T lymphocytes is reflected in altered nuclear protein interactions with IL-4 transcriptional regulatory element. J Invest Dermatol 1996; 106:1131–1136.
13. Akdis CA, Akdis M, Simon HU, Blaser K. Regulation of allergic inflammation by skin-homing T cells in allergic eczema. Int Arch Allergy Immunol 1999; 118:140–144.
14. Taha RA, Leung DY, Ghaffar O, Boguniewicz M, Hamid Q. In vivo expression of cytokine receptor mRNA in atopic dermatitis. J Allergy Clin Immunol 1998; 102:245–250.
15. Chan SC, Kim JW, Henderson WR, Hanifin JM. Altered prostaglandin E2 regulation of cytokine production in atopic dermatitis. J Immunol 1993; 151:3345–3352.
16. Ohmen JD, Hanifin JM, Nickoloff BJ, Rea TH, Wyzykowski R, Kim J, Jullien D, McHugh T, Nassif AS, Chan SC, et al. Overexpression of IL-10 in atopic dermatitis. Contrasting cytokine patterns with delayed-type hypersensitivity reactions. J Immunol 1995; 154:1956–1963.
17. Banerjee P, Xu XJ, Poulter LW, Rustin MH. Changes in CD23 expression of blood and skin in atopic eczema after Chinese herbal therapy. Clin Exp Allergy 1998; 28:306–314.
18. Ruzicka T, Gluck S. Cutaneous histamine levels and histamine releasability from the skin in atopic dermatitis and hyper-IgE-syndrome. Arch Dermatol Res 1983; 275:41–44.

19. Ring J, Thomas P. Histamine and atopic eczema. Acta Derm Venereol Suppl (Stockh) 1989; 144:70–77.

20. Heyer G. Abnormal cutaneous neurosensitivity in atopic skin. Acta Derm Venereol Suppl (Stockh) 1992; 176:93–94.

21. Toyoda M, Makino T, Kagoura M, Morohashi M. Immunolocalization of substance P in human skin mast cells. Arch Dermatol Res 2000; 292:418–421.

22. Sicherer SH, Sampson HA. Food hypersensitivity and atopic dermatitis: pathophysiology, epidemiology, diagnosis, and management. J Allergy Clin Immunol 1999; 104:S114–122.

23. Reekers R, Busche M, Wittmann M, Kapp A, Werfel T. Birch pollen-related foods trigger atopic dermatitis in patients with specific cutaneous T-cell responses to birch pollen antigens. J Allergy Clin Immunol 1999; 104:466–472.

24. Clark RA, Adinoff AD. The relationship between positive aeroallergen patch test reactions and aeroallergen exacerbations of atopic dermatitis. Clin Immunol Immunopathol 1989; 53:S132–140.

25. Roehr CC, Reibel S, Ziegert M, Sommerfeld C, Wahn U, Niggemann B. Atopy patch tests, together with determination of specific IgE levels, reduce the need for oral food challenges in children with atopic dermatitis. J Allergy Clin Immunol 2001; 107:548–553.

26. Breuer K, Wittmann M, Bosche B, Kapp A, Werfel T. Severe atopic dermatitis is associated with sensitization to staphylococcal enterotoxin B (SEB). Allergy 2000; 55:551–555.

27. Bunikowski R, Mielke M, Skarabis H, Herz U, Bergmann RL, Wahn U, Renz H. Prevalence and role of serum IgE antibodies to the *Staphylococcus aureus*-derived superantigens SEA and SEB in children with atopic dermatitis. J Allergy Clin Immunol 1999; 103:119–124.

28. Zollner TM, Wichelhaus TA, Hartung A, Von Mallinckrodt C, Wagner TO, Brade V, Kaufmann R. Colonization with superantigen-producing *Staphylococcus aureus* is associated with increased severity of atopic dermatitis. Exp Clin Allergy 2000; 30:994–1000.

29. Herz U, Bunikowski R, Mielke M, Renz H. Contribution of bacterial superantigens to atopic dermatitis. Int Arch Allergy Immunol 1999; 118:240–241.

30. Bunikowski R, Mielke ME, Skarabis H, Worm M, Anagnostopoulos I, Kolde G, Wahn U, Renz H. Evidence for a disease-promoting effect of *Staphylococcus aureus*-derived exotoxins in atopic dermatitis. J Allergy Clin Immunol 2000; 105:814–819.

31. Hariya T, Hirao T, Katsuyama M, Ichikawa H, Aihara M, Ikezawa Z. [A relationship between a psychosomatic and a skin condition in patients with atopic dermatitis]. Arerugi 2000; 49:463–471.

32. Schmid-Ott G, Jaeger B, Adamek C, Koch H, Lamprecht F, Kapp A, Werfel T. Levels of circulating CD8(+) T lymphocytes, natural killer cells, and eosinophils increase upon acute psychosocial stress in patients with atopic dermatitis. J Allergy Clin Immunol 2001; 107:171–177.

33. Imokawa G, Abe A, Jin K, Higaki Y, Kawashima M, Hidano A. Decreased level of ceramides in stratum corneum of atopic dermatitis: an etiologic factor in atopic dry skin? J Invest Dermatol 1991; 96:523–526.

34. Kondo H, Ichikawa Y, Imokawa G. Percutaneous sensitization with allergens through barrier-disrupted skin elicits a Th2-dominant cytokine response. Eur J Immunol 1998; 28:769–779.
35. Spergel JM, Mizoguchi E, Brewer JP, Martin TR, Bhan AK, Geha RS. Epicutaneous sensitization with protein antigen induces localized allergic dermatitis and hyperresponsiveness to methacholine after single exposure to aerosolized antigen in mice. J Clin Invest 1998; 101:1614–1622.
36. Spergel JM, Mizoguchi E, Oettgen H, Bhan AK, Geha RS. Roles of TH1 and TH2 cytokines in a murine model of allergic dermatitis. J Clin Invest 1999; 103:1103–1111.
37. Kondo K, Nagami T, Teramoto S. Differences in haematopoietic death among inbred strains of mice. In: Bond PV, Sugahara T, eds. Comparative Cellular and Species Radiosensitivity. 1969:20.
38. Festing MFW. Inbred Strains in Biomedical Research. London: Macmillan, 1979.
39. Matsuda H, Watanabe N, Geba GP, Sperl J, Tsudzuki M, Hiroi J, Matsumoto M, Ushio H, Saito S, Askenase PW, et al. Development of atopic dermatitis-like skin lesion with IgE hyperproduction in NC/Nga mice. Int Immunol 1997; 9:461–466.
40. Suto H, Matsuda H, Mitsuishi K, Hira K, Uchida T, Unno T, Ogawa H, Ra C. NC/Nga mice: a mouse model for atopic dermatitis. Int Arch Allergy Immunol 1999; 120(suppl 1):70–75.
41. Vestergaard C, Yoneyama H, Murai M, Nakamura K, Tamaki K, Terashima Y, Imai T, Yoshie O, Irimura T, Mizutani H, et al. Overproduction of Th2-specific chemokines in NC/Nga mice exhibiting atopic dermatitis-like lesions. J Clin Invest 1999; 104:1097–1105.
42. Matsumoto M, Ra C, Kawamoto K, Sato H, Itakura A, Sawada J, Ushio H, Suto H, Mitsuishi K, Hikasa Y, et al. IgE hyperproduction through enhanced tyrosine phosphorylation of Janus Kinase 3 in NC/Nga mice, a model for human atopic dermatitis. J Immunol 1999; 162:1056–1063.
43. Hiroi J, Sengoku T, Morita K, Kishi S, Sato S, Ogawa T, Tsudzuki M, Matsuda H, Wada A, Esaki K. Effect of tacrolimus hydrate (FK506) ointment on spontaneous dermatitis in NC/Nga mice. Jpn J Pharmacol 1998; 76:175–183.
44. Vestergaard C, Yoneyama H, Matsushima K. The NC/Nga mouse: a model for atopic dermatitis. Mol Med Today 2000; 6:209–210.
45. Kondo T, Shiomoto Y, Kondo T, Kubo S. The NOA mouse, a new hair-deficient mutant (A possible animal model of allergic dermatitis). Mouse Genome 1997; 95:698–700.
46. Watanabe O, Natori K, Tamari M, Shiomoto Y, Kubo S, Nakamura Y. Significantly elevated expression of PF4 (platelet factor 4) and eotaxin in the NOA mouse, a model for atopic dermatitis. J Hum Genet 1999; 44:173–176.
47. Broekman MJ, Handin RI, Cohen P. Distribution of fibrinogen, and platelet factors 4 and XIII in subcellular fractions of human platelets. Br J Haematol 1975; 31:51–55.
48. Kaplan KL, Broekman MJ, Chernoff A, Lesznik GR, Drillings M. Platelet alpha-granule proteins: studies on release and subcellular localization. Blood 1979; 53:604–618.
49. Moore S, Pepper DS, Cash JD. Platelet antiheparin activity. The isolation and charac-

terisation of platelet factor 4 released from thrombin-aggregated washed human platelets and its dissociation into subunits and the isolation of membrane-bound anti-heparin activity. Biochim Biophys Acta 1975; 379:370–384.

50. Rucinski B, Niewiarowski S, James P, Walz DA, Budzynski AZ. Antiheparin proteins secreted by human platelets. purification, characterization, and radioimmunoassay. Blood 1979; 53:47–62.

51. Ryo R, Nakeff A, Huang SS, Ginsberg M, Deuel TF. New synthesis of a platelet-specific protein: platelet factor 4 synthesis in a megakaryocyte-enriched rabbit bone marrow culture system. J Cell Biol 1983; 96:515–520.

52. Hsu CH, Chua KY, Huang SK, Chiang IP, Hsieh KH. Glutathione-S-transferase induces murine dermatitis that resembles human atopic dermatitis. Clin Exp Allergy 1996; 26:1329–1337.

53. Smith DB, Davern KM, Board PG, Tiu WU, Garcia EG, Mitchell GF. Mr 26,000 antigen of *Schistosoma japonicum* recognized by resistant WEHI 129/J mice is a parasite glutathione S-transferase. Proc Natl Acad Sci USA 1986; 83:8703–8707.

54. Smith DB, Rubira MR, Simpson RJ, Davern KM, Tiu WU, Board PG, Mitchell GF. Expression of an enzymatically active parasite molecule in *Escherichia coli: Schistosoma japonicum* glutathione S-transferase. Mol Biochem Parasitol 1988; 27: 249–256.

55. Davern KM, Tiu WU, Morahan G, Wright MD, Garcia EG, Mitchell GF. Responses in mice to Sj26, a glutathione S-transferase of *Schistosoma japonicum* worms. Immunol Cell Biol 1987; 65:473–482.

56. Herz U, Schnoy N, Borelli S, Weigl L, Kasbohrer U, Daser A, Wahn U, Kottgen E, Renz H. A human-SCID mouse model for allergic immune response bacterial superantigen enhances skin inflammation and suppresses IgE production. J Invest Dermatol 1998; 110:224–231.

57. de Weck AL. The Carl Prausnitz Memorial Lecture. What can we learn from the allergic zoo? Int Arch Allergy Immunol 1995; 107:13–18.

58. Griot-Wenk ME, Busato A, Welle M, Racine BP, Weilenmann R, Tschudi P, Tipold A. Total serum IgE and IgA antibody levels in healthy dogs of different breeds and exposed to different environments. Res Vet Sci 1999; 67:239–243.

59. Lian TM, Halliwell RE. Allergen-specific IgE and IgGd antibodies in atopic and normal dogs. Vet Immunol Immunopathol 1998; 66:203–223.

60. de Weck AL, Mayer P, Stumper B, Schiessl B, Pickart L. Dog allergy, a model for allergy genetics. Int Arch Allergy Immunol 1997; 113:55–57.

61. Becker AB, Chung F, McDonald DM, Frick OL, Gold WM. Cutaneous allergic response in atopic dogs: relationship of cellular and histamine responses. J Allergy Clin Immunol 1988; 81:441–448.

62. Guilford WG, Strombeck DR, Rogers Q, Frick OL, Lawoko C. Development of gastroscopic food sensitivity testing in dogs. J Vet Intern Med 1994; 8:414–422.

63. Ermel RW, Kock M, Griffey SM, Reinhart GA, Frick OL. The atopic dog: a model for food allergy. Lab Anim Sci 1997; 47:40–49.

64. Frank LA. Atopic dermatitis. Clin Dermatol 1994; 12:565–571.

65. Schwartzman RM, Rockey JH, Halliwell RE. Canine reaginic antibody. Characterization of the spontaneous anti-ragweed and induced anti-dinitrophenyl reaginic antibodies of the atopic dog. Clin Exp Immunol 1971; 9:549–569.

66. Nesbitt GH. Canine allergic inhalant dermatitis: a review of 230 cases. J Am Vet Med Assoc 1978; 172:55–60.

67. Halliwell RE. Atopic disease in the dog. Vet Rec 1971; 89:209–214.

68. Mason IS, Lloyd DH. The role of allergy in the development of canine pyoderma. J Small Anim Pract 1989; 30:216–218.

69. Willemse T. [Atopic dermatitis in dogs. Symptomatology and diagnosis]. Tierarztl Prax 1991; 19:96–101.

70. Willemse T. [Atopic dermatitis in dogs: new diagnostic criteria]. Tierarztl Prax 1990; 18:525–528.

71. Willemse T. Atopic skin disease: a review and a consideration of diagnostic criteria. J Small Anim Pract 1986; 27:771–778.

72. Jeffers JG, Shanley KJ, Meyer EK. Diagnostic testing of dogs for food hypersensitivity. J Am Vet Med Assoc 1991; 198:245–250.

73. Rosser EJ. Diagnosis of food allergy in dogs. J Am Vet Med Assoc 1993; 203:259–262.

74. August JR. Dietary hypersensitivity in dogs: cutaneous manifestations, diagnosis, and management. Compend Contin Educ Pract Vet 1985; 7:469–477.

75. Masuda K, Tsujimoto H, Fujiwara S, Kurata K, Hasegawa A, Taniguchi Y, Yamashita K, Yasueda H, DeBoer DJ, de Weck AL, et al. IgE-reactivity to major Japanese cedar (*Cryptomeria japonica*) pollen allergens (Cry j 1 and Cry j 2) by ELISA in dogs with atopic dermatitis. Vet Immunol Immunopathol 2000; 74:263–270.

76. Mueller RS, Burrows A, Tsohalis J. Comparison of intradermal testing and serum testing for allergen-specific IgE using monoclonal IgE antibodies in 84 atopic dogs. Aust Vet J 1999; 77:290–294.

77. Sture GH, Halliwell RE, Thoday KL, van den Broek AH, Henfrey JI, Lloyd DH, Mason IS, Ferguson E. Canine atopic disease: the prevalence of positive intradermal skin tests at two sites in the north and south of Great Britain. Vet Immunol Immunopathol 1995; 44:293–308.

78. Willemse A, Noordzij A, Rutten VP, Bernadina WE. Induction of non-IgE anaphylactic antibodies in dogs. Clin Exp Immunol 1985; 59:351–358.

79. Kunkle G, Horner S. Validity of skin testing for diagnosis of food allergy in dogs. J Am Vet Med Assoc 1992; 200:677–680.

80. Mueller RS, Cannon A, Reubl GH, Ihrke PJ. Serum and skin IgA concentrations in normal and atopic dogs. Aust Vet J 1997; 75:906–909.

81. Olivry T, Naydan DK, Moore PF. Characterization of the cutaneous inflammatory infiltrate in canine atopic dermatitis. Am J Dermatopathol 1997; 19:477–486.

82. Gross TL, Ihrke PJ, Walder EJ. Veterinary Dermatopathology. St. Mosby, Louis: 1992:114–116.

83. Wilkie JS, Yager JA, Eyre P, Parker WM. Morphometric analyses of the skin of dogs with atopic dermatitis and correlations with cutaneous and plasma histamine and total serum IgE. Vet Pathol 1990; 27:179–186.

84. Sinke JD, Thepen T, Bihari IC, Rutten VP, Willemse T. Immunophenotyping of skin-infiltrating T-cell subsets in dogs with atopic dermatitis. Vet Immunol Immunopathol 1997; 57:13–23.

85. Olivry T, Dean GA, Tompkins MB, Dow JL, Moore PF. Toward a canine model

of atopic dermatitis: amplification of cytokine-gene transcripts in the skin of atopic dogs. Exp Dermatol 1999; 8:204–211.

86. Braverman Y, Ungar-Waron H, Frith K, Adler H, Danieli Y, Baker KP, Quinn PJ. Epidemiological and immunological studies of sweet itch in horses in Israel. Vet Rec 1983; 112:521–524.

87. Larmi E, Reijula K, Hannuksela M, Pikkarainen S, Hassi J. Skin disorders and prick and patch test reactivity in Finnish reindeer herders. Derm Beruf Umwelt 1988; 36: 83–85.

88. Roosje PJ, Whitaker-Menezes D, Goldschmidt MH, Moore PF, Willemse T, Murphy GF. Feline atopic dermatitis. A model for Langerhans cell participation in disease pathogenesis. Am J Pathol 1997; 151:927–932.

89. Roosje PJ, van Kooten PJ, Thepen T, Bihari IC, Rutten VP, Koeman JP, Willemse T. Increased numbers of CD4+ and CD8+ T cells in lesional skin of cats with allergic dermatitis. Vet Pathol 1998; 35:268–273.

10
Pathophysiology of Pruritus

Sonja Ständer, Martin Steinhoff, and Thomas A. Luger
University of Muenster, Muenster, Germany

I. INTRODUCTION

Pruritus, regularly defined as an unpleasant sensation provoking the desire to scratch (1), is an essential feature of atopic dermatitis (AD) (2,3). Because of the high impact on life quality, most of the patients measure the severity of the eczema by the intensity of pruritus rather than by the appearance of skin lesions (4,5). Although pruritus is a cardinal symptom of atopic dermatitis, its neuromechanism is not fully understood. As a cutaneous sensory perception, itch is excited on neuropeptide-containing free nerve endings of unmyelinated nociceptor fibers. It is known that several mediators such as neuropeptides, proteases, or cytokines provoke itch by direct binding to itch receptors or indirectly via histamine release. Interestingly, some variations of this complex pathophysiology have been demonstrated in patients with atopic dermatitis.

II. SENSORY CUTANEOUS NERVES

A. Sensory Nerves

The skin is equipped with an effective communication and control system designed to protect the organism in a constantly changing environment. For this purpose a dense network of highly specialized afferent sensory and efferent autonomic nerve branches occurs in all cutaneous layers. The sensory system contains receptors for touch, temperature, pain, itch, and various other physical and chemical stimuli. The information is either processed in the central nervous system (CNS) or may directly elicit an inflammatory reaction by antidromic propagation of these impulses. The effector function of a nerve may be determined by secreted neuropeptides and the corresponding receptors of target structures (reviewed by Ref. 6). In addition, there is accumulating evidence that neuropeptides exert multiple effects on immunocompetent cells, suggesting a strong interaction between the nervous and the immune systems (7–9).

Micrographic recordings have clearly shown that the sensation of itch is transmitted by a subpopulation of unmyelinated C-polymodal nociceptive neurons (10,11). It is assumed that their terminals are free nerve endings located in the superficial dermis, epidermis, and around skin appendages. In humans, "free" nerve endings do not represent naked axons but remain covered by small cytoplasmic extensions of Schwann cells and a basement membrane that may show continuity with that of the epidermis (6). Multiple sensory modalities such as touch, temperature, pain, and itch may be attributed to the free nerve endings of polymodal C-fibers. However, some of the myelinated Aδ-fibers may account for particular subqualities of pain and itch. It can be hypothesized that pruritogenic agents specifically bind to itch receptors on the surface of chemosensitive nerve endings and thereby cause firing of axons. Since some weak mechanical and electrical stimuli often promote itch, whereas more intense injury evokes pain, it was previously believed that itch is an altered form of pain. However, recent investigations clearly demonstrate that itch and pain should be considered as independent sensory modalities (10,11).

B. Autonomic Nerves in the Skin

In contrast to sensory nerve fibers, the distribution of autonomic nerves is restricted to the dermis, innervating blood vessels, arteriovenous anastomoses, lymphatic vessels, glands, hair follicles, and stimulating immune cells to release neurotransmitters. Although autonomic nerves represent only a minority of cutaneous fibers that predominantly generate neurotransmitters such as acetylcholine (ACh) and catecholamines, recent observations revealed a potential role for neuropeptides released from sympathetic and parasympathetic neurons during cutaneous inflammation. Moreover, autonomic nerve fibers participate in the regulation of vascular effects in the skin by releasing ACh and vasoactive intestinal peptide (VIP) (12–16). In addition, muscarinic and nicotinergic acetylcholine receptor expression has been described on keratinocytes, melanocytes, fibroblasts, and lymphocytes indicating a regulatory role of both the autonomic and sensory nervous system in the pathophysiology of AD (reviewed in Refs. 17–20).

C. Nervous System in Atopic Dermatitis

Several investigators demonstrated that the number of cutaneous nerve fibers is altered in atopic skin lesions. An increase of sensory but decrease of adrenergic autonomic nerve fibers was observed (21), indicating a differential role of primary afferent and autonomic nerve fibers in pruritus pathophysiology. Therefore, immunohistochemical analysis of neuropeptide distribution in cutaneous nerve fibers were performed. Lesional atopic skin showed an increased number of neurofilament–, PGP 9.5–, Calcitonin gene–related peptide (CGRP)–, and substance P (SP)–positive nerve fibers in the papillary dermis (22), at the dermoepidermal junction (23,24), in the epidermis (21), and around sweat glands (25). One group additionally described the presence of neuropeptide Y (NPY) in dendritic epidermal cells (24), while another group was unable to reproduce these findings (21). In an semiquantitative analysis, Sugiura et al. (22) found different densities of PGP-positive peripheral nerves in early acute lesions of AD (2.5×10^3 $\mu m^2/\Delta s$), in subacute lesions (3.8×10^3 $\mu m^2/\Delta s$), in lichenified lesions (4.9×10^3 $\mu m^2/\Delta s$), and in prurigo lesions (7.1×10^3 $\mu m^2/\Delta s$) in comparison to noninvolved skin of patients with AD (2.0×10^3 $\mu m^2/\Delta s$). Hypertrophy of nerve fibers in atopic dermatitis is possibly stimulated by an increased release of nerve growth factor secreted by basal keratinocytes (26,27). Mihm et al. (28) described cutaneous myelinated nerves appearing demyelinated and sclerotic. However, other groups were not able to confirm these pathological changes upon light microscopic levels (23,29). Electron microscopic investigation of lesional skin revealed an increased content of hyperplastic nerve fibers with enlarged axons (22,23). Terminal Schwann cells seem to migrate closer to the epidermis as in normal controls (23). In addition, axons lost their surrounding cytoplasm of Schwann cells in some areas and may thus communicate directly with dermal cells (22). These axons contained many mitochondria and neurofilaments with abundant neurovesicles (22), confirming immunohistological findings. Finally, a higher immunoreactivity for most neuronal markers like CGRP and SP and altered nerve structures suggests that peripheral nerve fibers may play a role in the pathophysiology of itching in AD (24).

D. Central Transmission of Pruritus

Peripheral pruritogenic stimuli may be directly sensed as an inflammatory reaction by antidromic propagation of the impulses in the periphery or transferred to the CNS (6). Several observations are in favor of an important role of the CNS in modulating itch responses. First, intraventricular injection of morphine induces heavy itch responses. One major possibility are opioid receptors to mediate these effects, which are located on peripheral nerves and in the CNS (30,31). In support of this idea, it was shown that naloxone significantly inhibits itching in patients with different inflammatory dermatoses (32–34). The lower part of the medulla oblongata was proposed as an itch center, albeit direct evidence for this location is still lacking (35). Recent investigations suggested the left primary sensory cortex to be involved in central itch perception, as demonstrated by positron emission tomography (PET) (36). In addition, activation of motor-associated areas probably reflects the tendency to pruritofensive movements (36). In atopic dermatitis, a decreased ability of sensory nerves to signal itching to the CNS was suggested (37). In summary, the anatomy and physiology of the central perception and regulation of pruritus is still fragmentary and awaits further investigation.

III. NOCICEPTION IN ATOPIC SKIN

Itching reflects a distinct quality of cutaneous nociception elicited by chemical and other stimuli to neuronal receptors. Several studies demonstrated that itch in individuals with AD follows different pathways as compared to in nonatopic individuals. For example, while normal volunteers experience intense pruritus after injection of histamine or substance P, patients with AD only remark weak itch sensations. On the other hand, application of acetylcholine results in pruritus rather than pain in AD patient (Table 1; Fig. 1).

A. Histamine

Many mediators triggering itch have been investigated in AD. Among them, histamine has been a persistent candidate and has been the most thoroughly studied pruritogen for decades. About 80 years ago, Lewis reported that intradermal injections of histamine provoke redness, wheal, and flare (so-called triple response of neurogenic inflammation) accompanied by pruritus (38,39). Williams (40) suggested that histamine may play a role in the pathogenesis of AD since intramuscular histamine injections resulted in pruritus. Elevated histamine levels in both lesional and uninvolved skin in AD patients were also reported (41,42). However, recent investigations were not able to detect increased histamine levels in the skin (43). Uehara and Heyer (37,44–46) noticed reduced itch sensations in response to either intracutaneously injected or iontophoretically applied histamine when compared to nonatopic healthy subjects. Interestingly, histamine may induce not only itch but also perifocal alloknesis (itch elicited by a slight mechanical, otherwise nonitching stimulus). Furthermore, intradermally injected SP releases histamine and provokes diminished itch perception in patients with AD in comparison to healthy subject, which underlines the minor capacity of histamine to induce pruritus in AD (47). These conflicting results of elevated levels of histamine and diminished itching after histamine application may indicate either an intrinsic downregulation of neuronal H1-receptor density or affinity or an increased histamine degradation in atopic skin (48). Consequently, antihistamines are often not efficient in AD, as demonstrated in experimental studies as well as in double-blind, crossover trials. Recently, Rukwied et al. (49) demonstrated that pruritus induced by the mast cell degranulating substance compound 48/80 in AD patients could not be relieved by cetirizine H1 blockade. Wahlgren et al. (50) compared

Table 1 Mediators of Pruritus in Atopic Dermatitis

Substrate	Provocation of itch	Mechanism
Amine		
Histamine	+	Direct binding to itch receptor, neurogenic inflammation
Neuropeptides		
Substance P	+	Histamine liberator
Calcitonin gene–related peptide	+	Histamine liberator, increase of IL-8
Vasoactive intestinal peptide	+	Histamine liberator
Somatostatin	+	m.n.n.
Neurotensin	+	Histamine liberator
Acetylcholine	+	m.n.n.
Proteases		
Tryptase	+	Activates protease-activated receptor-2
Papain	+	m.n.n.
Chymase	+	m.n.n.
Opioid peptides		
Endorphins	+	Central and peripheral modulation
Enkephalins	+	of itch perception, histamine-
Morphine	+	independent
Eicosanoids		
Prostaglandins	(+)	Potentiate histamine-, serotonin-, papain-induced pruritus, lowered itch threshold
Leukotrienes	+	m.n.n.
Platelet-activating factor	+	Histamine liberator
Cytokines		
Interleukin-2	+	Possible release of various media-
Interleukin-6	−	tors
Interleukin-8	−	
Interferon-gamma	relief pruritus	m.n.n
Neurotrophin-4	+	m.n.n.
Eosinophils	+	Release mediators like PAF, leuko- trienes; histamine liberation?
Basophils	−	

−, No induction of itch; (+), induction of weak itch; +, clear induction of itch; m.n.n., mechanism not known.

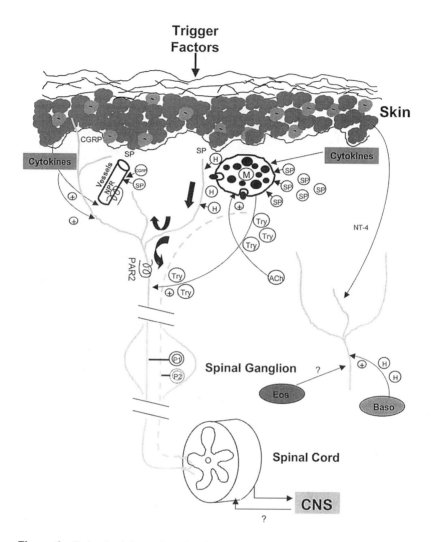

Figure 1 Pathophysiology of pruritus in atopic dermatitis. Trigger factors (see Table 2) may directly activate neuropeptide release from sensory nerves or indirectly by stimulating mediators (see Table 1) from mast cells or keratinocytes. Activation of primary afferent nerve fibers may either result in antidromic stimulation of neuropeptide release or will be processed to the central nervous system. Neuropeptides, proteases, or cytokines may provoke itch by direct binding to itch receptors or indirectly via histamine release from mast cells or basophils. ACh, Acetylcholine; Baso, basophils; CGRP, calcitonin gene–related peptide; CNS, central nervous system; Eos, eosinophils; H, histamine; M, mast cells; NPR, neuropeptide receptor; NT-4, neurotrophin-4; PAR2, proteinase-activated receptor-2; SP, substance P; Try, tryptase.

the antipruritic effect of H1 antagonist and placebo in AD patients and found no difference between these two agents. These results support the idea that other mediators such as proteases and cytokines may be involved in the pathophysiology of itch response during AD.

B. Neuropeptides

Several observations support the idea of an important role of neuropeptides in the pathophysiology of itching in various skin diseases (8,9,20,51). Neuropeptides such as SP, vasoactive intestinal polypeptide (VIP), somatostatin, and neurotensin provoke itch along with the characteristics of neurogenic inflammation such as erythema, wheal, and flare (52–55). SP induces itch responses in human and mice, which are probably mediated via activation of the neurokinin 1 receptor (NK1R) (56,57), supporting a direct effect of SP in mediating pruritus in vivo. In contrast, CGRP does not mediate pruritogenic effects (58,59). Opioids have also been demonstrated to induce pruritus, which can be blocked using naloxone, a μ-opioid receptor antagonist (60,61).

In patients with atopic dermatitis, alterations in the nerve fiber–containing neuropeptide profile could be demonstrated. Somatostatin-immunoreactive nerve fibers were decreased in AD patients (62). NPY-positive nerve fibers and Langerhans cells are increased as compared to healthy controls (21,24,62). Moreover, tissue concentrations of VIP were decreased while SP concentrations were increased in lesional skin of AD patients (63–65). In contrast, staining pattern for CGRP was not altered in comparison to controls (62). These observations support the idea that an imbalance of the cutaneous nervous system including nerve fibers, neuropeptides, and their receptors as well as neuropeptide-degrading enzymes may play a crucial role in the pathophysiology of pruritus in AD (66).

C. Acetylcholine

Acetylcholine is very likely to play an important role in producing itch sensations in patients suffering from atopic dermatitis. Acetylcholine is not only a neurotransmitter in glandular epithelium like eccrine sweat glands, it has also been shown to activate muscarinic receptors on cultured human keratinocytes and can be synthesized, released, and degraded by human keratinocytes in vitro (67,68). Interestingly, Scott (69) found increased ACh levels in biopsies of patients with AD, suggesting that increased production or release of acetylcholine is involved in the pathophysiology of pruritus in AD (69).

Recent investigations showed that intradermal application of acetylcholine elicits pruritus instead of pain in patients with AD (16,46). While all healthy control subjects reported on burning pain after ACh administration, patients with AD complained of pure itching that developed shortly after acetylcholine injection and lasted significantly longer than in controls (16). In addition, injection of ACh evoked pruritus in eczematous atopic lesions and intermingled burning as well as itching sensations in uninvolved areas (46), which underlines a different physiological pruritus pathway in lesional as compared to nonlesional or healthy skin. Combined intracutaneous injections of VIP and ACh induce weal, flare, and a dose-dependent pruritus in both lesional skin in AD and normal healthy controls (49,70). However, the subjective pruritus score did not differ between combined injections of VIP and ACh from ACh injections alone in patients with AD (49). These results suggest a predominant role of ACh over VIP and a cholinergic, histamine-independent mechanism in the pathophysiology of pruritus in AD. Finally, acetylcholine is a major neurotransmitter activating sweat glands, which may explain generalised itching during and after sweating in patients with AD.

D. Mast Cells, Proteinases, and Proteinase-Activated Receptors

A role for proteinases such as trypsin, chymotrypsin, and papain as pruritogenic agents has been proposed for over 40 years (71). Moreover, the pruritogenic effect and triple response of neurogenic inflammation induced by proteinases can be blocked by antihistamines (72), indicating an interaction of proteinases and mast cells in pruritus.

Intradermal injection of mast cell tryptase into human and rabbit skin results in pruritus, vasodilatation, and erythema, followed by leukocyte infiltration and local induration (73), suggesting a role for tryptase in cutaneous inflammation and itching. Importantly, tryptase but not chymase appears to be enhanced in lesional and nonlesional skin of patients with atopic dermatitis (74) and has been suggested to induce itch responses in human skin (49,75). Other studies support a role of tryptase in itch responses of patients with AD (74,76–78). Thus, tryptase may be an important regulator of inflammatory and itch responses in the skin of patients with atopic dermatitis. However, the mechanism by which tryptase mediates these effects in cutaneous target cells such as keratinocytes and endothelial cells is still uncertain.

Recently it has been demonstrated that tryptase mediates some of its cellular effects via activating a proteinase-activated receptor-2 (PAR-2). Tryptase activates PAR-2 on keratinocytes (79), dermal endothelial cells (M. Steinhoff and T. Luger, unpublished observation, 2001) and sensory nerves (75), thereby contributing to inflammatory effects of mast cells. Since tryptase is involved in pruritus, mast cells are important regulators of inflammatory and itch responses during atopic dermatitis, and PAR-2 immunoreactivity is enhanced in atopic dermatitis patients (M. Steinhoff and T. Luger, unpublished observation, 2001), it can be hypothesized that tryptase may activate PAR-2 in inflammatory conditions when there is mast cell infiltration and degranulation. Thus, PAR-2 may be involved in pruritus of patients with atopic dermatitis, explaining why AD patients show a rather weak response following treatment with antihistamines.

IV. CYTOKINES AND INFLAMMATORY CELLS INVOLVED IN PATHOGENESIS OF PRURITUS IN ATOPIC DERMATITIS

Cytokines are released from various cutaneous and immune cells during inflammation. Certain cytokines have been demonstrated to induce pruritus and activate neuropeptide release from sensory nerves in the skin of patients with atopic dermatitis (Fig. 1).

A. Interleukin-2

While interleukin (IL)-1 does not seem to correlate with itching, IL-2 is claimed to be a potent inducer of pruritus. As observed upon therapeutic application, high doses of recombinant IL-2, as given in cancer patients, frequently provoke redness and cutaneous itching (80). Furthermore, AD patients treated with oral cyclosporin A, a drug that inhibits the production of various cytokines including IL-2, experience attenuation of itch (81,82). Additionally, a single intracutaneous injection of IL-2 induced a low-intensity intermittent local itch with maximal intensity between 6 and 48 hours as well as erythema in both atopic and healthy individuals (83,84). Interestingly, in patients with AD, this reaction tends to appear earlier than in healthy controls. Moreover, bradykinin appears to enhance the effect of IL-2–induced pruritus on sensory nerves (85). Upon prick testing, supernatants of mitogen-stimulated leukocytes were pruritic in AD patients but not in controls, probably due to increased concentration of IL-2 and IL-6 (86). The mechanism for the induction of itch by IL-2 remains to be established, but the latency preceding the itch response after injection in AD patients suggests an indirect pruritogenic effect of IL-2 via other mediators.

B. Interleukin-6

IL-6 and IL-6 receptor are expressed in Schwann cells of the peripheral nerve (87), and IL-6–like immunoreactivity was increased in nerve fibers of patients with positive epicutaneous patch tests and prurigo nodularis (88), suggesting a role for this cytokine in pruritus. However, recent studies suggest that IL-6 does not play a major role for pruritus in AD (86,89,90). In accordance to that, in vitro studies with concavalin A–stimulated lymphocytes also failed to provoke itch responses (91).

C. Interleukin-8

Recently, various studies revealed increased levels of the proinflammatory chemokine IL-8 in lesional skin (92), plasma (93), and blood mononuclear cells (89,94), especially eosinophils (95) of AD patients. However, the capacity of IL-8 to induce pruritus is questionable since prick testing with IL-8 does not induce whealing or pruritus (89). Further studies will have to clarify the influence of IL-8 in the pathophysiology of pruritus.

D. Interferon gamma

Interferon gamma (IFN-γ) appears to have a beneficial effect on pruritus in AD (96). In a double-blind study, pruritus was reduced by 50% even 1–2 years after long-term treatment with recombinant human IFN-γ (97). It is well known that INF-γ production is profoundly diminished in peripheral blood mononuclear cells of AD patients (98), which may contribute to the development of pruritus. Although an important role of INF-γ in the pathophysiology of pruritus in AD is likely, the underlying mechanism by which low INF-γ levels induce pruritus, however, has to be identified.

E. Neurotrophin

Recent observations indicate that neurotrophin-4 (NT-4) may be involved in inflammatory and itch responses of patients with AD. NT-4 is a keratinocyte-derived agent, which is highly expressed under inflammatory conditions and which exerts growth-promoting effects on nerve cells. Accordingly, NT-4 expression was found to be significantly increased in lesional skin of patients with atopic dermatitis and in prurigo lesions of atopic dermatitis skin (99). Interestingly, NT-4 production can be induced by INF-γ, which itself is known to have a beneficial effect on pruritus. These findings suggest a close relationship between immune and neurotrophic factors in the pathophysiology of pruritus in AD.

F. Eosinophils

Although a role for eosinophils in the pathogenesis of AD is well established, their role in the pathophysiology of pruritus during AD is still an enigma. Eosinophils release factors which may have a direct pruritogenic effect such as PAF, leukotrienes, prostanoids, kinins, cytokines, and proteases (100–105). They may also exert an indirect itch response by activating mast cells to release histamine or proteinases from eosinophils. In summary, although some reports favor a role for eosinophils during pruritus in various diseases (100–102), direct evidence for a role of eosinophils in itch responses during AD is still lacking.

G. Basophils

In patients with AD, peripheral blood basophils are normal in number, but in vitro studies revealed abnormal function with increased or faster histamine releasability (106,107). However, Bull et al. demonstrated that basophils and basophil release of histamine do not contribute to induction of itch and erythema in patients with AD (108).

V. EXPERIMENTAL INDUCED PRURITUS IN ATOPIC DERMATITIS EXPLAINING NEW APPROACHES IN THE THERAPY

Platelet-activating factor (PAF) is a lipid mediator with a potent proinflammatory activity. PAF is released by several inflammatory cells such as mast cells, eosinophils, basophils, and neutrophils (74). PAF has been demonstrated to increase vascular permeability. Consequently, a wheal-and-flare reaction as well as pruritus resulted after intradermal injection, suggesting release of histamine by PAF (109). Several PAF antagonists have been developed so far, and preliminary results of a double-blind study applying a synthetic PAF antagonist topically demonstrated a statistically significant reduction of pruritus in patients with AD during the first 2 weeks of therapy (110). However, further studies will be needed to clarify the practicability of PAF antagonists upon daily use.

So far, the role of leukotrienes in the pathogenesis of pruritus is speculative, although there is increasing evidence of their relevance in elicitation itch. Andoh and Kuraishi (111) demonstrated that intradermal injected leukotriene E_4 is able to provoke scratching in mice. Additionally, a correlation of nocturnal itch and high urinary leukotriene E_4 levels was demonstrated, suggesting that increased production of leukotrienes may contribute to nocturnal itch induction in AD (112). Introductory studies showed a reduction of pruritus in patients with AD during treatment with the leukotriene receptor antagonists zafirlukast and zileuton (113–115).

Capsaicin, a naturally occurring alkaloid and the principal pungent of hot chili peppers, has been advocated to be antipruritic in various dermatoses (116,117). Repeated topical application of capsaicin releases and prevents specifically the reaccumulation of neuropeptides in unmyelinated, polymodal C–type cutaneous nerves. Capsaicin exerts its functions via binding to a capsaicin-specific receptor, i.e., the vanilloid receptor (VR1), which is located on free nerve endings (118). Receptor binding of capsaicin opens cation-specific ion channels, leads to depolarization of nerve fibers and release of secretory granules containing neuropeptides, such as SP, CGRP, VIP, and neurokinin A. Since nociceptive sensations are mediated by unmyelinated C-fibers, depletion of neuropeptides upon continuous application of capsaicin impedes the perception of pain and itch sensations (119). Consequently, topical application of capsaicin appears to be helpful in AD (120,121).

Morphine and opioids are known to play an intriguing part in itch elicited not only by histamine release from cutaneous mast cells (122), but also by a direct central and peripheral pruritogenic effect beside to their predominant role in pain (30–32,60,123,124). Generalized pruritus after systemic application of morphine is a rare side effect, but epidural or in particular paraspinal application of opioid analgesics frequently induce itching. Consequently, opiate receptor antagonists have been demonstrated to have an inhibitory effect on pruritus (33,34,61,125–127). Recent experiments revealed that the oral opiate antagonist naltrexone is more effective to suppress histamine-induced itch and alloknesis than the antihistamine cetirizine (46,128) in patients with AD. However, although β-endorphin serum levels were demonstrated to be significantly elevated in children with pruritic AD (129), results of a therapy with opiate receptor antagonists were not reproducible. While a few case reports demonstrated diminished pruritus using opiate antagonists naloxone and nalmefene (130), other groups could not reproduce these effects using nalmefene and nemexine in AD (34,131,132). Further controlled studies are needed to clarify their relevance to the treatment of atopic dermatitis.

VI. TRIGGERING FACTORS MODULATING PRURITUS PERCEPTION IN ATOPIC DERMATITIS

The skin of AD patients reveals a higher tendency to itch upon minimal provocation due to reduced itch threshold and prolonged itch duration to pruritic stimuli as compared to healthy skin (133–135). A series of pruritus-triggering factors are known (135), which release mast cell mediators or vasomotor and sweat reactions to cause itch, and all may be subject to emotional influences (134) (Table 2).

A. Epidermal Barrier

Xerosis of the skin in patients with AD reflects a disturbed epidermal barrier and is a well-known activator of pruritus in AD patients of all ages. An increased transepidermal water loss and a decreased ability of the stratum corneum to bind water was measured (136), which may result from incomplete arrangement of intercellular lipid lamellae in the stratum corneum (137,138). A decrease of water content below 10% seems to be crucial for induction of itch and scratching (139). This generalized dryness of the skin triggers pruritus by unknown mechanisms (136,137). One possibility may be that an impaired barrier function in the skin

Table 2 Triggering Factors Inducing and Aggravating Pruritus in Atopic Dermatitis

Trigger factors	Examples
Endogenous trigger factors	Perspiration (most common trigger factor in AD)
	Xerosis
	Cutaneous microvasculature
	Emotional stress
Exogenous irritants	Scratching
	Wool fibers
	Lipid solvents (soap, detergents)
	Disinfectants
Contact and aeroallergens	Dust mites
	Furry animals
	Pollens
	Molds
	Human dander
Microbial agents	Viral infections
	Staphylococcus aureus
	Pityrosporum yeast, *Candida*, dermatophytes
Food	Hot, spicy food
	Hot drinks
	Alcoholics

Source: Modified from Refs. 142, 200.

supports the entrance of irritants and itchy agents (140,141). Additionally, pH changes within the skin may activate itch receptors (118).

B. Sweating

Generalized itching initiated by any stimulus to sweating (thermal, emotional stimuli) is a typical hallmark and represents the most common trigger factor of itch in patients with AD (134,142,143). Interestingly, increased sweating in lichenified skin was observed in AD patients, suggesting a decreased threshold for sweat stimulation in chronic pruritic and altered skin (144). The underlying mechanism of sweat-induced pruritus remains to be explored, but there is increasing evidence that acetylcholine is involved. ACh induces eccrine sweating (6), is found to be increased in the skin of AD patients (69), and finally acts pruritogenic in AD patients (16).

C. Microcirculation

There is considerable evidence that the cutaneous microvasculature contributes to pruritus. Clinically, itching is mostly associated with erythema and hyperthermia. Most mediators for itching such as histamine, tryptase, ACh, SP, and prostaglandins are potent vasodilatators, rarely vasoconstrictors like NPY or catecholamines. Interestingly, while neuropeptide-induced itching does not vary between atopic and nonatopic patients, vascular responses obviously showed a significant difference between these two groups. Moreover, patients with AD were more susceptible to stress and showed increased vasodilatation as compared to controls (145).

D. Exogenous Factors

Pruritus produced by direct contact with wool in patients with AD is a characteristic and reproducible phenomenon (91,146). It is likely that the irritation is caused by the spiky nature of wool fiber itself while wearing wool garments close to the skin. Mechanical vibration seems not to be responsible for induction of itch, since it inhibits experimental, histamine-induced itch (147). Thicker wool fibers were found to provoke more intense itching than thinner fibers and an additional redness after application of wool samples (148). Other irritants like lipid solvents and disinfectants (149) may additionally contribute to aggravate xerosis. Contact and aeroallergens such as dust mites or pollens (reviewed in Ref. 142) may also provoke pruritus. Microbiological agents like bacteria (*Staphylococcus aureus*) or yeast may exacerbate both dermatitis and pruritus (135,142).

Pruritus and erythema may also be triggered by substances increasing blood flow, conduct vasodilatation, or release histamine. Among those, heat, hot and spicy foods, hot drinks, and alcohol are most likely to generate itch in AD patients (135,142,150). In early childhood, food allergies exacerbate eczematous skin lesions, although food allergies mostly resolve during aging in older children and adults (150).

E. Stress and Psychiatric Conditions

In general, itch can be induced or modified by cognitive stress perception like fatigue, anxiety, repressed emotions, as well as psychiatric diseases like depression (151–158). Consequently, in atopic dermatitis a correlation between the intensity of pruritus, scratching, and mental stress factors and psychiatric conditions have been demonstrated in experimental studies (153,154,159–161). Furthermore, AD patients experienced a more intensive pruritus in comparison to healthy persons and patients with psoriasis under equal study conditions (159). Consistently, upon clinical examinations up to 81% of AD patients acknowledge their pruritus to be aggravated by emotional stress (54). Relaxation therapies like autogenic training or hypnosis indirectly prove these findings by revealing a significant improvement of itching and eczema in AD patients (162,163). The mechanism of psychogen-triggered pruritus is unknown, but activation of the psychoneuroendocrine system is likely (8,9,153,154). Moreover, there is evidence from a recent study of a stress-induced pertubation of the epidermal barrier function resulting in inflammation and pruritus (164).

It is well established that animals respond to external noxious stimuli, resulting in alarm reaction followed by a resistance phase and potentially exhaustion of the biological system. In a rat model it was demonstrated that immobilization stress triggers mast cell degranulation, which was reduced by pretreatment with capsaicin (165). Thus, increased release of pruritogenic mediators by mast cells may result in scratching and skin lesions following stress tension (153). Pruritus intensity may also be increased by vasodilator responses and increased skin temperature upon emotional stress, as demonstrated by psychophysiological studies (134,166). Thus, stress is connected with production of mediators that influence several tissue organs including the skin (159). Neuropeptides such as SP, VIP, NPY, somatostatin, or CGRP released from sensory afferent nerves or neurotransmitters such as catecholamines and ACh generated by autonomic nerve fibers may be associated with emotional distress and cutaneous symptoms. For example, more pronounced release of neuropeptides like SP, CGRP, and neurotensin as well as vascular changes could be demonstrated during itching and scratching in AD patients as compared to normal controls (24,62,66). Furthermore, increased mast cell degranulation (165) and elevated count of blood granulocytes and leukocytes (167) were found in patients with AD upon stress stimuli. Finally, adrenaline may influence pruritus in a reverse mode. Patients with AD judge a preexisting pruritus to be less intensive in stress situations with high adrenaline levels (153,154,160).

VII. CLINICAL ASPECTS

The diagnosis of active AD cannot be made if there is no history of itching (2). There are several aspects defining pruritus in patients with AD. Besides pruritus associated with erythema, alloknesis and atmoknesis are often observed in atopic dermatitis, probably due to altered itch threshold. Many patients complain of nocturnal itch associated with sleep disturbance. All these types of pruritus may lead to a vigorous itch-scratch cycle.

A. Clinical Manifestation of Pruritus

It has long been debated whether itch precedes visible skin lesions or if erythema and accompanied inflammatory reaction appears first to evoke pruritus (140, 142,143). However, both theories can be assumed to fit with clinical observations and furthermore to maintain the itch-scratch cycle. It is well known that various triggering factors like stress result first in appearance of erythema followed by itch (143,168,169). Furthermore, itch may be followed by vasodilatation and inflammation due to scratching (140,142). However, pruritus in AD is regularly intense but intermittent with greater intensity in the evening and at night. Usually itching is generalized, but localized forms are also known with preferential appearance in flexures, wrist, face, and neck (170). As a consequence, permanent itch leads to an intense scratch behavior, and patients often resort to towels, combs, back-scratchers, brushes, and even scissors to combat pruritus (91,171). Interestingly, children with atopic dermatitis regularly pinch, knead, and roll their skin slowly instead of scratching or rubbing (G. Bonsmann, personal communication, 2001) (Fig. 2). Scratching is at times so vigorous that it evokes

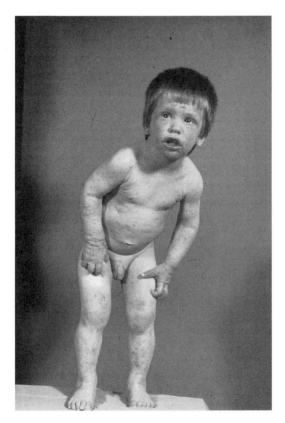

Figure 2   Child with atopic dermatitis and pruritus who pinches and kneads skin instead of scratching.

pain and an "antipruritic state" due to suppression of pruritus-conducting noci-ceptive C-fibers by pain-conducting A-fibers. Intense and permanent pinching, rubbing, and scratching causes many of the skin lesions observed in patients with AD (140,172) such as acute skin traumatization like excoriations, erosions, bleeding, and crusts. But secondary changes like lichenifications, nodules, pig-ment shift, and scars may also reflect chronic scratching (155,171). Now it is generally accepted that lichen simplex and prurigo nodularis, as often seen in AD, represent a cutaneous reaction pattern to repeated scratching (172). Interest-ingly, in areas not accessible to patients with AD like the upper back, unaffected skin without scratch artefacts appears leading to the so-called butterfly sign (140).

B. Alloknesis, Atmoknesis

Alloknesis is a phenomenon occurring in AD as well as other dermatoses and defines pruritus that is evoked by nonpruritogenic light stimuli (91). The clinical observation that once an itch has started in AD patients, it increases the liability of the surrounding skin resulting in itch is explainable by alloknesis. Another phenomenon is atmoknesis, defining pruritus caused by exposure to air or un-dressing, particularly notable in patients with AD. Alloknesis and atmoknesis both may result from an altered itch threshold (171). Regarding pruritus and alloknesis, 52% of patients with AD complain about itch without a rash in com-parison to 6% of nonatopic patients (143).

C. Nocturnal Itch

Several authors report on frequent sleep disturbances caused by nocturnal scratching (173–175). Upon scratch-monitor analysis and infrared video camera examination, a higher nocturnal scratch frequency in patients with severe AD was demonstrated resulting in serious sleep disturbance as compared to patients with moderate AD or healthy controls (173,174). Two types of scratching activity appeared, one during the time when patients were not asleep, with various scratching movements like rubbing or pinching. During sleep, scratch movements started abruptly, were monotonous and rhythmical, suggesting that scratch during sleep has the nature of a reflex. Most scratch movements appear during early and mid-night periods; rare movements were observed before daybreak, possibly due to physiological release of corticosteroids or melatonin (173,176,177). Finally, the scratching rate was reduced upon successful therapy (174,178).

D. Itch-Scratch Cycle

Severe pruritus in atopic dermatitis elicits reflectory scratching, often resulting in a vicious cycle of itch and scratch. Increased amounts of neuropeptides, cytokines, and other inflammatory mediators are released by scratching and contribute to aggravation of both itch and erythema (54,140,169). Thus, the itch-scratch cycle is perpetuated. Various other pruritogenic triggers like wool fibers additionally maintain the itch-scratch cycle (140,179). Furthermore, it was demonstrated that patients with AD developed conditioned scratch responses earlier than control subjects (179), which is in favor of an additional factor perpetuating the itch-scratch cycle. Patients with AD tend to frequently act out anger and hostility or other emotional stress by scratching, rather than by verbalizing their feelings (134,161,168,179,180). In addition, they are more likely to respond to minor signals and stimuli by scratching than nonatopic individuals, and many patients describe an emotionally disturbing event before occurrence of a flare reaction (54,181).

VIII.   THERAPEUTIC CONSIDERATIONS

A.   Nonspecific Antipruritic Modalities

Some general principles are helpful during therapy of pruritus of any origin, including atopic dermatitis (Table 3). First of all, elimination of identified provocative factors like wool fibers must be appreciated as the primary goal of the management (155,182,183). Furthermore, since scratching represents a trigger factor and maintains the itch-scratch cycle, it must be interrupted by educating the patient to control scratch behavior (184). For example, the behavior method of habit reversal can be employed (185). First, patients become aware of their scratching behavior by counting scratch movements. In a second step, they learn a new behavior by reacting to scratch impulses. Controlled physical exercise like gymnastics or ball games were demonstrated in a controlled study to teach patients to cope better with itch attacks (186). Scratch-induced skin damage caused by nocturnal scratch movements may be improved by wearing cotton gloves. To reduce sweating-induced itch, simple skin care such as cleaning by warm shower and application of ointment has been recommended (46). Cooling the skin with lotions (e.g., containing menthol) results in relief of itch (187). To combat skin dryness, application of hydrophilic emollients and bathing with oily bath additives is helpful (182,183). Topical anaesthetics are reported to be useful in pruritus (188), albeit no effect was observed in AD patients (189). Unspecific physical modalities are described to be beneficial like acupuncture (190), and cutaneous field stimulation (191,192). A new ethnomedical approach is the oral application of the Japanese traditional kampo medicine formula *Byakkokaninjinto*. Studies in NC mice, an animal model for atopic dermatitis, revealed a significant reduction of scratching activity, possibly due to a cooling effect on skin temperature (193). However, only one abstract reports a successful treatment with this substance so far (194).

Table 3 Therapeutic Strategies Combating Pruritus in Atopic Dermatitis

Therapeutical modalities	Examples
General principles	Interruption of itch-scratch cycle
	Elimination of provocative factors
	Skin care to reduce sweating-induced itch
Unspecific topical preparations	Emollients
	Lotions containing cooling additives, menthol
	Bathing with oily additives
Unspecific physical modalities	Physical exercise[a]
	Acupuncture
	Cutaneous field stimulation
Japanese traditional medicine	Kampo herbals
Anti-inflammatory therapy	Corticosteroids, t and o[a]
	Cyclosporin A, o[a]
	Tacrolimus, t[a]
	Ascomycins, t[a]
	Ultraviolet light
	Interferon gamma, i.c.[a]
	Macrolide antibiotics, o
Interfering with pathophysiol-	Capsaicin, t
ogy of pruritus in AD	Dinitrochlorobenzene, t
	Eicosapentaenoic acid, t
	Type 4 phosphodiesterase inhibitors, t
	Doxepin (but contact allergy upon long-term application), t
	PAF antagonists, t[a]
	Leukotriene antagonists, o (e.g., zafirlukast)
	Immunoglobulin therapy, i.v.
Contradictory results	Antihistamines, o
	Mycophenolat mofetil, o
	Opiate antagonists, o and i.v. (e.g., naltrexone)
No antipruritic effect	Topical anesthetics
	Nitrazepam, o

[a] As proven by randomized, controlled studies.
t, Topically; o, orally; i.c., intracutaneously; i.v., intravenously.

B. Specific Antipruritic Therapies

Although various symptomatic treatments were employed to relieve pruritus and scratching in patients with AD, no specific therapies are available as of yet (140). Since lesional AD skin shows a dense inflammatory cell infiltrate known to mediate or aggravate pruritus, anti-inflammatory therapies often result in cessation of pruritus. So far, most effective and consistent antipruritics remain systemic immunomodulators such as glucocorticoids, cyclosporin A, tacrolimus (FK 506), ascomycines (ASM 981), and ultraviolet light therapy (81,195–197) (Table 3). Moreover, there are no evident and efficient alternatives to topical application of corticosteroids for the control of acute episodes in atopic dermatitis (198–200). With reduction of skin lesions, a decreased itch intensity results, probably due to reduction of inflammatory cells and protection of depolarization of nerve fibers mediated directly by the steroid (201). Cyclosporin A (CyA), a cyclic polypeptide with potent immunosuppressive effects, has been reported to have an itch-relieving effect in various diseases, including atopic dermatitis. In a randomized study, CyA was demonstrated to significantly reduce itch intensity (81,202). After discontinuation of this therapy, pruritus recurred immediately, suggesting that CyA represents a symptomatic and not causal therapy of pruritus. Since oral cyclosporin A has demonstrated to be effective in atopic dermatitis, a topical CyA formulation has been developed to avoid systemic adverse effects. However, no significant improvement of atopic dermatitis was found upon clinical application (203). Recently, much interest has been drawn to tacrolimus (FK 506), an effective immunosuppressant drug that prevents rejection after organ transplantation. Although its mode of action is similar to that of CyA, its molecular weight is lower and its potency of inhibiting T-cell activation is 10–100 times higher. Topically applied tacrolimus appears to penetrate the skin sufficiently to effect local immunosuppression as inhibition of experimentally induced allergic contact dermatitis (204,205). Randomized studies also confirmed topical administration of 0.03–0.3% tacrolimus to be antipruritic in adults and even children (2–15 years) with AD (195,206–209). In controlled studies, ASM 981, belonging to the group of ascomycin macrolactam derivatives with high anti-inflammatory activity (210), reveals significant improvement of the ADSI score, especially of pruritus and excoriations (197,211). Since ascomycin induces inhibitory effects on the production of pro-inflammatory cytokines from T cells and mast cells (210), the specific improvement of pruritus suggests interference of ascomycin with the neuroimmunological network in the skin of patients with AD.

Mycophenolat mofetil (MMF) is a novel immunosuppressive drug that selectively inhibits lymphocyte proliferation. Uncontrolled studies with patients suffering from AD exhibit contradictory results. Some authors report on effective treatment of erythema and pruritus (212,213), while another found MMF to increase pruritus (214).

Treatment with IFN-γ has been shown to be effective not only for the improvement of erythema, excoriations, and lichenifications, but also of pruritus (97,215,216). In addition, this effect was maintained up to 2 years after therapy (97).

Arachidonic acid metabolites are released from mast cells and are involved in the onset of AD. It has been demonstrated that eicosapentaenoic acid (EPA) may inhibit the activity of arachidonic acid metabolites. A recent study reported topical EPA administration to significantly reduce pruritus in AD (217).

Studies concerning the pathophysiology of pruritus clearly demonstrated that different nociceptive mechanisms are involved in AD. Thus, conventional therapeutic modalities like antihistamines often fail to ameliorate pruritus in AD (202). This corresponds with the idea that histamine is not the major mediator of pruritus in AD (49). Placebo-controlled studies concerning the antipruritic effect of oral antihistamines have shown conflicting results in AD. In some studies, no superior effect was observed as compared to placebo (50,218,219), while others showed a significant antipruritic effect (46,220–222). In recent experimental studies, the H1 antihistamine cetirizine was demonstrated to focally reduce itch (46). However, an evidence-based review concerning the efficacy of antihistamines in relieving pruritus in atopic dermatitis concluded that little objective evidence exists for H1 antihistamines to demonstrate improvement of pruritus (223).

Other modalities also failed to show an antipruritic effect in AD. Moreover, a placebo-controlled study with nitrazepam was initiated claimed to reduce the nocturnal scratching behavior. However, the substance failed to influence the total duration of nocturnal scratching in patients with AD (224).

Topical application of the tricyclic antidepressant doxepin was suggested to have antipruritic effects because of its high affinity to H1 histamine receptors. In fact, 5% doxepin cream revealed improvement of histamine-induced and SP-mediated cutaneous responses but also evoked sedative effects in some patients (225,226). Unfortunately, doxepin was accompanied by contact allergies after long-term application (227).

Recently, oral administration of macrolide antibiotics was reported to have an antipruritic effect in atopic dermatitis, possibly due to their capacity to inhibit production of cytokines like IL-6 and IL-8 (228). Amelioration of pruritus has also been described under intravenous immunoglobulin therapy in a few cases of AD (229,230). As of yet, however, no controlled studies have been performed.

Lately, contact sensitization to dinitrochlorobenzene (DNCB) was claimed to significantly improve the clinical status of severe AD (231,232). There is also recent evidence that type 4 phosphodiesterase inhibitors have anti-inflammatory and antipruritic activities in patients with AD (233). Therapeutic modalities such as capsaicin (120,121), opiate antagonists (34,127), PAF antagonist (110), and leukotriene antagonists (113–115) appear to be promising new approaches in the therapy of atopic dermatitis but will have to prove their safety and practicability in further controlled studies. In conclusion, no completely effective and safe antipruritic agent has been successfully approved by controlled studies for the therapy of pruritus in atopic dermatitis so far. Further investigations are necessary to establish that antipruritic substances influence the centrally and peripherally altered itch perception in order to interfere with the complex pathophysiology of pruritus in atopic dermatitis.

REFERENCES

1. SS Rothman. Physiology of itching. Physiol Rev 21:357–381, 1941.
2. JM Hanifin, G Rajka. Diagnostic features of atopic dermatitis. Acta Derm Venereol (Stockh) 92(suppl):44–47, 1980.
3. CS Koblenzer. Itching and the atopic skin. J Allergy Clin Immunol 104:S109–113, 1999.
4. UW Schnyder. Neurodermatitis vom klinisch dermatologischen Standpunkt. Acta Allergol 16:463–474, 1961.
5. GBE Jemec, HC Wulf. Patient-physician consensus on quality of life in dermatology. Clin Exp Dermatol 21:177–179, 1996.
6. D Metze, T Luger. Nervous system in the skin. In: New basic science in dermatology: Biology of the skin. D Woodley, ed., London: Parthenon Publishing, Chapter 9, in press.
7. M Schmelz, K Michael, C Weidner, R Schmidt, HE Torebjork, HO Handwerker. Which nerve fibers mediate the axon reflex flare in human skin? Neuroreport 11: 645–648, 2000.
8. T Scholzen, CA Armstrong, NW Bunnett, TA Luger, JE Olerud, JC Ansel. Neuropeptides in the skin: interactions between the neuroendocrine and the skin immune system. Exp Dermatol 7:81–96, 1998.
9. M Steinhoff, C Armstrong, T Scholzen, T Luger, NW Bunnett, JC Ansel. Neurocutaneous control of inflammation. In: TB Fitzpatrick, DA Norris, TS Kupper, eds. Immune Mechanisms in Cutaneous Disease, 2nd ed. New York: Marcel Dekker Inc., in press.
10. HO Handwerker. Sixty years of C-fiber recordings from animal and human skin nerves: historical notes. Prog Brain Res 113:39–51, 1996.
11. M Schmelz, R Schmidt, A Bickel, HO Handwerker, HE Torebjork. Specific C-receptors for itch in human skin. J Neurosci 17:8003–8008, 1997.
12. A Kaji, H Shigematsu, K Fujita, T Maeda, S Watanabe. Parasympathetic innervation of cutaneous blood vessels by vasoactive intestinal polypeptide-immunoreactive and acetylcholinesterase-positive nerves: histochemical and experimental study on rat lower lip. Neuroscience 25:353, 1988.
13. C Advenier, P Devillier. Neurokinins and the skin. Allerg Immunol (Paris) 25:280–282, 1993.
14. SD Brain, TJ Williams. Inflammatory oedema induced by synergism between calcitonin gene-related peptide (CGRP) and mediators of increased vascular permeability. Br J Pharmacol 86:855–860, 1985.
15. J Wallengren, K Badendick, F Sundler, R Hakanson, E Zander. Innervation of the skin of the forearm in diabetic patients: relation to nerve function. Acta Derm Venereol 75:37–42, 1995.

16. G Heyer, M Vogelsang, OP Hornstein. Acetylcholine is an inducer of itching in patients with atopic dermatitis. J Dermatol 24:621–625, 1997.

17. KU Schallreuter. Epidermal adrenergic signal transduction as part of the neuronal network in the human epidermis. J Investig Dermatol Symp Proc 2:37–40, 1997.

18. M Röcken, K Schallreuter, H Renz, A Szentivanyi. What exactly is "atopy"? Exp Dermatol 7:97–104, 1998.

19. SA Grando. Biological functions of keratinocyte cholinergic receptors. J Investig Dermatol Symp Proc 2:41–48, 1997.

20. A Slominski, J Wortsman. Neuroendocrinology of the skin. Endocr Rev 21:457–487, 2000.

21. D Tobin, G Nabarro, HB de la Faille, WA van Vloten, SCJ van der Putte, HJ Schuurman. Increased number of immunoreactive nerve fibers in atopic dermatitis. J Allergy Clin Immunol 90:613–622, 1992.

22. H Sugiura, M Omoto, Hirota Y, K Danno, M Uehara. Density and fine structure of peripheral nerves in various skin lesions at atopic dermatitis. Arch Derm Res 289:125–131, 1997.

23. R Urashima, M Mihara. Cutaneous nerves in atopic dermatitis. A histological, immunohistochemical and electron microscopic study. Virchows Arch 432:363–370, 1998.

24. C Pincelli, F Fantini, P Massimi, G Girolomoni, S Seidenari, A Giannetti. Neuropeptides in skin from patients with atopic dermatitis: an immunohistochemical study. Br J Dermatol 122:745–750, 1990.

25. LS Osterle, T Cowen, MH Rustin. Neuropeptides in the skin of patients with atopic dermatitis. Clin Exp Dermatol 20:462–467, 1995.

26. KM Albers, DE Wright, BM Davis. Overexpression of nerve growth factor in epidermis of transgenic mice causes hypertrophy of peripheral nerve system. J Neurosci 14:1422–1432, 1994.

27. C Pincelli, C Sevignani, R Manfredini, A Grande, F Fantini, L Bracci-Laudiere, L Aloe, S Ferrari, A Cossarizza, A Giannetti. Expression and function of nerve growth factor and nerve growth factor receptor on cultured keratinocytes. J Invest Dermatol 103:13–18, 1994.

28. MC Mihm, NA Soter, HF Dvorak, KF Austen. The structure of normal skin and the morphology of atopic eczema. J Inv Dermatol 67:305–312, 1976.

29. PH Prose, E Sedlis. Morphologic and histochemical studies of atopic eczema in infants and children. J Inv Derm 34:149–165, 1960.

30. B Fjellner, Ö Hägermark. The influence of the opiate antagonist naloxone on experimental pruritus. Acta Derm Venereol 64:73–75, 1984.

31. C Stein. The control of pain in peripheral tissue by opioids. N Engl J Med 332:1685–1690, 1995.

32. JE Bernstein, RM Swift. Relief of intractable pruritus with naloxone. Arch Dermatol 115:1366–1367, 1979.

33. JA Summerfield. Naloxone modulates the perception of itch in man. Br J Clin Pharmacol 10:180–183, 1980.

34. D Metze, S Reimann, S Beissert, TA Luger. Efficacy and safety of naltrexone, an oral opiate receptor antagonist, in the treatment of pruritus in internal and dermatological diseases. J Am Acad Dermatol 41:533–539, 1999.

35. H Königstein. Experimental study of itch stimuli in animals. Arch Derm Syph 57: 829–849, 1948.
36. U Darsow, A Drzezga, M Fritsch, F Munz, F Weilke, P Bartenstein, M Schwaiger, J Ring. Processing of histamine-induced itch in the human cerebral cortex: a correlation analysis with dermal reactions. J Invest Dermatol 115:1029–1033, 2000.
37. G Heyer, OP Hornstein, HO Handwerker. Skin reactions and itch sensation induced by epicutaneous histamine application in atopic dermatitis and controls. J Invest Dermatol 93:492–496, 1989.
38. T Lewis. The Blood Vessels of the Human Skin and Their Responses. London: Shaw and Sons, 1927.
39. T Lewis, RT Grant, HM Marvin. Vascular reactions of the skin to injury. Heart 14:139–160, 1929.
40. DH Williams. Skin temperature reaction to histamine in atopic dermatitis (disseminated neurodermatitis). J Invest Dermatol 1:119–129, 1938.
41. HH Johnson, GA DeOreo, WP Lascheid, F Mitchell. Skin histamine levels in chronic atopic dermatitis. J Invest Dermatol 34:237–238, 1960.
42. L Juhlin. Localization and content of histamine in normal and diseased skin. Acta Derm Venereol (Stockh) 47:383–391, 1967.
43. T Ruzicka, S Glück. Cutaneous histamine levels in histamine releasability from the skin in atopic dermatitis and hyper-IgE syndrome. Arch Derm Res 275:41–44, 1983.
44. M Uehara. Reduced histamine reaction in atopic dermatitis. Arch Derm (Chic) 118: 244–245, 1982.
45. G Heyer, W Koppert, P Martus, HO Handwerker. Histamine and cutaneous nociception: histamine-induced responses in patients with atopic eczema, psoriasis and urticaria. Acta Derm Venereol (Stockh) 78:123–126, 1998.
46. GR Heyer, OP Hornstein. Recent studies of cutaneous nociception in atopic and non-atopic subject. J Dermatol 26:77–86, 1999.
47. G Heyer, OP Hornstein, HO Handwerker. Reactions to intradermally injected substance P and topically applied mustard oil in atopic dermatitis patients. Acta Derm Venerol (Stockh) 71:291–295, 1991.
48. G Heyer. Abnormal cutaneous neurosensitivity in atopic skin. Acta Derm Venereol (Stockh) 176(suppl):93–94, 1992.
49. R Rukwied, G Lischetzki, F McGlone, G Heyer, M Schmelz. Mast cell mediators other than histamine induce pruritus in atopic dermatitis patients: a dermal microdialysis study. Br J Derm 142:1114–1120, 2000.
50. CF Wahlgren, Ö Hägermark, R Bergström. The antipruritic effect of a sedative and a non-sedative antihistamine in atopic dermatitis. Br J Derm 122:545–551, 1990.
51. JC Ansel, AH Kaynard, CA Armstrong, J Olerud, N Bunnett, D Payan. Skin-nervous system interactions. J Invest Dermatol 106:198–204, 1996.
52. R Rukwied, G Heyer. Cutaneous reactions and sensations after intracutaneous injection of vasoactive intestinal polypeptide and acetylcholine in atopic eczema patients and healthy controls. Arch Dermatol Res 290:198–204, 1998.
53. G Heyer, FJ Ulmer, J Schmitz, HO Handwerker. Histamine-induced itch and allokenesis (itchy skin) in atopic eczema patients and controls. Acta Derm Venereol 75:348–352, 1995.

54. CF Wahlgren. Pathophysiology of itching in urticaria and atopic dermatitis. Allergy 47:65–75, 1992.

55. CF Wahlgren. Measurement of itch. Semin Dermatol 14:284, 1995.

56. T Andoh, T Nagasawa, M Satoh, Y Kuraishi. Substance P induction of itch-associated response mediated by cutaneous NK1 tachykinin receptors in mice. J Pharmacol Exp Ther 286:1140–1145, 1998.

57. TE Scholzen, M Steinhoff, P Bonaccorsi, R Klein, S Amadesi, P Geppetti, B Lu, NP Gerard, JE Olerud, TA Luger, NW Bunnett, EF Grady, CA Armstrong, JC Ansel. Neutral endopeptidase terminates substance P-induced inflammation in allergic contact dermatitis. J Immunol 166:1285–1291, 2001.

58. B Fjellner, Ö Hägermark. Studies on pruritogenic and histamine-releasing effects of some putative peptide neurotransmitters. Acta Derm Venereol (Stockh) 61:245–250, 1981.

59. F Fantini, C Pincelli, P Massimi, A Giannetti. Neuropeptide-like immunoreactivity in skin lesions of atopic dermatitis and psoriasis. Br J Dermatol 122:838–839, 1990.

60. B Fjellner, Ö Hägermark. Potentiation of histamine-induced itch and flare responses in human skin by the encephalin analogue FK 33-824, β-endorphin and morphine. Arch Derm Res 274:29–37, 1982.

61. JE Bernstein, RA Grinzi. Butorphanol-induced pruritus antagonized by naloxone. J Am Acad Dermatol 5:227–228, 1981.

62. C Pincelli, F Fantini, P Massimi, A Giannetti. Neuropeptide Y-like immunoreactivity in Langerhans cells from patients with atopic dermatitis. Int J Neurosci 51:219–220, 1990.

63. P Anand, DR Springall, MA Blank, D Sellu, JM Polak, SR Bloom. Neuropeptides in skin disease: increased VIP in eczema and psoriasis but not axillary hyperhidrosis. Br J Dermatol 124:547–549, 1991.

64. C Pincelli, F Fantini, P Romualdi, G Lesa, A Giannetti. Skin levels of vasoactive intestinal polypeptide in atopic dermatitis. Arch Dermatol Res 283:230–232, 1991.

65. F Fantini, C Pincelli, P Romualdi, A Donatini, A Giannetti. Substance P levels are decreased in lesional skin of atopic dermatitis. Exp Dermatol 1:127–128, 1992.

66. A Giannetti, F Fantini, A Cimitan, C Pincelli. Vasoactive intestinal polypeptide and substance P in the pathogenesis of atopic dermatitis. Acta Derm Venereol (Stockh) 176(suppl):90–92, 1992.

67. SA Grando, DA Kist, M Qui, MV Dahl. Human keratinocytes synthesize, secrete and degrade acetylcholine. J Invest Dermatol 101:32–36, 1993.

68. SA Grando, BD Zelickson, DA Kist. Keratinocyte muscarinic acetylcholine reports: immunolocalisation and partial characterization. J Invest Dermatol 104:95–100, 1995.

69. A Scott. Acetylcholine in normal and disease skin. Br J Dermatol 74:317–322, 1962.

70. R Rukwied, G Heyer. Administration of acetylcholine and vasoactive intestinal polypeptide to atopic eczema patients. Exp Dermatol 8:39–45, 1999.

71. W Shelley, R Arthur. The neurohistology and neurophysiology of the itch sensation in man. Arch Dermatol 76:296–323, 1957.

72. Ö Hägermark, G Rajka, U Bergvist. Experimental itch in human skin elicited by rat mast cell chymase. Acta Derm Venereol 52:125–128, 1972.

73. JE Bernstein. Capsaicin in dermatological disease. Semin Dermatol 7:304–309, 1988.

74. A Jarvikallio, A Naukkarinen, IT Harvima, ML Aalto, M Horsmanheimo. Quantitative analysis of tryptase- and chymase-containing mast cells in atopic dermatitis and nummular eczema. Br J Dermatol 136:871–877, 1997.

75. M Steinhoff, N Vergnolle, SH Young, M Tognetto, S Amadesi, HS Ennes, M Trevisani, MD Hollenberg, JL Wallace, GH Caughey, SE Mitchell, LM Williams, P Geppetti, EA Mayer, NW Bunnett. Agonists of proteinase-activated receptor 2 induce inflammation by a neurogenic mechanism. Nat Med 6:151–158, 2000.

76. IT Harvima, A Naukkarinen, RJ Harvima, M Horsmanheimo. Enzyme- and immunohistochemical localization of mast cell tryptase in psoriatic skin. Arch Dermatol Res 281:387–391, 1989.

77. A Naukkarinen, IT Harvima, ML Aalto, M Horsmanheimo. Mast cell tryptase and chymase are potential regulators of neurogenic inflammation in psoriatic skin. Int J Dermatol 33:366, 1994.

78. TE Damsgaard, AB Olesen, FB Sorensen, K Thestrup-Pedersen, PO Schiotz. Mast cells and atopic dermatitis. Stereological quantification of mast cells in atopic dermatitis and normal human skin. Arch Dermatol Res 289:256–260, 1997.

79. M Steinhoff, CU Corvera, MS Thoma, W Kong, BE McAlpine, GH Caughey, JC Ansel, NW Bunnett. Proteinase-activated receptor-2 in human skin: tissue distribution and activation of keratinocytes by mast cell tryptase. Exp Dermatol 8:282–294, 1999.

80. AA Gaspari, MT Lotze, SA Rosenberg, JB Stern, SI Katz. Dermatologic changes associated with interleukin 2 administration. JAMA 258:1624–1629, 1987.

81. CF Wahlgren, A Scheynius, Ö Hägermark. Antipruritic effect of oral cyclosporin A in atopic dermatitis. Acta Derm Venereol (Stockh) 70:323–329, 1990.

82. T van Joost, E Stolz, F Heule. Efficacy of low-dose cyclosporine in severe atopic skin disease. Arch Dermatol 123:166–167, 1987.

83. CF Wahlgren, M Tengvall Linder, Ö Hägermark, A Scheynius. Itch and inflammation induced by intradermally injected interleukin-2 in atopic dermatitis patients and healthy subjects. Arch Dermatol Res 287:572–580, 1995.

84. U Darsow, R Scharein, B Bromm, J Ring. Skin testing of the pruritogenic activity of histamine and cytokines (interleukin-2 and tumor necrosis factor-alpha) at the dermal-epidermal junction. Br J Dermatol 137:415–417, 1997.

85. HA Martin. Bradykinin potentiates the chemoresponsiveness of rat cutaneous C-fiber polymodal nociceptors to interleukin-2. Arch Physiol Biochem 104:229–238, 1996.

86. B Cremer, A Heimann, E Dippel, BM Czarnetzki. Pruritogenic effects of mitogen stimulated peripheral blood mononuclear cells in atopic eczema. Acta Derm Venerol (Stockh) 75:426–428, 1995.

87. C Grothe, K Heese, C Meisinger, K Wewetzer, D Kunz, P Cattini, U Otten. Expression of interleukin-6 and its receptor in the sciatic nerve and cultured Schwann cells: relation to 18-kD fibroblast growth factor-2. Brain Res 885:172–181, 2000.

88. K Nordlind, LB Chin, AA Ahmed, J Brakenhoff, E Theodorsson, S Liden. Immunohistochemical localization of interleukin-6-like immunoreactivity to peripheral

nerve-like structures in normal and inflamed human skin. Arch Dermatol Res 288: 431–435, 1996.

89. U Lippert, A Hoer, A Möller, I Ramboer, B Cremer, BM Henz. Role of antigen-induced cytokine released in atopic pruritus. Int Arch Allergy Immunol 116:36–39, 1998.

90. H Kanai, A Nagashima, E Hirakata, H Hirakata, S Okuda, S Fujimi, M Fujishima. The effect of azelastin hydrochloride on pruritus and leukotriene B4 in hemodialysis patients. Life Sci 57:207–213, 1995.

91. CF Wahlgren, Ö Hägermark, R Bergstrom. Patients' perception of itch induced by histamine, compound 48/80 and wool fibers in atopic dermatitis. Acta Derm Venereol 71:488–494, 1991.

92. M Sticherling, E Bornscheuer, JM Schröder, E Christophers. Immunohistochemical studies on NAP-1/IL-8 in contact eczema and atopic dermatitis. Arch Dermatol Res 284:82–85, 1992.

93. H Kimata, I Lindley. Detection of plasma interleukin-8 in atopic dermatitis. Arch Dis Child 70:119–122, 1994.

94. Y Hatano, K Katagiri, S Takayasu. Increased levels in vivo of mRNAs for IL-8 and macrophage inflammatory protein-1 alpha (MIP-1 alpha), but not of RANTES mRNA in peripheral blood mononuclear cells of patients with atopic dermatitis (AD). Clin Exp Immunol 117:237–243, 1999.

95. S Yousefi, S Hemmann, M Weber, C Holzer, K Hartung, K Blaser, HU Simon. IL-8 is expressed by human peripheral blood eosinophils. Evidence for increased secretion in asthma. J Immunol 154:5481–5490, 1995.

96. U Reinhold, S Kukel, J Brzoska, HW Kreysel. Systemic interferon gamma treatment in severe atopic dermatitis. J Am Acad Dermatol 29:58–63, 1993.

97. SR Stevens, JM Hanifin, T Hamilton, SJ Tofte, KD Cooper. Long-term effectiveness and safety of recombinant human interferon gamma therapy for atopic dermatitis despite unchanged serum IgE levels. Arch Dermatol 134:799–804, 1998.

98. U Reinhold, W Wehrmann, S Kukel, HW Kreysel. Evidence that defective interferon-gamma production in atopic dermatitis patients is due to intrinsic abnormalities. Clin Exp Immunol 79:374–379, 1990.

99. M Grewe, K Vogelsang, T Ruzicka, H Stege, J Krutmann. Neurotrophin-4 production by human epidermal keratinocytes: increased expression in atopic dermatitis. J Invest Dermatol 114:1108–1112, 2000.

100. JR Velaquez, P Lacy, R Moqbel. Replenishment of RANTES mRNA expression in activated eosinophils from atopic asthmatics. Immunology 99:591–599, 2000.

101. CA Akdis, M Akdis, A Trautmann, K Blaser. Immune regulation in atopic dermatitis. Curr Opin Immunol 12:641–646, 2000.

102. J Yamamoto, Y Adachi, Y Onoue, H Kanegane, T Miyawaki, M Toyoda, T Seki, M Morohashi. CD 30 expression on circulation memory CD4+ T cells as a Th2-dominated situation in patients with atopic dermatitis. Allergy 55:1011–1018, 2000.

103. BM Czarnetzki, M Csato. Comparative studies on human eosinophil migration towards platelet-activating factor and leukotriene B4. Int Arch Allergy Appl Immunol 88:191–193, 1989.

104. CE Sigal, FH Valone, MJ Holtzmann, EJ Goetzl. Preferential human eosinophil

chemotactic activity of the platelet-activating factor (PAF) 1-0-hexadecyl-2-acetyl-sn-glyceryl-3-phosphocholine (AGEPC). J Clin Immunol 7:179–184, 1987.

105. PF Weller, CW Lee, DW Foster, EJ Corey, KF Austen, RA Lewis. Generation and metabolism of 5-lipoxygenase pathway leukotriens by human eosinophils: predominant production of leukotriene C4. Proc Natl Acad Sci USA 80:7626–7630, 1983.

106. B Lebel, PY Venencie, JH Saurat, C Soubrane, J Paupe. Anti-IgE induced histamine release from basophils in children with atopic dermatitis. Acta Derm Venereol (Stockh) 92(suppl):57–59, 1980.

107. D von der Helm, J Ring, W Dorsch. Comparison of histamine release and prostaglandin E2 production of human basophils in atopic and normal individuals. Arch Derm Res 279:536–542, 1987.

108. HA Bull, PF Courtney, CB Bunker, MH Rustin, FL Pearce, PM Dowd. Basophil mediator release in atopic dermatitis. J Invest Dermatol 100:305–309, 1993.

109. B Fjellner, Ö Hägermark. Experimental pruritus evoked by platelet activating factor (PAF-acether) in human skin. Acta Derm Venereol (Stockh) 65:409–412, 1985.

110. D Abeck, T Andersson, E Grosshans, S Jablonska, K Kragballe, A Vahlquist, T Schmidt, P Dupuy, J Ring. Topical application of a platelet-activating factor (PAF) antagonist in atopic dermatitis. Acta Derm Venereol (Stockh) 77:449–451, 1997.

111. T Andoh, Y Kuraishi. Intradermal leukotriene B4, but not prostaglandin E2, induces itch-associated responses in mice. Eur J Pharmacol 353:93–96, 1998.

112. M Miyoshi, T Sakurai, S Kodama. Clinical evaluation of urinary leukotriene E4 levels in children with atopic dermatitis. Arerugi 48:1148–1152, 1999.

113. JA Carruci, K Washenik, A Weinstein, J Shupack, DE Cohen. The leukotriene antagonist zafirlukast as a therapeutic agent for atopic dermatitis. Arch Dermatol 134:785–786, 1998.

114. EJ Zabawski, MA Kahn, LJ Gregg. Treatment of atopic dermatitis with zafirlukast. Dermatol Online J 5:10, 1999.

115. DP Woodmanse, RA Simon. A pilot study examining the role of zileuton in atopic dermatitis. Ann Allergy Asthma Immunol 83:548–552, 1999.

116. JE Bernstein, LC Parish, M Rapaport, MM Rosenbaum, HH Roenigk. Effects of topically applied capsaicin on moderate and severe psoriasis vulgaris. J Am Acad Dermatol 15:504–507, 1986.

117. CN Ellis, B Berberian, VI Sulica, WA Dodd, MT Jarratt, I Katz, S Prawer, G Kruegger, IH Rex, JE Wolf. A double-blind evaluation of topical capsaicin in pruritic psoriasis. J Am Acad Dermatol 29:438–42, 1993.

118. Caterina MJ, Schumacher MA, Tominaga M, Rosen TA, Levine JD, Julius D. The capsaicin receptor: a heat-activated ion channel in the pain pathway. Nature 389: 816–824, 1997.

119. A Dray. Neuropharmacological mechanisms of capsaicin and related substances. Biochem Pharmacol 44:611–615, 1992.

120. S Reimann, T Luger, D Metze. Topische Anwendung von Capsaicin in der Dermatologie zur Therapie von Juckreiz und Schmerz. Hautarzt 51:164–172, 2000.

121. S Ständer, T Luger, D Metze: Effective treatment of prurigo nodularis with topical capsaicin. J Am Acad Dermatol 44:471–478, 2001.

122. DV Leung, EE Schneeberger, RS Gerha. The presence of IgE in macrophages and

dendritic cells infiltrating into the skin lesions of atopic dermatitis. Clin Immunol Immunopathol 42:328, 1987.

123. JA Summerfield. Pain, itch and endorphins. Br J Dermatol 105:725–726, 1981.
124. Ö Hägermark. Peripheral and central mediators of itch. Skin Pharmacol 5:1–8, 1992.
125. JP Penning, B Samson, AD Baxter. Reversal of epidural morphine-induced respiratory depression and pruritus with nalbuphine. Can J Anaesth 35:559–604,1988.
126. NV Bergasa, DW Alling, TL Talbot, MG Swain, C Yurdaydin, ML Turner, JM Schmitt, EC Walker, EA Jones. Effects of naloxone infusions in patients with the pruritus of cholestasis. A double-blind, randomized, controlled trial. Ann Intern Med 123:161–167, 1995.
127. D Metze, S Reimann, TA Luger. Effective treatment of pruritus with naltrexone, an orally active opiate antagonist. Ann NY Acad Sci 885:430–432, 1999.
128. GR Heyer, M Dotzer, TL Diepgen, HO Handwerker. Opiate and H1 antagonists effects on histamine induced pruritus and alloknesis. Pain 73:239–243, 1997.
129. S Georgala, KH Schulpis, ED Papaconstantinou, J Stratigos. Raised β-endorphin serum levels in children with atopic dermatitis and pruritus. J Dermatol Sci 8:125–128, 1994.
130. EW Monroe. Efficacy and safety of nalmefene in patients with severe pruritus caused by chronic urticaria and atopic dermatitis. J Am Acad Dermatol 21:135–136, 1989.
131. D Banerji, R Fox, M Seleznick, R Lockey. Controlled antipruritic trial of nalmefene in chronic urticaria and atopic dermatitis (abstr). J Allergy Clin Immunol 81:252, 1988.
132. JR Burch, PV Harrison. Opiates, sleep and itch. Clin Exp Dermatol 13:418–419, 1988.
133. G Rajka. Essential Aspects of Atopic Dermatitis. Berlin: Springer-Verlag, 1989, pp 57–69.
134. JM Hanifin. Pharmacophysiology of atopic dermatitis. Clin Rev Allergy 4:43–65, 1986.
135. MA Morren, B Przybilla, M Bamelis, B Heykants, A Reynaers, H Degreef. Atopic dermatitis: triggering factors. J Am Acad Dermatol 31:467–473, 1994.
136. Y Werner. The water content of the stratum corneum in patients with atopic dermatitis. Measurement with the corneometer CM 420. Acta Derm Venereol (Stockh) 66:281–284, 1986.
137. Y Werner, M Lindberg, B Forslind. Membrane-coating granules in "dry" non-eczematous skin of patients with atopic dermatitis. A quantitative electron microscopic study. Acta Derm Venereol (Stockh) 67:385–390, 1987.
138. M Fartasch, TL Diepgen. The barrier function in atopic dry skin. Disturbance of membrane-coating granule exocytosis and formation of epidermal lipids? Acta Derm Venereol (Stockh) 1992; 176(suppl):26–31.
139. Ö Hägermark. The pathophysiology of itch. In: Handbook of Atopic Eczema. Berlin: Springer-Verlag, 1991, pp 278–286.
140. CF Wahlgren. Itch and atopic dermatitis. J Dermatol 26:770–779, 1999.
141. T Yoshiike, Y Aikawa, J Sindhvananda, H Suto, K Nishimura, T Kawamoto, H Ogawa. Skin barrier defect in atopic dermatitis: increased permeability of the stratum corneum using dimethylsulfoxide and theophylline. J Dermatol Sci 5:92–96, 1993.

142. VS Beltrani. The clinical spectrum of atopic dermatitis. J Allergy Clin Immunol 104:S87–98, 1999.
143. JM Hanifin. Basic and clinical aspects of atopic dermatitis. Ann Allergy 52:386–393, 1984.
144. J Rovensky, O Saxl. Differences in the dynamics of sweat secretion in atopic children. J Invest Dermatol 43:171–176, 1964.
145. DT Graham, S Wolf. The relation of eczema to attitude and vascular reactions of the human skin. J Lab Clin Med 42:238, 1953.
146. N Bendsoe, A Bjornberg, H Asnes. Itching from wool fibers in atopic dermatitis. Contact Derm 17:21–22, 1987.
147. A Ekblom, B Fjellner, P Hansson. The influence of mechanical vibratory stimulation and transcutaneous electrical nerve stimulation on experimental pruritus induced by histamine. Acta Physiol Scand 122:361–367, 1984.
148. AA Fisher. Nonallergic "itch" and "prickly" sensation to wool fibers in atopic and nonatopic persons. Cutis 58:323–324, 1996.
149. D Hogan, C Danaker, HI Maibach. Contact dermatitis risk factors and rehabilitation. Semin Dermatol 31:467–473, 1994.
150. SH Sicherer, HA Sampson. Food hypersensitivity and atopic dermatitis: pathophysiology, epidemiology, diagnosis, and management. J Allergy Clin Immunol 104: 114–122, 1999.
151. RD Griesemer. Emotionally triggered disease in a dermatological practice. Psychiatr Ann 8:49–56, 1978.
152. V Niemeier, J Kupfer, U Gieler. Observations during an itch-inducing lecture. Dermatol Psychosom 1:15–18, 2000.
153. B Fjellner, BB Arnetz, Eneroth P, Kallner A. Pruritus during standardized mental stress. Relationship to psychoneuroendocrine and metabolic parameters. Acta Dermatol Venerol 65:199–205, 1985.
154. B Fjellner, BB Arnetz. Psychological predictors of pruritus during mental stress. Acta Derma Venereol (Stockh) 65:504–508, 1985.
155. D Metze, S Reimann, T Luger. Juckreiz—Symptom oder Krankheit? Berlin: Springer-Verlag, 1997, pp 77–86.
156. CS Koblenzer. Psychologic and Psychiatric Aspects of Itching. New York: McGraw-Hill, 1994, pp 347–365.
157. MA Gupta, AK Gupta, NJ Schork, CN Ellis. Depression modulates pruritus perception. A study of pruritus in psoriasis, atopic dermatitis and chronic idiopathic urticaria. Psychosom Med 56:36–40, 1994.
158. FE Cormia. Experimental histamine pruritus I. Influence of physical and psychological factors on threshold reactivity. J Invest Dermatol 19:21–34, 1952.
159. BB Arnetz, B Fjellner, P Eneroth, A Kallner. Endocrine and dermatological concomitants of mental stress. Acta Derm Venereol Suppl (Stockh) 156:9–12, 1991.
160. H Buhk, FA Muthny. Psychophysiologische und psychoneuroimmunologische Ergebnisse zur Neurodermitis. Hautarzt 48:5–11, 1997.
161. N Hermanns, OB Scholz. Kognitive Einflüsse auf einen histamininduzierten Juckreiz und Quaddelbildung bei der atopischen Dermatitis. Verhaltensmod Verhaltensmed 13:171–194, 1992.
162. A Ehlers, U Stangier, U Gieler. Treatment of atopic dermatitis: a comparison of

psychological and dermatological approaches to relapse prevention. J Consult Clin Psychol 63:624–635, 1995.
163. PD Shenefelt. Hypnosis in dermatology. Arch Dermatol 136:393–399, 2000.
164. A Garg, MM Chren, LP Sands, MS Matsui, KD Marenus, KR Feingold, PM Elias. Psychological stress perturbs epidermal permeability barrier homeostasis. Arch Dermatol 137:53–59, 2001.
165. LK Singh, X Pang, N Alexacos, R Letourneau, TC Theoharides. Acute immobilization stress triggers skin mast cell degranulation via corticotropin releasing hormone, neurotensin, and substance P: a link to neurogenic skin disorders. Brain Behav Immunity 13:225–239, 1999.
166. K Münzel, R Schandry. Atopisches Ekzem: psychophysiologische Reaktivität unter standardisierter Belastung. Hautarzt 41:606–611, 1990.
167. A Schwarzer, OB Scholz. Auswirkungen unterschiedlicher Aktivierungsbedingungen auf Patienten mit atopischer Dermatitis. Verhaltensmod Verhaltensmed 11:45–58, 1990.
168. DT Graham, S Wolf. The relation of eczema to attitude and to vascular reactions of the human skin. J Lab Clin Med 42:238–254, 1953.
169. DY Leung. The immunologic basis of atopic dermatitis. Clin Rev Allergy 11:447–469, 1993.
170. G Heyer, W Magerl. Pruritus als Leit-und Leidsymptom beim atopischen Ekzem-Patienten—klinische und neurophysiologische Untersuchungen. Berlin: BMV, 1991, pp 145–159.
171. JD Bernhard. Pruritus in Skin Diseases. New York: McGraw-Hill, 1994, pp 44–48.
172. RW Goldblum, WN Piper. Artificial lichenification produced by a scratching machine. J Invest Dermatol 22:405–415, 1954.
173. K Endo, H Sumitsuji, T Fukuzumi, J Adachi, T Aoki. Evaluation of scratch movements by a new scratch-monitor to analyze nocturnal itching in atopic dermatitis. Acta Derma Venereol (Stockh) 77:432–435, 1997.
174. T Ebata, H Aizawa, R Kamide, M Niimura. The characteristics of nocturnal scratching in adults with atopic dermatitis. Br J Dermatol 141:82–86, 1999.
175. T Aoki, H Kushimoto, E Kobayashi, Y Ogushi. Computer analysis of nocturnal scratch in atopic dermatitis. Acta Derm Venereol (Stockh) 92(suppl):33–37, 1980.
176. B Heubeck, A Schonberger, OP Hornstein. Sind Verschiebungen des zirkadianen Cortisolrhythmus ein endokrines Symptom des atopischen Ekzems? Hautarzt 39:12–17, 1988.
177. W Schwarz, N Birau, OP Hornstein, B Heubeck, A Schonberger, C Meyer, J Gottschalk. Alterations of melatonin secretion in atopic dermatitis. Acta Dermatol Venereol (Stockh) 68:224–229, 1988.
178. R Felix, S Shuster. A new method for the measurement of itch and the response to treatment. Br J Dermatol 93:303–311, 1975.
179. JM Jordan, FA Whitlock. Emotions and the skin: the conditioning of scratch responses in cases of atopic dermatitis. Br J Dermatol 86:574–585, 1972.
180. IH Ginsburg, JH Prystowsky, DS Kornfeld, H Wolland. Role of emotional factors in adults with atopic dermatitis. Int J Dermatol 32:656–660, 1993.

181. H Musaph. Itching and Scratching: Psychodynamics in Dermatology. Philadelphia:
      FA Davis Co, 1964.
182. EN Charleswoth. Practical approaches to the treatment of atopic dermatitis. Allergy
      Proc 15:269–274, 1994.
183. HA Bueller, JD Bernhard. Review of pruritus therapy. Dermatol Nurs 10:101–107,
      1998.
184. WW van der Schaar, H Lamberts. Scratching for the itch in eczema; a psychoder-
      matologic approach. Ned Tijdschr Geneeskd 141:2049–2051, 1997.
185. L Melin, T Frederiksen, P Norén, BG Swebilius. Behavioural treatment of
      scratching in patients with atopic dermatitis. Br J Dermatol 115:467–474, 1986.
186. OP Hornstein, K Gall, B Salzer, M Rupprecht. Controlled physical exercise in pa-
      tients with chronic neurodermatitis. Dtsch Zeitschr Sportmed 49:39–45, 1998.
187. H Fruhstorfer, M Hermanns, L Latzke. The effects of thermal stimulation on clini-
      cal and experimental itch. Pain 24:259–269, 1986.
188. D Vieluf, C Matthias, J Ring. Trockene juckende Haut—ihre Behandlung mit einer
      neuen Polidocanol-Harnstoff-Zubereitung. Dermatologica 169:53–59, 1992.
189. E Weishaar, C Foster, M Dotzer, G Heyer. Experimentally induced pruritus and
      cutaneous reactions with topical antihistamine and local analgesics in atopic ec-
      zema. Skin Pharmacol 10:183–190, 1997.
190. T Lundeberg, L Bondesson, M Thomas. Effect of acupuncture on experimental
      induced itch. Br J Dermatol 117:771–777, 1987.
191. H Bjorna, B Kaada. Succesful treatment of itching and atopic eczema by transcuta-
      neous nerve stimulation. Acupunct Electrother Res 12:101–112, 1987.
192. HJ Nilsson, A Levinsson, J Schouenborg. Cutaneous field stimulation (CFS): a new
      powerful method to combat itch. Pain 71:49–55, 1997.
193. C Thoda, H Sugahara, Y Kuraishi, K Komatsu. Inhibitory effect of Byakko-ka-
      ninjin-to on itch in a mouse model of atopic dermatitis. Phytother Res 14:192–
      194, 2000.
194. H Onda. The treatment of atopic dermatitis by Kampo medicines. J Tradit Med
      14:245–251, 1997.
195. JM Hanifin, MR Ling, R Langley, D Breneman, E Rafal. Tacrolimus ointment for
      the treatment of atopic dermatitis in adult patients. Part I, efficacy. J Am Acad
      Dermatol 44:S28–S38, 2001.
196. J Jekler, O Larkö. Combined UVA-UVB versus UVB phototherapy for atopic der-
      matitis: a paired-comparison study. J Am Acad Dermatol 22:49–53, 1990.
197. T Luger, EJM van Leent, M Graeber, S Hedgecock, M Thurston, A Kandra, J
      Berth-Jones, J Bjerke, E Christophers, J Knop, AC Knulst, M Morren, A Morris,
      S Reitamo, J Roed-Petersen, E Schoepf, K Thestrup-Petersen, PGM van der Valk,
      JD Bos. SDZ ASM 981: an emerging safe and effective treatment for atopic derma-
      titis. Br J Dermatol 144:788–794, 2001.
198. C Hoare, A Li Wan Po, H Williams. Systemic review of treatment for atopic ec-
      zema. Health Technol Assess 4:1–191, 2000.
199. A Aliaga, M Rodriguez, M Armijo, J Bravo, A Lopez Avila, JM Mascaro, J Fer-
      rando, R Del Rio, R Lozano, A Balaguer. Double-blind study of prednicarbate
      versus flucortin butyl ester in atopic dermatitis. Int J Dermatol 35:131–132, 1996.
200. JM Maloney, MR Morman, DM Stewart, MD Tarp, JJ Brown, R Rajagopalan.

Clobetasol propionate emollient 0.05% in the treatment of atopic dermatitis. Int J Dermatol 37:128–144, 1998.

201. G Yosipovitch, C Szolar, XY Hui, H Maibach. High-potency topical corticosteroid rapidly decreases histamine-induced itch but not thermal sensation and pain in human beings. J Am Acad Dermatol 35:118–120, 1996.

202. CF Wahlgren. Itch and atopic dermatitis: clinical and experimental studies. Acta Dermato-Venereol Suppl 165:1–53, 1991.

203. MA DeRie, MM Meinardi, JD Bos. Lack of efficacy of topical cyclosporin A in atopic dermatitis and allergic contact dermatitis. Acta Derm Venereol (Stockh) 71: 452–454, 1991.

204. AI Lauerma, Maibach HI, H Granlund, P Erkko, M Kartamaa, S Stubb. Inhibition of contact allergy reactions by topical FK 506. Lancet 340:556, 1992.

205. AB Fleischer. Treatment of atopic dermatitis: role of tacrolimus ointment as a topical noncorticosteroidal therapy. J Allergy Clin Immunol 104:S126–130, 1999.

206. A Paller, LF Eichenfield, DY Leung, D Stewart, M Appell. A 12-week study of tacrolimus ointment for the treatment of atopic dermatitis in pediatric patients. J Am Acad Dermatol 44:S47–S57, 2001.

207. S Kang, AW Lcuky, D Pariser, I Lawrence, JM Hanifin. Long-term safety and efficacy of tacrolimus ointment for the treatment of atopic dermatitis in children. J Am Acad Dermatol 44:S58–S64, 2001.

208. M Boguniewicz, VC Fiedler, S Raimer, ID Lawrence, DY Leung, JM Hanifin. A randomized, vehicle-controlled trial of tacrolimus ointment for treatment of atopic dermatitis in children. Pediatric tacrolimus study group. J Allergy Clin Immunol 102:637–644, 1998.

209. T Ruzicka, T Bieber, E Schöpf, A Rubins, A Dobozy, JD Bos, S Jablonska, I Ahmed, K Thestrup-Pedersen, F Daniel, A Finzi, S Reitamo. A short-term trial of tacrolimus ointment for atopic dermatitis. N Engl J Med 337:816–821, 1997.

210. M Grassberger, T Baumruker, A Enz, P Hiestand, T Hultsch, F Kalthoff, W Schuler, M Schulz, FJ Werner, A Winiski, B Wolff, G Zenke. A novel anti-inflammatory drug, SDZ ASM 981, for the treatment of skin diseases: in vitro pharmacology. Br J Dermatol 141:264–273, 1999.

211. EJ Van Leent, M Graber, M Thurston, A Wagenaar, PI Spuls, JD Bos. Effectiveness of the ascomycin macrolactam SDZ ASM 981 in the topical treatment of atopic dermatitis. Arch Dermatol 134:805–809, 1998.

212. M Grundmann-Kollmann, HC Korting, S Behrens, U Leiter, G Krahn, R Kaufmann, RU Peter, M Kerscher. Successful treatment of severe refractory atopic dermatitis with mycophenolate mofetil. Br J Dermatol 141:175–176, 1999.

213. K Neuber, I Schwartz, G Itschert, AT Dieck. Treatment of atopic eczema with oral mycophenolate mofetil. Br J Dermatol 143:385–391, 2000.

214. ER Hansen, S Buus, M Deleuran, KE Andersen. Treatment of atopic dermatitis with mycophenolate mofetil. Br J Dermatol 143:1324–1326, 2000.

215. JM Hanifin, LC Schneider, DY Leung, CN Ellis, HS Jaffe, AE Izu, LR Bucalo, SE Hirabayashi, SJ Tofte, G Cantu-Gonzales, H Milgrom, M Boguniewicz, KD Cooper. Recombinant interferon gamma therapy for atopic dermatitis. J Am Acad Dermatol 28:189–197, 1993.

216. JG Jang, JK Yang, HJ Lee, JY Yi, HO Kim, CW Kim, TY Kim. Clinical improve-

ment and immunohistochemical findings in severe atopic dermatitis treated with interferon gamma. J Am Acad Dermatol 42:1033–1040, 2000.

217. T Watanabe, Y Kuroda. The effect of a newly developed ointment containing eicosapentaenoic acid and docosahexaenoic acid in the treatment of atopic dermatitis. J Med Invest 46:173–177, 1999.

218. BM Henz, P Metzenauer, E O'Keefe, T Zuberbier. Differential effects of new-generation H1-receptor antagonists in pruritic dermatoses. Allergy 53:180–183, 1998.

219. J Berth-Jones, RAC Graham-Brown. Failure of terenadine in relieving the pruritus of atopic dermatitis. Br J Dermatol 121:635–637, 1989.

220. V Doherty, DGH Sylvester, CTC Kennedy, SG Harvey, JG Calthrop, JR Gibson. Treatment of itching in atopic eczema with antihistamines with a low sedative profile. Br Med J 298:96, 1989.

221. M Hannuksela, K Kalimo, K Lammintausta, K Turjanmaa, E Vajionen, PJ Coulie. Dose ranging study: cetirizine in the treatment of atopic dermatitis in adults. Ann Allergy 70:127–133, 1993.

222. TA Luger, T Ruzicka. Therapie juckender Dermatosen. In: Stuttgart: Georg Thieme Verlag, pp 51–72, 1999.

223. PA Klein, RAF Clark. An evidence-based review of the efficacy of antihistamines in relieving pruritus in atopic dermatitis. Arch Dermatol 135:1522–1525, 1999.

224. T Ebata, H Izumi, H Aizawa, R Kamide, M Niimura. Effects of nitrazepam on nocturnal scratching in adults with atopic dermatitis: a double-blind placebo-controlled crossover study. Br J Dermatol 138:631–634, 1998.

225. RA Sabroe, CT Kennedy, CB Archer. The effects of topical doxepin on responses to histamine, substance P, and prostaglandin E2 in human skin. Br J Dermatol 137: 386–390, 1997.

226. LA Drake, LE Millikan and the doxepin study group. The antipruritic effect of 5% doxepin cream in patients with eczematous dermatitis. Arch Dermatol 131:1403–1408, 1995.

227. WB Shelley, ED Shelley, NY Talanin. Self-potentiating allergic contact dermatitis caused by doxepin hydrochloride cream. J Am Acad Dermatol 34:143–144, 1996.

228. K Tamaki. Antipruritic effect of macrolide antibiotics. J Dermatol 27:66–67, 2000.

229. H Kimata. High dose gammaglobulin treatment for atopic dermatitis. Arch Dis Child 70:107–113, 1998.

230. EW Gelfand, LP Landwehr, B Esterl, B Mazer. Intravenous immune globulin: an alternative therapy in steroid-dependent allergic diseases. Clin Exp Immunol 104(suppl):61–66, 1996.

231. LB Mills, LJ Mordan, HL Roth, EE Winger, WL Epstein. Treatment of severe atopic dermatitis by topical immune modulation using dinitrochlorobenzene. J Am Acad Dermatol 42:687–689, 2000.

232. Y Yoshizawa, H Matusi, S Izaki, K Kitamura, HI Maibach. Topical dinitrochlorobenzene therapy in the treatment of refractory atopic dermatitis: systemic immunotherapy. J Am Acad Dermatol 42:258–262, 2000.

233. JM Hanifin, SC Chan, JB Cheng, SJ Tofte, WR Henderson, DS Kirby, ES Weiner. Type 4 phosphodiesterase inhibitors have clinical and in vitro anti-inflammatory effects in atopic dermatitis. J Invest Dermatol 107:51–56, 1996.

11

Cellular Aspects of Atopic Dermatitis: Overview

Haydee M. Ramirez, Kefei Kang, Seth R. Stevens, and Kevin D. Cooper
University Hospitals of Cleveland and Case Western Reserve University, Cleveland, Ohio

I. INTRODUCTION

Atopic dermatitis (AD) is a common inflammatory skin disease with increasing worldwide prevalence estimated at more than 10% in children (1,2). Recent studies of schoolchildren in Oregon reveal a surprisingly high (17.2%) prevalence of this disease (3). Ongoing studies are elucidating novel pathophysiological mechanisms which are leading to steady improvements in treatment. In this overview, we will discuss cellular-mediated immunological pathomechanisms of this extremely common yet simultaneously complicated disorder. Emphasis will be given to the role played by antigen-presenting cells (APCs), T cells, keratinocytes, eosinophils, and basophils/mast cells in the pathophysiology of AD. Further details can be found in the corresponding chapters in this section.

II. BASELINE ABNORMALITIES

A. Barrier Function

The most common clinical manifestations of AD are itchiness and dry skin. These two symptoms lead to scratching and trauma-induced inflammation (Figs. 1, 2). It is well accepted that skin barrier function is impaired in individuals with AD, which may be intrinsic or due to low-grade spongiotic dermatitis even in uninvolved skin (4). Abnormalities in neuropeptides, skin innervation, or tissue re-

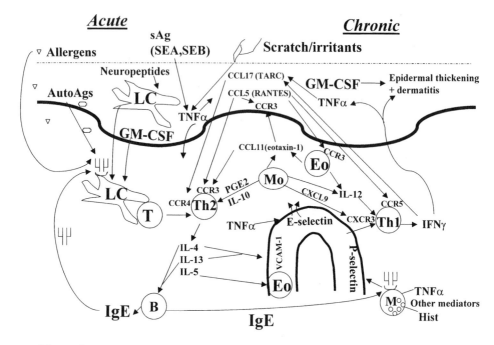

Figure 1 General view of cellular-mediated immunopathogenesis in atopic dermatitis. In AD, Langerhans cells in the epidermis are capable of capturing and presenting allergens and autoantigens, in the context of MHC molecules on the LC surface. This presentation leads to activation of T cells in the draining lymph nodes. LC function can also be modulated by neuropeptides, such as calcitonin gene–related peptide (CGRP). Increased monocyte cAMP-PDE results in increased secretion of PGE2 and IL-10, which directs T-cell differentiation toward Th2 (CCR3+, CCR4+), in conjunction with IL-4, IL-5, and IL-13 overexpression. Th2 cells are recruited to the skin preferentially with the help of chemokines, such as CCL17 (thymus and activation regulated chemokine, TARC) CCL-11 (eotaxin-1) and CCL5 (RANTES). B cells produce IgE with the help of IL-4 and IL-13 secreted from Th2 cells. Activated keratinocytes (which can also be stimulated by nonspecific irritants, such as scratching) produce TNFα, and mast cells release high quantities of TNFα, IL-4, and IL-13, which enhance the expression of P-selectin, E-selectin, and VCAM-1 on endothelial cells. Upregulated expression of adhesion molecules vigorously recruits T cells and especially eosinophils from blood into the dermis. Eosinophils are markedly elevated in AD peripheral blood and in both the epidermis and dermis. Overexpressed GM-CSF in the thickened epidermis sustains LCs and eosinophils as well. Eosinophils and monocytes are the source of IL-12, Mig, and RANTES and may participate in the pathogenesis of chronic lesion development in disease, in which expression of IFNγ is noticeably increased.

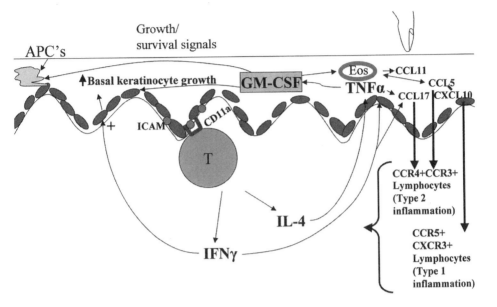

Figure 2   Model for the interaction of growth and survival cytokine/chemokine signaling. Perturbation of the skin (e.g., scratch injury) can lead to keratinocyte release of a number of cytokines. One of the principal growth factors released by keratinocytes is GM-CSF, which is upregulated in response to cytokines such as IL-1, TNFα, and IFNγ. This growth factor promotes the proliferation of APCs, keratinocytes themselves, and eosinophils. After reaching the epidermis, eosinophils can produce the chemoattractant chemokine CCL5, a ligand for CCR3 and CCR5, and CCL11, an additional ligand for CCR3. Keratinocytes are also activated via the T-cell cytokines IFNγ and IL-4, which can potentiate IFNγ and TNFα induction of CXCR3 ligands, such as CXCL10, which is important for Type 1 inflammation. IFNγ and TNFα production can also stimulate keratinocyte production of CCL17, a ligand for CCR4 important in Type 2 inflammation. Keratinocytes play a potential role in T-cell retention via ICAM-1 expression, which is upregulated following IFNγ exposure.

sponsiveness to adrenergic neurological tone may also be implicated in both barrier maintenance and immunological hyperactivity. Poor barrier function can favor the production of inflammatory cytokines associated with Type 2 immune responses.

B. Trigger Factors

Several trigger factors are relevant to AD. The most important factors are allergens and bacterial products.

1. Allergens

Aeroallergens such as dust mites, pollen, and mold have been implicated in AD exacerbations. Food allergens such as cow's milk, eggs, peanut, and soy play a pathogenic role in some patients with AD, especially children (5). IgE autoantibodies have been found to cross-link autoallergens (human proteins) that are structurally and immunologically similar with the exogenous allergens in severe and chronic AD (6).

2. Microbial Factors

There is an increased incidence of *Staphylococcus aureus* colonization in patients with AD compared with non-AD patients. *S. aureus* has been cultured and found in affected skin in more than 90% of patients with AD (7). Because both *S. aureus* and streptococci can produce superantigens, which can activate Langerhans cells (LCs) and other cells (monocytes/macrophages, T cells, and keratinocytes) in a nonspecific manner, these bacteria are believed to be acting as key modulators of the inflammatory cascade in AD skin. Cytokines such as tumor necrosis factor alpha (TNFα), produced by activated cells, can induce endothelial cell production of adhesion molecules such as E-selectin, P-selectin, and vascular cell adhesion molecule (VCAM-1) and contribute to this inflammatory cascade in AD skin (8,9) (Figs. 1, 2). Evidence supporting the role of superantigens produced by *S. aureus* in AD includes the observation that T cells in AD skin bear superantigen-reactive T-cell receptors. These T cells express superantigen receptors to a greater extent than is found in the systemic circulation (10).

C. Cell-Mediated Immunopathogenesis

The skin is rich in cells embryologically derived from bone marrow. A key proof of the concept that marrow-derived cells are critical for the maintenance of AD lesions was the early discovery that the skin rash in patients with Wiskott-Aldrich syndrome, an X-linked syndrome with the triad of AD-like symptoms—skin lesions, thrombocytopenia, and susceptibility to infections—resolved following bone marrow transplantation. This phenomenon was attributed to the correction of the underlying immunological defect (11). Conversely, allergen-specific IgE-mediated hypersensitivity may be transferred with allogeneic bone marrow transplantation from an atopic individual to one who is nonatopic (12). These two examples support the notion that bone marrow–derived cells mediate AD. Improvement of clinical symptoms in response to cyclosporin A, tacrolimus, and ascomycin also clearly document the immune pathogenesis of AD (13,14).

D. Antigen-Presenting Cells

APCs represent an important population of bone marrow–derived cells in the skin. They are major histocompatibility complex (MHC) II molecule–bearing accessory cells, which have the capacity to present antigen to antigen-specific T cells.

In normal skin, there is compartmentalization of the LC phenotype with epidermal LCs demonstrating high CD1a, absent CD1b, absent CD36, and low FcεRIα. By contrast, dermal LCs demonstrate low CD1a, positive CD1b, and absent CD36 with low FcεRIα (15–17). In AD lesional skin, however, LCs express both CD1a and CD1b as well as CD36, CD32, and high FCεRI (18,19) (Fig. 3). These LCs have been termed inflammatory dendritic epidermal cells

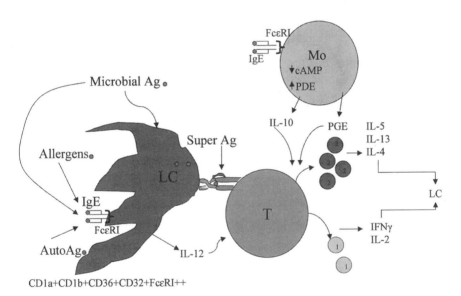

Figure 3 APC T-cell Type 1 and 2 interactions. Most important in APC reactions of AD is the presence and upregulation of the high-Fcε receptor, FcεRI, which is critical for AD patients because it binds IgE. Allergens such as microbes, dust mites, and human dander, which act as autoantigens, are processed inside the APCs, where they are then presented to the T-cell receptor along with coactivation by APC release of IL-12. Superantigens such as staphylococcal enterotoxins binding to the lateral wall of MHC peptide–antigen binding groove activates T cells nonspecifically. In the early phase of disease, Type 2 T cells predominate under the influence of PGE and IL-10 production by monocytes. Type 2 T cells express IL-5, IL-13, and IL-4, which further induces FcεRI expression on LCs. Production of T cells shifts to a Type 1 T cell, which produces IFNγ and IL-2 as the disease progresses and becomes chronic.

(IDECs) (19,20) and are present in both the epidermis and dermis of AD skin (18). The functional consequences of this aberrant phenotype are still not entirely understood, but they are associated with heightened APC activity for autoreactive T cells (18), facilitation of antigen processing and presentation of IgE-detected allergens (21), and increased calcium flux upon FcεRIα ligation (22) relative to normals (16). Phenotyping of epidermal dendritic cells (DCs) by Oppel et al. allowed for the distinction between extrinsic and intrinsic forms of AD. Analysis of CD36 expression on DCs and the percentage of CD1a+ epidermal DCs showed that FcεRI expression was more characteristic of extrinsic AD than that of intrinsic AD (23).

LC high-affinity IgE receptor may represent a key link between allergens and antigen-specific T cells. In this model, IgE bound to its receptor on LCs captures antigen, facilitates internalization and processing, and finally presents the antigen as a peptide fragment of the original allergen in the peptide-binding groove of the appropriate MHC molecules on the surface of such IgE-binding APCs. The APC, with its processed allergenic fragment, then interacts with specific antigen receptors on T cells. This antigen-focusing system allows for T-cell activation at much reduced antigen concentrations (24). Some IgE-detected proteins are, in fact, self-proteins expressed in the epidermis; this may explain the autoreactive T-cell–stimulating capability of APCs (6,25). This T-cell activation results in the subsequent production of cytokines.

E. Lymphocytes

In AD, increased levels of activated T cells are observed. Normally, the majority of postthymic naive T-cells begin as Th0 type cells with the potential to become differentiated to either Type 1 or Type 2 after activation by APCs and infiltration into the skin. After activation by APC, Th0, which previously produced neither Type 1 nor Type 2 lymphokine, undergo further differentiation to become Type 1 or Type 2 cells.

Important interleukins (IL) produced by APC and T-cell interaction are IL-1 and IL-2, which induce T-cell activation and growth. Activated T cells produce a number of other lymphokines of relevance: IFNγ has pleiotropic effects on many cell types. IFNγ inhibits the proliferation of Th2 cells and expression of the IL-4 receptor on T cells (26) as well as IgE synthesis. IL-4 and IL-13 act as B-cell growth factors and can upregulate VCAM-1 (8) and E-selectin from endothelial cells. IL-5 acts as a B-cell differentiation factor and stimulates eosinophils. T-cell differentiation events during initial activation can determine whether the immunological environment favors the development of Th1 or Th2 type cells, which produce differing relative amounts of these lymphokines (Figs. 1, 3).

T-cell surface glycoproteins are differentially expressed during maturation. With certain exceptions, as T cells become dedicated to either a helper/regulatory phenotype (CD4) or a cytotoxic/suppressor phenotype (CD8), they express dis-

Table 1 Nomenclature for Selected Chemokines and Their Receptors Dysregulated in AD

Chemokine	Source	Receptor
CCL11 (Eotaxin-1)	Lymphocytes Monocytes Keratinocytes Fibroblasts	CCR3
CCL5 (RANTES)	Keratinocytes Lymphocytes Eosinophils	CCR1, CCR3, CCR5
CCL17 (TARC)	Keratinocytes	CCR4
CXCL9 (Mig)	Monocytes Neutrophils	CXCR3
CXCL10 (IP-10)	Monocytes Neutrophils Eosinophils	CXCR3

tinctly different cell surface molecules. The CD4 T cells are further subdivided into two groups, Th1 and Th2, based upon distinct lymphokine profiles. Because of the observation that CD8+ T cells can also secrete distinct patterns of regulatory cytokines, the terms Type 1 and Type 2 cells have come to supplement the use of Th1 and Th2. Type 1 T cells are involved in cell-mediated immunity against viral, fungal, and mycobacterial infections, produce lymphokines such as IFNγ, TNF, IL-2, and IL-17, in conjunction with APCs producing IL-12, and are chemoattracted by CCR5 and CXCR3 ligands such as CCL5 (RANTES—Regulated on Activation, Normal T-cell Expressed and Secreted) and CXCL9-10 (i.e., Mig, IP-10) (27). (Fig 2) (Table 1). By contrast, Type 2 cells are associated with clearing helminthic infections and allergic inflammation, promoting humoral immunity, and enabling B-cell function by secreting IL-4, IL-13, and IL-5. Whereas immunoglobulins produced under the influence of Type 1 cytokines fix complement, Type 2 cytokines induce immunoglobulin production that does not fix complement (i.e., IgE and IgG4). Type 2 T-cell differentiation is promoted by IL-10 and prostaglandin E (PGE), and leukocytes involved in such reaction are chemoattracted by CCR3 and CCR4 chemokines (Fig. 2). These self-sustaining loops of inflammation can propagate the distinct inflammatory processes that are contained in AD lesions.

F. IgE

Elevated levels of IgE produced by B cells in AD are induced by IL-4 and IL-13. IL-4 and IL-13 are the only cytokines that induce germline transcription at the Cε axon and promote isotype switching to IgE (28). Both IL-4 and IL-13 inhibit Th1 cytokine production and upregulate CD23 on monocytes and B cells.

IgE may also contribute to the regulation of the high affinity receptor, FcεRI, on LCs. IgE binds to and stabilizes surface FcεRI. This leads to inhibition of receptor internalization and an accumulation of newly synthesized FcεRI on the cell surface (29).

IgE has also been linked to autoreactivity in atopic dermatitis. In a study by Valenta et al., human serum from 12 of 20 patients with pronounced skin lesions was found to have self-reactive IgE antibodies (Abs), suggesting that IgE autoimmunity occurs frequently in atopic dermatitis patients and that this may be of pathogenic relevance (21). Valenta et al. suggested two possible pathomechanisms for self-reactive IgE Abs: first, that autoallergens may cross-link effector cell-bound IgE autoantibodies and release inflammatory mediators, leading to immediate-type sensitivity reactions; second, that IgE-mediated presentation of autoallergens may activate autoreactive T cells, causing release of proinflammatory cytokines, contributing further to this cascade in an allergic tissue reaction (6).

G. Keratinocytes

Keratinocytes actively participate in the pathogenesis of AD by producing a number of cytokines and chemokines (Fig. 2) (30,31). GM-CSF and TNFα expression are markedly enhanced by keratinocytes after activation and are elevated in AD epidermis (Fig. 2). These keratinocyte-derived cytokines interact with the Type 1 lymphokine IFNγ as well as the Type 2 lymphokine IL-4 to induce a variety of inflammatory chemokines (Fig. 2). GM-CSF is important for LC and APC growth and survival, possibly explaining the expansion of LCs and IDECs in AD, while TNF is critical for APC/dendritic cell differentiation (32) (Fig 2).

CCL5 is upregulated by TNFα, and its expression is increased in AD (Figs. 1,2) (33). CCL5, together with GM-CSF and CCL11, are important eosinophil-attracting chemokines (34). In addition, CCL5 acts not only as a chemoattractant but also as an eosinophil activator in the skin of AD patients (35), while GM-CSF promotes eosinophilic survival in AD skin (36,37).

Chemokine CCL17 (TARC—Thymus and Activation-Regulated Chemokine) has been found in the keratinocytes of AD lesional skin (38) and, like CCL5, can be induced by IFNγ and TNFα (39). CCL17 attaches to Type 2 cells via the CCR4 receptor. An upregulation of skin homing surface molecules CLA+CCR4+ on lymphocytes has been shown in peripheral blood from AD patients (38) (Fig. 2).

H. Eosinophils

Eosinophil counts are elevated in AD and undergo activation. Substances released from degranulated eosinophils such as major basic protein (MBP), cationic protein, and eosinophil-derived neurotoxin are toxic and induce tissue injury in AD. MBP is distributed throughout the AD dermis and is capable of degranulating mast cells (15). Eosinophils are induced by the Type 2 cytokines IL-4, GM-CSF, and IL-5. The ability of eosinophils to secrete IL-12 upon exposure to Type 2 cytokines is thought to play a role in the emergence of Type 1 T cells in more chronic lesions of AD (40).

Eosinophils are targeted by the chemokine CCL11 (eotaxin). CCL11 acts as a potent chemoattractant to eosinophils and basophils. Eotaxin is produced by eosinophils, lymphocytes, monocytes, and basophils; its receptor, CCR3, is expressed by eosinophils, basophils, and preferentially expressed on activated Type 2 T cells (41). This may be a mechanism by which a positive feedback loop sustains a Type 2 response in AD lesions (Fig. 2).

I. Basophils/Mast Cells

Both basophils and mast cells originate from bone marrow progenitors. Basophils complete their maturation before being released from bone marrow into the circulation. In contrast, mast cells complete their maturation after migrating into tissues. Both cells express high-affinity FcεRI on their cell membranes. IgE crosslinking with FcεRI on the cells results in histamine release, causing immediate hypersensitivity. The spontaneous histamine release by basophils is increased in AD. The presence of mast cells in the chronic lesions may be relevant to the acute flare-ups associated with AD.

III. BIPHASIC FEATURES OF ATOPIC DERMATITIS

Although the early acute phase of AD is predominantly Type 2 driven, later, Type 1 T cells also participate (Fig. 1).

IL-4 is made predominantly in the initial phase by Type 2 T cells and shifts to a Th1/Th0 response in the late and chronic phase associated with IFNγ-producing T cells as well.

The biphasic nature of this disease was also shown using patch test studies in skin from patients with AD. Patch tests of the skin are considered to be an in vivo model of AD, as they are similar to atopic eczema both clinically and histologically. Analysis of T-cell cytokine expression during the development of atopy patch-test lesions revealed that in the early phase (within 24 hours) of inflammation, AD patients showed a positive patch-test reaction having an increase in IL-4 mRNA and protein after which IL-4 expression declined with time (48, 72, 96 hours after allergen application). In contrast, increased IFN-γ mRNA expression was not detected in 24-hour patch-test lesions but was strongly overexpressed at later time points (>48 hours). This expression was not seen in patients who were not atopic (42,43).

Because differentiation of T cells to Type 1 has been shown to be induced by IL-12, IL-12 was subsequently studied in AD. A peak in IL-12 expression was observed to precede the elevation of IFNγ mRNA expression in evolving dust mite allergen–induced patch test lesions (43–45), and IL-12 mRNA is also observed to be increased in chronic skin lesions of patients with AD (46). IL-12 detection was observed with infiltration by macrophages and eosinophils (47). Thus, IL-12 production in AD lesions by macrophages, APCs, or eosinophils, combined with chemokines attracting Type 1 T cells with CCR5 and CXCR3 receptors, may lead to IFNγ production in chronic lesions. These lesions are associated with epidermal hyperplasia. IFNγ-producing T cells, dependent upon both IFNγ and GM-CSF, are capable of inducing noncycling resting basal epidermal stem cells to enter cell cycle and start multiplying, resulting in epidermal keratinocyte growth (48,49) (Fig. 2).

Early in lesional skin, perivascular infiltrates of lymphocytic cells have cutaneous lymphocyte antigen (CLA) on their surface. This Ag acts as a homing device, leading these cells to specifically target skin, their desired place of action. These lymphocytes consist mainly of memory T cells, being CD3, CD4, and CD45 RO, which suggests a previous encounter with an offending antigen. Mast cells from different tissues irrespective of their protease phenotype may exhibit functional differences in their responses to non–IgE-dependent activators and pharmacological modulators of activation. Mast cells are increased in number at lesional sites of AD.

IV. SUMMARY

We have discussed briefly the aspects involved in AD cellular immunology. We now understand the importance of the skin and its function as a barrier against offending environmental insults as well as the threat by skin flora to a person with AD whose barrier function is compromised. In AD, Langerhans cells, monocytes/macrophages, T and B cells, keratinocytes, eosinophils, and mast cells are activated with cytokines largely involving T cell Type 2 (initial, early, and acute phase) and Type 1 (chronic and late phase). The presence of high-affinity IgE receptors that are important to the presentation of allergens and antigen are upregulated in AD. These high-affinity receptors participate in the inflammatory cascades of AD. The roles of chemokines in skin homing cells that allow proper trafficking of these complexes to their proper tissue destination are also upregulated in AD. In the following chapters, the reader will have the opportunity to learn about the function of many of these cells. It is our hope that this brief overview gives more insight into the etio-pathogenesis of this disease and how medical therapeutics for this disease can be most effective.

ACKNOWLEDGMENTS

We are grateful to Thomas S. McCormick, Ph.D., for his excellent assistance in the creation of this chapter.

REFERENCES

1. Schultz Larsen F, Diepgen T, Svensson A. The occurrence of atopic dermatitis in north Europe: an international questionnaire study. J Am Acad Dermatol 1996; 34: 760–764.
2. Schultz Larsen F. Atopic dermatitis: a genetic-epidemiologic study in a population-based twin sample. J Am Acad Dermatol 1993; 28:719–723.
3. Laughter D, Istvan JA, Tofte SJ, Hanifin JM. The prevalence of atopic dermatitis in Oregon schoolchildren. J Am Acad Dermatol 2000; 43:649–655.
4. Uehara M. Clinical and histological features of dry skin in atopic dermatitis. Acta Derm Venereol (Stockh) 1985; 114(suppl):82–86.
5. Sampson HA. Food allergy. Part 1: immunopathogenesis and clinical disorders. J Allergy Clin Immunol 1999; 103:717–728.
6. Valenta R, Seiberler S, Natter S, Mahler V, Mossabeb R, Ring J, Stingl G. Autoallergy: a pathogenetic factor in atopic dermatitis? J Allergy Clin Immunol 2000; 105: 432–437.
7. Leyden JJ, Marples RR, Kligman AM. *Staphylococcus aureus* in the lesions of atopic dermatitis. Br J Dermatol 1974; 90:525–530.
8. Etter H, Althaus R, Eugster HP, Santamaria-Babi LF, Weber L, Moser R. IL-4 and IL-13 downregulate rolling adhesion of leukocytes to IL-1 or TNF-alpha-activated endothelial cells by limiting the interval of E- selectin expression. Cytokine 1998; 10:395–403.
9. Schnyder B, Lugli S, Feng N, Etter H, Lutz RA, Ryffel B, Sugamura K, Wunderli-Allenspach H, Moser R. Interleukin-4 (IL-4) and IL-13 bind to a shared heterodimeric complex on endothelial cells mediating vascular cell adhesion molecule-1 induction in the absence of the common gamma chain. Blood 1996; 87:4286–4295.
10. Strickland I, Hauk PJ, Trumble AE, Picker LJ, Leung DY. Evidence for superantigen involvement in skin homing of T cells in atopic dermatitis. J Invest Dermatol 1999; 112:249–253.
11. Saurat J-H. Eczema in primary immune deficiencies. Clues to the pathogenesis of atopic dermatitis with special reference to the Wiskott Aldrich syndrome. Dermatovenereology 1985; 114:125–128.
12. Agosti JM, Sprenger JD, Lum LG, Witherspoon RP, Fisher LD, Storb R, Henderson WR, Jr. Transfer of allergen-specific IgE-mediated hypersensitivity with allogeneic bone marrow transplantation. N Engl J Med 1988; 319:1623–1628.
13. Taylor RS, Cooper KD, Headington JT, Ho V, Ellis CN, Voorhees JJ. Cyclosporine therapy for severe atopic dermatitis. J Am Acad Dermatol 1989; 21:580–583.
14. Hanifin JM, Chan S. Biochemical and immunologic mechanisms in atopic dermatitis: new targets for emerging therapies. J Am Acad Dermatol 1999; 41:72–77.

15. Cooper KD. Atopic dermatitis: recent trends in pathogenesis and therapy. Prog Dermatol 1993; 27:1–16.
16. Shibaki A, Ohkawara A, Shimada S, Ra C, Aiba S, Cooper KD. Expression, but lack of calcium mobilization by high-affinity IgE Fc epsilon receptor I on human epidermal and dermal Langerhans cells. Exp Dermatol 1996; 5:272–278.
17. Wollenberg A, Wen S, Bieber T. Langerhans cell phenotyping: a new tool for differential diagnosis of inflammatory skin diseases. Lancet 1995; 346:1626–1627.
18. Taylor RS, Baadsgaard O, Hammerberg C, Cooper KD. Hyperstimulatory CD1a$^+$CD1b$^+$CD36$^+$ Langerhans cells are responsible for increased autologous T lymphocyte reactivity to lesional epidermal cells of patients with atopic dermatitis. J Immunol 1991; 147:3794–3802.
19. Wollenberg A, Kraft S, Hanau D, Bieber T. Immunomorphological and ultrastructural characterization of Langerhans cells and a novel, inflammatory dendritic epidermal cell (IDEC) population in lesional skin of atopic eczema. J Invest Dermatol 1996; 106:446–453.
20. Wollenberg A, Wen S, Bieber T. Phenotyping of epidermal dendritic cells: clinical applications of a flow cytometric micromethod. Cytometry 1999; 37:147–155.
21. Valenta R, Maurer D, Steiner R, Deiberler S, Sperr WR, Valent P, Spitzauer S, Kapiotis S, Smolen J, Stingl G. Immunoglobulin E response to human proteins in atopic patients. J Invest Dermatol 1996; 107:203–208.
22. Jurgens M, Wollenberg A, Hanau D, de la Salle H, Bieber T. Activation of human epidermal Langerhans cells by engagement of the high affinity receptor for IgE. J Immunol 1995; 22:5184–5189.
23. Oppel T, Schuller E, Gunther S, Moderer M, Haberstok J, Bieber T, Wollenberg A. Phenotyping of epidermal dendritic cells allows the differentiation between extrinsic and intrinsic forms of atopic dermatitis. Br J Dermatol 2000; 143:1193–1198.
24. Maurer D, Fiebiger E, Reininger B, Wolff-Winiski B, Jouvin M-H, Kilgus O, Kinet J-P, Stingl G. Expression of functional high affinity immunoglobulin E receptors (Fc epsilon RI) on monocytes of atopic individuals. J Exp Med 1994; 179:745–750.
25. Seiberler S, Natter S, Hufnagl P, Binder BR, Valenta R. Characterization of IgE-reactive autoantigens in atopic dermatitis. 2. A pilot study on IgE versus IgG subclass response and seasonal variation of IgE autoreactivity. Int Arch Allergy Immunol 1999; 120:117–125.
26. Leung DY. Atopic dermatitis: new insights and opportunities for therapeutic intervention. J Allergy Clin Immunol 2000; 105:860–876.
27. Loetscher P, Pellegrino A, Gong JH, Mattioli I, Loetscher M, Bardi G, Baggiolini M, Clark-Lewis I. The ligands of CXC chemokine receptor 3, I-TAC, Mig, and IP10, are natural antagonists for CCR3. J Biol Chem 2001; 276:2986–2991.
28. Oettgen HC, Geha RS. IgE in asthma and atopy: cellular and molecular connections. J Clin Invest 1999; 104:829–835.
29. Kraft S, Wessendorf JH, Hanau D, Bieber T. Regulation of the high affinity receptor for IgE on human epidermal Langerhans cells. J Immunol 1998; 161:1000–1006.
30. Girolomoni G, Pastore S. The role of keratinocytes in the pathogenesis of atopic dermatitis. J Am Acad Dermatol 2001; 45:S25–S28.
31. Pastore S, Mascia F, Giustizieri ML, Giannetti A, Girolomoni G. Pathogenetic mechanisms of atopic dermatitis. Arch Immunol Ther Exp 2000; 48:497–504.

32. Romani N, Gruner S, Brang D, Kampgen E, Lenz A, Trockenbacher B, Konwalinka G, Fritsch PO, Steinman RM, Schuler G. Proliferating dendritic cell progenitors in human blood. J Exp Med 1994; 180:83–93.

33. Giustizieri ML, Mascia F, Frezzolini A, De Pita O, Chinni LM, Giannetti A, Girolomoni G, Pastore S. Keratinocytes from patients with atopic dermatitis and psoriasis show a distinct chemokine production profile in response to T cell-derived cytokines. J Allergy Clin Immunol 2001; 107:871–877.

34. Schroder JM, Mochizuki M. The role of chemokines in cutaneous allergic inflammation. Biol Chem 1999; 380:889–896.

35. Kapp A, Zeck-Kapp G, Czech W, Schopf E. The chemokine RANTES is more than a chemoattractant: characterization of its effect on human eosinophil oxidative metabolism and morphology in comparison with IL-5 and GM-CSF. J Invest Dermatol 1994; 102:906–914.

36. Mehregan DR, Fransway AF, Edmonson JH, Leiferman KM. Cutaneous reactions to granulocyte-monocyte colony-stimulating factor. Arch Dermatol 1992; 128:1055–1059.

37. Leiferman KM. A role for eosinophils in atopic dermatitis. J Am Acad Dermatol 2001; 45:S21–S24.

38. Vestergaard C, Bang K, Gesser B, Yoneyama H, Matsushima K, Larsen CG. A Th2 chemokine, TARC, produced by keratinocytes may recruit CLA+CCR4+ lymphocytes into lesional atopic dermatitis skin. J Invest Dermatol 2000; 115:640–646.

39. Vestergaard C, Kirstejn N, Gesser B, Mortensen JT, Matsushima K, Larsen CG. IL-10 augments the IFN-gamma and TNF-alpha induced TARC production in HaCaT cells: a possible mechanism in the inflammatory reaction of atopic dermatitis. J Dermatol Sci 2001; 26:46–54.

40. Grewe M, Czech W, Morita A, Werfel T, Klammer M, Kapp A, Ruzicka T, Schopf E, Krutmann J. Human eosinophils produce biologically active IL-12: implications for control of T cell responses. J Immunol 1998; 161:415–420.

41. Luster AD. Chemokines—chemotactic cytokines that mediate inflammation. N Engl J Med 1998; 338:436–445.

42. Thepen T, Langeveld-Wildschut EG, Bihari IC, van Wichen DF, Van Reijsen FC, Mudde GC, Bruijnzeel-Koomen CA. Biphasic response against aeroallergen in atopic dermatis showing a switch from an initial TH2 response to a TH1 response in situ: an immunocytochemical study. J Allergy Clin Immunol 1996; 97:828–837.

43. Grewe M, Walther S, Gyufko K, Czech W, Schopf E, Krutmann J. Analysis of the cytokine pattern expressed in situ in inhalant allergen patch test reactions of atopic dermatitis patients. J Invest Dermatol 1995; 105:407–410.

44. Werfel T, Morita A, Grewe M, Renz H, Wahn U, Krutmann J, Kapp A. Allergen specificity of skin-infiltrating T cells is not restricted to a type-2 cytokine pattern in chronic skin lesions of atopic dermatitis. J Invest Dermatol 1996; 107:871–876.

45. Junghans V, Gutgesell C, Jung T, Neumann C. Epidermal cytokines IL-1beta, TNF-alpha, and IL-12 in patients with atopic dermatitis: response to application of house dust mite antigens. J Invest Dermatol 1998; 111:1184–1188.

46. Hamid Q, Naseer T, Minshall EM, Song YL, Boguniewicz M, Leung DY. In vivo expression of IL-12 and IL-13 in atopic dermatitis. J Allergy Clin Immunol 1996; 98:225–231.

47. Nutku E, Zhuang Q, Soussi-Gounni A, Aris F, Mazer BD, Hamid Q. Functional expression of IL-12 receptor by human eosinophils: il-12 promotes eosinophil apoptosis. J Immunol 2001; 167:1039–1046.

48. Bata-Csorgo Z, Cooper KD, Ting KM, Voorhees JJ, Hammerberg C. Fibronectin and $\alpha 5$ integrin regulate keratinocyte cell cycling. J Clin Invest 1998; 101:1509–1518.

49. Bata-Csorgo Z, Hammerberg C, Voorhees JJ, Cooper KD. Kinetics and regulation of human keratinocyte stem cell growth in short-term primary ex vivo culture. Cooperative growth factors from psoriatic lesional T lymphocytes stimulate proliferation among psoriatic uninvolved, but not normal, stem keratinocytes. J Clin Invest 1995; 95:317–327.

12
Keratinocytes

Giampiero Girolomoni and Saveria Pastore
Istituto Dermopatico dell'Immacolata, IRCCS, Rome, Italy

Alberto Giannetti
University of Modena and Reggio Emilia, Modena, Italy

I. INTRODUCTION

Keratinocytes support the initiation and amplification of skin inflammatory and immune responses through the regulated expression of an array of mediators. Keratinocytes cultured from nonlesional skin of atopic dermatitis (AD) patients produce higher amounts of certain cytokines and chemokines compared to keratinocytes cultured from nonatopic subjects. Exaggerated release of these factors can be important for enhanced recruitment as well as sustained survival and activation of inflammatory cells, including dendritic cells and T lymphocytes. Recent evidence indicates that AD keratinocytes have a dysregulated activity of activator protein (AP)-1 transcription factors, which can help to explain the abnormal expression of granulocyte-macrophage colony-stimulating factor (GM-CSF) and other cytokines and suggests the existence of molecular mechanisms targeting atopic inflammation to the skin of AD patients. In this chapter we outline current knowledge supporting the concept that keratinocytes actively contribute to the pathogenesis of AD.

II. KERATINOCYTES ACTIVELY PARTICIPATE IN THE AMPLIFICATION OF SKIN INFLAMMATORY RESPONSES

Keratinocytes are the most abundant cell type of the epidermis and can be induced by different stimuli to initiate a program of expression of a variety of molecules active in modulating skin immune responses. Recent acquisitions have also demonstrated that any perturbation of the epidermal permeability barrier represents per se an effective mechanism leading to cutaneous inflammation, since the cytokines and growth factors released by keratinocytes as autocrine regulators of barrier homeostasis can also favor the development of inflammatory reactions (1). The contribution and mechanisms of impaired skin barrier function to AD pathogenesis has been addressed in previous chapters. Among the environmental factors, ultraviolet radiation, irritants, bacteria-derived products, and reactive haptens have been identified as triggers of the inflammatory activities of keratinocytes.

However, the most thoroughly investigated keratinocyte-activating factors are cytokines, especially those secreted by T lymphocytes. Indeed, resting keratinocytes express functional receptors for and are sensitive to T-cell–derived cytokines and can thus actively participate in the amplification of skin inflammatory reactions induced by T cells. T lymphocytes play a fundamental role in the pathogenesis of chronic skin disorders such as AD, allergic contact dermatitis to haptens, and psoriasis. In these conditions, infiltrating T lymphocytes release cytokines, which stimulate keratinocytes to express soluble and membrane mediators with a primary role in the recruitment, retention, and activation of T cells and other leukocytes in the skin.

Interferon (IFN)-γ is the best characterized proinflammatory cytokine for keratinocytes. IFN-γ–producing T-cell clones dominate psoriasis and allergic contact dermatitis lesions (2) but also intervene in the establishment of chronic AD lesions (3). After exposure to IFN-γ, keratinocytes express on their surface the adhesion molecule intercellular adhesion molecule (ICAM)-1, crucial for T-cell retention in the epidermis (4,5). Basal and suprabasal keratinocytes of chronic AD lesions express ICAM-1 (Fig. 1), although not to the extent observed in allergic contact dermatitis or psoriasis, and this expression can be an indicator of the presence of some IFN-γ–releasing T cells in the underlying infiltrate. Moreover, IFN-γ upregulates MHC class I molecules, induces de novo synthesis of mature MHC class II molecules, and upregulates Fas expression, thus rendering keratinocytes sensitive to Fas-mediated lysis (6,7). IFN-γ induces keratinocyte expression of cytokines with a well-recognized role in skin inflammation, including interleukin (IL)-1α, IL-1 receptor antagonist (IL-1ra), tumor necrosis factor (TNF)-α, and GM-CSF (8), and a variety of chemokines active in T-cell attraction, including interferon-induced protein of 10 kDa (IP-10/CXCL10), IFN-inducible T-cell α-chemoattractant (I-TAC/CXCL11), monokine induced by IFN-γ (Mig/CXCL9), and monocyte chemoattractant protein (MCP)-1/CCL2 (9).

The efficiency of IFN-γ in activating keratinocytes is enhanced by co-treatment with other cytokines, such as TNF-α and IL-17 (5,9). During chronic inflammatory diseases, TNF-α is released throughout the epidermis by activated keratinocytes and by infiltrating leukocytes (10), and, in turn, TNF-α is very

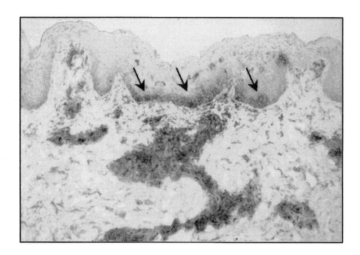

Figure 1 ICAM-1 is expressed by basal keratinocytes in chronic AD lesions. Frozen sections from chronic AD lesions were incubated with anti-ICAM-1 monoclonal antibody and stained with an indirect immunoperoxidase system. ICAM-1 is expressed by endothelial cells, the vast majority of the dermal infiltrate, and by basal keratinocytes (arrows), especially in those areas overlying the inflammatory infiltrate.

effective in inducing IL-8/CXCL8 and RANTES/CCL5 expression in keratinocytes (5). Among T-cell–derived cytokines abundantly released in the skin in the course of AD, IL-4 has been characterized as an active contributor to keratinocyte activation only recently (9,11). Cells expressing IL-4 can be detected even in the uninvolved skin of patients with AD, and their number increases prominently in acute and chronic lesions (12). Keratinocytes express functional IL-4 receptor, and although IL-4 alone has a modest capacity to induce cytokine release by keratinocytes, it effectively reinforces the activity of other T-cell–derived proinflammatory cytokines. In particular, IL-4 potentiates IFN-γ and TNF-α in the induction of CXCR3 agonist chemokines such as IP-10 and Mig and hence elicits T-lymphocyte attraction into the inflamed skin (9).

III. KERATINOCYTES FROM AD PATIENTS PRODUCE AUGMENTED AMOUNTS OF GM-CSF AND OTHER PROINFLAMMATORY CYTOKINES

GM-CSF is readily produced by epithelial cells in response to autocrine IL-1α and TNF-α and to the T-cell–derived cytokines IFN-γ, IL-4, and IL-17 (8,11,13).

GM-CSF promotes the proliferation and survival of keratinocytes, T cells, eosinophils, monocytes, and dendritic cell precursors. In addition, GM-CSF can favor the recruitment and activation of monocytes, basophils, eosinophils, and dendritic cells, thus providing powerful mechanisms for the initiation and perpetuation of inflammation. In the context of atopic diseases, a prominent increased expression of GM-CSF has been documented in nasal and bronchial epithelial cells of rhinitis and asthma patients, respectively (14–17), as well as in peripheral blood mononuclear cells of AD patients (18). We have shown that GM-CSF is overexpressed in keratinocytes of AD lesions and that keratinocytes cultured from nonlesional skin of adult AD patients produce higher levels of GM-CSF, both basally and in response to IL-1α, IFN-γ, or phorbol esters (PMA), when compared to keratinocytes from nonatopic individuals (Fig. 2) (8,13). In addition, supernatants from atopic keratinocytes are able to strongly stimulate mononuclear cell proliferation in a GM-CSF–dependent manner, and conditioned medium from PMA-treated AD keratinocytes, together with exogenous IL-4, can support phenotypical and functional differentiation of peripheral blood monocytes into dendritic cells. These findings could explain the persistence of a heavy infiltrate of "inflammatory" dendritic cells in AD skin (13). Other than GM-CSF, AD keratinocytes release higher amounts of TNF-α (Fig. 2), IL-1α, and IL-1 receptor antagonist following IFN-γ stimulation (8). In the context of chronic AD lesions,

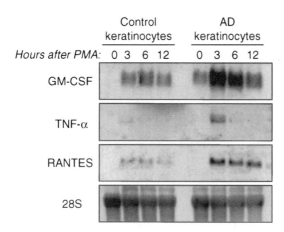

Figure 2 Keratinocytes cultured from AD patients express higher amounts of GM-CSF, TNF-α, and RANTES mRNA compared to keratinocytes from healthy control. Northern blot analysis of keratinocyte cultures prepared from a nonatopic, healthy individual and normal-appearing skin of a patient with AD. Cells were left untreated or stimulated with 10 ng/mL phorbol ester (PMA) for 3–12 hours.

keratinocyte overresponse to IFN-γ may serve as a further amplification mechanism to enhance disease severity (3).

IV. CONTRIBUTION OF KERATINOCYTES TO THE RECRUITMENT OF INFLAMMATORY CELLS IN AD

The lymphocytic infiltrate of AD consists predominantly of dendritic cells and memory CD4+ T cells (12). Essentially all T cells infiltrating the skin lesions express the cutaneous lymphocyte-associated antigen (CLA), which functions as a skin homing receptor for T lymphocytes by mediating T-lymphocyte rolling over E-selectin expressed by activated endothelial cells. More recently, chemokine receptors have been indicated as important regulators of the tissue targeting of T lymphocytes. In line with this concept, it has been shown that skin-seeking CLA+ T cells co-express the CCR4 receptor, the ligand for TARC (thymus and activation regulated chemokine, CCL17) and MDC (macrophage-derived chemokine, CCL22) (19). CCR4 is also preferentially expressed by Th2 compared to Th1 lymphocytes (20). Keratinocytes offer numerous chemotactic signals for the attraction of T lymphocytes in lesional AD skin. In acute and, to a lesser extent, chronic AD lesions, enhanced keratinocyte expression of IL-16 mRNA has been associated with increased numbers of skin-infiltrating CD4+ cells (21), and IL-16 has been shown to exert chemotactic activity towards different CD4+ cells, including CD4+ T cells and CD4-bearing eosinophils (22). Keratinocytes of the lesional epidermis can also contribute to the selective recruitment of CCR4+ lymphocytes through the production of TARC (23). MCP-1 is another chemokine strongly expressed by basal keratinocytes of lesional AD skin and effective towards T cells, monocytes, and dendritic cells (24). Recently, the chemokine named cutaneous T-cell–attracting chemokine (CTACK/CCL27) has been characterized, which could be involved in the attraction of T lymphocytes into AD lesional skin. CTACK is constitutively produced by keratinocytes, can be potently induced by stimulation with TNF-α and IL-1β in synergism (25), and preferentially attracts a specific, yet undefined, subset of the CLA+ memory T cells (26).

If activated Th2 cells may dictate the initiation phase of AD, subsequently local inflammation will attract and activate infiltrating cells such as eosinophils, dendritic cells, and macrophages to produce IL-12, which leads to the expansion of Th1 cells. Eventually, IFN-γ–producing T cells may be responsible for the chronic phase of AD and disease severity (3). Keratinocytes could contribute relevantly to this partial lymphocyte switch through the release of RANTES/CCL5. Basal keratinocytes of lesional AD skin are committed to neosynthesizing RANTES, which can be detected at high levels also in skin scales of AD patients (27). Via the interaction with CCR3, RANTES may play a role in the early recruitment of Th2 cells and eosinophils, but it is also a powerful chemoattractant for dendritic cells and monocytes; however, in chronic lesions, RANTES can also attract Th1 cells through CCR5 (28,29). In vitro experiments indicated that keratinocytes cultured from nonlesional skin of AD patients responded to stimulation with IFN-γ, TNF-α, or PMA with significant higher levels of RANTES secretion, when compared to keratinocytes from healthy controls or psoriatic patients (Fig. 2) (24).

In line with the evidence that keratinocytes are committed to an increased synthesis of this chemokine is the recent observation that AD patients carry a functional mutation, responsible for a much higher transcriptional activity of RANTES promoter (30). In acute and chronic AD lesions, keratinocytes have recently been reported to synthesize eotaxin/CCL11 and MCP-4/CCL13, particularly active chemokines in eosinophil attraction and activation (31). However, no significant staining for eotaxin could be found in the keratinocytes of AD skin in a previous work, while its expression was observed in mononuclear cells, eosinophils, as well as in fibroblasts (32). Moreover, in vitro studies indicated that cytokine-activated fibroblasts are major sources of eotaxin and MCP-4 in the lesional skin (33,34).

V. DYSREGULATED ACTIVATION OF AP-1 TRANSCRIPTION FACTORS MAY BE IMPLICATED IN THE ENHANCED EXPRESSION OF SPECIFIC CYTOKINES IN AD KERATINOCYTES

Functional polymorphisms in the regulatory/coding regions of clusters of cytokine genes have been found in atopic patients, which could be implicated in the overproduction of cytokines and chemokines observed in AD keratinocytes (30,35). Furthermore, an altered response to inflammatory stimuli could confer specific tissue targeting of the atopic syndromes.

In our search for a molecular mechanism underlying abnormal cytokine production in AD keratinocytes, we have examined GM-SCF expression following PMA stimulation (36). A similar GM-CSF mRNA decay kinetics in keratinocytes from both nonatopic and AD subjects indicated that GM-CSF mRNA overexpression in AD keratinocytes was not due to reduced mRNA degradation. Conversely, GM-CSF gene transcriptional activity was significantly stronger in AD keratinocytes, both in unstimulated and in PMA-stimulated conditions, and it was correlated with higher nuclear levels of functional AP-1 complexes. A higher expression level of c-Jun and a more pronounced PMA-induced phosphorylation of JunB and c-Fos were observed. Although the activity of AP-1 depends on complex promoter- and tissue-specific cooperation with other transcription factors, an amplification of its function could seriously affect a variety of AP-1-

mediated processes. In particular, AP-1 binding sites are located in the promoters of a vast array of cytokines and chemokines, including IL-1, TNF-α, and RANTES (37,38). The mechanisms that underlie the selective, excessive activation of c-Jun, JunB, and c-Fos in AD keratinocytes are presently unknown. However, it is possible that abnormal function of diacylglycerol (DAG)–dependent protein kinase C (PKC) isoforms contributes to enhanced AP-1 activation (39). In fact, the epidermis of AD patients is characterized by a marked decrease in the content of ceramides, which causes a dysfunction in the cutaneous permeability barrier (40). Ceramides can compete with the activating binding of DAGs on distinct PKC isozymes and interfere with PKC functions (41). A defect in ceramide generation could therefore result in enhanced PKC activation and thus excessive AP-1 activation. A constitutive, abnormal activation of signal transducer and activator of transcription (STAT)-1 associated with an increased expression of its specific target genes has been selectively detected in bronchial epithelial cells of atopic asthmatic patients, predisposing these subjects to excessive IFN-γ–mediated airway inflammation (42). This observation is consistent with the hypothesis that a dysregulated signal transduction in epithelial cells or other resident cells could underlie an exaggerated response to inflammatory stimuli in atopic subjects and be involved in the specific tissue targeting of the atopic inflammation.

VI. CONCLUDING REMARKS

Keratinocytes can participate to the pathogenesis of skin inflammatory diseases through the production of numerous inflammatory signals, which amplify and sustain skin inflammation. It is likely that genetic abnormalities affect the constitutive and induced production of mediators by AD keratinocytes through complex patterns involving inflammatory genes themselves and/or signal transduction pathways. A better understanding of the molecular bases of this abnormal behavior may ultimately afford the identification of novel targets for specific and effective therapeutic intervention.

REFERENCES

1. PM Elias, LC Wood, KR Feingold. Epidermal pathogenesis of inflammatory dermatoses. Am J Contact Dermatitis 10:119–126, 1999.
2. JD Bos, MA De Rie. The pathogenesis of psoriasis: immunological facts and speculations. Immunol Today 20:40–46, 1999.
3. M Grewe, CA Bruijnzeel-Koomen, E Schopf, T Thepen, AG Langeveld-Wildschut, T Ruzicka, J Krutmann. A role for Th1 and Th2 cells in the immunopathogenesis of atopic dermatitis. Immunol Today 19:359–361, 1998.

4. C Albanesi, S Pastore, E Fanales-Belasio, G Girolomoni. Cetirizine and hydrocortisone differentially regulate ICAM-1 expression and chemokine release in cultured human keratinocytes. Clin Exp Allergy 28:101–109, 1998.

5. C Albanesi, A Cavani, G Girolomoni. IL-17 is produced by nickel-specific T lymphocytes and regulates ICAM-1 expression and chemokine production in human keratinocytes: synergistic and antagonist effects with IFN-γ and TNF-α. J Immunol 162:494–502, 1999.

6. C Albanesi, A Cavani, G Girolomoni. Interferon-γ-stimulated human keratinocytes express the genes necessary for the production of the peptide-loaded MHC-class II molecule. J Invest Dermatol 110:138–142, 1998.

7. C Traidl, S Sebastiani, C Albanesi, HF Merk, P Puddu, G Girolomoni, A Cavani. Disparate cytotoxic activity of nickel-specific CD8+ and CD4+ T cell subsets against keratinocytes. J Immunol 165:3058–3064, 2000.

8. S Pastore, S Corinti, M La Placa, B Didona, G Girolomoni. Interferon-γ promotes exaggerated cytokine production in keratinocytes cultured from patients with atopic dermatitis. J Allergy Clin Immunol 101:538–544, 1998.

9. C Albanesi, C Scarponi, S Sebastiani, A Cavani, M Federici, O De Pità, P Puddu, G Girolomoni. IL-4 enhances keratinocyte expression of CXCR3 agonistic chemokines. J Immunol 165:1395–1402, 2000.

10. BJ Nickoloff, Y Naidu. Perturbation of epidermal barrier function correlates with initiation of cytokine cascade in human skin. J Am Acad Dermatol 30:535–546, 1994.

11. C Albanesi, C Scarponi, A Cavani, M Federici, F Nasorri, G Girolomoni. Interleukin-17 is produced by both Th1 and Th2 lymphocytes, and modulates interferon-γ- and interleukin-4-induced activation of human keratinocytes. J Invest Dermatol 115:81–87, 2000.

12. DYM Leung. Atopic dermatitis: new insights and opportunities for therapeutic interventions. J Allergy Clin Immunol 105:860–876, 2000.

13. S Pastore, E Fanales-Belasio, C Albanesi, LM Chinni, A Giannetti, G Girolomoni. Granulocyte/macrophage colony-stimulating factor is overproduced by keratinocytes in atopic dermatitis. J Clin Invest 99:3009–3017, 1997.

14. M Marini, E Vittori, J Hollemborg, S Mattoli. Expression of the potent inflammatory cytokines, GM-CSF, IL-6, and IL-8 in bronchial epithelial cells of patients with asthma. J Allergy Clin Immunol 89:1001–1009, 1992.

15. AR Sousa, RN Paston, SJ Lane, J Nakhosteen, TH Lee. Detection of GM-CSF in asthmatic bronchial epithelium and decrease by inhaled corticosteroids. Am Rev Respir Dis 147:1557–1561, 1993.

16. M Nonaka, R Nonaka, M Jordana, J Dolovich. GM-CSF, IL-8, IL-1R, TNF-αR and HLA-DR in nasal epithelial cells in allergic rhinitis. Am J Respir Crit Care Med 153:1675–1681, 1996.

17. MA Calderón, JL Devalia, AJ Prior, RJ Sapsford, RJ Davies. A comparison of cytokine release from epithelial cells cultured from nasal biopsy specimens of atopic patients with and without rhinitis and nonatopic subjects without rhinitis. J Allergy Clin Immunol 99:65–76, 1997.

18. DL Bratton, Q Hamid, M Boguniewicz, DE Doherty, JM Kailey, DYM Leung.

Granulocyte/macrophage colony-stimulating contributes to enhanced monocyte survival in chronic atopic dermatitis. J Clin Invest 95:211–218, 1995.

19. JJ Campbell. The chemokine receptor CCR4 in vascular recognition by cutaneous but not intestinal memory T cells. Nature 400:776–780, 1999.

20. T Imai, M Nagira, S Takagi, M Kakizaki, M Nishimura, J Wang, PW Gray, K Matsushima, O Yoshie. Selective recruitment of CCR4-bearing Th2 cells toward antigen-presenting cells by the CC chemokine thymus and activation-regulated chemokine and macrophage-derived chemokine. Int Immunol 11:81–88, 1999.

21. S Laberge, O Ghaffar, M Boguniewicz, DM Center, DJ Leung, Q Hamid. Association of increased CD4+ T-cell infiltration with increased IL-16 gene expression in atopic dermatitis. J Allergy Clin Immunol 102:645–650, 1998.

22. DM Center, H Kornfeld, WW Cruikshank. Interleukin-16 and its function as a CD4 ligand. Immunol Today 17:476–481, 1996.

23. C Vestergaard, K Bang, B Gesser, H Yoneyama, K Matsushima, C Grønhøj Larsen. A Th2 chemokine, TARC, produced by keratinocytes may recruit CLA+CCR4+ lymphocytes into lesional atopic dermatitis skin. J Invest Dermatol 115:640–646, 2000.

24. M Giustizieri, F Mascia, A Frezzolini, O De Pità, LM Chinni, A Giannetti, G Girolomoni, S Pastore. Keratinocytes from patients with atopic dermatitis and psoriasis show a distinct chemokine production profile in response to T cell-derived cytokines. J Allergy Clin Immunol 107:871–877, 2001.

25. B Homey, W Wang, H Soto, ME Buchanan, A Wiesenborn, D Catron, A Müller, TK McClanahan, M-C Dieu-Nosjean, R Orozco, T Ruzicka, P Lehmann, E Oldham, A Zlotnik. Cutting edge: the orphan chemokine receptor-2 (GPR-2, CCR10) binds the skin associated chemokine CCL27 (CTACK/ALP/ILC). J Immunol 164:3465–3470, 2000.

26. J Morales, B Homey, AP Vicari, S Hudak, E Oldham, J Hedrick, R Orozco, NG Copeland, NA Jenkins, A Zlotnik. CTACK, a skin-associated chemokine that preferentially attracts skin-homing memory T cells. Proc Natl Acad Sci 96:14470–14475, 1999.

27. J-M Schroeder, N Noso, M Sticherling, E Christophers. Role of eosinophil-chemotactic CC chemokines in cutaneous inflammation. J Leukoc Biol 59:1–5, 1996.

28. A Zlotnik, O Yoshie. Chemokines: a new classification and their role in immunity. Immunity 12:121–127, 2000.

29. S Ying, L Taborda-Barata, Q Meng, Humbert, AB Kay. The kinetics of allergen-induced transcription of messenger RNA for monocyte chemotactic protein-3 and RANTES in the skin of human atopic subjects: relationship to eosinophil, T cell, and macrophage recruitment. J Exp Med 181:2153–2159, 1995.

30. RG Nickel, V Casolaro, U Wahn, K Beyer, KC Barnes, BS Plunkett, LR Freidhoff, C Sengler, JR Plitt, RP Schleimer, L Caraballo, RP Naidu, PN Levett, TH Beaty, S-K Huang. Atopic dermatitis is associated with a functional mutation of the promoter of the C-C chemokine RANTES. J Immunol 164:1612–1616, 2000.

31. RA Taha, EM Minshall, DYM Leung, M Boguniewicz, A Luster, S Muro, M Toda, QA Hamid. Evidence for increased expression of eotaxin and monocyte chemotactic protein-4 in atopic dermatitis. J Allergy Clin Immunol 105:1002–1007, 2000.

32. N Yawalkar, M Uguccioni, J Schärer, J Braunwalder, S Karlen, B Dewald, LR Braathen, M Baggiolini. Enhanced expression of eotaxin and CCR3 in atopic dermatitis. J Invest Dermatol 113:43–48, 1999.

33. M Mochizuki, J Bartels, AI Mallet, E Christophers, J-M Schroeder. IL-4 induces eotaxin: a possible mechanism of selective eosinophil recruitment in helminth infection and atopy. J Immunol 160:60–68, 1998.

34. H Petering, R Höchstetter, D Kimming, R Smolarski, A Kapp, J Elsner. Detection of MCP-4 in dermal fibroblasts and its activation of the respiratory burst in human eosinophils. J Immunol 160:555–558, 1998.

35. SJ Ono. Molecular genetics of allergic diseases. Annu Rev Immunol 18:347–366, 2000.

36. S Pastore, ML Giustizieri, F Mascia, A Giannetti, K Kaushansky, G Girolomoni. Dysregulated activation of activatorr protein 1 in keratinocytes of atopic dermatitis patients with enhanced expression of granulocyte/macrophage-colony stimulating factor. J Invest Dermatol 115:1134–1143, 2000.

37. PJ Barnes, IM Adcock. Transcription factors and asthma. Eur Respir J 12:221–234, 1998.

38. VC Foletta, DH Segal, DR Cohen. Transcriptional regulation in the immune system: all roads lead to AP-1. J Leukoc Biol 63:139–152, 1998.

39. SE Rutberg, E Saez, A Glick, AA Dlugosz, BM Spiegelman, SH Yuspa. Differentiation of mouse keratinocytes is accompanied by PKC-dependent changes in AP-1 proteins. Oncogene 13:167–176, 1996.

40. Y Murata, J Ogata, Y Higaki, M Kawashima, Y Yada, K Higuchi, T Tsuchiya, S Kawaminami, G Imokawa. Abnormal expression of sphingomyelin acylase in atopic dermatitis: an etiologic factor for ceramide deficiency? J Invest Dermatol 106:1242–1249, 1996.

41. MJ Jones, AW Murray. Evidence that ceramide selectively inhibits protein kinase C-α translocation and modulates bradykinin activation of phospholipase D. J Biol Chem 270:5007–5013, 1995.

42. D Sampath, M Castro, DC Look, MJ Holtzman. Constitutive activation of epithelial signal transducer and activator of transcription (STAT) pathway in asthma. J Clin Invest 103:1353–1361, 1999.

13
T Cells in Atopic Dermatitis

Thomas Werfel and Alexander Kapp
Hannover Medical University, Hannover, Germany

I. INTRODUCTION

Atopic dermatitis (AD) is a chronic eczematous skin disease, which often begins early in infancy and runs a course of remissions and exacerbations. T lymphocytes, which represent the majority of skin-infiltrating cells, play a prominant role in this skin disease (1–4). A number of studies point to the fact that AD may be a systemic disease which is reflected by some abnormalities of T-lymphocyte numbers and circulation functions.

II. T LYMPHOCYTES IN PERIPHERAL BLOOD

Patients suffering from AD have increased levels of activated circulating T cells and increased levels of L-selectin and the secretory IL-2R, which are markers for lymphocyte activation and which correlate with disease severity (5–8). In addition, Wu et al. (9) recently described a significant reduction of the telomere length in all T-cell subsets from atopic dermatitis patients compared with normal individuals. The authors concluded that the increased telomerase activity and shortened telomere length indicates that T lymphocytes in atopic dermatitis are chronically stimulated and have an increased cell turnover in vivo (9).

The number of CD4+ cells is increased, and CD8+ suppressor/cytotoxic lymphocytes are decreased in peripheral blood. However, psychological stress has recently been shown to lead to significantly higher increases in the number of circulating CD8+ T lymphocytes in AD patients compared to healthy controls (10).

The role of CD8+ T cells is not well defined for atopic dermatitis yet. It it has been shown, however, that CD8+ T cells that had been isolated from the circulation expressing the skin-homing molecule cutaneous lymphocyte-associated antigen (CLA) are as potent as CLA + CD4+ T cells in induction of IgE and enhancement of eosinophil survival, which suggests that these cells have more than bystander functions in AD (11).

III. HISTOLOGY AND IMMUNOHISTOLOGY OF AD: PREDOMINANCE OF SKIN-INFILTRATING T CELLS

The skin lesions of AD are histologically characterized by an infiltration of lymphocytes, monocytes/macrophages, fully granulated mast cells, eosinophils, dermal dendritic cells, and epidermal Langerhans cells (12,13). Cells of mononuclear lineages predominate in skin lesions. Mononuclear cells and eosinophil granulocytes can be found mainly in the dermis (14–16), Langerhans cells with specific IgE bound to FcεRI on their surface in the epidermis (17,18).

The mononuclear infiltrate in lesional skin of atopic dermatitis is similar to that of allergic contact dermatitis, a T-cell–mediated allergic skin disease characterized by a delayed-type hypersensitivity (DTH) reaction, when stained with immunohistochemical techniques. CD4+ T-helper cells dominate the cellular infiltrate in atopic dermatitis (1,19). The CD4/CD8 ratio of dermis infiltrating T cells is similar to that in peripheral blood.

Many intralesional T cells show signs of activation as defined by the membrane expression of IL-2Rα and HLA-DR molecules (2). T cells invading lesional skin in AD can further be distinguished by CD45R0, a marker of T-memory cells suggesting a previous encounter with antigen or allergen (20), and by CLA (21). CLA defines the subset of skin-homing T cells that binds to E-selectin, an adhesion molecule expressed by endothelial cells in inflamed tissues during the first step of leukocyte extravasation (22–24).

IV. T-CELL CYTOKINES IN ATOPIC DERMATITIS: GENERAL ASPECTS

Activated T lymphocytes secrete a variety of cytokines, which have effects on the inflammatory reaction in lesional skin. An important cytokine (probably a major target of anti-inflammatory drugs like corticosteroids or macrolactams) is interleukin (IL)-2. IL-2 is a very efficient activator of surrounding resting T lymphocytes, which may perpetuate the local cellular reaction. It may increase the clinical reaction since intradermal injection of this cytokine can cause intense pruritus (25). In contrast to findings in murine systems, the production of IL-2 is not restricted to Th1 lymphocytes in human beings. Th1 and Th2 cytokines have been investigated in great detail in AD during the last 10 years. Th1 cells are defined by the secretion mainly of IFN-γ in men. In contrast, Th2 cells are defined by the production of IL-4, IL-5, and/or IL-13. Both T-cell subsets secrete IL-3 and GM-CSF in addition to IL-2 (2). A major function of the Th2 cytokine IL-4 is displayed on B lymphocytes: IL-4 functions as an IgE isotype switching factor on these cells (26). Moreover, it upregulates important membrane molecules such as CD40, IL-4R, and CD23 on B cells (2,3). The analysis of mitogen and allergen-stimulated T cells from peripheral blood demonstrated a dysregulation of IL-4 and IFN-γ secretion with an overproduction of IL-4 in patients suffering from AD (27,28).

V. Th1 AND Th2 CYTOKINES IN LESIONAL SKIN

Th1 and Th2 cytokines may contribute to the pathogenesis of local skin inflammation in AD, with the relative contribution of each cytokine dependent on the duration of the skin lesion. In previous studies, the majority of allergen-specific T cells derived from skin lesions that had been provoked in patients with the extrinsic variant of AD by epicutaneous application of inhalant allergens was found to produce predominantly Th2 cytokines such as IL-4 or IL-5. This was considered to be a specific feature reflecting immune dysregulation in AD (29,30). Polarized type 2 cytokine patterns were confined to atopy patch test sites since allergen-specific T cells in the blood of the same patients secreted both type 1 and type 2 cytokines (29). Later, allergen-specific T-cell clones from spontaneous AD lesions showed that these cells differ from allergen-specific T cells isolated from inhalant allergen patch test lesions by virtue of their capacity to produce IFN-γ as well (31). This study extended previous findings at the mRNA level as well as at the protein level, which had shown shown that expression of IFN-γ rather than of IL-4 predominates in spontaneous or older patch test lesions in AD (32,33). Importantly, treatment of patients that resulted in improvement of lesions has been correlated with downregulation of IFN-γ expression in the skin, but not of IL-4 (32).

IFN-γ may have a number of profound effects on the perpetuation and enhancement of the inflammatory reaction in the skin in atopic dermatitis (e.g., induction of MHC class I and class II molecules, of adhesion molecules such as ICAM-1, induction of cytotoxic responses) (2). A recent observation pointed out that IFN-γ–secreting T lymphocytes induce apoptosis in keratinocytes by first upregulating the FAS receptor on these cells and then delivering a lethal hit via the FAS ligand, which is either expressed on the membrane of skin-infiltrating

T cells or secreted by these cells. Keratinocyte apoptosis was demonstrated in situ in lesional skin, in normal human and in a cultured skin-equivalent, which was exposed to activated T cells (34).

VI. FACTORS CONTRIBUTING TO THE Th1 OR TO THE Th2 MILIEU IN AD

A number of factors may be involved in the switch from Th2 to Th1 in older lesions. IL-12 appears to be a predominant mediator (Fig. 1). This molecule has recently been found to be produced not only by constitutive cells (e.g., keratinocytes, dendritic cells, dermal macrophages) of the skin but also by eosinophils, an effector cell population actively involved in the eczematous skin reaction (35). The reason for the relative lack of expression of IL-12 shown on the mRNA level by in situ hybridization in acute skin lesions (36) is not completely understood.

In vitro induction of IL-12 in resting monocytes requires two signals: a "priming signal," which can be delivered by IFN-γ or GM-CSF, and "second signal," which can be provided by a wide range of substances (e.g., TNF-α, CD40 ligand, or LPS). Recent findings showed that the incubation of resting (unprimed) cells with substances of the latter group leads to an inability of these cells to respond to further stimulation with an expression of IL-12, probably via an intracellular ERK-dependant signal-transducing pathway (37,38). One may therefore speculate that infiltrating CD40L+ T cells act as a second signal and lead to a refractory state of constitutive cells in the skin with respect to IL-12 production at the beginning of an eczematous skin reaction (38).

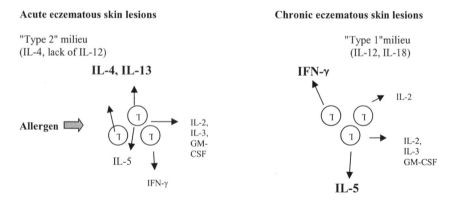

Figure 1 Cytokine pattern in acute versus chronic eczematous skin lesions.

IL-18 is another cytokine that functions in parallel to IL-12 and which is probably involved in the switch of the cytokine pattern towards Th1 during chronification of AD (39). This cytokine activates the IFN-γ promotor at an activator protein-1–binding site (40). Little is known yet about the expression of IL-18 in acute versus chronic skin.

The molecule that is the strongest inducer of a type 2 cytokine milieu is IL-4 itself. This cytokine is produced by skin-infiltrating T cells, but it may also come from mast cells, basophils, or eosinophils during an eczematous skin reaction. The high frequency of IL-4–producing T cells in the skin is not necessarily associated with atopy since mRNA for IL-4 and T cells expressing IL-4 are found in nickel-induced patch test reactions as well (41–43). Thus, IL-4 secretion seems to be related to this particular type of skin lesion (i.e., patch test lesion or acute eczema).

In acute eczema IL-4 may induce a variety of local responses such as the induction of the adhesion molecule VCAM-1 on endothelial cells or of Fc receptors on eosinophils. A recent finding which may be important for the regulation of the local cutaneous inflammatory reaction is the induction of apoptosis in eosinophils by IL-4 (44), which is otherwise delayed in AD (45). Importantly, IL-4 inhibits the expression of the IL-12β2 subunit on T cells, which is the binding and signal-transducing component of the IL-12 receptor (46). Furthermore, IL-4 as well as proinflammatory cytokines like IL-1, tumor necrosis factor (TNF), and interferons may stimulate the production of eotaxin (47), which is involved in the chemoattraction of eosinophils and possibly of Th2 lymphocytes.

In conclusion, many findings suggest a compartimentalization of IL-4 production in acute eczematous reactions irrespective of the nature of the allergen (i.e., environmental protein or haptenized protein) provoking cutaneous eczema in humans. There seem to be variations in the kinetics of the expression of Th2 cytokines in acute versus chronic lesions, as the number of IL-5–expressing cells increases during chronification (48). The rise in IL-5 expression during the transition from acute to chronic AD likely plays a role in the prolongation of eosinophil survival and function (45,49).

Other cytokines that are differentially expressed in acute versus chronic AD skin lesions are summarized in Table 1 (36,48). Interstingly, the expression of some these cytokines is paralleld by their corresponding cytokine receptors in acute versus chronic skin lesions (50).

VII. MECHANISM OF ADHESION OF T CELLS IN AD

Lymphocytes circulate through three different types of compartments in the human body that can be divided into primary, secondary, and tertiary lymphoid organs. In order to arrive in these organs the lymphocytes express adhesion mole-

Table 1 Expression of Cytokines and Cytokine Receptors
in Acute Versus Chronic Lesions of Atopic Dermatitis

	Acute skin lesion	Chronic skin lesion
Cytokines		
IL-4	+ +	−
IL-5	+	+ +
IL-12[a]	−	+ +
IL-16	+ +	+
IFN-y	+	+ +
GM-CSF	+	+ +
Cytokine receptors		
IL4R-α	+ +	+
IL5R-α	+	+ +
GM-CSFR-α	+	+ +

[a] Not produced by T cells.
Source: Refs. 29–33, 36, 48.

cules which are more or less specific for the target organ. The mechanism of
lymphocyte invasion into the tissues is thought to resemble that of monocytes and
neutrophils, being a multistep process involving attachment and rolling through
selectin-carbohydrate interactions, activation through chemoattractant-receptor
interactions, and firm adhesion through intergrin-immunoglobulin family interactions (24).

More than 80% of skin-infiltrating T lymphocytes express the CLA molecule (21). This molecule has been intensively studied with respect to inflammatory skin responses in men during the last years. The CLA epitope is characterized
by specific binding to a monoclonal antibody named HECA-452 (21). CLA consists of a sialyl Lewis-x carbohydrate and corresponds to a posttranslational modification of the P-selectin glycoprotein ligand 1 (51). CLA expression is dependent
on the activity of α(1,3)-fucosyltransferase (FucT-VII), which is critical in the
fucosylation needed for the functional E-selectins (52). With respect to AD the
expression of CLA has been found to be regulated through superantigen induction
of IL-12, which is probably also mediated through 1,3-fucosyltransferase VII
(53). IL-12 and/or staphylococcal superantigen stimulation upregulated CLA expression on Th2 in a recent study. On stimulation with IL-12, CLA was expressed
also on the surface of T-cell clones, which represented non–skin-related antigen-
specific T cells, which suggests that skin-selective homing is not restricted to
functional and phenotypic T-cell subsets (54).

Santamaria Babi et al. (23), who investigated proliferative responses to allergens by circulating T-lymphocyte subpopulations, observed a mite-specific response in AD patients sensitized to house dust mite dependent on the subset expressing CLA. In contrast, in sensitized patients with allergic asthma bronchial house dust mite–dependent proliferation was found in the CLA-negative subset (23). This observation points to an immunological mechanism which may target allergen-specific T cells to the skin in AD. CLA+ T cells isolated from the circulation showed signs of in vivo activation such as the expression of CD25, CD40 ligand, or HLA-DR. Intracellular cytokine staining immediately after purification revealed that these cells contain high amounts of IL-13 and IL-5 but only small amounts of IL-4 or IFN-γ (55).

Besides the interaction between CLA and E-selectin, additional binding between VLA-4 and VCAM-1 and between LFA-1 and ICAM-1 are necessary for the migration of T-memory cells across activated endothelium into the skin (56).

VIII. THE ROLE OF T-CELL–ATTRACTING MOLECULES AND THEIR REGULATION IN AD

Chemokines are small proteins that play a major role in controlling leukocyte trafficking (57,58). They are divided into subgroups according to a cystein-cystein motif with varying numbers of amino acids between the cystein residues; thus there are four subgroups: CC, CXC, CX3C, and C. The receptors for the chemokines are subdivided in the same manner- CCR1-9, CXCR1-5, and CX3CR1 (59).

Recently it has been demonstrated that the chemokine receptors are expressed in a specific manner between Th1-type and Th2-type lymphocytes, with CCR5 and CXCR3 preferentially being expressed on Th1-type lymphocytes and CCR3, CCR4 and CCR8 on Th2-type lymphocytes (60–62). However, the selective expression of these receptors on Th2 cells still is a matter of debate since CCR4 was reported to be expressed on activated Th1 cells as well (63), and we and others were unable to find significant higher binding of anti-CCR3 antibodies to well established IL-4–secreting T-cell clones (unpublished observations). Nevertheless, there are some well-controlled observations that suggest that these receptors may indeed be involved in chemoattraction of T cells into lesional skin of AD.

Vestergaard et al. recently found that in the peripheral blood of AD patients there is a significant upregulation of CLA+CCR4+ cells compared with normal controls (64). It has been shown that in peripheral blood the lymphocytes expressing CCR4 include all the cells expressing CLA and a subset of other systemic memory lymphocytes, but not intestinal T lymphocytes ($\alpha 4\beta 7+$) (65). In addition, the staining of serial sections of skin biopsies from AD patients demonstrated that the lymphocytes invading the dermis or the epidermis are CCR4+. As thymus and activation-regulated chemokine (TARC) induces chemotaxis of CCR4+ cells (62), these results indicate that TARC may be an important chemoattractant for the CLA + CCR4+ cells and thereby skin-homing lymphocytes in AD. The CC chemokine TARC is an 8 kDa chemokine, which has been found to be expressed by dendritic cells differentiated from monocytes with granulocyte-macrophage colony-stimulating factor, IL-3, and IL-4 (66). Other recent studies showed that (1) TARC is produced in endothelial cells of the venules of chronic inflamed human skin (65), (2) TARC is produced abundantly in the basal keratinocytes of lesional skin in a murine model of AD (67), and (3) TARC can be produced by a keratinocytic cell line and possibly by keratinocytes in human skin (64).

Eotaxin, a CC chemokine, is a potent chemoattractant and activator of eosinophils and basophils (49,58,68). Recent reports suggest that it also an attractant for Th2 lymphocytes (61,69). Eotaxin is produced by various cell types including eosinophils, lymphocytes, macrophages, chondrocytes, fibroblasts, smooth muscle cells, and endothelial and epithelial cells (59). The activities of eotaxin are mediated by binding to the chemokine receptor CCR3, which has been been found on eosinophils, basophils, dendritic cells, and Th2 lymphocytes (61,68–70). Besides influencing eosinophil recruitment and activation, eotaxin may thus contribute to the selective infiltration of Th2 subsets in acute lesional as well as nonlesional AD skin. A marked enhancement of CCR3 mRNA and immunoreactivity was detected in nonlesional AD skin as compared with normal skin. This led to the suggestion that activation of CCR3-positive cells, especially in nonlesional AD skin, may trigger the development of eczematous lesions. As shown by the analysis of consecutive sections, the pattern of eotaxin and CCR3 immunoreactivity partly corresponded to that of CD3+ cells (71).

A recently described CC chemokine, cutaneous T-cell–attracting chemokine (CTACK/CCL 27), which is produced in the skin of both humans and mice, attracts a subset of the CLA+ memory T cells (72). The CTACK receptor was named CRP-2 or CCR10, and it appears that this molecule is prefentially expressed on CLA+ cells (73).

The CLA+ subset of memory T cells also expresses CCR6 (74), and many skin-infiltrating cells were also found to be CCR6+ in a recent study (75). The authors also found that immunostaining of LARC/CCL20, a ligand of CCR6, was weak in normal skin tissues but strongly augmented in lesional skin tissues with atopic dermatitis. The authors concluded that epidermal keratinocytes produce LARC/CCL20 upon stimulation with proinflammatory cytokines and attract CCR6-expressing memory/effector T cells into the dermis of inflamed skin of atopic dermatitis (75).

There is some evidence for degradation of the complement component C3 (which can be produced by human keratinocytes and macrophages in human skin) in eczematous skin lesions, which leads to the deposition of C3 fragments at the basement membrane (76,77) and probably to the generation of the chemotactic small C3a fragment. In a recent study we investigated the expression of the high-affinity receptor for C3a (C3aR) in human T lymphocytes using receptor-specific antibodies (78). C3aR expression was detected in CD4(+) and CD8(+) blood- or skin-derived T-cell clones from birch pollen–sensitized patients with atopic dermatitis. No significant difference in C3aR expression in CD4(+) or CD8(+) TCCs was observed. In contrast to C3a(desArg), C3a led to a transient calcium flux in TCCs expressing the C3aR, whereas C3aR-negative TCCs were unreactive. Circulating T cells from patients suffering from severe atopic dermatitis and other inflammatory skin diseases expressed the C3aR, whereas no expression of C3aR was found in unstimulated T lymphocytes from patients with mild inflammatory skin diseases or from healthy individuals. Type I IFNs were identified as upregulators of C3aR expression in vitro in freshly isolated or cloned T lymphocytes (78). These data point to a possible biological function of the chemoattractant C3a in atopic dermatitis.

Moreover, it has been shown that IL-8 induces transendothelial migration of CLA+ T cells (79). IL-16, a chemoattractant for CD4+ T cells, was also found to be highly expressed in acute in comparison to chronic AD skin lesions (80). In summary, these results demonstrate that the process of attracting CLA+ T cells into the skin is complicated and complex and that overlapping signals rather than a single signal could be responsible for the attraction of T cells.

IX. ALLERGEN SPECIFICITY OF T CELLS IN AD

The contribution of aeroallergens to the pathogenesis of AD has been extensively studied. In addition to immediate reactions, many patients react to aeroallergen after epicutaneous application with a late eczematous skin lesions (81,82). These resemble histopathologically delayed-type hypersensitivity reactions similar to allergic contact dermatitis (83).

From the model of the so-called atopy patch test (i.e., a patch test with aeroallergens in AD), experimental evidence was provided that Langerhans cells are able to present allergen to T cells via IgE bound on high-affinity receptors for IgE (18,84).

Proliferative responses can often be elicited in blood lymphocytes with inhalant allergens, which indicates the presence of a specific T-cell–mediated hypersensitivity in AD. The clinical relevance of these findings was confirmed by the observation that proliferative responses to these antigens are significantly higher in patients with positive patch test reactions to the corresponding allergens than in nonreactive patients with AD (85). As described above, an allergen-specific response was observed in patients with AD in the subset expressing the skin-homing molecule CLA (23,86,87), which points to an immunological mechanism that targets allergen-specific T cells to the skin in AD. Direct evidence for the presence of skin-infiltrating, inhalant allergen-specific T cells in AD came from the analysis of T-cell clones (TCC), which had been generated from biopsies of patch test lesions (29,30) and later from spontaneous lesions (31) in AD.

Bohle et al. investigated T-cell lines and clones that had been established within a period of up to 4 years from the same patients with AD (88). With the help of a T-cell–tracing protocol in which oligonucleotides specific for the TCR β-chain hypervariable junctional region were used as tools to identify each particular TCC, they demonstrated that some pollen- and house dust mite–specific TCC with a Th2-like cytokine production pattern in vitro could be identified as long-lived memory T cells in vivo. They concluded that allergen-specific TCC can persist for years and provided evidence for this finding both in blood and in the skin of atopic dermatitis.

Besides inhalant allergens, foods are well-established trigger factors of atopic dermatitis. There are now some studies addressing the role of food-specific T lymphocytes in these patients.

The expansion of peripheral blood derived CLA+ T cells in response to casein was described for children with milk-induced eczema, which directly points to an involvement of food-specific T lymphocytes in a subgroup of children with atopic dermatitis (86). In addition, we observed significant differences in the proliferative response of blood lymphocytes between patients who reacted to milk with worsening of atopic dermatitis and control groups and were able to generate casein-specific T-cell clones from the blood of these patients (89–92). Higher proliferative responses to casein—the major protein fraction in cow's milk and thus the main protein source in the alimentation of many human beings—were observed both in atopic children and in adults reacting with worsening of eczema to oral provocation. Whereas casein-specific TCC displayed a Th2 cytokine pattern in milk-response children with atopic dermatitis, casein-specific TCC from adolescents or adults were found to express a Th1 cytokine pattern in our studies (89,91).

Schade et al. (93) used an antigen-specific culturing system with autologous B cells as antigen-presenting cells to establish cow's milk protein-specific T-cell clones derived from PBMCs in infants with AD in a recent study. Analysis of antigen-specific cytokine production confirmed that the response was Th2 skewed in infants with cow's milk allergy. In contrast, infants with atopic dermatitis but without cow's milk allergy had a Th1-skewed response, with high levels of IFN-γ and low levels of IL-4, IL-5, and IL-13. The authors concluded that food allergy in infants with AD is associated with production of Th2 cytokines by circulating antigen-specific CD4+ T cells, whereas tolerance to food antigens is associated with low levels of these cytokines in infants (93).

The immune responses to casein were further studied with cultured PBMC and dermal lymphocytes from adult patients reacting to cow's milk with a deterioration of eczema using a limiting dilution protocol. The average frequencies of proliferating T lymphocytes both from peripheral blood and lesional skin were in the same range when casein or an extract of *Der.p.* was added to the cultures (91,92). A food (peanut allergen)–specific T-cell response was also described for lesional skin in an infant suffering from from AD (94).

The role of foods that cross-react with birch pollen allergens was investigated in adolescents and adults with atopic dermatitis who were highly sensitized to birch pollen antigens (87). In contrast to the majority of birch pollen–sensitized individuals, these patients belonged to the group of one third of all sensitized patients who did not suffer from immediate symptoms to birch pollen–related foods. They did therefore not maintain a birch pollen–related elimination diet prior to this study. A subpopulation of the birch pollen–sensitized patients reacted with a marked deterioration of their eczema upon oral provocation with pollen-related foods, and this clinical reaction was associated with a specific T-cell–mediated immune response to birch pollen antigens: the rate of CLA+ blood lymphocytes from food-responsive patients—but not from nonresponders—increased significantly upon in vitro stimulation with birch pollen antigens. Frequency analysis revealed higher growth rates of lymphocytes in limiting dilution assays in the presence of birch pollen antigens when skin-derived lymphocytes from responders were compared to cells from nonresponders. Finally, the proportion of specific T-cell clones generated from limiting dilution cultures of the skin was significantly higher when we compared cells from reactive patients to cells from nonreactive patients (87).

X. THE ROLE OF AUTOANTIGENS, STAPHYLOGENIC PROTEINS, AND *PITYROSPORUM OVALE*

By the use of limiting dilution cultures, allergen-specific T cells have been shown to represent only a minority (1–5%) of infiltrating T cells in lesional skin (29,31). Therefore, other factors that lead to the activation of T cells at the site of inflammation are probably involved in the pathogenesis of atopic dermatitis.

A. T-Cell Responses to Autoantigens

Several studies have shown that human skin dander can trigger immediate hypersensitivity reactions in the skin of patients with AD, which suggests an IgE-dependent immune reaction. In 1963, a proliferative response to human skin extracts was reported by Hashem et al. (95). Valenta et al. (96) reported that the majority of sera from patients with severe AD contain IgE antibodies directed against human proteins. This group cloned some autoantigens that they detected in IgE immune complexes of AD sera. Although the autoantigen-specific T-cell response has not been characterized, these findings may lead to the hypothesis that T-cell–mediated responses to autoantigens are involved in the maintenance of chronic inflammatory skin reactions in AD patients with low or absent specific responses to conventional allergens (96).

B. T-Cell Responses to Staphylogenic Proteins

Infections with *Staphylococcus aureus* have been studied extensively as possible trigger factors of AD. These bacteria can be detected on the skin of more than 90% of all AD patients (97,98). Exotoxines are detectable in up to two thirds of all cultures containing *S. aureus* generated from skin swabs in AD (99). Both autologous and allogeneic and even xenogeneic antigen-presenting cells are able to stimulate up to 25% of the T-cell pool in the presence of superantigens, which are strong mitogens even at a concentration of 10^{-10} M (100). On the other hand, a "conventional" allergen that undergoes classical antigen presentation may stimulate about 0.1% of allergen-specific T cells in a MHC-restricted fashion via their T-cell receptors.

Different pathways of T-lymphocyte activation may be involved after stimulation with different concentrations of exotoxins in patients with atopic dermatitis. The influence of exotoxins on T-cell proliferation and production of lymphokines seems to be dependent on their concentration. In the nanogram range and more, TSST-1 induces a strong proliferation of PBMC with an increase in IFN-γ secretion and consequently causes an inhibition of the synthesis of total IgE. At picogram and femtogram concentrations, TSST-1 leads to lower IFN-γ production and promotes polyclonal B-cell activation via bridging the TCR and the MHC class II on B cells with an increase in total IgE (101). In a humanized SCID mouse model, where hu-PBMC were administered intraperitoneally followed by an intradermal injection of autologous PBMC, the epidermal application of both SEB (50 ng) and mite allergens together elicited a profound dermal and epidermal inflammation, whereas the application of SEB alone resulted in a weaker inflammation. Mite allergens alone had no effect, although the donor was sensitized to mites. Intraperitoneal application of SEB and mite allergen together resulted in an inhibition of total and specific IgE synthesis of peritoneal PBMC (102). These data indicate that exotoxins at higher concentrations induce a strong proliferation of T cells and favor a Th1-like cytokine profile.

Different groups have shown that exotoxins can exacerbate cutaneous lesions of atopic dermatitis acting as superantigens. T cells of patients with atopic dermatitis expressing certain TCR-Vβ chains are activated upon incubation with staphylococcal superantigens in the skin. Strickland et al. demonstrated that colonization with toxigenic *S. aureus* strains is associated with an expansion of T cells expressing the appropriate TCR-Vβ chains among the CLA+ T-cell subsets in the peripheral blood (103). Similarly, patients with active atopic dermatitis had a higher percentage of cells positive for the TCR Vβ2 and Vβ5.1 in the CLA+, but not in the CLA− subset. Furthermore, the authors found an increased proportion of HLA-DR+ cells in the compartment expressing CLA and TCR Vβ5.1 in patients with active atopic dermatitis (104). Leung et al. demonstrated that staphylococcal exotoxins were able to upregulate the expression of the cutaneous homing receptor CLA on normal PBMC by induction of IL-12. Furthermore, selective TCR Vβ-chains were induced (53). These findings indicate that exotoxins may contribute to the pathogenesis of atopic dermatitis by increasing the frequency of superantigen-reactive T cells able to migrate to AD lesions.

In some patients with atopic dermatitis, preferential expression of certain TCR Vβ chains were also found in lesional skin. The pattern of TCR Vβ expression was heterogeneous among patients and were related to different exotoxins in one patient (105). Neuber et al. found that most of the T cells detected in lesional skin were TCR Vβ3+, and PBMC from patients with atopic dermatitis showed a significantly higher proliferation and IL-5 secretion than healthy individuals after stimulation with monoclonal antibodies against TCR Vβ3 and TCR Vβ8 (106).

A shift in the intradermal TCR-Vβ repertoire corresponding to the respective superantigen was found in lesional skin of children with atopic dermatitis by immunohistochemical staining (107). Skin biopsy specimens obtained from SEB-treated areas demonstrated a selective accumulation of T cells expressing staphylococcal enterotoxin B (SEB)–reactive TCR-Vβ elements in patients with atopic dermatitis and healthy individuals (108). Different groups showed that disease activity in children colonized with toxigenic *S. aureus* strains is higher than in patients colonized with nontoxigenic strains, which underlines the clinical importance of these data (107,109).

In addition, superantigens might enhance the specific T-cell response to aeroallergens in patients with atopic dermatitis by the recruitment of superantigen-reactive T cells bearing the appropriate TCR-Vβ elements in the skin, which are specific to aeroallergens.

Leung et al. (110) first proposed that superantigens may exacerbate AD by acting as a new group of allergens, since specific IgE to SEA, SEB, and TSST-1 could be detected in the sera from 57% of AD patients, most of whom were identified as carriers of toxigenic *S. aureus* strains. Basophils of these patients were found to release histamine upon incubation with the respective toxin, which points to a functional role of these antibodies in patients with atopic dermatitis (110).

Recently we showed that adults suffering from atopic dermatitis who are sensitized to the SEB have a higher disease activity as assessed clinically and by determination of eosinophil protein mediators in serum and urine as in vitro parameters of inflammation (111). Our results are concordant with the findings of Nomura et al., who demonstrated a correlation between IgE anti-SEB levels and severity of atopic dermatitis in children and adolescents (112). Additionally, Bunikowski et al. found a relationship between a sensitization to staphylococcal enterotoxins A and B, found in 34% of children with atopic dermatitis, and the severitity of atopic dermatitis (113). One can speculate that staphyloccal exotoxins may exacerbate skin lesions in atopic dermatitis through the same mechanism that is now widely accepted for inhalant allergens: the presence of exotoxins on the skin could lead to a release of proinflammatory mediators from cutaneous mast cells and a subsequent pruritus and scratching. Perhaps more importantly, the toxins may bind to specific IgE on the surface of Langerhans cells, thus leading to a facilitated allergen presentation and to the activation of eotaxin-specific T lymphocytes.

In a recent publication Campbell et al. demonstrated that children under 7 years with atopic dermatitis more frequently have IgG antibodies to SEB—and thus a T-cell–dependent specific immune response—than normal controls. In addition, atopic children have higher levels of SEB-specific IgG than controls (114). This suggests that the increased titers of SEB-specific IgG are caused by increased superantigen exposure, i.e., colonization with SEB-producing strains.

To investigate the extent to which staphylococcal exotoxins activate T cells as superantigens or as allergens, we generated exotoxin-reactive T-cell lines (TCL) from lesional skin and blood of adult patients who suffered from a long-standing severe atopic dermatitis and who were colonized with exotoxin-reactive *S. aureus* strains. We not only found a superantigen-mediated T-cell response but also an allergen-specific T-cell response to staphylococcal exotoxins in TCL from lesional skin and blood of patients with atopic dermatitis, who were colonized with toxigenic *S. aureus* strains (K. Breuer et al., unpublished).

C. T-Cell Responses to *Pityrosporum ovale*

In addition to *S. aureus*, the saprophyte *Pityrosporum ovale* is believed to elicit a specific immune response and thus provoke eczema in the face and neck of AD patients (115). The yeast *Malassezia furfur*, also known as *Pityrosporum orbiculare (ovale)*, is part of the normal microflora of the human skin but has also been associated with different skin diseases, including atopic dermatitis. More than 50% of atopic dermatitis patients have positive skin tests and specific IgE to *M. furfur* extracts. However, the pathophysiological role of these IgE-mediated reactions in the development of the disease remains unknown. An enhanced lymphocyte proliferative response to *P. ovale* antigens was detected in

AD patients with manifestations of the skin disease in the above localizations, and specific T-cell clones could be established from lesional skin of these patients (116). A number of allergens from *Pityrosporum ovale* have now been selectively cloned, which will enable studies of specific T-cell responses in more detail (117).

XI. COMPARISON OF T-LYMPHOCYTE CHARACTERISTICS IN INTRINSIC VERSUS EXTRINSIC AD

AD is most often associated with the existence of environmental-allergen specific IgE. This variant is now often called the ''extrinsic'' form of AD. As described above, there is increasing evidence that T-cell responses to environmental allergens are important for the pathogenesis of AD. Elevated IgE was, however, found only in 60–80% of all AD patients, which is therefore not a strong prerequisite of atopic dermatitis (118,119).

The extrinsic variant of AD has been differentiated from an ''intrinsic'' variant, which has been found in 20% of diseases with the typical clinical appearance of AD but without specific IgE in studies of the 1970s and 1980s. Recent data from Schäfer et al., coming from a multicenter cross-sectional study of approximately 4,000 5–6-year-old preschool children, point to a dramatic increase in the intrinsic type of AD: only 50.4% of children with eczema in West Germany and 36.5% of diseased children in East Germany reacted positively in skin prick tests to conventional allergens (120). Although the intrinsic variant is defined by the lack of environmental or food-specific IgE, it might be associated with circulating and skin-infiltrating T lymphocytes expressing a distinct functional phenotype.

The rate of positive patch test reactions to inhalant allergens such as house dust mite has not yet been determined in a sufficiently large group of patients with intrinsic-type AD, and no data are available about putative allergen-specific T cells in the intrinsic variant so far. Previous studies have, however, consistently found small subpopulations of AD patients reacting to inhalant allergens in patch tests without displaying a specific IgE response to these allergens (82,85).

In previous studies applying oral provocation tests in adult AD patients, no correlation between specific lymphocyte proliferation and specific IgE was found (91). A lack of correlation between specific IgE and the clinical response to food has been reported for food-responsive AD (121,122). This indicates that an IgE-independent mechanism may be involved in the eczematous reacton to food in some patients stressing the pathophysiological role of allergen-specific T lymphocytes in AD and a putative role of T- cell–mediated food-specific reactions also in the intrinsic type of AD.

Akdis et al. (123) showed that the staphylococcal superantigen SEB induces a significant proliferation of T lymphocytes derived from lesional skin of patients with both the extrinsic and the intrinsic form of atopic dermatitis in a dose-dependent manner. In contrast to T lymphocytes derived from the skin of patients with the extrinsic form of AD, cells from patients with intrinsic AD failed to produce significant amounts of IL-13 upon incubation with SEB, which would therefore be unable to offer help to B cells to produce specific IgE in these patients (123). The characterization of the cytokine pattern of skin- infiltrating cells further showed that IL-4 is not secreted by skin-infiltrating T lymphocytes in both types of AD. In contrast, IL-5 was found to be expressed in both the intrinsic and extrinsic types of AD. Skin-derived T lymphocytes from the intrinsic type of AD generally expressed lower IL-13 than T cells from the extrinsic type, which points to a different immune mechanism in the skin in spite of the common clinical morphology of the different variants of AD (123).

A lack of IL-4 but a high IL-5 secretion of blood lymphocytes from patients with the intrinsic variant of AD was described by Kägi et al. (124). High IL-5 production may well explain the blood eosinophilia and the delayed apoptosis of blood eosinophils observable in both variants of the disease (45). In addition

Table 2 Immunological Findings in Intrinsic and Extrinsic Variants of AD

Parameter	Intrinsic variant	Extrinsic variant
Blood		
IgE	normal	⇑⇑
Eosinophils	⇑⇑	⇑⇑
Survival of eosinophils	⇑⇑	⇑⇑
Soluble IL-2R	⇑⇑	⇑⇑
CD4+ T lymphocytes	⇑	⇑
HLA DR+ lymphocytes	⇑	⇑
IL-2R+ lymphocytes	⇑	⇑
CD23+ B lymphocytes	—	⇑
IL-4–secreting T cells	—	⇑
IL-5–secreting T cells	⇑	⇑
IL-13–secreting T cells	⇑	⇑
IFN-γ–secreting T cells	⇑	⇑
Skin (spontaneous lesions)		
IL-4–secreting T cells	—	—
IL-5–secreting T cells	⇑	⇑
IL-13–secreting T cells	⇑	⇑⇑
IFN-γ–secreting T cells	⇑	⇑

to IL-5 secretion, Kägi et al. found a similar activation pattern of IL-2R+ and HLA DR+ blood lymphocytes in both forms of AD (124). The only membrane molecule of circulating lymphocytes that was exclusively increased in the extrinsic variant of AD was the (IL-4–regulated) low-affinity Fc receptor for IgE (CD23) on B lymphocytes. Table 2 summarizes some immunological findings in the intrinsic and the extrinsic variants of AD (123–127).

Immunohistological studies on skin-infiltrating cells in both variants of AD revealed that the majority of the cells represented CLA+CD4+ and CD8+ cells, suggesting an important role for T cells in both groups (122). The CD4/CD8 ratios between blood and skin appeared to be similar, suggesting that both CD4+ and CD8+ T subpopulations are equally recruited into the inflammatory sites of both variants.

Future studies should elucidate whether allergen-specific, superantigen- or auto-reactive T lymphocytes are sufficient to elevate eczematous reactions in the absence of specific IgE or whether other factors play a major role in the etiopathology of this variant of AD.

REFERENCES

1. A Kapp. Atopic dermatitis—the skin manifestation of atopy. Clin Exp Allergy 25: 210–219, 1995.
2. U Herz, R Bunikowski, H Renz. Role of T cells in atopic dermatitis. New aspects on the dynamics of cytokine production and the contribution of bacterial superantigens. Int Arch Allergy Immunol 115:179–190, 1998.
3. DY Leung. Atopic dermatitis: new insights and opportunities for therapeutic intervention. J Allergy Clin Immunol 105:860–876, 2000.
4. T Werfel, A Kapp. Environmental and other major provocation factors in atopic dermatitis. Allergy 53:731–739, 1998.
5. A Kapp, P Neuner, J Krutmann, TA Luger, E Schopf. Production of interleukin-2 by mononuclear cells in vitro in patients with atopic dermatitis and psoriasis. Comparison with serum interleukin-2 receptor levels. Acta Derm Venereol 71:403–406, 1991.
6. A Kapp, A Piskorski, E Schopf. Elevated levels of interleukin 2 receptor in sera of patients with atopic dermatitis and psoriasis. Br J Dermatol 119:707–710, 1988.
7. MN Dworzak, G Froschl, D Printz, C Fleischer, U Potschger, G Fritsch, H Gadner, W Emminger. Skin-associated lymphocytes in the peripheral blood of patients with atopic dermatitis: signs of subset expansion and stimulation. J Allergy Clin Immunol 103:901–906, 1999.
8. Y Shimada, S Sato, M Hasegawa, TF Tedder, K Takehara. Elevated serum L-selectin levels and abnormal regulation of L-selectin expression on leukocytes in atopic dermatitis: soluble L-selectin levels indicate disease severity. J Allergy Clin Immunol 104:163–168, 1999.
9. K Wu, N Higashi, ER Hansen, M Lund, K Bang, K Thestrup-Pedersen. Telomerase

activity is increased and telomere length shortened in T cells from blood of patients with atopic dermatitis and psoriasis. J Immunol 165:4742–4747, 2000.

10. G Schmid-Ott, B Jaeger, C Adamek, H Koch, F Lamprecht, A Kapp, T Werfel. Levels of circulating CD8 T lymphocytes, natural killer cells, and eosinophils increase upon acute psychosocial stress in patients with atopic dermatitis. J Allergy Clin Immunol 107:171–177, 2001.

11. Akdis M, Simon HU, Weigl L, Kreyden O, Blaser K, Akdis CA. Skin homing (cutaneous lymphocyte-associated antigen-positive) CD8+ T cells respond to superantigen and contribute to eosinophilia and IgE production in atopic dermatitis. J Immunol 163:466–475, 1999.

12. NA Soter. Morphology of atopic eczema. Allergy 44:16–19, 1989.

13. JD Bos, ID van Garderen, SR Krieg, LW Poulter. Different in situ distribution patterns of dendritic cells having Langerhans (T6+) and interdigitating (RFD1+) cell immunophenotype in psoriasis, atopic dermatitis, and other inflammatory dermatoses. J Invest Dermatol 87:358–361, 1986.

14. A Gondo, NTY Saeki. Challenge reactions in atopic dermatitis after percutaneous entry of mite allergen. Br J Dermatol 115:485–493, 1986.

15. PL Bruijnzeel, PH Kuijper, A Kapp, RA Warringa, S Betz, CA Bruijnzeel-Koomen. The involvement of eosinophils in the patch test reaction to aeroallergens in atopic dermatitis: its relevance for the pathogenesis of atopic dermatitis. Clin Exp Allergy 23:97–109, 1993.

16. Y Tanaka, S Anan, H Yoshida. Immunohistochemical studies in mite-induced patch test site in atopic dermatitis. J Dermatol Sci 1:361–368, 1990.

17. T Bieber, H de la Salle, A Wollenberg, J Hakimi, R Chizzonite, J Ring, D Hanau, C de la Salle. Human epidermal langerhans cells express the high affinity receptor for immunoglobulin E (FceRI). J Exp Med 175:1285–1290, 1992.

18. GC Mudde, R Bheekha, CA Bruijnzeel-Koomen. IgE-mediated antigen presentation. Allergy 50:193–199, 1995.

19. CB Zachary, MH Allen, DM MacDonald. In situ quantification of T-lymphocyte subsets and Langerhans cells in the inflammatory infiltrate of atopic eczema. Br J Dermatol 112:149–156, 1985.

20. JD Bos, C Hagenaars, PK Das, SR Krieg, WJ Voorn, ML Kapsenberg. Predominance of "memory" T cells (CD4+, CDw29+) over "naive" T cells (CD4+, CD45R+) in both normal and diseased human skin. Arch Dermatol Res 281:24–30, 1989.

21. LJ Picker, SA Michie, LS Rott, EC Butcher. A unique phenotype of skin-associated lymphocytes in humans. Preferential expression of the HECA-452 epitope by benign and malignant T cells at cutaneous sites. Am J Pathol 136:1053–1068, 1990.

22. EL Berg, T Yoshino, LS Rott, MK Robinson, RA Warnock, TK Kishimoto, LJ Picker. The cutaneous lymphocyte antigen is a skin lymphocyte homing receptor for the vascular lectin endothelial cell-leukocyte adhesion molecule 1. J Exp Med 174:1461–1466, 1991.

23. LF Santamaria Babi, LJ Picker, MT Perez Soler, K Drzimalla, P Flohr, K Blaser, C Hauser. Circulating allergen-reactive T cells from patients with atopic dermatitis and allergic contact dermatitis express the skin-selective homing receptor, the cutaneous lymphocyte-associated antigen. J Exp Med 181:1935–40, 1995.

24. TA Springer. Traffic signals for lymphocyte recirculation and leukocyte emigration. The multistep paradigm. Cell 76:301–314, 1994.

25. CF Wahlgren, M Tengvall Linder, O Hagermark, A Scheynius. Itch and inflammation induced by intradermally injected interleukin-2 in atopic dermatitis patients and healthy subjects. Arch Dermatol Res. 287:572–580, 1995.

26. DA Lehmann, AA Lehmann, RL Coffmann. Interleukin-4 causes Isotype switching to IgE in T cell stimulated clonal B cell cultures. J Exp Med 168:853–862, 1988.

27. K Jujo, H Renz, J Abe, EW Gelfand, DYM Leung. Decreased gamma interferon and increased interleukin 4 production promote IgE synthesis in atopic dermatitis. J Allergy Clin Immunol 90:323–330, 1992.

28. P Parronchi, D Macchia, MP Picchini, P Biswas, C Simonelli, E Maggi, M Ricci, AA Ansari, S Romagnani. Allergen- and bacterial antigen-specific T cell clones established from atopic donors show a different profile of cytokine production. Proc Natl Acad USA 88:4538–4542, 1991.

29. N Sager, A Feldmann, G Schilling, P Kreitsch, C Neumann. House dust mite-specific T cells in the skin of subjects with atopic dermatitis: Frequency and lymphokine profile in the allergen patch test. J Allergy Clin Immunol 89:801–810, 1992.

30. FC van Reijsen, CA Bruijnzeel-Koomen, FS Kalthoff, E Maggi, S Romagnani, JK Westland, GC Mudde. Skin derived aeroallergen-specific T-cell clones of Th2 phenotype in patients with atopic dermatitis. J Allergy Clin Immunol 90:184–193, 1992.

31. T Werfel, A Morita, M Grewe, H Renz, U Wahn, J Krutmann, A Kapp. Allergen-specificity of skin-infiltrating T-cells is not restricted to a type 2 cytokine pattern in chronic skin lesions of atopic dermatitis. J Invest Dermatol 107:871–876, 1996.

32. M Grewe, K Gyufko, E Schöpf, J Krutmann. Lesional expression of interferon-γ in atopic eczema. Lancet 343:25–26, 1994.

33. T Thepen, EG Langeveld-Wildschut, IC Bihari, CF van Wichen, FC van Reijsen, GC Mudde, CA Bruijnzeel-Koomen. Bi-phasic response against aeroallergen in atopic dermatitis showing a switch from initial TH2 response into an TH1 response in situ. An immunocyto-chemical study. J Allergy Clin Immunol 97:828–837, 1996.

34. A Trautmann, M Akdis, D Kleemann, F Altznauer, HU Simon, T Graeve, M Noll, EB Brocker, K Blaser, CA Akdis. T cell-mediated Fas-induced keratinocyte apoptosis plays a key pathogenetic role in eczematous dermatitis. J Clin Invest 106: 25–35, 2000.

35. M Grewe, W Czech, A Morita, T Werfel, M Klammer, A Kapp, T Ruzicka, E Schöpf, J Krutmann. Human eosinophils produce biologically active IL-12: implications for the control of T-cell responses. J Immunol 161:415–420, 1998.

36. Q Hamid, T Naseer, EM Minshall, YL Song, M Boguniewicz, DY Leung. In vivo expression of IL-12 and IL-13 in atopic dermatitis. J Allergy Clin Immunol 98: 225–231, 1996.

37. Wittmann M, Larsson VA, Schmidt P, Begemann G, Kapp A, Werfel T. Suppression of interleukin-12 production by human monocytes after preincubation with lipopolysaccharide. Blood 94:1717–1726, 1999.

38. M Wittmann, P Kienlin, G Begemann, A Kapp, T Werfel. The sequence of stimuli determines the amount of IL-12 produced by human monocytes. Int Arch Allergy Immunol 124:218–220, 2001.

39. S Stoll, H Jonuleit, E Schmitt, G Müller, H Yamauchi, M Kurimoto, J Knop, AH Enk. Production of functional IL-18 by different subtypes of murine and human dendritic cells (DC): DC-derived IL-18 enhances IL-12 dependent Th1 development. Eur J Immunol 28:3231–3239, 1998.

40. CA Dinarello. IL-18: a Th1-inducing, proinflammatory cytokine and new member of the IL-1 family. J Allergy Clin Immunol 103:11–24, 1999.

41. T Werfel, M Hentschel, A Kapp, H Renz. Dichotomy of blood and skin-derived interleukin-4 producing allergen specific T-cells and restricted Vβ repertoire in nickel mediated contact dermatitis. J Immunol 158:2500–2505, 1997.

42. JC Szepietowski, RC McKenzie, SG Keohane, RD Aldridge, JA Hunter. Atopic and non-atopic individuals react to nickel challenge in a similar way. A study of the cytokine profile in nickel-induced contact dermatitis. Br J Dermatol 137:195–200, 1997.

43. M Wittmann, J Neumman, P Kienlin, B Eilers, A Kapp, T Werfel. Evidence for a similar cytokine pattern expressed in allergic and atopic dermatitis. Int Arch Allergy Immunol 124:346–348, 2001.

44. B Wedi, U Raap, H Lewrick, A Kapp. Interleukin-4 induced apoptosis in peripheral blood eosinophils. J Allergy Clin Immunol 102:1013–1020, 1998.

45. B Wedi, U Raap, H Lewrick, A Kapp. Delayed eosinophil programmed cell death in vitro: A common feature of inhalant allergy and extrinsic and intrinsic atopic dermatitis. J Allergy Clin Immunol 100:536–543, 1997.

46. L Rogge, L Barberis-Maino, M Biffi, N Passini, DH Presky, U Gubler, F Sinigaglia. Selective expression of an interleukin-12 receptor component by human T helper 1 cells. J Exp Med 185:825–831, 1997.

47. M Mochizuki, J Bartels, AI Mallet, E Christophers, JM Schröder. IL-4 induces eotaxin: a possible mechanism of selective eosinophil recruitment in helminth infection and atopy. J Immunol 160:60–68, 1998.

48. Q Hamid, M Boguniewicz, DY Leung. Differential in situ cytokine gene expression in acute versus chronic atopic dermatitis. J Clin Invest 94:870–876, 1994.

49. J Elsner, A Kapp. Regulation and modulation of eosinophil effector functions. Allergy 54:15–26, 1999.

50. RA Taha, DY Leung, O Ghaffar, M Boguniewicz, Q Hamid. In vivo expression of cytokine receptor mRNA in atopic dermatitis. J Allergy Clin Immunol. 102:245–250, 1998.

51. RC Fuhlbrigge, JD Kiefer, D Amerding, TS Kupper. Cutaneous lymphocyte antigen is a specialized form of PSGL-1 expressed on skin homing T cells. Nature 389:978–981, 1997.

52. AJ Wagers, CM Waters, LM Stoolman, GS Kansas. Interleukin 12 and interleukin 4 control T cell adhesion to endothelial selectins through opposite effects on alpha 1, 3-fucosyltransferase VII gene expression. J Exp Med 188:2225–2231, 1998.

53. DY Leung, M Gately, A Trumble, B Ferguson-Darnell, PM Schlievert, LJ Picker. Bacterial superantigens induce T cell expression of the skin-selective homing recep-

tor, the cutaneous lymphocyte-associated antigen, via stimulation of interleukin 12 production. J Exp Med 181:747–753, 1995.

54. M Akdis, S Klunker, M Schliz, K Blaser, CA Akdis. Expression of cutaneous lymphocyte-associated antigen on human CD4(+) and CD8(+) Th2 cells. Eur J Immunol 30:3533–3541, 2000.

55. M Akdis, CA Akdis, L Weigl, R Disch, K Blaser. Skin-homing, CLA$^+$ memory T cells are activated in atopic dermatitis and regulate IgE by an IL-13-dominated cytokine pattern. IgG4 counter-regulation by CLA-memory T-cells. J Immunol 159:4611–4619, 1997.

56. LF Santamaria Babi, R Moser, MT Perez Soler, LJ Picker, K Blaser, C Hauser. The migration of skin-homing T cells across cytokine-activated human endothelial cell layers involves interaction of the cutaneous lymphocyte-associated antigen (CLA), the very late antigen-4 (VLA-4) and the lymphocyte function-associated antigen-1 (LFA-1). J Immunol 154:1543–1550, 1995.

57. M Baggiolini. Chemokines and leukocyte traffic. Nature 392:565–568, 1998.

58. J Elsner, A Kapp. Activation on human eosiniphils by chemokines. Chem Immunol 76:177–207, 2000.

59. AD Luster. Chemokine-chemotactic cytokines that mediate inflammation. N Engl J Med 338:436–45, 1998.

60. R Bonecchi, G Bianchi, PP Bordignon, D D'Ambrosio, R Lang, A Borsatti, S Sozzani, P Allavena, PA Gray, A Mantovani, F Sinigaglia. Differential expression of chemokine receptors and chemotactic responsiveness of type 1 T helper cells (Th1s) and Th2s. J Exp Med 187:129–134, 1998.

61. F Sallusto, D Lenig, CR Mackay, A Lanzavecchia. Flexible programs of chemokine receptor expression on human polarized T helper 1 and 2 lymphocytes. J Exp Med 187:875–883, 1998.

62. T Imai, M Nagira, S Takagi, M Kakizaki, M Nishimura, J Wang, PW Gray, K Matsushima, O Yoshie. Selective recruitment of CCR4-bearing Th2 cells toward antigen-presenting cells by the CC chemokine thymus and activation-regulated chemokine and macrophage-derived chemokine. Int Immunol 11:81–88, 1999.

63. D D'Ambrosio, A Iellem, R Bonecchi, D Mazzeo, S Sozzani, A Mantovani, F Sinigaglia. Selective up-regulation of chemokine receptors CCR4 and CCR8 upon activation of polarized human type 2 Th cells. J Immunol 161:5111–5115, 1998.

64. C Vestergaard, K Bang, B Gesser, H Yoneyama, K Matsushima, C Grønhøj Larsen. A Th2 chemokine, TARC, produced by keratinocytes may recruit CLA+CCR4+ lymphocytes into lesional atopic dermatitis skin. J Invest Dermatol 115:640–646, 2000.

65. JJ Campbell, G Haraldsen, J Pan, J Rottman, S Qin, P Ponath, DP Andrews, R Warnke, N Ruffing, N Kassam, L Wu, EC Butcher. The chemokine receptor, CCR, 4 in vascular recognition by cutaneous but not intestinal memory, T-cells. Nature 400:776–780, 1999.

66. S Hashimoto, T Suzuki, H Dong, N Yamazaki, K Matsushima. Serial analysis of gene expression in human monocytes and macrophages. Blood 94:837–844, 1999.

67. C Vestergaard, H Yoneyama, M Murai et al. Overproduction of Th2 CC chemo-

kines TARC and MDC in the skin of the NC/Nga mouse correlates with exacerbation of atopic dermatitis like lesions. J Clin Invest 104:1097–1105, 1999.

68. PD Ponath, S Qin, DJ Ringler, I Clark-Lewis, J Wang, N Kassam, H Smith, X Shi, JA Gonzalo, W Newman, JC Guitierrez-Ramos, CR Mackay. Cloning of the human eosinophil chemoattractant, eotaxin. Expression, Receptor binding, and functional properties suggest a mechanism for the selective recruitment of eosinophils. J Clin Invest 97:604–612, 1996.

69. BO Gerber, MP Zanni, M Uguccioni, M Lötscher, CR Mackay, WJ Pichler, N Yawalkar, M Baggiolini, B Moser. Functional expression of the eotaxin receptor CCR3 in T lymphocytes co-localizing with eosinophils. Curr Biol 7:836–843, 1997.

70. A Rubbert, C Combadiere, M Ostrowski, J Arthos, M Dybul, E Machado, MA Cohn, JA Hoxie, PM Murphy, AS Fanci, D Weissmann. Dendritic cells express multiple chemokine receptors used as coreceptors for HIV entry. J Immunol 160: 3933–3941, 1998.

71. N Yawalkar, M Uguccioni, J Schärer, J Braunwalder, S Karlen, B Dewald, LR Braathen, M Baggiolini. Enhanced expression of eotaxin and CCR3 in atopic dermatitis. J Invest Dermatol 113:43–48, 1999.

72. J Morales, B Homey, AP Vicari, S Hudak, E Oldham, J Hedrick, R Orozco, NG Copeland, NA Jenkins, LM Mc Evoy, A Zlotnik. CTACK. a skin-associated chemokine that preferentially attracts skin-homing memory T cells. Proc Natl Acad Sci USA 96:14470–14475, 1999.

73. B Homey, W Wang, H Soto, ME Buchanan, A Wiesenborn, D Catron, A Müller, TK McClanahan, MC Dieu-Nosjean, R Orozco, T Ruzicka, P Lehmann, E Oldham, A Zlotnik. The orphan chemokine receptor G protein-coupled receptor-2 (CRP-2. CCR10) binds the skin-associated chemokine CCL27 (CTACK/ALP/ILC). J Immunol 164:3465–3470, 2000.

74. F Liao, RL Rabin, CS Smith, G Sharma, TB Nutman, JM Farber. CC-chemokine receptor 6 is expressed on diverse memory subsets of T cells and determines responsiveness to macrophage inflammatory protein 3 alpha. J Immunol 162:186–194, 1999.

75. T Nakayama, R Fujisawa, H Yamada, T Horikawa, H Kawasaki, K Hieshima, D Izawa, S Fujiie, T Tezuka, O Yoshie. Inducible expression of a CC chemokine liver- and activation-regulated chemokine (LARC)/macrophage inflammatory protein (MIP)-3alpha/CCL20 by epidermal keratinocytes and its role in atopic dermatitis. Int Immunol 13:95–103, 2001.

76. J Ring, T Senter, RC Cornell, CM Arroyave, EM Tan. Complement and immunoglobulin deposits in the skin of patients with atopic dermatitis. Br J Dermatol 99: 495–501, 1978.

77. L Secher, H Permin, F Juhl. Immunofluorescence of the skin in allergic diseases: an investigation of patients with contact dermatitis, allergic vasculitis and atopic dermatitis. Acta Derm Venereol 58:117–120, 1978.

78. T Werfel, K Kirchhoff, M Wittmann, G Begemann, A Kapp, F Heidenreich, O Götze, J Zwirner. Activated human T lymphocytes express a functional C3a receptor. J Immunol 165:6599–6605, 2000.

79. LF Santamaria Babi, B Moser, MT Perez Soler, R Moser, P Lötscher, B Villiger,

K Blaser, C Hauser. The interleukin-8 receptor B and CXC chemokines can mediate transendothelial migration of human skin homing T cells. Eur J Immunol 26:2056–2061, 1996.

80. S Laberge, O Ghaffar, M Boguniewicz, DM Center, DY Leung, Q Hamid. Association of increased CD4+ T-cell infiltration with increased IL-16 gene expression in atopic dermatitis. J Allergy Clin Immunol 102:645–650, 1998.

81. EB Mitchel, MD Chapman, F Pope, S Crow, S Jouhal, TAE Platts Mills. Basophils in allergen-induced patch test sites in atopic dermatitis. Lancet i:127–130, 1982.

82. U Darsow, D Vieluf, J Ring. Evaluating the relevance of aeroallergen sensitization in atopic eczema with the atopy patch test: a randomized, double-blind multicenter study. Atopy Patch Test Study Group. J Am Acad Dermatol 40:187–193, 1999.

83. S Reitamo, K Visa, K Kahonen, K Kyhk, S Stubb, OP Salo. Eczematous reactions in atopic patients caused by epicutaneous testing with inhalent allergens. Br J Dermatol 114:303–309, 1986.

84. GC Mudde, FC von Reijsen, GJ Boland, GC Gast, PL Bruijnzeel, CA Bruijnzeel-Koomen. Allergen presentation by epidermal Langerhans cells from patients with atopic dermatitis is mediated by IgE. Immunology 69:335–341, 1990.

85. A Wistokat-Wülfing, P Schmidt, U Darsow, J Ring, A Kapp, T Werfel. Atopy patch test reactions are associated with T lymphocyte-mediated allergen-specific immune responses in atopic dermatitis. Clin Exp Allergy 29:513–521, 1999.

86. KJ Abernathy-Carver, HA Sampson, LJ Picker, DYM Leung. Milk-induced eczema is associated with the expansion of T cells expressing cutaneous lymphocyte antigen. J Clin Invest 95:913–918, 1995.

87. R Reekers, M Busche, M Wittmann, A Kapp, T Werfel. Birch pollen related food trigger atopic dermatitis with specific cutaneous T-cell responses to birch pollen antigens. J Allergy Clin Immunol 104:466–472, 1999.

88. B Bohle, H Schwihla, HZ Hu, R Friedl-Hajek, S Sowka, F Ferreira, H Breiteneder, CA CA Bruijnzeel-Koomen, RA de Weger, GC Mudde, C Ebner, FC Van Reijsen. Long-lived Th2 clones specific for seasonal and perennial allergens can be detected in blood and skin by their TCR-hypervariable regions. J Immunol 160:2022–2027, 1998.

89. R Reekers, K Beyer, N Niggemann, U Wahn, J Freihorst, A Kapp, T Werfel. The role of circulating food antigen specific lymphocytes in food allergic children with atopic dermatitis. Br J Dermatol 135:935–941, 1996.

90. T Werfel, G Ahlers, M Boeker, A Kapp. Detection of a κ-casein specific lymphocyte response in milk-responsive atopic dermatitis. Clin Exp Allergy 26:1380, 1996.

91. T Werfel, G Ahlers, M Boeker, A Kapp, C Neumann. Milk-responsive atopic dermatitis is associated with a casein-specific lymphocyte response in adolescent and adult patients. J Allergy Clin Immunol 99:124–133, 1997.

92. T Werfel, G Ahlers, M Boeker, A Kapp. Characterization of specific T-cell responses to food antigens in atopic dermatitis (AD). In: J Ring, D Vieluf, H Behrendt, eds. New Trends in Allergy IV. Berlin: Springer Verlag, 1997, pp 233–236.

93. RP Schade, AG Van Ieperen-Van Dijk, FC Van Reijsen, C Versluis, JL Kimpen, EF Knol, CA Bruijnzeel-Koomen, E Van Hoffen. Differences in antigen-specific T-cell responses between infants with atopic dermatitis with and without cow's

milk allergy: relevance of TH2 cytokines. J Allergy Clin Immunol 106:1155–1162, 2000.

94. FC van Reijsen, A Felius, EA Wauters, CA Bruijnzeel-Koomen, SJ Koppelman. T-cell reactivity for a peanut-derived epitope in the skin of a young infant with atopic dermatitis. J Allergy Clin Immunol 101:207–209, 1998.

95. N Hashem, E Sedlis, K Hirschhorn, E Emmet Holt. Infantile eczema: evidence of autoimmunity to human skin. Lancet 2:269–270, 1963.

96. R Valenta, S Seiberler, S Natter, V Mahler, R Mossabeb, J Ring, G Stingl. Autoallergy: a pathogenetic factor in atopic dermatitis? J Allergy Clin Immunol 105:432–437, 2000.

97. JE Leyden, RR Marples, AM Kligman. Staphylococcus aureus in the lesions of atopic dermatitis. Br J Dermatol 90:525–530, 1974.

98. R Lever, K Hadley, D Downey, R MacKie. Staphylococcal colonization in atopic dermatitis and the effect of topical mupirocin therapy. Br J Dermatol 119:189–198, 1988.

99. JP McFadden, WC Noble, RDR Camp. Superantigenic exotoxin-secreting potential of staphylococci isolated from atopic eczematous skin. Br J Dermatol 128:631–632, 1993.

100. R Carlsson, H Fischer, HO Sjogren. Binding of staphylococcal enterotoxin A to accessory cells is a requirement for its ability to activate human T cells. J Immunol 140:2484–2488, 1988.

101. MF Hofer, MR Lester, PM Schlievert, DYM Leung. Upregulation of IgE synthesis by staphylococcal toxic shock syndrome toxin-1 in peripheral blood mononuclear cells from patients with atopic dermatitis. Clin Exp Allergy 25:1218–1227, 1995.

102. U Herz, N Schnoy, S Borelli, L Weigl, U Käsbohrer, A Daser, U Wahn, E Kottgen, H Renz. A human-SCID mouse model for allergic immune responses: bacterial superantigen enhances skin inflammation and suppresses IgE production. J Invest Dermatol 110:224–231, 1998.

103. I Strickland, PJ Hauk, A Trumble, LJ Picker, DY Leung. Evidence for superantigen involvement in skin homing of T cells in atopic dermatitis. J Invest Dermatol 112:249–253, 1999.

104. MJ Torres, FJ Gonzales, JL Corza, MD Giron, MJ Carvajal, V Garcia et al. Circulating CLA+ lymphocytes from children with atopic dermatitis contain an increased percentage of cells bearing staphylococcal-related T-cell receptor variable segments. Clin Exp Allergy 28:1264–1272, 1998.

105. SJ Ha, HJ Lee, DG Byun, JW Kim. Expression of T cell receptor Vb chains in lesional skin of atopic dermatitis. Acta Dermatol Venereol Stockh 78:424–427, 1998.

106. K Neuber, C Löliger, I Köhler, J Ring. Preferential expression of T-cells receptor Vb-chains in atopic ekzema. Acta Dermatol Venereol Stockh 76:214–218, 1996.

107. R Bunikowski, M Mielke, H Skarabis, M Worm, I Anagnostopoulos, G Kolde, U Wahn, H Renz. Evidence for a disease-promoting effect of Staphylococcus aureus-derived exotoxins in atopic dermatitis. J Allergy Clin Immunol 105:814–909, 2000.

108. L Skov, JV Olsen, R Giorno, PM Schlievert, O Baadsgaard, DYM Leung. Application of staphylococcal enterotoxin B on normal and atopic skin induces up-regula-

tion of T cells by a superantigen-mediated mechanism. J Allergy Clin Immunol 105:820–826, 2000.

109. TM Zöllner, TA Wichelhaus, A Hartung, C von Mallinckrodt, TO Wagner, V Brade, R Kaufmann. Colonization with superantigen-producing *Staphylococcus aureus* is associated with increased severity of atopic dermatitis. Clin Exp Allergy 30:994–1000, 2000.

110. DYM Leung, R Harbeck, P Bina, R Reiser, E Yang, DA Norris, JM Hanifin, HA Sampson. Presence of IgE antibodies to staphylococcal exotoxins on the skin of patients with atopic dermatitis. J Clin Invest 92:1374–1380, 1993.

111. K Breuer, M Wittmann, B Bösche, A Kapp, T Werfel. Severe atopic dermatitis is associated with sensitization to staphylococcal enterotoxin B (SEB). Allergy 55: 551–555, 2000.

112. I Nomura, K Tanaka, H Tomita, T Katsunama, Y Ohya, N Ikeda, T Takeda, H Saito, A Akasawa. Evaluation of staphylococcal exotoxin and its specific IgE in childhood atopic dermatitis. J Allergy Clin Immunol 104:441–446, 1999.

113. R Bunikowski, M Mielke, H Skarabis, U Herz, RL Bergmann, U Wahn, H Renz. Prevalence and role of serum IgE antibodies to *S. aureus*-derived superantigens SEA and SEB in children with atopic dermatitis. J Allergy Clin Immunol 103:119–124, 1999.

114. DE Campbell, AS Kemp. Production of antibodies to staphylococcal superantigens in atopic dermatitis. Arch Dis Child 79:400–404, 1998.

115. A Waersted, N Hjorth. Pityrosporum orbiculare: A pathogenic factor for atopic dermatitis of the face, scalp, and neck? Acta Dermatol Venereol Suppl 114:146–148, 1985.

116. M Tengvall Linder, C Johansson, A Zargari, A Bengtsson, I van der Ploeg, B Harfast, A Scheynius. Detection of Pityrosporum orbiculare reactive T cells from skin and blood in atopic dermatitis and characterization of their cystokine profiles. Clin Exp Allergy 26:1286–1297, 1996.

117. M Lindborg, CGM Magnusson, A Zargari, M Schmidt, A Scheynius, R Crameri, P Whitley. Selective cloning of allergens from the skin colonizing yeast *Malassezia furfur* by phage surface display technology. J Invest Dermatol 113:156–161, 1999.

118. B Wüthrich. Atopic dermatitis flare provoked by inhalant allergens. Dermatologica 178:51–53, 1989.

119. Wüthrich. Serum IgE in atopic dermatitis. Clin Allergy 8:241–248, 1978.

120. T Schäfer, U Kramer, D Vieluf, D Abeck, H Behrendt, J Ring. The excess of atopic eczema in East Germany is related to the intrinsic type. Br J Dermatol 143:992–998, 2000.

121. DJ Atherton, M Sewell, JF Soothhill, RS Wells, CED Chilvers. A double-blind controlled crossover trial of an antigen avoidance diet in atopic eczema. Lancet 1: 401–403, 1978.

122. DJ Hill, AM Hosking, CS Hosking, IL Hidson. Clinical manifestations of cow's milk allergy in childhood. II: The diagnostic value of skin tests and RAST. Clin Allergy 18:481–490, 1988.

123. CA Akdis, M Akdis, D Simon, B Dibbert, M Weber, S Gratzl, O Kreyden, R Disch, B Wüthrich, K Blaser, HU Simon. T cells and T cell-derived cytokines as patho-

genic factors in the non-allergic form of atopic dermatitis. J Invest Dermatol 113: 628–634, 1999.

124. MK Kägi, B Wüthrich, E Montano, J Barandun, K Blaser, C Walker. Differential cytokine profiles in peripheral blood lymphocyte supernatants and skin biopsies from patients with different forms of atopic dermatitis, psoriasis and normal individuals. Int Arch Allergy Immunol 10:332–340, 1994.

125. C Walker, MK Kägi, P Ingold, P Braun, K Blaser, CA Bruijnzeel-Koomen, B Wüthrich. Atopic dermatitis: correlation of peripheral blood T cell activation, eosinophilia and serum factors with clinical severity. Clin Exp Allergy 23:145–153, 1993.

126. B Wüthrich, H Joller-Jemelka, U Helfenstein, PJ Grob. Levels of soluble interleukin-2 receptors correlate with the severity of atopic dermatitis. Dermatologica 181: 92–97, 1990.

127. MK Kägi, H Joller-Jemelka, B Wüthrich. Correlation of eosinophils, eosinophil cationic protein and soluble interleukin-2 receptor with the clinical activity of atopic dermatitis. Dermatology 185:88–92, 1992.

14

Antigen-Presenting Cells

Andreas Wollenberg
University of Munich, Munich, Germany

Thomas Bieber
University of Bonn, Bonn, Germany

I. INTRODUCTION AND BACKGROUND

Atopic dermatitis (AD) is a chronic inflammatory skin disease clinically and histologically highly similar to allergic contact dermatitis (20,41). Because of this similarity, the putative pathophysiological relationship between classical IgE-mediated allergic reactions occurring in atopic individuals, i.e., allergic rhinitis and allergic asthma bronchiale, and eczematous skin lesions in AD remains elusive. Our current understanding of allergic reactions in the skin, particularly in the field of eczematous skin diseases, implies that this kind of cellular infiltrate, mainly composed of T cells, has to be initiated and/or sustained by antigen-presenting cells (APC). As a rule, T cells require efficient stimulation by APC in order to become effector cells and to be implicated in a pathophysiological process. Thus, it is assumed that APC play a key role in driving the inflammatory reaction in AD lesions (8). Recently, it has been proposed to subdivide AD into two distinct forms: the "extrinsic" or "allergic" form (occurring in the context of sensitization toward environmental allergens) and the "intrinsic" or "nonallergic" form (occurring in the absence of any typical atopical background) (61). Based on the above, APC should be involved in both forms of AD. In this chapter we will focus on the role of professional APC, i.e., monocytes and dendritic cells (DC), including epidermal Langerhans cells (LC), since most progress has been made in recent years in understanding the putative role of these APC in the extrinsic/allergic form of AD.

II. IDENTIFICATION OF APC IN AD SKIN

In the human system, many cell types have been shown to be capable of antigen presentation. Depending on the more or less inflammatory environment of the skin, many cell types, such as epidermal LC, inflammatory dendritic epidermal cells (IDEC), dermal dendritic cells, skin macrophages, B cells, and even keratinocytes, may bear an antigen-presenting capacity. However, differences between a capacity for primary and secondary immune responses as well as quantitative differences in the strength of the established immune response must be considered.

Dendritic cells are a morphologically and functionally defined but growing family of cells, which may be found in small percentages in most organs of the human body (3,47) and may be further divided into myeloid and lymphoid types. Dendritic cells are the most efficient of all APC and are capable of the initiation of both primary and secondary immune responses.

A. Langerhans Cells

Langerhans cells are the exclusive DC population of the normal, uninflamed human epidermis and are capable of initiating primary and secondary immune responses. Of all DC subtypes of the human body, LC are the most intensively investigated cell population and are thus regarded as paradigmatic DC. LC are defined as bone marrow–derived, epidermally located, dendritically shaped, antigen-presenting cells, which contain Birbeck granules and express CD1a and class II molecules (57). In the epidermis, LC form a close network with their dendrites, which may be regarded as a first barrier of the immune system towards the environment. All antigens penetrating the human body as well as locally produced self-antigens have to pass this first immunological wall of defense.

The medical student Paul Langerhans (1847–1888) first described the "high level clear cells of the epidermis" in 1868 when he performed a gold chloride stain according to Cohnheim on human skin sections (31). Routine light microscopic examination shows the LC as a clear cell in the basal and suprabasal layer of the epidermis.

LC may be identified by immunohistological staining of their surface molecules HLA-DR and CD1a. With this technique, the dendrites of LC are easily detected between the keratinocytes. The strength of immunohistochemistry lies in the preservation of the tissue architecture and the relative distribution patterns of the cells inside the skin, whereas the lack of quantitative analysis is its main weakness. In normal human skin, LC are homogeneously distributed at a density of about $450/mm^2$ along the entire body; only palms and soles have lower cell densities of about $60/mm^2$ (6). In normal human skin, the LC frequency varies between 0.5 and 2% of all epidermal cells.

In addition to immunohistochemistry, the immunophenotype of LC has been extensively characterized by flow cytometry. This very sensitive technique allows for quantitative analysis, but it is restricted to trypsin-resistant structures. In freshly isolated LC, the phenotype has been thoroughly investigated. A variety of immunoglobulin receptors, MHC class I and class II molecules, and multiple adhesion molecules are the immunophenotypic hallmark of normal LC. The non-classical MHC class Ib molecule CD1a is regarded as the most specific LC marker for normal human skin available at present. This does not apply to inflammatory skin conditions, since another CD1a-expressing, inflammatory dendritic epidermal cell (IDEC) population (56) is present in the epidermis (see below). Table 1 gives an overview of some relevant markers expressed on LC from normal and inflamed human skin. The differentiation between normal and inflamed human skin is important, since the immunophenotype of the LC is subjected to highly complex regulatory mechanisms: (a) freshly isolated LC change their phenotype (and function) during short-term culture towards highly stimulatory dendritic cells; (2) the inflammatory microenvironment alters the immunophenotype of the LC in situ; (3) in some skin diseases, e.g., AD, a subset of membrane receptors is subject to disease-specific regulation (60).

Table 1 Expression of Surface Molecules on CD1a Expressing Cells in the Inflamed Epidermis, Shown Semiquantitatively for LC and IDEC[a]

	LC	IDEC
CD1a	+++	+/++
CD1b	φ	+/++
CD11a	φ	++
CD11b	φ/±	+++
CD11c	+	+++
VLA4α	+	+/++
FcεRI	φ/++	+/+++
FcεRII	φ/+	φ/++
FcγRI	φ	++
FcγRII	++	++/+++
FcγRIII	φ	φ/+
CD36	φ/+	++/+++
CD80	φ/±	φ/+
CD86	φ/±	φ/+
LAG/Langerin	++	φ

[a] While some surface markers show a rather stable expression, others are subjected to strong regulatory signals from the epidermal micromilieu.

The ultrastructural features of LC include a clear cytoplasm, a lobulated nucleus, and the complete absence of desmosomes, melanosomes, or Merkel cell granules. Electron microscopic detection of the LC-specific, racket-shaped cytoplasmic Langerhans cell granules with their characteristic, trilamellar handle, better known as Birbeck granules (BG), is the most specific identification technique for LC. BG were described first in 1961 by Michael S. Birbeck, a British scientist who studied the ultrastructure of LC in vitiligo (12). The function of BG is unclear at present, but some data suggest a role in antigen processing by the LC (24). The LC granule antigen CD207, also known as LAG antigen, is a protein of unknown function, which is exclusively present inside Birbeck granules and may be detected by the monoclonal anti-LAG antibody (28). More recently another BG-specific marker, the so-called Langerin, has been characterized (50,51). LAG and Langerin fail to stain the interstitial-type DC, e.g., IDEC, but exclusively label the BG-positive LC. Cytoplasmic immunostaining of LAG and surface staining of Langerin are frequently used to quantify or simply demonstrate the presence of BG without the need to perform electron microscopy. The absolute specificity of BG for LC was questioned by the recent demonstration of BG-like structures in EDTA-treated platelets (25), as well as by the observation of complete BG absence inside all LC from a perfectly healthy individuum (37). However, BG are still regarded as the most specific LC-identifying feature.

LC take up intact protein antigens or protein-coupled low molecular weight haptens, which enter the endocytic pathway and are cleaved inside the cell by limited digestion into small peptides. These peptides are loaded as a rule onto MHC II or in some instances onto MHC II complexes for antigen presentation to T cells. LC and DC take up extracellular fluid by means of different processes: (1) the fluid phase uptake is based on the engulfment of extracellular space by the plasma membrane and subsequent translocation of the created endosomes into the endocytic pathway of the cell; (2) in receptor-mediated endocytosis, the cell is preferentially taking up those molecules binding to specific membrane-bound receptors, such as the mannose receptor or high-affinity receptor for IgE (see below). The latter mechanism is assumed to play a central pathogenetic role in IgE-mediated atopic skin disease, namely AD (7).

Migration of LC into the T-cell areas of the lymph nodes is a prerequisite for initiation of primary immune responses by LC. This migration is associated with a maturation from a good antigen-processing but badly presenting cell type into a badly processing but extremely well antigen-presenting cell. Isolation and short-term culture of LC initiates a similar maturation cascade in vitro, as has been shown in the mouse and human systems (43,45). Once migrating through the lymph vessels, LC are identified as veiled cells. With further migration into the paracortical area of the lymph node, the veiled cells are now identified as interdigitating reticulum cells. LC may be driven out of the epidermis by application of contact allergen via induction of the key cytokines IL-1 β or TNF-α (17,21).

The cell surface molecules involved in the initiation of immune responses may roughly be grouped into three categories: molecules involved in cell-cell adhesion (e.g., ICAM1), molecules dealing with peptide presentation (e.g., MHC molecules), and molecules delivering costimulatory signals (e.g., CD80 or CD86 and CD28). The presence of costimulatory molecules is necessary to direct the immune system towards an immune response and not tolerance induction. However, LC present in normal human skin do not express CD80 or CD86 but acquire these molecules during their migration and maturation process (46).

B. Inflammatory Dendritic Epidermal Cells

Inflammatory dendritic epidermal cells are a non-LC, dendritic cell population, which accumulates inside the inflammatory epidermis of AD and other inflammatory skin diseases. They are defined by a moderate CD1a but high CD11b expression and a lack of the LC-specific BG (56). The immunophenotype of IDEC has been extensively studied, and with adhesion molecules, MHC class II molecules, and costimulatory molecules, the essential structures for DC function have been identified. IDEC have been observed for many years by different research groups (2,4,48,49), but ultrastructural and immunophenotypic delineation of these two cell types in atopic dermatitis has been achieved only recently (56). The ontogenesis of IDEC is unclear, but there is indirect evidence for a monocyte-derived origin of these cells. Some key features of epidermal DC in AD lesions, such as in situ IgE binding and expression of the high-affinity IgE receptor, are shared by IDEC and LC (60).

Epidermal cell suspensions of lesional and nonlesional human skin of more than 800 skin biopsies have been analyzed for the presence of IDEC. As a rule, all inflammatory skin diseases associated with a lymphohistiocytic skin infiltrate are associated with the occurrence of IDEC in the epidermis. AD, psoriasis vulgaris, allergic contact eczema, mycosis fungoides, lichen planus, as well as the more uncommon diseases Dorfman-Chanarin syndrome, Oid-Oid disease, and others, exhibit variable percentages of IDEC inside the epidermis. The more severe the lesion and the longer the disease duration, the higher the percentage of IDEC that can be expected. Normal human skin does not contain significant numbers of IDEC.

The immunophenotype of IDEC has been thoroughly investigated and includes Fc receptors, MHC molecules, adhesion molecules, chemokine receptors, costimulatory molecules, the thrombospondin receptor CD36, and the mannose receptor. An extended phenotype of these cells, as compared to LC, is given in Table 1. Based on the results of these experiments, IDEC resemble the immunophenotype of immature myeloid dendritic cells of the interstitial type (3). In contrast to LC, which bear a relatively constant immunophenotype, the expression of some surface receptors on IDEC are highly variable. These variations have been shown to be related to the underlying skin disease. The highest levels of the high-affinity IgE-receptor expression on IDEC were seen in AD, allowing for a diagnostic application of a standardized DC phenotyping procedure. In a retrospective analysis of 75 skin samples, AD was detected with a high sensitivity and specificity out of all other inflammatory skin diseases by calculation of the FcεRI/FcγRII expression ratio on epidermal DC (59). Most interestingly, extrinsic/allergic AD but not intrinsic/nonallergic AD could be detected with this technique, thus arguing against a simple substitution of aeroallergens by skin-derived autoantigens such as the recently identified HomS1 (39). In addition, the high expression of the two Fc receptors for IgG, CD32 and CD64, is a diagnostic hallmark of psoriasis vulgaris (55). Overall, from a phenotypic point of view, IDEC from intrinsic and extrinsic forms of AD differ mainly with respect to their FcεRI expression, while the expression of other surface molecules, e.g., CD36, CD1b, CD11b, CD80, and CD86, is not significantly different.

The ultrastructure of IDEC shows a clear cytoplasm, a lobulated nucleus, but no BG, melanosomes, Merkel cell granules or desmosomes (56). The lack of BG or LAG/Langerin-reactivity is a key feature of IDEC and allows the ultra-structural delineation of IDEC from LC (56). Close to the cell membrane, there are areas with numerous coated pits, coated and uncoated vesicules, which appear to be fusing with endosomes, thus witnessing the endocytotic activity (A. Wollenberg et al., unpublished).

At present, there is only indirect evidence for the function of IDEC. Earlier work with epidermal cell suspensions isolated from lesional AD skin identified a hyperstimulatory role for the epidermal DC towards their autologous T cells, as shown by ^{3}H-thymidine incorporation assays (35). A special morphological/maturation state of the epidermal LC was assumed in this paper, but no differentiation between LC and IDEC was made.

Following immunohistological and flow cytometric detection of the mannose receptor on IDEC but not LC, functional analysis of pinocytosis and receptor-mediated endocytosis by epidermal DC was performed in a standardized technique modified from Sallusto et al. (44). Mannose receptor–independent uptake of the fluorescent dye lucifer yellow by pinocytosis was seen in both LC and IDEC, whereas mannose receptor–mediated endocytosis was essentially limited to IDEC and immature monocyte-derived dendritic cells (A. Wollenberg et al., unpublished).

C. Other Antigen-Presenting Cells

The concept of the skin immune system (SIS), as proposed by Bos (13), includes further cell types with antigen-presenting capacity, which will not be discussed here in depth due to space limitation. One cell type with a long history of investigation, especially in atopic dermatitis, are the macrophages of the mononuclear infiltrate (32). Macrophages have been demonstrated to produce IL-10 in UV-induced dermatitis solaris (27). In vitro, IL-10 prevents the maturation of mono-cytes into dendritic cells but favors the generation of macrophages (1). Another important cell type, the dermal dendritic cells, have mostly been characterized in skin lesions of psoriasis vulgaris. Dermal dendritic cells isolated from psoriatic plaques were much more effective stimulators of spontaneous T-cell proliferation in the absence of exogenous mitogen as compared with either psoriatic blood-derived DC or dermal DC derived from normal human skin (36,38).

III. Ige-BINDING STRUCTURES ON APC IN AD

The emergence of extrinsic/allergic AD (i.e., a cell-mediated inflammation) in atopic patients (i.e., individuals prone to increased IgE production and to devel-oping IgE-mediated hypersensitivity reactions) remained puzzling until in the mid-1980s. The first indication of the presence of an IgE-binding receptor on epidermal LC came from studies by Bruijnzeel-Koomen et al. (14). Their obser-vation, that Langerhans cells from patients with AD but not healthy individuals carried IgE molecules, pointed towards an involvement of an IgE-binding struc-ture in the disease. At that time, not only epidermal LC but also dermal DC and macrophages were shown to bear IgE and thus were suspected to play a role in AD (5,32). Thus, a new pathophysiological concept was proposed in which LC and/or other IgE-bearing APC would trigger an eczematous inflammation (15). At least three different IgE-binding structures are known in the human system, all of which have subsequently been demonstrated on LC: the high-affinity recep-tor for IgE (FcεRI) (9,52), the low-affinity receptor for IgE (FcεRII/CD23) (11), and the IgE-binding protein εBP (now called galectin-3) (54).

IV. THE HIGH-AFFINITY RECEPTOR FOR IgE ON SKIN DC: MOLECULAR STRUCTURE, REGULATION, AND FUNCTIONAL CHARACTERIZATION

Epidermal LC and IDEC are known to express all three IgE-binding structures. Thus, the identity of the relevant IgE-binding structure of cutaneous DC was unclear for years until we and others demonstrated the presence of FcεRI on LC (9,52).

A. Molecular Structure of FcεRI on APC

The presence of FcεRI has been reported on several types of human professional APC other than LC, i.e., monocytes (34), blood DC (33), and IDEC (56). Interestingly, FcεRI has not been found on APC in mice of any strain. Lacking the classical β-chain, FcεRI on APC displays a different structure from that on mast cells or basophils. Consequently, FcεRI on human APC is composed of an IgE-binding α-chain and two disulfide linked γ-chains (8). This trimeric α,2γ structure retains all the minimal features required for a functional receptor on APC, as discussed below.

B. Expression of FcεRI on APC

On APC, FcεRI expression is highly variable. Concerning monocytes, some authors report that the receptor expression may be related to atopy (34), while others found at least low levels of FcεRI on monocytes in all individuals (42). In a recent study we explored the expression of FcεRI and other surface markers on monocytes in a large panel of donors including nonatopics, atopic patients with allergic rhinitis, and patients with both extrinsic/allergic and intrinsic/nonallergic forms of AD. We showed a significant correlation between the status of the patient and the expression of distinct markers such as FcεRI, CD40, or IL-4R on monocytes (N. Novak et al., unpublished), supporting the concept of distinct stage of maturation of monocytes in atopic individuals. Whether this variability is also found in blood DC (33) still remains to be explored in a large number of individuals. So far, the issue of variability of receptor expression has been best investigated in epidermal LC and monocyte-derived DC. For example, it is nearly undetectable on the surface of epidermal LC in about 10% of the population, and the expression is usually low on LC isolated from normal skin of nonatopic individuals (7). In contrast, FcεRI expression is dramatically enhanced on LC and IDEC in lesional skin of AD (56,60). Interestingly, the amount of receptor expressed on LC/IDEC isolated from lesional skin correlates to the serum IgE level of the patients (56,60). In other skin diseases, FcεRI expression is also increased, but to a much lesser extent, again suggesting that distinct mediators present in AD may contribute to a dramatic upregulation of this receptor on LC and IDEC, thereby increasing the binding sites for IgE. Based on this observation, we developed a new diagnostic tool that makes it possible to establish the diagnosis of AD (59,60) and to clearly distinguish between extrinsic/allergic and intrinsic/nonallergic forms of AD (39).

Insights into the mechanisms regulating the FcεRI expression in LC have shown that the IgE-binding α-chain is constitutively expressed intracellularly and its surface expression is controlled by the variable expression of the γ-chain (30). Further detailed analysis by confocal laser microscopy and biochemistry on monocyte-derived DC have confirmed that the lack of association with the γ-chain is responsible for a segregation of the α-chain in the endoplasmic reticulum (ER) and that these structures are incompletely processed in terms of glycosylation (S. Kraft et al., unpublished).

C. Activation of APC via FcεRI

Aggregation of FcεRI on normal monocytes and LC does not lead to Ca^{2+} mobilization, whereas LC isolated from AD or monocytes that have been allowed to adhere to plastic clearly respond with an increase in free intracellular Ca^{2+} despite the absence of the β-chain (26,34). Investigation of the activation cascade initiated by FcεRI-ligation on APC suggests that, for mast cells and basophils, activation of protein-tyrosine kinases of the src and the syk families are mandatory proximal events in the signal transduction activation cascade. In APC with low surface expression, receptor ligation leads to a limited activation of the signal transduction cascade resulting in an inefficient phosphorylation of PLC-γ (S. Kraft et al., unpublished), which explains the lack of Ca^{2+} mobilization in LC from nonatopic individuals (26). Finally, cross-linking with anti-CD45 mAb prior to FcεRI aggregation leads to a diminution of the Ca^{2+} mobilization in LC from atopic individuals (10). This indicates the role of the protein-tyrosine phosphatase (PTPase) CD45 in the initiation of the signal transduction.

The investigation of transcription factors putatively mediating FcεRI-induced gene regulation has just begun. In general, members of the NF-κB family are known to regulate APC function and differentiation, with special importance for the RelB subunit in DC generation. In addition, Ikaros and PU.1 have also been shown to be essential factors for DC differentiation, whereas Oct-2 is upregulated by differentiation towards macrophages. Recently, FcεRI has been demonstrated to induce NF-κB activation via IκB-α serine phosphorylation and degradation in monocytes and DC (S. Kraft et al., unpublished). Inhibitors of NF-κB activation such as NAC or TPCK can suppress FcεRI-induced TNF-α and MCP-1 release. Interestingly, similarly to the observation mentioned above, in human LC NF-κB activation can only be observed when high amounts of FcεRI are present. In addition, the composition of NF-κB complexes differs between monocytes, monocyte-derived DC (MoDC) and LC, suggesting a cell-type specific regulation. Moreover, the transcription factor NFAT is induced upon FcεRI ligation in human APC (S. Kraft et al., unpublished).

D. Roles of FcεRI on APC in the Generation of the Inflammatory Reaction: Facts and Speculations

Based on the signal transduction cascade and the activation of transcription factors mentioned above, one may speculate that FcεRI ligation on APC triggers the synthesis and release of mediators that may initiate or modulate local inflammatory reactions, as has been demonstrated for mast cells. Thus, FcεRI/IgE-mediated allergen uptake and subsequent antigen presentation has been considered a key event in the pathogenesis of atopic dermatitis (8). Using this uptake machinery, APC may, in the presence of antigen-specific IgE, increase their presenting capacity up to 100-fold (33). The observation that the presence of FcεRI-expressing LC/IDEC, bearing IgE molecules, is a prerequisite to provoking eczematous lesions observed after application of aeroallergens to the skin of atopic patients strongly supports this concept (C. Bruynzeel-Kommen, personal communication). Therefore, IgE receptors are the connecting link between the specificity gaining IgE molecules and the APC. However, FcεRI seems to play the major role in these phenomenona. It should be noted that FcεRI expressed on circulating monocytes may have other functions, mainly in regulating their survival and differentiation outcome (29).

Following the presentation of allergens to T cells, allergen-specific B cells in the periphery may be activated to produce high amounts of allergen-specific IgE. This IgE may then in turn bind to the FcεRI on the antigen-presenting cells, closing a vicious circle of facilitated antigen presentation (Fig. 1). The intermittent or continuous supply of aeroallergens or autoantigens to the process of facilitated antigen presentation may define the pathophysiological basis of the recurrent or self-perpetuating course of atopic dermatitis frequently seen in untreated patients (53). Moreover, it has been proposed, based on the model of atopy patch test, that AD is a biphasic disease where IL-4–producing Th2 cells predominate in the very early phase (up to 48 hours), after which a switch to IFN-γ–producing Th1 cells occurs under the influence of locally produced IL-12 (22). Either de novo infiltrating eosinophils (23) and/or IDEC (which in contrast to eosinophils

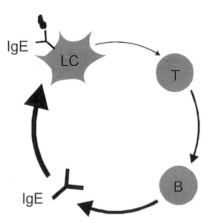

Figure 1   Langerhans cells take up intact protein allergens, process them into peptides, and present those to T cells, activating B cells, leading to a production of allergen-specific IgE. This IgE binds to the surface of the antigen-presenting cell, thereby enhancing the allergen-specific antigen-presenting capacity of the Langerhans cells about 100-fold and starting the vicious circle of antigen presentation.

persist in the inflammatory infiltrate of AD) are good candidates for this task. This would explain how the skin lesions ultimately resemble classical allergic contact dermatitis.

The successful application of aeroallergens such as cat dander in the recently standardized atopy patch test (18,19) shows that it is possible to provoke eczematous skin lesions by sole external application of aeroallergens to the normal atopic skin. Based on the facilitated antigen presentation model of AD, the need for identification of the individual provocation factors in each patient calls for diagnostic procedures based on the allergen-specific IgE. Cat dander, house dust mite allergens, and a variety of food allergens may be sucessfully avoided following a thoroughly undertaken prick test in vitro IgE diagnostic evaluation and confirmation of relevancy by oral provocation tests where applicable. These phenomena are summarized in Fig. 2, where the putative initial role of LC is depicted followed by the amplifying action of IDEC.

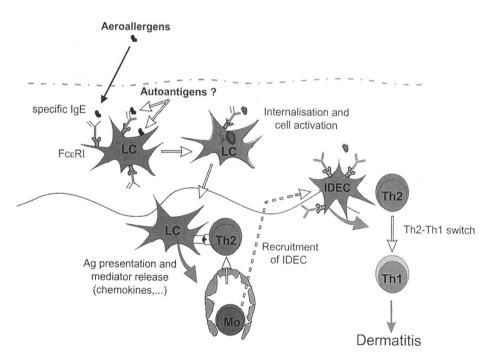

Figure 2 Possible scenario involving FcεRI-expressing Langerhans cells (LC) and subsequently inflammatory dendritic epidermal cells (IDEC) in the pathogenesis of AD lesions.

V. SKIN APC AS THERAPEUTIC TARGETS IN AD

In spite of the still elusive pathogenesis of AD, it is tempting to speculate on skin DC as potential targets for a therapy of AD. Most of these strategies are designed to interfere with the cellular integrity of DC or their functional capacity to process or present antigen.

The induction of skin DC apoptosis by UV light or corticosteroids or biochemical, more cell specific targets inducing apoptosis in skin DC is an attractive strategy, but it interferes with both wanted and unwanted immune responses induced by DC. The same holds true for all strategies interfering with the general capacity of DC to internalize, process, and present antigen, such as pinocytosis, peptide loading, MHC expression, adhesion or costimulatory molecule expression. Another potential strategy is to interfere with the chemokine and chemokine receptor–based cell-trafficking system, targeting the DC into the skin and back to the lymph nodes. Some relevant chemokine receptors have recently been identified (16).

IgE-mediated facilitated antigen presentation of aero-, food, and autoallergens is regarded a central pathogenetic event in atopic dermatitis (8). Hence, another potential srategy is to interfere with this process. This may be accomplished by downregulation of the FcεRI on lesional LC and IDEC or by interfering with the binding of IgE to its receptor by anti-FcεRI antibodies or FcεRI antagonists. The selectivity of this approach to IgE-mediated responses seems to be an advantage over the other, more general strategies mentioned above.

Inhibition of cytokine production or skin DC maturation might be another worthwhile therapeutic strategy. Finally, immunomodulatory drugs such as tacrolimus may lead to phenotypic and functional alteration of LC and IDEC if applied topically to lesional AD skin (58). In addition, these drug effects have been studied in vitro, where it has been shown that they profoundly affect the maturation and stimulatory activity of LC (40).

VI. FUTURE PERSPECTIVES

The clinical, histological, and immunohistological aspects of AD imply that, as in allergic contact dermatitis, APCs are needed to drive the inflammatory reaction in this disease. Although recent progress has made it possible to better characterize the different types of APC putatively involved in the pathogenesis of AD, further ex vivo and in vitro studies on the precise contribution of LC, DC, and monocyte/macrophages are urgently needed in order to assign the place of these pieces in the context of the complex pathophysiological puzzle of AD. Current progress in the techniques designed to generate and reproduce in vitro those APCs found in the normal and lesional skin of AD will doubtlessly greatly enhance our knowledge on the respective role of these cells in this chronic inflammatory condition. The answer to the still numerous open questions on the APCs in AD will also hopefully clarify the issue of whether extrinsic/allergic and intrinsic/nonallergic forms of AD are to be considered as relatives in a family of eczematous diseases in the genetically complex atopic background.

REFERENCES

1. Allavena P, Piemonti L, Longoni D, Bernasconi S, Stoppacciaro A, Ruco L, Mantovani A. IL-10 prevents the differentiation of monocytes to dendritic cells but promotes their maturation to macrophages. Eur J Immunol 28:359–369, 1998.

2. Baadsgaard O, Gupta AK, Taylor RS, Ellis CN, Voorhees JJ, Cooper KD. Psoriatic epidermal cells demonstrate increased numbers and function of non-Langerhans antigen presenting cells. J Invest Dermatol 92:190–195, 1989.

3. Banchereau J, Steinman RM. Dendritic cells and the control of immunity. Nature 392:245–252, 1998.

4. Bani D, Moretti S, Pimpinelli N, Gianotti B. Differentiation of monocytes into Langerhans cells in human epidermis. An ultrastructural study. In: Thivolet J, Schmitt D, eds. The Langerhans Cell. London: John Libbey, 1988, pp 75–83.

5. Barker JN, Alegre VA, MacDonald DM. Surface-bound immunoglobulin E on antigen-presenting cells in cutaneous tissue of atopic dermatitis. J Invest Dermatol 90:117–121, 1988.

6. Berman B, Chen VL, France DS, Dotz WI, Petroni G. Anatomical mapping of epidermal Langerhans cell densities in adults. Br J Dermatol 109:553–558, 1983.

7. Bieber T. Fc epsilon RI on human Langerhans cells: a receptor in search of new functions. Immunol Today 15:52–53, 1994.

8. Bieber T. FceRI-expressing antigen-presenting cells: new players in the atopic game. Immunol Today 18:311–313, 1997.

9. Bieber T, de la Salle H, Wollenberg A, Hakimi J, Chizzonite R, Ring J, Hanau D, de la Salle C. Human epidermal Langerhans cells express the high affinity receptor for immunoglobulin E (Fc epsilon RI). J Exp Med 175:1285–1290, 1992.

10. Bieber T, Jürgens M, Wollenberg A, Strobel I, Hanau D, de la Salle H. Characterization of the phosphotyrosine phosphatase CD45 on human Langerhans cells. Eur J Immunol 25:317–321, 1995.

11. Bieber T, Rieger A, Neuchrist C, Prinz J, Rieber E, Boltz-Nitulescu G, Scheiner O, Kraft D, Ring J, Stingl G. Induction of FceR2/CD23 on human epidermal Langerhans cells by human recombinant interleukin-4 and gamma interferon. J Exp Med 170:309–314, 1989.

12. Birbeck MS, Breathnach AS, Everall JD. An electron microscopic study of basal melanocyte and high level clear cells (Langerhans cells) in vitiligo. J Invest Dermatol 37:51–63, 1961.

13. Bos JD. Skin Immune System (SIS). Boca Raton: CRC Press, 1997.

14. Bruijnzeel-Koomen C, van Wichen DF, Toonstra J, Berrens L, Bruijnzeel PL. The presence of IgE molecules on epidermal Langerhans cells in patients with atopic dermatitis. Arch Dermatol Res 278:199–205, 1986.

15. Bruijnzeel-Koomen CA, Fokkens WJ, Mudde GC, Bruijnzeel PL. Role of Langerhans cells in atopic disease. Int Arch Allergy Appl Immunol 90 Suppl 1:51–56, 1989.

16. Charbonnier AS, Kohrgruber N, Kriehuber E, Stingl G, Rot A, Maurer D. Macrophage inflammatory protein 3alpha is involved in the constitutive trafficking of epidermal Langerhans cells. J Exp Med 190:1755–1768, 1999.

17. Cumberbatch M, Dearman RJ, Kimber I. Interleukin 1 beta and the stimulation of Langerhans cell migration: comparisons with tumor necrosis factor alpha. Arch Dermatol Res 289:277–284, 1997.

18. Darsow U, Vieluf D, Ring J. Atopy patch test with different vehicles and allergen concentrations: an approach to standardization. J Allergy Clin Immunol 95:677–684, 1995.

19. Darsow U, Vieluf D, Ring J. Evaluating the relevance of aeroallergen sensitization in atopic eczema with the atopy patch test: a randomized, double-blind multicenter study. Atopy Patch Test Study Group. J Am Acad Dermatol 40:187–193, 1999.

20. Eckert F. Histopathological and immunohistological aspects of atopic dermatitis. In: Ruzicka T, Ring J, Przybilla B, eds. Handbook of Atopic Dermatitis. Berlin: Springer, 1991, pp 127–131.

21. Enk AH, Angeloni VL, Udey MC, Katz SI. An essential role for Langerhans cell-derived IL-1 beta in the initiation of primary immune responses in skin. J Immunol 150:3698–3704, 1993.

22. Grewe M, Bruijnzeel-Koomen CA, Schöpf E, Thepen T, Langeveld-Wildschut AG, Ruzicka T, Krutmann J. A role for Th1 and Th2 cells in the immunopathogenesis of atopic dermatitis. Immunol Today 19:359–361, 1998.

23. Grewe M, Czech W, Morita A, Werfel T, Klammer M, Kapp A, Ruzicka T, Schopf E, Krutmann J. Human eosinophils produce biologically active IL-12: implications for control of T cell responses. J Immunol 161:415–420, 1998.

24. Hanau D, Fabre M, Schmitt D, Stampf J, Garaud J, Bieber T, Grosshans E, Benezra C, Cazenave J. Human epidermal Langerhans cells internalize by receptor-mediated endocytosis T6 (CD1 "NA1/34") surface antigen. Birbeck granules are involved in the intracellular traffic of the T6 antigen. J Invest Dermatol 89:172–177, 1987.

25. Hanau D, Gachet C, Schmitt D, Ohlmann P, Brisson C, Fabre M, Cazenave J. Ultrastructural similarities between epidermal Langerhans cell Birbeck granules and the surface-connected canalicular system of EDTA-treated human blood platelets. J Invest Dermatol 97:756–762, 1991.

26. Jürgens M, Wollenberg A, Hanau D, de la Salle H, Bieber T. Activation of human epidermal Langerhans cells by engagement of the high affinity receptor for IgE, FceRI. J Immunol 155:5184–5189, 1995.

27. Kang K, Hammerberg C, Meunier L, Cooper KD. CD11b+ macrophages that infiltrate human epidermis after in vivo ultraviolet exposure potently produce IL-10 and represent the major secretory source of epidermal IL-10 protein. J Immunol 153:5256–5264, 1994.

28. Kashihara M, Masamichi U, Horiguchi Y, Furukawa F, Hanaoka M, Imamura S. A

Monoclonal antibody specifically reactive to human Langerhans cells. J Invest Dermatol 87:602–607, 1986.

29. Katoh N, Kraft S, Wessendorf JH, Bieber T. The high-affinity IgE receptor (FcepsilonRI) blocks apoptosis in normal human monocytes. J Clin Invest 105:183–190, 2000.

30. Kraft S, Weβendorf JHM, Hanau D, Bieber T. Regulation of the high affinity receptor for IgE on human epidermal Langerhans cells. J Immunol 161:1000–1006, 1998.

31. Langerhans P. Über die Nerven der menschlichen Haut. Arch Pathol Anatom 44: 325–337, 1868.

32. Leung DY, Schneeberger EE, Siraganian RP, Geha RS, Bhan AK. The presence of IgE on macrophages and dendritic cells infiltrating into the skin lesion of atopic dermatitis. Clin Immunol Immunopathol 42:328–337, 1987.

33. Maurer D, Fiebiger E, Ebner C, Reininger B, Fischer GF, Wichlas S, Jouvin M-H, Schmitt-Egenolf M, Kraft D, Kinet J-P, Stingl G. Peripheral blood dendritic cells express FceRI as a complex composed of FceRIa and FceRIg-chains and can use this receptor for IgE-mediated allergen presentation. J Immunol 157:607–616, 1996.

34. Maurer D, Fiebiger E, Reininger B, Wolff-Winiski B, Jouvin M, Kilgus O, Kinet J, Stingl G. Expression of functional high affinity immunoglobulin E receptors (FceRI) on monocytes of atopic individuals. J Exp Med 179:747–750, 1994.

35. Meunier L, Gonzalez RA, Cooper KD. Heterogeneous populations of class II MHC+ cells in human dermal cell suspensions. Identification of a small subset responsible for potent dermal antigen-presenting cell activity with features analogous to Langerhans cells. J Immunol 151:4067–4080, 1993.

36. Mitra RS, Judge TA, Nestle FO, Turka LA, Nickoloff BJ. Psoriatic skin-derived dendritic cell function is inhibited by exogenous IL-10. Differential modulation of B7-1 (CD80) and B7-2 (CD86) expression. J Immunol 154:2668–2677, 1995.

37. Mommaas M, Mulder A, Vermeer BJ, Koning F. Functional human epidermal Langerhans cells that lack Birbeck granules. J Invest Dermatol 103:807–810, 1994.

38. Nestle FO, Turka LA, Nickoloff BJ. Characterization of dermal dendritic cells in psoriasis—autostimulation of T lymphocytes and induction of Th1 type cytokines. J Clin Invest 94:202–209, 1994.

39. Oppel T, Schuller E, Günther S, Moderer M, Haberstok J, Bieber T, Wollenberg A. Phenotyping of epidermal dendritic cells allows the differentiation between extrinsic and intrinsic form of atopic dermatitis. Br J Dermatol 143:1193–1198, 2000.

40. Panhans-Groβ A, Novak N, Kraft S, Bieber T. Human epidermal Langerhans cells are targets for the immunosuppressive macrolide tacrolimus (FK506). J Allergy Clin Immunol 107:345–352, 2001.

41. Rajka G. Essential Aspects of Atopic Dermatitis. Berlin: Springer, 1989.

42. Reischl IG, Corvaia N, Effenberger F, Wolff Winiski B, Kromer E, Mudde GC. Function and regulation of Fc epsilon RI expression on monocytes from non-atopic donors. Clin Exp Allergy 26:630–641, 1996.

43. Romani N, Lenz A, Glassel H, Stanzl H, Majdic O, Fritsch P, Schuler G. Cultured human Langerhans cells resemble lymphoid dendritic cells in phenotype and function. J Invest Dermatol 93:600–609, 1989.

44. Sallusto F, Cella M, Danieli C, Lanzavecchia A. Dendritic cells use macropinocytosis and the mannose receptor to concentrate macromolecules in the major histo-

compatibility complex class II compartment: downregulation by cytokines and bacterial products. J Exp Med 182:389–400, 1995.

45. Schuler G, Steinman RM. Murine epidermal Langerhans cells mature into potent immunostimulatory dendritic cells in vitro. J Exp Med 161:526–546, 1985.

46. Schuller E, Teichmann B, Haberstok J, Moderer M, Bieber T, Wollenberg A. In situ-expression of the costimulatory molecules CD80 and CD86 on Langerhans cells and inflammatory dendritic epidermal cells (IDEC) in atopic dermatitis. Arch Derm Res. In press.

47. Steinman RM. The dendritic cell system and its role in immunogenicity. Annu Rev Immunol 9:271–296, 1991.

48. Taylor RS, Baadsgaard O, Hammerberg C, Cooper KD. Hyperstimulatory CD1a+CD1b+CD36+ Langerhans cells are responsible for increased autologous T lymphocyte reactivity to lesional epidermal cells of patients with atopic dermatitis. J Immunol 147:3794–3802, 1991.

49. Teunissen MBM, Kapsenberg ML, Bos JD. Langerhans cells and related skin dendritic cells. In: Bos JD, ed. Skin Immune System (SIS). Boca Raton: CRC Press, 1997, pp 59–83.

50. Valladeau J, Duvert-Frances V, Pin JJ, Dezutter-Dambuyant C, Vincent C, Massacrier C, Vincent J, Yoneda K, Banchereau J, Caux C, Davoust J, Saeland S. The monoclonal antibody DCGM4 recognizes Langerin, a protein specific of Langerhans cells, and is rapidly internalized from the cell surface. Eur J Immunol 29:2695–2704, 1999.

51. Valladeau J, Ravel O, Dezutter-Dambuyant C, Moore K, Kleijmeer M, Liu Y, Duvert-Frances V, Vincent C, Schmitt D, Davoust J, Caux C, Lebecque S, Saeland S. Langerin, a novel C-type lectin specific to Langerhans cells, is an endocytic receptor that induces the formation of Birbeck granules. Immunity 12:71–81, 2000.

52. Wang B, Rieger A, Kilgus O, Ochiai K, Maurer D, Födinger D, Kinet J, Stingl G. Epidermal Langerhans cells from normal human skin bind monomeric IgE via FcεRI. J Exp Med 175:1353–1365, 1992.

53. Wollenberg A, Bieber T. Atopic dermatitis: from the genes to skin lesions. Allergy 55:205–213, 2000.

54. Wollenberg A, de la Salle H, Hanau D, Liu FT, Bieber T. Human keratinocytes release the endogenous β-galactoside-binding soluble lectin eBP which binds to Langerhans cells where it modulates their binding capacity for IgE glycoforms. J Exp Med 178:777–785, 1993.

55. Wollenberg A, Haberstok J, Schuller E, Teichmann B, Bieber T. Upregulation of Fcg receptors on epidermal dendritic cells is specific for psoriasis vulgaris. Arch Dermatol Res 291:153, 1999.

56. Wollenberg A, Kraft S, Hanau D, Bieber T. Immunomorphological and ultrastructural characterization of Langerhans cells and a novel, inflammatory dendritic epidermal cell (IDEC) population in lesional skin of atopic eczema. J Invest Dermatol 106:446–453, 1996.

57. Wollenberg A, Schuller E. Langerhans Zellen und Immunantwort. In: Plewig G, Wolff H, eds. Fortschritte der praktischen Dermatologie und Venerologie. Berlin: Springer, 1999, pp 41–48.

58. Wollenberg A, Sharma S, von Bubnoff D, Geiger E, Haberstok J, Bieber T. Topical

tacrolimus (FK506) leads to profound phenotypic and functional alterations of epidermal antigen-presenting dendritic cells in atopic dermatitis. J Allergy Clin Immunol 107:519–525, 2001.

59. Wollenberg A, Wen S, Bieber T. Langerhans cell phenotyping: a new tool for differential diagnosis of inflammatory skin diseases. Lancet 346:1626–1627, 1995.

60. Wollenberg A, Wen S, Bieber T. Phenotyping of epidermal dendritic cells—clinical applications of a flow cytometric micromethod. Cytometry 37:147–155, 1999.

61. Wüthrich B. Atopic dermatitis flare provoked by inhalant allergens. Dermatologica 178:51–53, 1989.

15
Mast Cells and Basophils

Naotomo Kambe, Anne-Marie Irani, and Lawrence B. Schwartz
Virginia Commonwealth University, Richmond, Virginia

I. INTRODUCTION

Mast cells and basophils are generally recognized as the principal cell types to initiate IgE-dependent, type I immediate hypersensitivity reactions. More recently, mast cells have been implicated as participants in innate immunity, additional aspects of acquired immunity, and tissue remodeling (Fig. 1). Mast cells originate from bone marrow progenitors but complete their maturation in tissues where they then reside. Basophils also originate from bone marrow progenitors but complete their maturation before being released from the bone marrow into the circulation, where they reside until called into tissues at sites of inflammation, particularly during the late phase of IgE-mediated immediate hypersensitivity reactions and during the early phase of cell-mediated, delayed-type hypersensitivity reactions. Mast cells and basophils are the only two cell types that constitutively express substantial quantities of the high-affinity, tetrameric receptor for IgE (FcϵRI) and store histamine in their secretory granules. These two cell types are distinguished from one another by their respective pathways for growth, differentiation, and survival; patterns of cell-surface adhesion, cytokine and chemokine receptors; responses to non–IgE-dependent agonists; secretory granule proteoglycans and proteases; and morphologies. For example, nuclei of peripheral blood basophils have deeply divided lobes, whereas those of mast cells in normal tissues are rounded.

Atopic dermatitis is a genetically influenced chronic inflammatory disorder of the skin characterized by persistent pruritus that leads to scratching and lichenification. Atopic dermatitis is commonly seen in association with allergic rhinitis and asthma in families or individuals, suggesting that it is a cutaneous form of

285

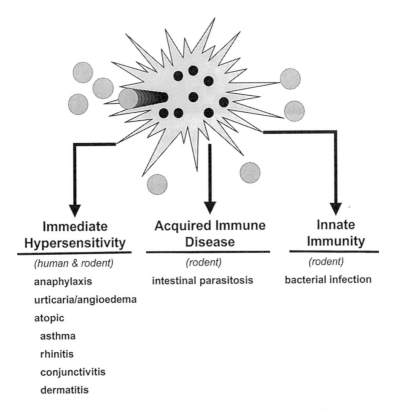

Immediate Hypersensitivity	**Acquired Immune Disease**	**Innate Immunity**
(human & rodent)	*(rodent)*	*(rodent)*
anaphylaxis	intestinal parasitosis	bacterial infection
urticaria/angioedema		
atopic		
asthma		
rhinitis		
conjunctivitis		
dermatitis		

Figure 1 Immunological effector roles of mast cells and basophils. Mast cells and basophils are the primary effector cells in immediate hypersensitivity reactions, but they also may participate in innate immune defense and in acquired immunity against certain microbes.

allergic disease. Although the participation of mast cells and basophils in allergic disorders is well established, their significance in atopic dermatitis still remains unclear. An experimental allergen challenge of an IgE-sensitized host reveals two phases to the subsequent immediate hypersensitivity reaction. The early phase of the IgE-dependent reaction (beginning 5–30 minutes postchallenge), depending on the target tissue and distribution of allergen, involves local edema, smooth muscle contraction, vasodilation, and increased permeability of postcapillary venules. These events represent the characteristic features of acute urticaria, but not of atopic dermatitis. The late phase of an immediate hypersensitivity reaction (4–12 hours postchallenge) involves the recruitment and activation of basophils, eosinophils, and other cell types. These late reactions can persist for at least 2 days in the challenged site, but eventually appear to completely resolve.

Topical applications of allergen repeated daily for 6 days can result in an increased number of mast cells (1). Thus, chronic allergic inflammation can result from prolonged allergen exposure and may contribute to the pathophysiology of atopic dermatitis.

Several studies suggest a relationship between atopic dermatitis and mast cells and basophils. First, in lichenified lesions of atopic dermatitis, the total number of mast cells may be increased (Fig. 2A, B), while in the acute phase of atopic dermatitis, mast cells are fragmented or degranulated but not notably

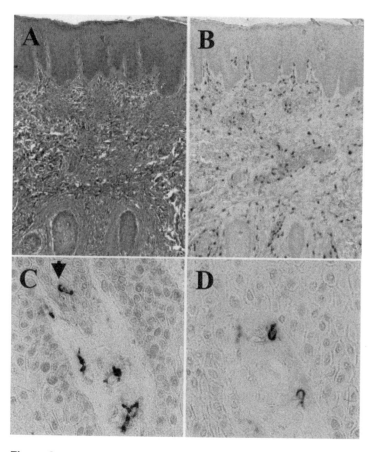

Figure 2 Mast cells in lesional skin of atopic dermatitis. Sequential sections of lichenified skin were stained with hematoxylin and eosin (A) and labeled with anti-tryptase mAb (B). Mast cells are difficult to identify in the hematoxylin and eosin-stained section, while immunohistochemistry for tryptase clearly reveals mast cell hyperplasia at this site. (C) Four MC_{TC} cells are seen, one of which has penetrated into the epidermis (arrow). (D) Three MC_T cells are observed in the dermis near the basement membrane.

increased in number (2–4). No significant correlation between clinical severity scores and mast cell numbers was found (5). Second, patients suffering from atopic dermatitis have markedly elevated levels of serum IgE. Mast cells and basophils are well-known target cells for this molecule, because they express abundant amounts of FcεRI on their surfaces. Third, certain genes associated with atopy are also expressed by mast cells. The β-subunit of FcεRI on chromosome 11q13 is linked to atopy, the state of enhanced IgE responsiveness (6,7). DNA sequences from atopic individuals show three base-pair substitutions converting Ile 181 to Leu 181. Although initially no such linkage was found in 95 English eczema families (8), linkage did emerge with later analyses (9). A significant association between the *Bst*XI polymorphism in mast cell chymase on chromosome 14q11 and eczema has been reported (10–12).

This chapter will focus on biology of human mast cells and basophils and the potential involvement of these cells in the pathogenesis of atopic dermatitis.

II. DIFFERENTIATION OF BASOPHILS AND MAST CELLS

Mast cells and basophils were initially thought to be developmentally related by virtue of their shared characteristic features, including metachromasia of their secretory granules, FcεRI on their surfaces, and histamine in their secretory granules. Both mast cells and basophils originate from hematopoietic stem cells, but they follow divergent pathways of differentiation. Basophils, like most myeloid cells, complete their differentiation in the bone marrow prior to entering the systemic circulation and develop largely under the influence of interleukin (IL)-3, a process that is augmented by transforming growth factor (TGF)-β. In contrast, mast cells destined to reside in peripheral tissues will leave the bone marrow as an immature mononuclear progenitor, probably with multipotential capabilities, enter the circulation still without characteristic secretory granules and surface FcεRI expression, but complete their differentiation into mature mast cells only after arriving in peripheral tissues such as lung, bowel, dermis, and nasal and conjunctival mucosa, largely under the influence of stem cell factor (SCF).

A. Murine Mast Cell Development

The evidence that tissue mast cells are derived from hematopoietic cells was first shown by using *bg^J/bg^J* mice (13). This beige mouse has a disorder similar to human Chediak-Higashi syndrome, characterized by marked enlargement of lysosomes and specific granules in various cell types. Transplantation of *bg^J/bg^J* mice bone marrow cells into irradiated +/+ mice resulted in the development of mast cells containing *bg^J/bg^J*-type giant granules. The origin of mast cells was also shown by in vitro suspension culture systems (14–18). When cells derived from hematopoietic tissues of mice were cultured with growth factors from stimulated T cells or with culture medium from a mouse myelomonocytic leukemia cell line WEHI-3, cells morphologically identified as mast cells appeared. Later, IL-3 was identified as the mast cell growth factor in the culture medium of WEHI-3 cells (19) and stimulated T cells (20). In suspension culture with IL-3, a large number of mast cells can be generated from murine hematopoietic progenitor cells. The importance of IL-3 for murine mast cell development in vivo also has been examined. Substantial IL-3–dependent hyperplasia of mast cells in the intestine after parasite infection has been observed for wild-type but not T cell–deficient (21) or IL-3–deficient mice (22). In the latter case, basophils were also deficient, but basal levels of mast cells were normal in both cases.

Genetically mast cell–deficient mice, named W/W^v (defective Kit) and Sl/Sl^d (defective SCF, also called Kit ligand), were identified by Kitamura and co-workers (23,24). These mice are anemic and also deficient in germ cells, melano-cytes, and intestinal cells of Cajal. In spite of the mast cell depletion in nonin-flamed tissues from W and Sl mutant mice, bone marrow–derived mast cells can be generated in vitro when bone marrow–derived progenitors are cultured with IL-3, and mast cells also can appear at tissue sites of inflammation. Fibroblasts derived from normal $+/+$ mouse embryos express SCF and thus can support the survival of bone marrow-derived mast cells derived from $+/+$ mice and those from Sl/Sl^d mice, but not those from W/W^v mice. W/W^v mice have been used to study the involvement of mast cells in various disease models, including anaphy-laxis and allergic airway inflammation (25).

B. Human Mast Cell Development

Human mast cells differentiate under the influence of SCF (26–28). In contrast to rodent mast cells, IL-3 has little, if any, influence on the differentiation of human mast cells other than to expand the pool of hematopoietic progenitor cells.

Human mast cells originate from CD34+ bone marrow–derived progenitor cells (29). Using sorted cells isolated from cord blood or peripheral blood, mast cell progenitors were further characterized as multipotential cells positive for CD34 and CD38 (30) or for CD34, CD13, and Kit (31). However, less mature CD34+/CD38- precursor cells (32) did not give rise to mast cells when cultured with SCF, indicating a need for additional factors at this early stage of hematopoi-esis. CD13, a membrane-bound zinc-dependent metalloprotease also known as aminopeptidase N, was originally recognized as a marker for subsets of normal and malignant myeloid cells (33) and later as a cell activation marker associated with proliferation. Thus, the early steps of hematopoietic commitment to a mast cell lineage still need further clarification.

Why mast cells fail to develop in the bone marrow where SCF clearly affects the development of other cell types is an enigma. Either the bone marrow microenvironment lacks an accessory factor present in peripheral sites or the microenvironment contains additional factors that are not permissive for mast cell development to occur. The latter seems in part to be the case, because both granulocyte-macrophage colony-stimulating factor (GM-CSF) (34) and IL-4 (34,35) appear to diminish SCF-dependent development of mast cells from progenitors in vitro but have little effect on more mature mast cells.

C. Growth Factors That Affect Human Mast Cell Development

Unlike other myelocytes, which stop expressing Kit as they mature, mast cells express increasing amounts of Kit as they develop. SCF, the ligand for Kit, exerts various effects on mast cells throughout their development, including differentiation, survival, chemotaxis, activation, and priming. SCF is the only growth factor that by itself supports the growth and differentiation in vitro of human mast cells from hematopoietic precursors in bone marrow and peripheral blood (28), cord blood (27,36), and fetal liver (26,37). These in vitro–derived human cultured mast cells now make possible further investigation about human mast cell characterization and their function, about the effect of cytokines on mast cell proliferation and development and receptor expression during the maturation process. Removal of SCF from cultured mast cells (38) results in their apoptosis. Certain gain of function mutations in human Kit (39) are associated with systemic mastocytosis. However, less commonly, loss of function mutations in Kit (40) are also associated with this disease characterized by mast cell hyperplasia, perhaps indicating that there are factors other than Kit involved in mastocytosis. A different group of activating Kit mutations are associated with intestinal stromal cell tumors in which interstitial cells of Cajal are transformed (41).

IL-4 effects on human mast cells are pleiotropic. Human mast cell numbers are diminished by IL-4 after culturing progenitor cells obtained from peripheral blood, cord blood, and fetal liver with SCF (38,42,43). The ability of IL-4 to downregulate expression of Kit may help to explain the ability of this cytokine to attenuate mast cell development under some circumstances (38,42). On the other hand, IL-4 induces FcεRI expression on developing fetal liver–derived and cord blood–derived mast cells (43,44), enhances SCF-dependent proliferation of intestinal preparations of mast cells activated through FcεRI (45), and enhances the survival of cord blood–derived mast cells after withdrawal of SCF (46). For cord blood–derived mast cells obtained with the combination of SCF and IL-6, IL-4 did not affect total mast cell numbers in one study but did induce their homotypic aggregation and enhance the percentage of chymase-positive mast cells (47). Enhancement by IL-4 of the chymase-positive mast cells also was observed for those derived from fetal liver (43). Using mast cells derived from fetal liver and cord blood progenitors cultured with SCF alone, IL-4 was shown to induce apoptosis only in the cord blood–derived mast cells, and this apoptotic effect on mast cells could be abolished if the cells were cultured with IL-6 in addition to SCF (35). IL-13, like IL-4 but with a weaker effect, downregulates Kit expression and upregulates adhesion molecule expression on HMC-1 cells, but has a negligible effect on SCF-dependent mast cell development from cord blood progenitors (48).

IL-6 has diverse effects on the development of human mast cells in vitro. IL-6 has been reported to both enhance (36) and attenuate (49) mast cell numbers obtained from cultures of cord blood progenitors and block IL-4–mediated apoptosis of cord blood-derived mast cells developed with SCF alone (35). IL-6 can enhance the percentage of mast cells expressing chymase (49).

IL-10, in rodent systems, stimulates mast cell growth when added to other mast cell growth factors, including IL-3, SCF, and IL-4 (50). IL-10 also increases cellular levels of the β-chymases, mouse mast cell protease (mMCP)-1, and mMCP-2, principally by stabilizing the corresponding mRNA molecules (51–53). With human cells IL-10 alone did not promote the survival of cord blood–derived (46) or fetal liver–derived (54) mast cells.

D. Mast Cell Heterogeneity

Like lymphocytes and other hematopoietic cells, mast cell subtypes have also been described that display variations in their morphological, biochemical, and functional properties. In mice, mast cells are often divided into connective tissue and mucosal mast cells. Connective tissue mast cells predominate in the skin, peritoneal cavity, and muscular propria of the stomach and express heparin proteoglycan; mucosal mast cells predominate in the mucosal layer of the gastrointestinal tract and express chondroitin sulfate proteoglycan. These different proteoglycan compositions probably account for differences in histochemical staining patterns. Both cell types can be stained by Alcian blue, but only those with heparin are stained with Safranin, a red dye, or Berberine sulfate, a fluorescent label.

In humans, two types of mast cells have been identified based on their protease composition (Fig. 3) (55). MC_{TC} cells contain tryptase, chymase, mast cell carboxypeptidase, and cathepsin G–like protease in their secretory granules. MC_T cells also contain tryptase in their granules but lack these other proteases. MC_{TC} cells are the predominant mast cell type in small bowel submucosa and in normal and urticaria pigmentosa skin as well as skin of atopic dermatitis, whereas MC_T cells are the predominant type found in the small bowel mucosa and normal airway and appear to be selectively recruited near the surface of the airway during seasonal allergic disease. Of possible interest is the selective attenuation in numbers of MC_T cells in the small bowel of patients with end-stage immunodeficiency diseases (56). Mast cells from different tissues, irrespective of their protease phenotype, may exhibit functional differences in their response to non–IgE-depen-

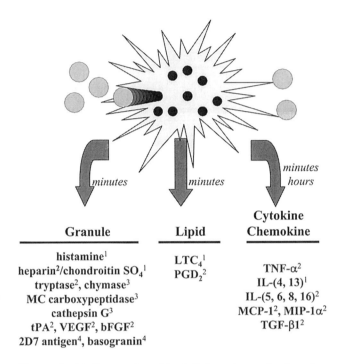

Granule	Lipid	Cytokine Chemokine
histamine[1] heparin[2]/chondroitin SO_4[1] tryptase[2], chymase[3] MC carboxypeptidase[3] cathepsin G[3] tPA[2], VEGF[2], bFGF[2] 2D7 antigen[4], basogranin[4]	LTC_4[1] PGD_2[2]	TNF-α[2] IL-(4, 13)[1] IL-(5, 6, 8, 16)[2] MCP-1[2], MIP-1α[2] TGF-β1[2]

Figure 3 Mediators released by IgE-dependent activation of mast cells and basophils. Superscripts indicate cell types as follows: both mast cells and basophils[1], MC_T and MC_{TC} cells[2], MC_{TC} cells[3], and basophils alone[4].

dent activators and pharmacological modulators of activation. The selected participation of basophils and different types of mast cells in various clinical conditions as well as the duration, intensity, and tissue distribution of a particular response will depend on various characteristics of the agonist, immunological sensitivity of the host, the target tissue involved, and any underlying pathology.

E. Effect of Microenvironment on Mast Cell Phenotype

In murine systems, the microenvironment influences the phenotype of the mast cells. When immature bone marrow–derived mast cells from wild-type mice are transferred into the peritoneal cavity of mast cell–deficient W/W^v mice, the histamine content increased more than 20-fold and the proteoglycan class changed from chondroitin sulfate to heparin. The phenotypic change also occurred in the opposite direction (57). In contrast, after injection of a single connective tissue type of mast cell from the peritoneal cavity of a wild-type mouse into the stomach wall of a W/W^v mouse, mast cells with phenotypic features of mucosal mast cells appeared in the mucosa and of connective tissue mast cells in the muscularis propria (57,58). Similarly, immature bone marrow–derived mast cells cocultured with mouse 3T3 fibroblasts developed a connective tissue mast cell–like phenotype, becoming Safranin and carboxypeptidase A positive (59). SCF alone induces this phenotypic maturation of bone marrow–derived mast cells into connective tissue mast cell–like cells (60). However, because Kit-deficient mast cells that develop in inflammatory skin lesions of W/W^v mice have the connective tissue mast cell phenotype (61), factors other than SCF may influence mast cell development in mice. For example, nerve growth factor in association with IL-3 results in a connective tissue mast cell–like phenotype (62). However, the developmental pathway(s) of human mast cells may not parallel those of the mouse.

In humans, conditions that influence the selective development or recruitment of MC_{TC} and MC_T cells are not yet understood. SCF-dependent in vitro–derived mast cells generally are immature and express tryptase but little if any chymase. Cytokines such as IL-4 (63), IL-6 (49), and NGF (64) have been reported to induce modest levels of chymase expression. However, fetal liver–derived mast cells express chymase mRNA but not chymase protein, suggesting that the level of regulation of chymase expression in such cells may be beyond gene expression. On the other hand, chymase expression in vivo may be regulated at the level of gene expression, because MC_T cells isolated from lung appear to lack chymase mRNA as well as chymase protein.

In vivo observations suggest that MC_{TC} and MC_T cells develop along distinct pathways. Patients with inherited severe combined immunodeficiency disease and acquired immunodeficiency syndrome, both end-stage, exhibited marked and selective decreases in MC_T cell concentrations in the small bowel, whereas the concentration and distribution of MC_{TC} cells were unaffected (56). This suggests that the recruitment, development, or survival of MC_T cells is dependent on functional T lymphocytes and that MC_{TC} cell development proceeds independently. Also, an ultrastructural analysis of immature mast cells in various tissues indicated that at the time granules first form, they form either as MC_T or MC_{TC} cells (65).

Potential chemokine-dependent pathways for recruitment of mast cells or mast cell progenitors into tissues have been suggested. Chemokines are small proteins involved in the recruitment of various leukocytes by interacting with specific chemokine receptors. The presence of the CXCR2 chemokine receptor for IL-8 on HMC-1 cells (66) and on relatively mature cord blood–derived mast cells (67) and CCR3, CCR5, CXCR2, and CXCR4 on developing cord blood–derived mast cells (67) has been reported. Of potential interest is CCR3, which is expressed on eosinophils, basophils, and a subset of T cells with Th2-like features. CCR3 binds eotaxin, eotaxin-2, RANTES, and monocyte chemotactic proteins (MCP)-2 to -4. When tissue sections were subjected to immunohistochemical staining, high percentages of CCR3-expressing mast cells were found in the skin and in the intestinal submucosa; much lower percentages were found in the intestinal mucosa and in lung, suggesting preferential expression of CCR3 by MC_{TC} cells (68). Thus, selective chemokines may play an important role in the tissue distribution of different types of human mast cells.

III. MEDIATORS

Mast cells and basophils contain numerous potent and biologically active mediators that can exert many different effects in inflammation at sites of their activation. Mediators secreted by activated mast cells and basophils can be divided into those stored in secretory granules prior to cell activation and those that are newly generated after an activation signal. The former include histamine, proteoglycans, proteases, and certain cytokines; the latter include metabolites of arachidonic acid, cytokines, and chemokines, as summarized in Figure 3.

A. Histamine

Histamine, the sole biogenic amine in human mast cells and basophils, is the only preformed mediator of the cells with direct potent vasoactive and smooth muscle spasmogenic effects. Histamine, β-imidazolylethylamine, is formed from histidine by histidine decarboxylase and then stored in secretory granules. With degranulation, histamine is released, diffuses rapidly, and is metabolized within minutes after release, suggesting that it is destined to act quickly and locally. Human mast cells and basophils contain 1–3 pg of histamine per cell. Mast cells account for nearly all the histamine stored in normal tissues, with the exception of the glandular stomach and central nervous system. Histamine concentrations of about 0.1 M are estimated to exist inside secretory granules, whereas concentrations of about 2 nM exist in plasma. The amount of histamine present in circulating basophils, if released, could raise plasma histamine levels about 500-fold, so great care must be exercised to avoid disrupting basophils when collecting blood for a plasma histamine determination.

Histamine exerts its biological and pathobiological effects through its interaction with cell-specific receptors designated H1, H2 and H3, which were initially defined with the recognition of specific agonists and antagonists. H1 (69) and H2 (70) receptors each have seven regions predicted to span the plasma membrane and are G protein–coupled receptors. H1 receptors are blocked by chlorpheniramine, H2 receptors are blocked by cimetidine, and H3 receptors are blocked by thioperamide. Examples of receptor-specific agonists include 2-methylhistamine at H1 receptors, dimaprit at H2 receptors, and α-methylhistamine at H3 receptors.

Effects of histamine mediated by H1 receptors include enhanced permeability of postcapillary venules, vasodilation, contraction of bronchial and gastrointestinal smooth muscle, and increased mucus secretion at mucosal sites. Increased vasopermeability will facilitate the tissue deposition of factors from plasma that may be important for tissue growth and repair and deposition of foreign material or immune complexes that result in tissue inflammation. Histamine by an H1 receptor–dependent mechanism in rodents also activates endothelial cells to transfer P-selectin from internal Weibel-Palade bodies to the cell surface, where neutrophil rolling is thereby enhanced (71,72). H1 receptor knock-out mice exhibit modest neurological alterations but show no developmental abnormalities (73).

H2 receptor agonists stimulate gastric acid secretion by parietal cells. H2 agonists also inhibit secretion by cytotoxic lymphocytes and granulocytes, augment suppression by T lymphocytes, enhance epithelial permeability across human airways, stimulate chemokinesis of neutrophils and eosinophils and expression of eosinophil C3b receptors, and activate endothelial cells to release a potent inhibitor of platelet aggregation, PGI_2 (prostacyclin).

The combined effects of H1 receptor– and H2 receptor–mediated activities of histamine are required for the full expression of vasoactivity. For example, the "triple response" caused by an intradermal injection of histamine, namely a central erythema within seconds (histamine arteriolar vasodilation), followed by circumferential erythema (axon reflex vasodilation mediated by neuropeptides) and a central weal (histamine vasopermeability, edema) peaking at about 15 minutes, is mostly blocked by H1 receptor antagonists but is completely blocked only with a combination of H1 and H2 receptor antagonists (74). Analogous results have been observed for the tachycardia, widened pulse pressure, diastolic hypotension, flushing, and headaches resulting from intravenous infusion of histamine (75).

Stimulation of H3 receptors affect neurotransmitter release and histamine formation in the central and peripheral nervous system. They are postulated but not proven to be involved in cross-talk between mast cells and peripheral nerves. Bronchial hyperreactivity in atopics with asthma to irritant stimuli may in part be mediated by histamine-mediated neurogenic hyperexcitability.

B. Proteoglycans

The presence of highly sulfated proteoglycans in secretory granules of mast cells and basophils results in metachromasia when these cells are stained with basic dyes. The intracellular proteoglycans present in mast cells are heparin and chondroitin sulfate E. Chondroitin sulfate A is the predominant type in human basophils and eosinophils. Among bone marrow–derived cells, heparin is selectively expressed by mast cells and resides in the secretory granules of all mature human mast cells (76), but only in connective tissue mast cells in rodents. Glial cells are also capable of producing heparin (77). When mast cells are activated to degranulate, heparin proteoglycan is exocytosed along with other granule constituents in a complex with positively charged proteases, likely to include tryptase and chymase.

Proteoglycans are composed of glycosaminoglycan side chains, repeating unbranched disaccharide units of a uronic acid and hexosamine moieties that are variably sulfated, which are covalently linked to a single-chain protein core via a specific trisaccharide-protein linkage region consisting of -Gal-Gal-Xyl-Ser. The average number of sulfate residues per respective disaccharide is 2.5, 1.5, and 1.0. The characteristic susceptibility of heparin to nitrous acid is due to attack at the N-sulfate residue; chondroitin sulfates lack this residue and are resistant to nitrous acid. On the other hand, the same peptide core is associated with heparin and chondroitin sulfate proteoglycans, and both proteoglycan types may reside in the same cell, even on the same peptide core. In humans the core protein is 17,600 daltons in size and contains a glycosaminoglycan attachment region of 18 amino acids, where two to three glycosaminoglycans of about 20,000 daltons are attached.

The biological functions of endogenous mast cell proteoglycans are somewhat speculative. These proteoglycans bind to histamine, neutral proteases, and acid hydrolases at the acidic pH inside mast cell secretory granules and may facilitate processing of the enzymes as well as uptake and packaging of these mediators into the secretory granules. The stabilizing effect of heparin and, to a lesser degree, chondroitin sulfate E on human tryptase activity may be crucial for the full expression of mast cell–mediated events. Heparin and, to a lesser extent, chondroitin sulfate E express anticoagulant, anticomplement, antikallikrein, and Hageman factor autoactivation activities. The anticoagulant activities of human and commercial porcine heparin are similar and depend on a specific pentasaccharide sequence. Heparin neutralizes the ability of eosinophil-derived major basic protein to kill schistosomula and enhances the binding of fibronectin to collagen. Heparin protects and facilitates basic fibroblast growth factor activity, which appears to reside in cutaneous mast cells (78), and modulates the cell adhesion properties of matrix proteins such as vitronectin, fibronectin, and laminin. Binding of heparin to L- and P-selectins inhibits inflammation (79), perhaps by blocking leukocyte rolling. However, when heparin is saturated with tryptase and other mast cell proteases, these activities may be attenuated. Disrupting the gene encoding glucosaminyl N-deacetylase/N-sulfotransferase-2 (NDST-2) (80,81) in mice yields mast cells exhibiting large vacuolated granules that were deficient in histamine and protease activities. In this NDST-2 knock-out mouse, only those mast cells that normally produce heparin, the so-called connective tissue mast cells, were affected, but coagulation-related problems were not noted.

C. Proteases

Proteases are enzymes that cleave peptide bonds, and certain ones are the dominant protein components of secretory granules in human and rodent mast cells. Basophils, compared to mast cells, are deficient in secretory granules protease activity. Some of these enzymes serve as selective markers that distinguish mast cells from other cell types, including basophils, and different mast cell subpopulations from one another.

1. Tryptase

Trypsin-like activity was first associated with human mast cells by histoenzymatic stains (82–84). Abundant and releasable trypsin-like activity was found in human lung mast cells in 1981 (85), followed by purification to homogeneity of the enzyme accounting for >90% of this activity, which was named tryptase (86). The enzyme was found to be a tetramer that spontaneously and irreversibly reverted to inactive monomers at neutral pH in a physiological salt solution unless stabilized by heparin or dextran sulfate (87,88). In 1998, the crystal structure of lung-derived tryptase was solved (89), confirming the tetrameric structure and the length of the heparin-binding groove previously predicted (87). Two heparin grooves per tetramer were found, each spanning the two adjacent subunits bound to one another only through weak hydrophobic interactions. All of the active sites faced into the small, central pore of the planar tetramer, thereby restricting inhibitor and substrate access (90). Because tryptase is selectively concentrated in mast cell secretory granules, it has also been studied as a clinical marker of mast cell–mediated diseases.

    Several cDNAs for human tryptase have been cloned (91–93). Tryptase genes are clustered on the short arm of human chromosome 16 (92,94). They have been divided mainly into two types, α-tryptase and β-tryptase, each encoding a 30-amino-acid leader sequence and a 245-amino-acid catalytic portion. α-Tryptases show ~90% sequence identity to β-tryptases. Defining differences appear to include Arg^{-3} and Gly^{215} in β-tryptases and Gln^{-3} and Asp^{215} in α-tryptases. Each α- and β-tryptase has several subtypes. αI- and αII-tryptases and βI-, βII-, and βIII- tryptases show at least 98% identity within types. Each of these tryptase genes is organized into six exons and five introns. By comparison, mouse mast cell tryptases mMCP-6 and mMCP-7 (95,96), syntenic on mouse chromosome 17, have amino acid sequences 71% identical to one another, each of which shows ~75% sequence identity and a similar exon/intron organization to the human enzymes. Human α- and β-tryptases are more closely related to one another than to known nonhuman tryptases (97). Although some ambiguity still remains in the number of tryptase genes per human haploid chromosome, at least one or two of the three β-tryptase subtypes, at least one of the two α-tryptase subtypes, and one pseudotryptase gene appear to reside on human chromosome 16.

Confusion arose when the term tryptase was applied to other trypsin-like serine proteases (Fig. 4). These include trypsin-like enzymes in natural killer and cytotoxic T cells (NK tryptases) (98–100), a MOLT-4 T-helper-cell line (tryptase TL₂) (101), and lung Clara cells (tryptase Clara) (102). However, these enzymes do not show sufficient sequence homology or comparable biochemical properties to the mast cell tryptase family to be in the same family. A family of serine protease genes has been cloned near the tryptase locus on human chromosome 16 and mouse chromosome 17 and referred to as transmembrane tryptases because of a predicted transmembrane region near the C terminus and trypsin-like substrate specificity (103). Again, these enzyme appear to be biochemically and immunologically distinct from α- and β-tryptases. Herein the term tryptase will be used only for the α- and β-tryptases of human mast cells.

Purified recombinant αI-protryptase and βII-protryptase were used to study processing to the active enzyme(s) (104,105). βII-Protryptase was processed in two proteolytic steps. First, autocatalytic intermolecular cleavage at Arg^{-3} occurred optimally at acidic pH and in the presence of heparin or dextran sulfate. Second, the remaining pro'dipeptide was removed by dipeptidyl peptidase I, a cysteine peptidase found in most hematopoietic cells with an acidic pH optimum. The mature peptide spontaneously formed enzymatically active tetramers, a process that seemed to require heparin or dextran sulfate. This processing mechanism might explain why tryptase and heparin are co-expressed in human mast cells

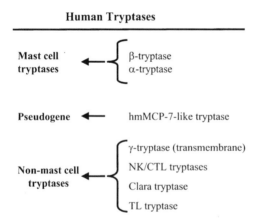

Figure 4 Proteases assigned the name tryptase are divided into those that are selectively expressed by mast cells, a pseudogene that appears not to be expressed, and those that are not selectively expressed by mast cells. The latter group are biochemically and immunologically distinct from mast cell tryptases.

and in mast cells of many other species. Two studies in mice assessed the impact of heparin on processing of mouse tryptases by disrupting the gene encoding glucosaminyl NDST-2 (80,81). In one study those mast cells that normally produce heparin were markedly deficient in histamine and in chymase and tryptase enzymatic activities (80), suggesting that processing of certain mouse chymases and mouse tryptases were suboptimal in the absence of heparin.

On the other hand, a biological processing mechanism for αprotryptase is still undefined. The presence of Gln^{-3} in αI-protryptase, instead of Arg^{-3} in β-tryptase, precludes optimal autocatalytic processing. Failure to process αI-protryptase to αI-pro'tryptase might explain why human mast cells appear to spontaneously secrete enzymatically inactive α-protryptase, while βII-tryptase is stored in their secretory granules. Recombinant human αI-protryptase with an enterokinase peptide cleavage site inserted next to the mature portion was processed in vitro to a catalytically active enzyme (106), bypassing the need for a natural processing step. The resultant α-tryptase exhibited relatively little enzymatic activity against small synthetic substrates and no fibrinogen-cleaving activity.

The quantity of catalytically active tryptase per mast cell (10–35 pg) (107) is dramatically higher than the levels of proteases found in other cell types, such as neutrophils ($\sim$1–3 pg of elastase and of cathepsin G per cell). What regulates tryptase activity after its release into the extracellular milieu is uncertain, because the enzyme is resistant to classical biological inhibitors of serine proteases (90).

A new possibility was raised after it was observed that lung and βII-tryptases degraded fibrinogen $\sim$50-fold faster at pH 6 than at 7.4 (108). A similar acidic pH optimum was noted for processing of βII-protryptase (104) and for cleavage of low molecular weight kininogen (109) by lung-derived tryptase. Release of β-tryptase at sites of acidic pH, such as foci of inflammation and areas of poor vascularity, might be optimal for the enzyme, while diffusion away from such sites would result in reduced proteolytic activity. Such a mechanism would tend to limit the activity of β-tryptase to its local tissue site of release.

Catalytically active tetrameric tryptase loses enzymatic activity and converts to monomers at neutral pH and physiological ionic strength in the absence of a stabilizing molecule like heparin. Placing inactive tryptase monomers (formed at neutral pH) into an acidic environment leads to the complete reassociation of these monomers into a catalytically active tetramer (110). Thus, at the acidic pH optimum for proteolysis, β-tryptase catalytic activity is stabilized, and inactive tryptase monomers theoretically could reassociate into catalytically active tetramers.

The biological activities of enzymatically active tryptase are not obvious from the involvement of mast cells in diseases such as mastocytosis, anaphylaxis, urticaria, and asthma. The most relevant biological substrate(s) of tryptase remain uncertain, though many potential ones have been evaluated, primarily in vitro. Predicted biological outcomes might include anticoagulation, fibrosis and fibrolysis, kinin generation and destruction, cell surface protease–activated receptor (PAR)-2 activation, enhancement of vasopermeability, angiogenesis, inflammation, and airway smooth muscle hyperreactivity. Showing the importance of these potential activities in vivo remains a challenge. The emerging availability of pharmacological inhibitors of tryptase, and preliminary studies suggesting they attenuate the bronchial response to an allergen challenge may facilitate identification of the most important biological substrates.

2. Chymase

Chymase is one of two principal enzymes accounting for the chymotrypsin-like activity present in human cutaneous mast cells. The enzyme was purified from human skin (111), and the corresponding gene cloned and localized to human chromosome 14 (112). Chymase was selectively localized to a subpopulation of mast cells by enzymatic (113) and immunohistochemical techniques (55). These MC_{TC} cells obtained from skin contain ~4.5 pg of chymase per cell.

Human chymase is a monomer of 30,000 daltons whose crystal structure has been solved (114). Its chymotryptic substrate specificity prefers the motif nX-Pro-(Phe,Tyr,Trp)-Y-Y, where $n \geq 6$, X is any amino acid, and Y is any amino acid except Pro (115). Like tryptase, chymase is a serine esterase that is stored fully active in mast cell secretory granules, presumably bound to heparin and chondroitin sulfate E. Heparin facilitates processing of prochymase to active chymase by dipeptidyl peptidase I (116) and either attracts or repels potential chymase substrates based on ionic forces (117). Unlike tryptase, chymase stability is not substantially affected by heparin and its activity is inhibited by classical biological inhibitors of serine proteinases, such as α_1-antichymotrypsin, α_1-proteinase inhibitor, and α_2-macroglobulin (118). Neither chymotrypsin-like enzymatic activity nor chymase mRNA were detected in lung MC_T cells (119).

Potential biological activities of chymase, like those of tryptase, are based on in vitro observations. Chymase is a potent activator of angiotensin I, inactivates bradykinin and PAR-1 receptors (120), and attacks the lamina lucida of the basement membrane at the dermal-epidermal junction of human skin. The potential importance of angiotensin II generation by mast cell chymase in humans is of great interest. Chymase potently stimulates mucus production from glandular cells in vitro (121), suggesting a similar role in asthma and allergic rhinitis, where release of chymase in proximity to glandular tissue might be involved in the state of hypersecretion. Biologically active Kit can be released from the cell surface by chymase (122). Processing of type I procollagen by chymase to collagen-like fibrils has been demonstrated in vitro (123) and may relate to the finding of chymase-containing mast cells at sites of fibrosis in places such as rheumatoid synovium (124).

3. Cathepsin G

Human mast cell cathepsin G, like chymase, is a serine-class neutral protease with chymotryptic substrate specificity that is found in a subset of mast cells as well as in neutrophils and monocytes. The enzyme resides with chymase in MC_{TC} cells (125) and exhibits a molecular weight of 30,000 daltons. Like chymase, it stimulates mucous glandular secretion (121), of possible importance in allergic asthma and rhinitis.

4. Mast Cell Carboxypeptidase

Human mast cell carboxypeptidase resides with chymase and cathepsin G in secretory granules of MC_{TC} cells (126). Stored fully active, when released it cleaves the carboxy terminal His^9-Leu^{10} bond of angiotensin I and behaves like a zinc-dependent exopeptidase. Human mast cells dispersed from skin contain 5–16 pg of carboxypeptidase per cell. Human mast cell carboxypeptidase is a monomer with a molecular weight of 34,500 daltons (127). Based on analysis of the cDNA-derived amino-acid sequence and gene structure (128), the human enzyme is more homologous to human pancreatic carboxypeptidase B than A, but the catalytic site is more homologous to human pancreatic carboxypeptidase A, as are its substrate specificities for carboxy-terminal Phe and Leu residues.

5. Other Proteases and Enzymes

Tissue-type plasminogen activator has been identified in tissue-derived mast cells (129), potentially complementing mast cell antithrombotic and anticoagulant activities with the fibrinolytic properties of this protease. Mast cells also concentrate various acid hydrolases in their secretory granules, perhaps reflecting the lysosomal origin of this organelle, including β-galactosidase, aryl sulfatase, and β-hexosaminidase, the latter enzyme serving as a marker to evaluate degranulation of dispersed preparations of mast cells (85).

Matrix metalloproteinase-9 (MMP-9), a gelatinase B, has been identified in cord blood–derived mast cells, and by immunohistochemistry, human skin, lung, and synovial mast cells are strongly positive for MMP9 (130). Because MMPs can promote the degradation of extracellular matrix, they are believed to play a role in the pathogenesis of certain disorders associated with tissue remodeling. Studies in dog mast cells suggest that SCF increases expression, whereas TGF-β downregulates expression of pro-gelatinase B (131), while in mice SCF downregulates MMP-9 (132). Thus, external agents may influence the fibrolytic versus fibrotic capabilities of this cell type.

D. Lipids

Human mast cells purified from lung incorporate exogenous arachidonic acid into neutral lipids and phospholipids and store these lipids in membranes and cytoplasmic lipid bodies. Liberation of the arachidonic acid destined for oxidative metabolism, as shown in mice, is dependent upon cytosolic phospholipase A_2 (133). In general, oxidation of arachidonic acid occurs through the cyclooxygenase (COX) pathway to prostaglandins (PGs) and thromboxanes (TXs), or the 5-, 12-, or 15-lipoxygenase (LO) pathways to monohydroxyl fatty acids, leukotrienes (LTs) that include both LTB_4 and the sulfidopeptides LTC_4, LTD_4, and LTE_4, formerly known as slow-reacting substances of anaphylaxis (SRS-A), and lipoxins. Platelet-activating factor, made by acetylating the lysophospholipid remaining after arachidonic acid departs, has not been shown to be a major secretory product of human mast cells and basophils. The major eicosanoid products secreted by activated mast cells and basophils are summarized in Figure 3.

Activation of human mast cells obtained from lung, skin, and intestine results in PGD_2 production through the activity of PGD synthase and in LTC_4 production through the activity of LTC synthase in weight ratios of approximately 5:1, respectively. Smaller amounts of LTB_4 isomers are also produced. Ratios of these metabolites cannot be used to distinguish MC_T from MC_{TC} cell activation. In contrast, activation of peripheral blood basophils obtained from normal human subjects results in LTC_4, but not PGD_2 production. However, cells other than mast cells and basophils produce PGD_2 (e.g., platelets and certain antigen-presenting cells) and LTC_4 (e.g., eosinophils). Both leukotriene and prostaglandin production by activated mast cells can be blocked without altering release of granule mediators and cytokines.

The biological importance of mast cell– and basophil-derived products of arachidonic acid metabolism has gained support with the advent of inhibitors of 5-LO and the cysLT1 receptor (134) for LTD_4, both of which are helpful in atopic and in aspirin-induced asthma, each condition also involving activation of mast cells as well as eosinophils, another major source of LTC_4. Of potential clinical interest was the finding that dexamethasone can upregulate 5-LO levels and LTC_4 production by HMC-1 cells in vitro (135). A metabolite of PGD_2 is elevated in the urine of patients with active systemic mastocytosis. The importance of PGD_2 production in the subgroup of these patients with recurrent hypotensive episodes was suggested when administration of aspirin inhibited generation of the PGD_2 metabolite and led to clinical improvement (136). PGD_2 is produced by mast cells during both the immediate and late phases of immediate hypersensitivity reactions, where COX-1 is responsible for PGD_2 production during the early phase, COX-2 during the late phase (137,138). The ability of PGD_2 to activate human eosinophils (139) and to play a role during induction of allergic airway disease in mice (140) suggest its potential importance in human allergic diseases at sites of mast cell–dependent inflammation.

E. Cytokines and Chemokines

There is no doubt that mast cells and basophils represent important sources of inflammatory mediators during acute, IgE-dependent reactions. Moreover, recent findings indicate that mast cells and basophils also can contribute to both the late-phase inflammation and the chronic tissue changes as potentially significant sources of several cytokines. Human mast cells and basophils, when activated, produce a diverse array of cytokines and chemokines (Fig. 3). These include tumor necrosis factor (TNF)-α, IL-3, -4, -5, -6, -8, -10, -13, and -16, lymphotactin, MCP-1, TGF-β1, and monocyte inflammatory peptide (MIP)-1α by mast cells, and at least IL-4 and IL-13 by basophils. In some cases cytokines may be stored in secretory granules and released with other preformed mediators. Mast cells have been noted to be the dominant IL-4–positive cell in allergic nasal mucosa (141), while basophils are the dominant IL-4–positive cell in the asthmatic airway 24 hours after allergen challenge (142) and in allergen-challenged peripheral blood cells (143). Cytokines also can be newly generated and released hours after mast cells or basophils are activated. These cytokines serve to recruit and activate other cell types, thereby amplifying the host response during immediate hypersensitivity events. For example, endothelial cells are activated by various mediators to recruit eosinophils and other cell types during the late phase response of immediate hypersensitivity reactions. Mast cells can thereby be involved in sustaining allergic inflammation hours after granule exocytosis is finished.

Interestingly, levels of FcεRI expression on mast cells and basophils can be regulated by IgE levels in vivo and in vitro in both mice (144, 145) and humans (43,146,147). Because this process also can increase the ability of mast cells to produce IL-4, IL-13, and MIP-1α, all of which can promote IgE production from plasma cells, IgE-dependent upregulation of FcεRI expression may also be part of a positive feedback mechanism for further production of IgE (148) and thereby promote allergic reactions associated with high levels of IgE. In addition, mast cells have been reported to be able to express CD40 ligand on their surface (149), an important co-stimulatory factor for the B-cell switch to IgE production.

IV. ACTIVATION AND REGULATED SECRETION

A. FcεRI-Mediated Activation

Mast cells and basophils are thought to play an important role in allergic disorders, primarily as a result of their expression of a high-affinity IgE receptor, FcεRI, that binds the Fc region of monomeric IgE with high specificity and affinity ($Ka = 10^9 M^{-1}$). At least under some circumstances, many other potential effector cells such as Langerhans cells, monocytes and macrophages, circulating dendritic cells, and eosinophils also may express small numbers of this receptor. In addition, another cell surface receptor, CD23, binds IgE, albeit with lower affinity ($Ka = 10^6 M^{-1}$). The expression of CD23 is widely distributed on B and T cells, monocytes, eosinophils, Langerhans cells, and platelets. However, the FcεRI expressed on mast cells and basophils is the principal molecule through which IgE exerts its characteristic biological function: the release of various kinds of inflammatory mediators.

The complete FcεRI receptor is composed of four subunits, α, β, and two γ chains, which appear to float on the cell surface in lipid-based domains called rafts (150). The α chain contains the extracellular IgE binding domain. Only the β chain crosses the plasma membrane four times and has both N- and C-termini protruding into the cytoplasm. Each β and two disulfide-linked ã chains, located primarily in the membrane and cytoplasm, have one special intracytoplasmic activation motif composed of a twice-repeated Tyr-X-X-Leu sequence, designated as ITAM, or immunoreceptor tyrosine activation motif. In humans, the presence of the β chain, though not essential for surface receptor expression or signal transduction, markedly amplifies phosphorylation of the γ chains and signal transduction, thereby increasing the magnitude of cell activation and host response (151,152). The γ chains are shared with the CD16 and FcεRIII receptors of natural killer cells and may substitute for the T-cell receptor ζ chain.

Mast cells and basophils undergo regulated degranulation when FcεRI are dimerized by multivalent antigen or anti-receptor antibody. The earliest biochemical events involved in signal transduction after FcεRI aggregation are tyrosine phosphorylation of ITAMs. The C-terminal of the β subunit of FcεRI is constitutively associated with Src-family protein tyrosine kinases (PTKs) such as Lyn. ITAMs located in the β- and γ-subunits of FcεRI are phosphorylated by Lyn within seconds after receptor cross-linking. These ITAMs, when doubly phosphorylated, provide docking sites for the cytoplasmic PTK, Syk, which has SH-2 domains that recognize such motifs. Syk is then phosphorylated by Lyn and possibly by itself (153–155). The Syk dependence of IgE-mediated signal transduction in humans appears to be clinically relevant, because patients whose basophils have low levels of Syk expression are nonreleasers to FcεRI cross-linking. Incubation of basophils with IL-3 induces Syk expression and, when FcεRI is cross-linked, degranulation and IL-4 production and VCAM-1 binding (156,157).

These early events also are regulated by signal inhibitory regulatory proteins (SIRPs) that contain ITIMs, immunotyrosine inhibition motifs. For example, SIRPα is expressed in human mast cells and has been shown in mice to act in part by recruiting SH-2–bearing protein tyrosine phosphatases (SHP-1 and -2) that dephosphorylate ITAMs on β and γ chains of FcεRI, thereby downregulating signal transduction and mediator release (158). CD45, a protein tyrosine phosphatase, promotes mediator release; mast cells from mice that are deficient in this enzyme do not exhibit IgE-dependent activation (159).

Later events in the signal transduction pathway are mediated by phosphorylated Syk, which then recruits other signal transduction molecules, such as Btk in mice, though perhaps not in human mast cells (160). Defective Btk in mice attenuates degranulation and cytokine production by activated mast cells as well as the anaphylactic response of the animal (161,162). SLP-76 is an adapter protein known to be a substrate for both ZAP-70 and Syk. In SLP-76 knock-out mice, mast cells undergo phosphorylation of Syk with FcεRI cross-linking but do not release mediators (163). The activation signal is finally transmitted to pathways involving phospholipase C (PLC)γ, MAP kinase, protein kinase C, and phosphotidyl inositol (PI)-3 kinase.

Degranulation of mast cells and basophils is associated with activation of small G proteins that cause actin polymerization and actin relocalization (164,165). Metabolism of phospholipids, which mostly reside in secretory granules, occurs early during the secretory response, is necessary for the later secretion of lipid mediators and may be important for regulated secretion to ensue. Generation of inositol triphosphate (IP$_3$) and diacylglycerol after FcεRI receptor aggregation results in release of calcium from the endoplasmic reticulum. This in turn stimulates calcium-dependent isoforms of protein kinase C and may directly facilitate fusion of lipid bilayers as exocytosis proceeds. A cytoplasmic calcium sensor called synaptotagmin II also influences exocytosis by mast cells (166).

B. Activation by Nonimmunological Reagents

Regulated secretion by mast cells and basophils also may be induced by nonimmunological agonists. Multivalent lectins, like bivalent concanavalin A, cross-link membrane FcεRI or IgE. Calcium ionophores activate by directly translocating calcium.

The secretory response to some nonimmunological reagents varies between mast cells isolated from different tissues. Basic biomolecules such as compound 48/80, C3a, C5a, morphine, codeine, mellitin, eosinophil-derived major basic protein, and various neuropeptides such as substance P, vasoactive intestinal peptide (VIP), somatostatin, and calcitonin gene–related protein (CGRP) activate human mast cells isolated from skin, but are inactive against mast cells derived from most other tissues. Mast cells from heart respond to C5a, but not to substance P (167). In contrast, basophils respond to C5a and C3a, but not to the neuropeptides, compound 48/80, morphine, and codeine. The desArg derivatives of C3a and C5a are inactive on skin mast cells but still show limited agonist activity against basophils. Whether these basic peptides activate mast cells and basophils by stereospecific receptor interactions or by ionic perturbations of membrane components is not clear (168). Differences in the secretory response between mast cells isolated from different tissues may relate in part to microenvironmental influences. For example, the rat mucosal mast cell line RBL-2H2 reversibly acquires responsiveness to substance P when cocultured with 3T3 fibroblasts without otherwise changing its phenotype.

Basophils also can be activated as well as primed to better respond to antigen by IL-3, an interleukin that does not affect human mast cell activation. The differences between basophils and mast cells with respect to their non–IgE-mediated pathways of activation, in theory, could lead to the activation of one cell type in the absence of the other. Basophils, like eosinophils but in contrast to mast cells, express surface FcαR and can be activated by an IgA-dependent pathway (169,170). The peptide f-Met-Leu-Phe activates human basophils, but not mast cells. HIV-1 gp120 activates IgE-armed basophils to secrete IL-4 and IL-13 (171), of possible interest to immediate hypersensitivity reactions commonly observed in HIV-infected individuals. Immunological activation of mast cells can be enhanced by adenosine (172), possibly through the adenosine A2b receptor in humans (173). In contrast, mediator release from human basophils is inhibited by adenosine. ATP also can enhance mediator release from activated mast cells by binding to the P2Y surface purinoreceptor expressed on human lung mast cells (174).

Various histamine-releasing factors derived from monocytes, lymphocytes, platelets, and neutrophils also have been described that are of potential clinical significance. The protein termed p23, for example, has been shown to have IgE-dependent histamine, cytokine, and LTC_4-releasing activity on basophils, an effect on mast cells being uncertain (175,176). Chemokines, initially discovered because of their abilities to attract predominantly monocytes or neutrophils, include potent basophil histamine-releasing and -attracting agents (177). Active chemokines include MCP-1 to -4, RANTES, MIP-1α and -1β, eotaxin and eotaxin-2, and ecalectin. Most of these chemokines affect eosinophils as well as basophils. The presence of the chemokine receptor CCR3 on basophils and eosinophils dovetails with the cellular specificity of these CC class chemokines (178). However, a further level of complexity was revealed for MCP-1, which when intact preferentially activates basophils over eosinophils but, after the N-terminal amino acid is removed, preferentially activates eosinophils over basophils. In contrast to the effects of these chemokines on basophils, mast cell mediator release appears to be unaffected (179,180), even though human mast cells express CCR3 (67,68). However, human mast cells appear to be capable of producing both MCP-1 and MIP-1α (148,181), suggesting a mechanism in which basophils may be recruited to and activated at tissue sites of mast cell activation.

V. CLINICAL MARKERS OF MAST CELLS AND BASOPHILS

Analysis of the cellular infiltration found in the skin of atopic dermatitis patients has provided important clues for understanding the pathogenesis of this disorder. The involvement of mast cells and basophils can be addressed in terms of both cell numbers and cell activation. Antibodies developed against cell-specific surface or granule components provide an immunohistological means for detecting these cells in tissues with greater sensitivity and specificity than classic dye-based histological stains.

A. Immunohistochemistry

The most selective surface marker phenotype for all human mast cells is the co-expression of high levels of Kit and FcεRI. This pattern is readily demonstrated on dispersed mast cells by flow cytometry. Tryptase serves as a granule marker for all human mast cells; the >100-fold smaller amounts present in basophils typically provide an adequate differential for distinguishing these two cell types from one another. Mast cells are difficult to identify in tissue specimens stained with hematoxylin and eosin (Fig. 2A), while tryptase provides a more sensitive and specific immunohistochemical marker for mast cells. Antitryptase immunohistochemistry reveals mast cell hyperplasia at sites of lichenification in atopic dermatitis (Fig. 2B). Monoclonal antibodies (mAbs) against chymase and mast cell carboxypeptidase serve to identify the MC_{TC} type of mast cell, because no other normal cell type appears to express these products. No specific marker for the MC_T type of mast cell has been found, these cells being identified by the presence of tryptase in the absence of chymase.

By using metachromatic stains, the total number of mast cells has been shown to be increased in lichenified lesions of atopic dermatitis. In the acute phase of atopic dermatitis of four patients, MC_{TC} cells identified by immunohistochemistry, as in skin of normal subjects, were reported to be the predominant mast cell type. However, unlike skin of normal subjects, a substantial population (1–17%) of the mast cells displayed an MC_T phenotype (Fig. 2D) (3). These findings were confirmed by another study, which demonstrated that in the upper dermis of nonlesional and lesional atopic dermatitis skin, only 80% of tryptase-positive cells displayed chymase enzyme activity, whereas all the skin mast cells of normal control subjects contained chymase (4). Whether chymase inside mast cells is inhibited in vivo or simply as a result of processing tissue bathed in high levels of serum-derived protease inhibitors remains to be clarified. Within the epidermis of atopic dermatitis, a few lesional samples were reported to contain chymase-positive cells (Fig. 2C) (3), a feature not seen in skin of healthy controls. In another report, mast cells were observed in the epidermis of 3 of 10 specimens of noninvolved skin from the upper arm of atopic dermatitis patients (182). However, the potential significance of epidermal mast cells is unclear.

Although an $Fc\epsilon RI^+/Kit^-$ surface phenotype or $Fc\epsilon RI^+/tryptase^-$ surface/granule phenotype has been considered to selectively represent basophils, the abilities of activated monocytes, eosinophils, and antigen-presenting cells such as Langerhans cells to express $Fc\epsilon RI$ make this consideration problematic, particularly at sites of inflammation (183). Two mAbs (184,185) that recognize components of basophil secretory granules but do not label other cell types, including mast cells and eosinophils, identify basophils in tissues by immunohistochemistry. The respective antigens are called 2D7 antigen and basogranin. Using such mAbs, basophil influx during the late phase of allergic reactions was shown to occur in the skin (186–188), lung (189,142,188), and nose (190). Basophil numbers were about fivefold lower than eosinophils, but appeared to account for a substantial portion of the IL-4–producing cells.

B. Serum Tryptase Levels

Immunoassays for cell-specific, releasable, and preformed granule mediators provide a more precise measure of either local or systemic activation of a particular cell type than is possible by either clinical criteria or documentation of antigen-specific IgE. Most mAbs against human tryptase recognize both α- and β-tryptase products, whereas one mAb called G5 (linear epitope) recognizes β-tryptase but not α-protryptase (Fig. 5). This is of clinical relevance because α-protryptase appears to be continuously secreted by human mast cells, and its levels in blood thereby serve as a measure of mast cell number. In contrast, β-tryptase is stored in secretory granules and is released only during granule exocytosis; its levels serve as a measure of mast cell activation.

Systemic mastocytosis is associated with mast cell hyperplasia in skin lesions (urticaria pigmentosa), liver, spleen, lymph nodes, and bone marrow (191). The disorder is subdivided into those with indolent mastocytosis, systemic mastocytosis associated with a hematological disorder, and aggressive systemic mastocytosis (192). In a study of tryptase levels in subjects with biopsy-diagnosed mastocytosis, most of those with systemic mastocytosis indicated by a bone marrow biopsy (35 of 42) had levels of total tryptase of >20 ng/mL and ratios of total tryptase to β-tryptase of >20 (193). Normal subjects ($n = 55$) had total tryptase levels of <14 ng/mL (194). This suggested a specificity of >98% and a sensitivity of 83% for total tryptase levels when compared to a bone marrow biopsy. However, among the seven subjects with systemic mastocytosis and a

Tryptase Immunoassays

Tryptase Type Recognized	β-Tryptase (B12/G5 mAbs)	Total Tryptase (B12/G4 mAbs)
	mature β	pro/mature α & β
Normal Serum (ng/ml)	<1	1 – 15
Systemic Anaphylaxis (acute)	>1 *(TOTAL/β ratio < 10*	↑
Systemic Mastocytosis (nonacute)	≠↑ *TOTAL/β ratio > 20*	≥20

Figure 5 Characteristics of the total tryptase and β-tryptase immunoassays for mast cell tryptases measured in serum or plasma. β-Tryptase is preferentially measured when the G5 mAb is used for detection, while both immature and mature forms of α and β tryptases are measured when the G4 mAb is used for detection. The B12 mAb is used for capture in both sandwich immunoassays.

serum total tryptase level below 20 ng/mL, all had total tryptase levels between 10 and 20 ng/mL, three had ambiguous bone marrow readings, and another had the bone marrow biopsy performed 5 years before the serum sample was collected. Most subjects with local cutaneous mast cell disease (10 of 13) had levels similar to normal controls (1–11 ng/mL; ratios ≤ 11). Among the three subjects with serum total tryptase levels above this range, one was an infant with diffuse cutaneous mastocytosis, and another had no bone marrow biopsy performed. The indolent group with urticaria pigmentosa and no evidence of systemic involvement had levels of total tryptase in the normal range. Thus, the level of total tryptase appears to distinguish those with local versus systemic disease. However, the absolute level of total tryptase did not predict clinical severity, suggesting that factors other than the mast cell burden alone are important in systemic mastocytosis.

β-Tryptase levels in serum or plasma are elevated in most subjects with systemic anaphylaxis of sufficient severity to result in hypotension (195). β-Tryptase is released from mast cells in parallel with histamine (85) but diffuses more slowly than histamine, presumably due to its association with the macromolecular protease-proteoglycan complex. During insect sting–induced anaphylaxis β-tryptase levels in the circulation are maximal 15–120 minutes after the sting, while histamine levels peak at about 5 minutes and decline to baseline by 15–30 minutes (196,197). Peak β-tryptase levels decline with a half-life of 1.5–2.5 hours.

In insect sting–induced systemic anaphylaxis, the ratios of total tryptase to β-tryptase were less than 6 in 16 of 17 subjects, being 23 in the one outlier (194). Thus, when β-tryptase is detectable in serum, a total to β-tryptase ratio of ≤10 suggests systemic anaphylaxis. Mast cells also have been implicated in anaphylactic reactions to cyclooxygenase inhibitors by finding elevated levels of β-tryptase in blood (196). In cases of clinical anaphylaxis with a normal level of β-tryptase, pathogenetic mechanisms without mast cell activation should be considered. These might include basophil activation or complement anaphylatoxin generation.

An analysis of serum samples from patients with atopic dermatitis revealed no elevation of total or β-tryptase (unpublished data). However, this does not rule out local cutaneous increases in either mast cell number or mast cell activation. The dermal microdialysis technique may offer the ability to better assess local mediator production in lesional and nonlesional sites of atopic dermatitis (198).

VI. MAST CELLS AND BASOPHILS AS THERAPEUTIC TARGETS IN ATOPIC DERMATITIS

The mediators for pruritus in atopic dermatitis are still unknown. While histamine is the crucial mediator of pruritus in type I allergic reactions, particularly in urticaria where H1 receptor blockade effectively abolishes itch and improves the skin condition, there is some controversy about the role of histamine in atopic dermatitis. Some authors report a significant reduction of pruritus by histamine H1-blockers (199–201), but others find no antipruritic effect or only a marginal effect probably due to sedative effects (202,203). Interestingly, the direct cutaneous application of histamine results in a lower itch rating (204) and smaller axon reflex flares in atopic dermatitis patients than control subjects (205), suggesting that histamine is not a crucial mediator for itch in atopic dermatitis (206). Pharmacological responsiveness of mast cells varies depending on the tissue source and differs from that of basophils. Disodium cromoglycate and nedocromil, both used for the treatment of allergic asthma, rhinitis, and conjunctivitis, are weak inhibitors of lung mast cell activation but are ineffective against mast cells from skin and intestine.

Topical corticosteroids are the most established treatment for atopic dermatitis. Dexamethasone in vitro inhibits mediator secretion by human basophils, but not by human lung-derived mast cells. Dexamethasone also inhibits SCF-induced development of mast cells from fetal liver cells but shows no appreciable effect on developed mast cells (207). In vivo, local instillation of nasal glucocorticosteroids over a prolonged period of time diminished mediator release during the immediate response to nasal allergen challenge, perhaps due to the capacity for local steroids to diminish mast cell concentrations as demonstrated in the synovium (208), skin (209), and rectal mucosa (210) or to the prevention of the superficial migration of mast cells that apparently occurs in atopic subjects during the allergy season (211,212).

Macrolide immunosuppressants are potent immunosuppressive drugs that act primarily on T cells by inhibiting cytokine gene activation. Cyclosporin A and tacrolimus (FK-506) produce rapid and long-lasting inhibition of IgE-dependent histamine release from human basophils and skin- and lung-derived mast cells (213–215). Rapamycin interferes with the inhibitory activity of FK-506 by competing for the same FK-binding protein, but by itself does not inhibit mast cell or basophil activation. Oral treatment with cyclosporin A has proven to be effective in atopic dermatitis (216), perhaps due both to its inhibitory effects on T cells as well as mast cells and basophils. Topical treatment with tacrolimus also appears to provide effective treatment of atopic dermatitis (217).

VII. SUMMARY

Mast cells and basophils, the two principal effector cells of immediate hypersensitivity, also appear to be involved in atopic dermatitis. Mast cells are increased in number at lesional sites. Occasionally mast cells penetrate into epidermis in these lesions. Mast cells in lesions may also exhibit an MC_T phenotype. Basophils are difficult to observe with metachromatic stains in sites of inflammation, but appear to be present by immunohistochemistry that targets basophil-specific markers. By virtue of the high levels of antigen-specific IgE also present, mast cells and basophils are armed and capable of discharging their mediators upon encountering antigen. However, the pruritic component of atopic dermatitis is most of the time minimally dependent on histamine, unlike urticaria. Also, the inflammatory components clearly involve multiple cell types. Thus, the role and importance in atopic dermatitis of mast cells and basophils may vary at different stages of the disease. As we learn more about these cell types, develop better markers for them, and obtain therapeutic agents more precisely targeted at them, their contributions to atopic dermatitis will be understood with greater precision.

REFERENCES

1. EB Mitchell, J Crow, G Williams, TA Platts-Mills. Increase in skin mast cells following chronic house dust mite exposure. Br J Dermatol 114:65–73, 1986.
2. M Mihm Jr, N Soter, H Dvorak, KF Austen. The structure of normal skin and the morphology of atopic eczema. J Invest Dermatol 67:305–312, 1976.
3. AA Irani, HA Sampson, LB Schwartz. Mast cells in atopic dermatitis. Allergy 44 (suppl 9):31–34, 1989.

4. A Järvikallio, A Naukkarinen, IT Harvima, ML Aalto, M Horsmanheimo. Quantitative analysis of tryptase- and chymase-containing mast cells in atopic dermatitis and nummular eczema. Br J Dermatol 136:871–877, 1997.

5. TE Damsgaard, AB Olesen, FB Sorensen, K Thestrup-Pedersen, PO Schiotz. Mast cells and atopic dermatitis. Stereological quantification of mast cells in atopic dermatitis and normal human skin. Arch Dermatol Res 289:256–260, 1997.

6. AJ Sandford, T Shirakawa, MF Moffatt, SE Daniels, C Ra, JA Faux, RP Young, Y Nakamura, GM Lathrop, WO Cookson. Localisation of atopy and beta subunit of high-affinity IgE receptor (Fc epsilon RI) on chromosome 11q [see comments]. Lancet 341:332–334, 1993.

7. T Shirakawa, A Li, M Dubowitz, JW Dekker, AE Shaw, JA Faux, C Ra, WO Cookson, JM Hopkin. Association between atopy and variants of the beta subunit of the high-affinity immunoglobulin E receptor [see comments]. Nat Genet 7:125–129, 1994.

8. R Coleman, RC Trembath, JI Harper. Chromosome 11q13 and atopy underlying atopic eczema. Lancet 341:1121–1122, 1993.

9. HE Cox, MF Moffatt, JA Faux, AJ Walley, R Coleman, RC Trembath, WO Cookson, JI Harper. Association of atopic dermatitis to the beta subunit of the high affinity immunoglobulin E receptor [see comments]. Br J Dermatol 138:182–187, 1998.

10. XQ Mao, T Shirakawa, T Yoshikawa, K Yoshikawa, M Kawai, S Sasaki, T Enomoto, T Hashimoto, J Furuyama, JM Hopkin, K Morimoto. Association between genetic variants of mast-cell chymase and eczema [see comments] [published erratum appears in Lancet 349(9044):64, 1997]. Lancet 348:581–583, 1996.

11. XQ Mao, T Shirakawa, T Enomoto, S Shimazu, Y Dake, H Kitano, A Hagihara, JM Hopkin. Association between variants of mast cell chymase gene and serum IgE levels in eczema [published erratum appears in Human Hered 48(2):91, 1998]. Human Heredity 48:38–41, 1998.

12. K Tanaka, H Sugiura, M Uehara, H Sato, T Hashimoto-Tamaoki, J Furuyama. Association between mast cell chymase genotype and atopic eczema: comparison between patients with atopic eczema alone and those with atopic eczema and atopic respiratory disease. Clin Exp Allergy 29:800–803, 1999.

13. Y Kitamura, M Shimada, K Hatanaka, Y Miyano. Development of mast cells from grafted bone marrow cells in irradiated mice. Nature 268:442–443, 1977.

14. S Hasthorpe. A hemopoietic cell line dependent upon a factor in pokeweed mitogen-stimulated spleen cell conditioning medium. J Cell Physiol 105:379–384, 1980.

15. GJ Nabel, SJ Galli, AM Dvorak, HF Dvorak, H Cantor. Inducer T lymphocytes synthesize a factor that stimulates proliferation of cloned mast cells. Nature 291:332–334, 1981.

16. K Nagao, K Yokoro, SA Aaronson. Continuous lines of basophil mast cells derived from normal mouse bone marrow. Science 212:333–335, 1981.

17. JW Schrader, SJ Lewis, I Clark-Lewis, JG Culvenor. The persisting (P) cell: histamine content, regulation by a T cell-derived factor, origin from a bone marrow precursor, and relationship to mast cells. Proc Natl Acad Sci USA 78:323–327, 1981.

18. YP Yung, R Eger, G Tertian, MA Moore. Long-term in vitro culture of murine mast cells. II. Purification of a mast cell growth factor and its dissociation from TCGF. J Immunol 127:794–799, 1981.

19. JN Ihle, JR Keller, S Oroszlan, LE Henderson, TD Copeland, FW Fitch, MB Prystowsky, E Goldwasser, JW Schrader, EW Palaszynski, M Dy, B Lebel. Biologic properties of homogeneous interleukin 3. I. Demonstration of WEHI-3 growth factor activity, mast cell growth factor activity, p cell-stimulating factor activity, colony-stimulating factor activity, and histamine-producing cell- stimulating factor activity. J Immunol 131:282–287, 1983.

20. T Yokota, F Lee, D Rennick, C Hall, N Arai, T Mosmann, G Nabel, H Cantor, K Arai. Isolation and characterization of a mouse cDNA clone that expresses mast-cell growth- factor activity in monkey cells. Proc Natl Acad Sci USA 81:1070–1074, 1984.

21. EJ Ruitenberg, A Elgersma. Absence of intestinal mast cell response in congenitally athymic mice during *Trichinella spiralis* infection. Nature 264:258–260, 1976.

22. CS Lantz, J Boesiger, CH Song, N Mach, T Kobayashi, RC Mulligan, Y Nawa, G Dranoff, SJ Galli. Role for interleukin-3 in mast-cell and basophil development and in immunity to parasites. Nature 392:90–93, 1998.

23. Y Kitamura, K Hatanaka. Decrease of mast cells in W/W^v mice and their increase by bone marrow transplantation. Blood 52:447–452, 1978.

24. Y Kitamura, S Go. Decreased production of mast cells in Sl/Sl^d anemic mice. Blood 53:492–497, 1979.

25. J Wedemeyer, M Tsai, SJ Galli. Roles of mast cells and basophils in innate and acquired immunity. Curr Opin Immunol 12:624–631, 2000.

26. AA Irani, G Nilsson, U Miettinen, SC Craig, LK Ashman, T Ishizaka, KM Zsebo, LB Schwartz. Recombinant human stem cell factor stimulates differentiation of mast cells from dispersed human fetal liver cells. Blood 80:3009–3021, 1992.

27. H Mitsui, T Furitsu, AM Dvorak, AA Irani, LB Schwartz, N Inagaki, M Takei, K Ishizaka, KM Zsebo, S Gillis, T Ishizaka. Development of human mast cells from umbilical cord blood cells by recombinant human and murine c-kit ligand. Proc Natl Acad Sci USA 90:735–739, 1993.

28. P Valent, E Spanblöchl, WR Sperr, C Sillaber, KM Zsebo, H Agis, H Strobl, K Geissler, P Bettelheim, K Lechner. Induction of differentiation of human mast cells from bone marrow and peripheral blood mononuclear cells by recombinant human stem cell factor/*kit*-ligand in long-term culture. Blood 80:2237–2245, 1992.

29. M Rottem, T Okada, JP Goff, DD Metcalfe. Mast cells cultured from the peripheral blood of normal donors and patients with mastocytosis originate from a CD34$^+$/Fcε RI$^-$ cell population. Blood 84:2489–2496, 1994.

30. D Kempuraj, H Saito, A Kaneko, K Fukagawa, M Nakayama, H Toru, M Tomikawa, H Tachimoto, M Ebisawa, A Akasawa, T Miyagi, H Kimura, T Nakajima, K Tsuji, T Nakahata. Characterization of mast cell-committed progenitors present in human umbilical cord blood. Blood 93:3338–3346, 1999.

31. AS Kirshenbaum, JP Goff, T Semere, B Foster, LM Scott, DD Metcalfe. Demonstration that human mast cells arise from a progenitor cell population that is CD34(+), c-kit(+), and expresses aminopeptidase N (CD13). Blood 94:2333–2342, 1999.

32. LW Terstappen, S Huang, M Safford, PM Lansdorp, MR Loken. Sequential generations of hematopoietic colonies derived from single nonlineage-committed CD34+CD38- progenitor cells. Blood 77:1218–1227, 1991.

33. CI Civin. Human monomyeloid cell membrane antigens. Exp Hematol 18:461–467, 1990.

34. ZM Du, YL Li, HZ Xia, AM Irani, LB Schwartz. Recombinant human granulocyte-macrophage colony-stimulating factor (CSF), but not recombinant human granulocyte CSF, down- regulates the recombinant human stem cell factor-dependent differentiation of human fetal liver-derived mast cells. J Immunol 159:838–845, 1997.

35. CA Oskeritzian, Z Wang, JP Kochan, M Grimes, Z Du, HW Chang, S Grant, LB Schwartz. Recombinant human (rh)IL-4-mediated apoptosis and recombinant human IL-6-mediated protection of recombinant human stem cell factor-dependent human mast cells derived from cord blood mononuclear cell progenitors. J Immunol 163:5105–5115, 1999.

36. H Saito, M Ebisawa, H Tachimoto, M Shichijo, K Fukagawa, K Matsumoto, Y Iikura, T Awaji, G Tsujimoto, M Yanagida, H Uzumaki, G Takahashi, K Tsuji, T Nakahata. Selective growth of human mast cell induced by *Steel* factor, IL-6, and prostaglandin E_2 from cord blood mononuclear cells. J Immunol 157:343–350, 1996.

37. N Kambe, M Kambe, HW Chang, A Matsui, HK Min, M Hussein, CA Oskerizian, J Kochan, AMA Irani, LB Schwartz. An improved procedure for the development of human mast cells from dispersed fetal liver cells in serum-free culture medium. J Immunol Meth 240:101–110, 2000.

38. G Nilsson, U Miettinen, T Ishizaka, LK Ashman, AM Irani, LB Schwartz. Interleukin-4 inhibits the expression of Kit and tryptase during stem cell factor-dependent development of human mast cells from fetal liver cells. Blood 84:1519–1527, 1994.

39. H Nagata, AS Worobec, CK Oh, S Tannenbaum, Y Suzuki, DD Metcalfe. Identification of a point mutation in the catalytic domain of the proto-oncogene c-*kit* in peripheral blood mononuclear cells of patients who have mastocytosis with an associated hematologic disorder. Proc Natl Acad Sci USA 92:10560–10564, 1995.

40. BJ Longley, Jr., DD Metcalfe, M Tharp, XM Wang, L Tyrrell, SZ Lu, D Heitjan, YS Ma. Activating and dominant inactivating c-*kit* catalytic domain mutations in distinct clinical forms of human mastocytosis. Proc Natl Acad Sci USA 96:1609–1614, 1999.

41. S Hirota, K Isozaki, Y Moriyama, K Hashimoto, T Nishida, S Ishiguro, K Kawano, M Hanada, A Kurata, M Takeda, GM Tunio, Y Matsuzawa, Y Kanakura, Y Shinomura, Y Kitamura. Gain-of-function mutations of c-*kit* in human gastrointestinal stromal tumors. Science 279:577–580, 1998.

42. C Sillaber, H Strobl, D Bevec, LK Ashman, JH Butterfield, K Lechner, D Maurer, P Bettelheim, P Valent. IL-4 regulates c-*kit* proto-oncogene product expression in human mast and myeloid progenitor cells. J Immunol 147:4224–4228, 1991.

43. HZ Xia, ZM Du, S Craig, G Klisch, N Noben-Trauth, JP Kochan, TH Huff, AM Irani, LB Schwartz. Effect of recombinant human IL-4 on tryptase, chymase, and Fcε receptor type I expression in recombinant human stem cell factor-dependent fetal liver-derived human mast cells. J Immunol 159:2911–2921, 1997.

44. H Toru, C Ra, S Nonoyama, K Suzuki, J Yata, T Nakahata. Induction of the high-

affinity IgE receptor (FcεRI) on human mast cells by IL-4. International Immunology 8:1367–1373, 1996.

45. SC Bischoff, G Sellge, A Lorentz, W Sebald, R Raab, MP Manns. IL-4 enhances proliferation and mediator release in mature human mast cells. Proc Natl Acad Sci USA 96:8080–8085, 1999.

46. M Yanagida, H Fukamachi, K Ohgami, T Kuwaki, H Ishii, H Uzumaki, K Amano, T Tokiwa, H Mitsui, H Saito, Y Iikura, T Ishizaka, T Nakahata. Effects of T-helper 2-type cytokines, interleukin-3 (IL- 3), IL-4, IL-5, and IL-6 on the survival of cultured human mast cells. Blood 86:3705–3714, 1995.

47. H Toru, T Kinashi, C Ra, S Nonoyama, J Yata, T Nakahata. Interleukin-4 induces homotypic aggregation of human mast cells by promoting LFA-1/ICAM-1 adhesion molecules. Blood 89:3296–3302, 1997.

48. G Nilsson, K Nilsson. Effects of interleukin (IL)-13 on immediate-early response gene expression, phenotype and differentiation of human mast cells. Comparison with IL-4. Eur J Immunol 25:870–873, 1995.

49. T Kinoshita, N Sawai, E Hidaka, T Yamashita, K Koike. Interleukin-6 directly modulates stem cell factor-dependent development of human mast cells derived from CD34(+) cord blood cells. Blood 94:496–508, 1999.

50. L Thompson-Snipes, V Dhar, MW Bond, TR Mosmann, KW Moore, DM Rennick. Interleukin 10: a novel stimulatory factor for mast cells and their progenitors. J Exp Med 173:507–510, 1991.

51. N Ghildyal, DS Friend, CF Nicodemus, KF Austen, RL Stevens. Reversible expression of mouse mast cell protease 2 mRNA and protein in cultured mast cells exposed to IL-10. J Immunol 151:3206–3214, 1993.

52. N Ghildyal, HP McNeil, MF Gurish, KF Austen, RL Stevens. Transcriptional regulation of the mucosal mast cell-specific protease gene, MMCP-2, by interleukin 10 and interleukin 3. J Biol Chem 267:8473–8477, 1992.

53. N Ghildyal, HP McNeil, S Stechschulte, KF Austen, D Silberstein, MF Gurish, LL Somerville, RL Stevens. IL-10 induces transcription of the gene for mouse mast cell protease-1, a serine protease preferentially expressed in mucosal mast cells of *Trichinella spiralis*-infected mice. J Immunol 149:2123–2129, 1992.

54. M Kambe, N Kambe, C Oskeritzian, NM Schechter, LB Schwartz. IL-6 attenuates apoptosis, while neither IL-6 nor IL-10 affect the numbers or protease phenotype of fetal liver-derived human mast cells. Clin Exp Allergy 31:1077–1085, 2001.

55. AA Irani, NM Schechter, SS Craig, G DeBlois, LB Schwartz. Two types of human mast cells that have distinct neutral protease compositions. Proc Natl Acad Sci USA 83:4464–4468, 1986.

56. AM Irani, SS Craig, G DeBlois, CO Elson, NM Schechter, LB Schwartz. Deficiency of the tryptase-positive, chymase-negative mast cell type in gastrointestinal mucosa of patients with defective T lymphocyte function. J Immunol 138:4381–4386, 1987.

57. Y Kanakura, H Thompson, T Nakano, T Yamamura, H Asai, Y Kitamura, DD Metcalfe, SJ Galli. Multiple bidirectional alterations of phenotype and changes in proliferative potential during the in vitro and in vivo passage of clonal mast cell populations derived from mouse peritoneal mast cells. Blood 72:877–885, 1988.

58. T Nakano, T Sonoda, C Hayashi, A Yamatodani, Y Kanayama, T Yamamura, H
     Asai, T Yonezawa, Y Kitamura, SJ Galli. Fate of bone marrow-derived cultured
     mast cells after inracutaneous, intraperitoneal and intracenous transfer into geneti-
     cally mast cell deficient W/W^v mice. Evidence that cultured mast cells can give
     rise to both connective tissue type and mucosal mast cells. J Exp Med 162:1025–
     1043, 1985.
59. F Levi-Schaffer, KF Austen, PM Gravallese, RL Stevens. Coculture of interleukin
     3-dependent mouse mast cells with fibroblasts results in a phenotypic change of
     the mast cells [published erratum appears in Proc Natl Acad Sci USA 83(20):7805,
     1986]. Proc Natl Acad Sci USA 83:6485–6488, 1986.
60. M Tsai, LS Shih, GF Newlands, T Takeishi, KE Langley, KM Zsebo, HR Miller,
     EN Geissler, SJ Galli. The rat c-kit ligand, stem cell factor, induces the development
     of connective tissue-type and mucosal mast cells in vivo. Analysis by anatomical
     distribution, histochemistry, and protease phenotype. J Exp Med 174:125–131,
     1991.
61. JR Gordon, SJ Galli. Phorbol 12-myristate 13-acetate-induced development of
     functionally active mast cells in W/W^v but not Sl/Sl^d genetically mast cell-deficient
     mice. Blood 75:1637–1645, 1990.
62. H Matsuda, Y Kannan, H Ushio, Y Kiso, T Kanemoto, H Suzuki, Y Kitamura.
     Nerve growth factor induces development of connective tissue-type mast cells in
     vitro from murine bone marrow cells. J Exp Med 174:7–14, 1991.
63. H Toru, M Eguchi, R Matsumoto, M Yanagida, J Yata, T Nakahata. Interleukin-
     4 promotes the development of tryptase and chymase double-positive human mast
     cells accompanied by cell maturation. Blood 91:187–195, 1998.
64. SY Tam, M Tsai, M Yamaguchi, K Yano, JH Butterfield, SJ Galli. Expression of
     functional TrkA receptor tyrosine kinase in the HMC-1 human mast cell line and
     in human mast cells. Blood 90:1807–1820, 1997.
65. SS Craig, NM Schechter, LB Schwartz. Ultrastructural analysis of maturing human
     T and TC mast cells in situ. Lab Invest 60:147–157, 1989.
66. G Nilsson, JA Mikovits, DD Metcalfe, DD Taub. Mast cell migratory response to
     interleukin-8 is mediated through interaction with chemokine receptor CXCR2/
     interleukin-8RB. Blood 93:2791–2797, 1999.
67. H Ochi, WM Hirani, Q Yuan, DS Friend, KF Austen, JA Boyce. T helper cell type
     2 cytokine-mediated comitogenic responses and CCR3 expression during differen-
     tiation of human mast cells in vitro. J Exp Med 190:267–280, 1999.
68. P Romagnani, A De Paulis, C Beltrame, F Annunziato, V Dente, E Maggi, S Ro-
     magnani, G Marone. Tryptase-chymase double-positive human mast cells express
     the eotaxin receptor CCR3 and are attracted by CCR3-binding chemokines. Am J
     Pathol 155:1195–1204, 1999.
69. K Yamauchi, R Sato, Y Tanno, Y Ohkawara, K Maeyama, T Watanabe, K Satoh,
     M Yoshizawa, S Shibahara, T Takishima. Nucleotide sequence of the cDNA encod-
     ing L-histidine decarboxylase derived from human basophilic leukemia cell line,
     KU-812- F. Nucleic Acids Res 18:5891–5891, 1990.
70. I Gantz, M Schaffer, J DelValle, C Logsdon, V Campbell, M Uhler, T Yamada.
     Molecular cloning of a gene encoding the histamine H2 receptor [published erratum

appears in Proc Natl Acad Sci USA 88(13):5937, 1991]. Proc Natl Acad Sci USA 88:429–433, 1991.

71. H Asako, I Kurose, R Wolf, S DeFrees, ZL Zheng, ML Phillips, JC Paulson, DN Granger. Role of H1 receptors and P-selectin in histamine-induced leukocyte rolling and adhesion in postcapillary venules. J Clin Invest 93:1508–1515, 1994.

72. P Kubes, S Kanwar. Histamine induces leukocyte rolling in post-capillary venules. A P-selectin-mediated event. J Immunol 152:3570–3577, 1994.

73. I Inoue, K Yanai, D Kitamura, I Taniuchi, T Kobayashi, K Niimura, T Watanabe, T Watanabe. Impaired locomotor activity and exploratory behavior in mice lacking histamine H1 receptors. Proc Natl Acad Sci USA 93:13316–13320, 1996.

74. I Robertson, MW Greaves. Responses of human skin blood vessels to synthetic histamine analogues. Br J Clin Pharmacol 5:319–1978.

75. M Kaliner, JH Shelhamer, EA Ottesen. Effects of infused histamine: correlation of plasma histamine levels and symptoms. J Allergy Clin Immunol 69:283–289, 1982.

76. SS Craig, A-MA Irani, DD Metcalfe, LB Schwartz. Ultrastructural localization of heparin to human mast cells of the MC_{TC} and MC_T types by labeling with antithrombin III-gold. Lab Invest 69:552–561, 1993.

77. SE Stringer, M Mayer-Proschel, A Kalyani, M Rao, JT Gallagher. Heparin is a unique marker of progenitors in the glial cell lineage. J Biol Chem 274:25455–25460, 1999.

78. JA Reed, AP Albino, NS McNutt. Human cutaneous mast cells express basic fibroblast growth factor. Lab Invest 72:215–222, 1995.

79. RM Nelson, O Cecconi, WG Roberts, A Aruffo, RJ Linhardt, MP Bevilacqua. Heparin oligosaccharides bind L- and P-selectin and inhibit acute inflammation. Blood 82:3253–3258, 1993.

80. E Forsberg, G Pejler, M Ringvall, C Lunderius, B Tomasini-Johansson, M Kusche-Gullberg, I Eriksson, J Ledin, L Hellman, L Kjellen. Abnormal mast cells in mice deficient in a heparin-synthesizing enzyme. Nature 400:773–776, 1999.

81. DE Humphries, GW Wong, DS Friend, MF Gurish, WT Qiu, CF Huang, AH Sharpe, RL Stevens. Heparin is essential for the storage of specific granule proteases in mast cells. Nature 400:769–772, 1999.

82. H Chiu, D Lagunoff. Histochemical comparison of vertebrate mast cells. Histochem J 4:135–144, 1972.

83. GC Glenner, LA Cohen. Histochemical demonstration of species-specific trypsin-like enzyme in mast cells. Nature (London) 185:846–847, 1960.

84. VK Hopsu, GG Glenner. A histochemical enzyme kinetic system applied to the trypsin-like amidase and esterase activity in human mast cells. J Cell Biol 17:503–510, 1963.

85. LB Schwartz, RA Lewis, D Seldin, KF Austen. Acid hydrolases and tryptase from secretory granules of dispersed human lung mast cells. J Immunol 126:1290–1294, 1981.

86. LB Schwartz, RA Lewis, KF Austen. Tryptase from human pulmonary mast cells. Purification and characterization. J Biol Chem 256:11939–11943, 1981.

87. SC Alter, DD Metcalfe, TR Bradford, LB Schwartz. Regulation of human mast

cell tryptase. Effects of enzyme concentration, ionic strength and the structure and negative charge density of polysaccharides. Biochem J 248:821–827, 1987.

88. LB Schwartz, TR Bradford. Regulation of tryptase from human lung mast cells by heparin. Stabilization of the active tetramer. J Biol Chem 261:7372–7379, 1986.

89. PJ Pereira, A Bergner, S Macedo-Ribeiro, R Huber, G Matschiner, H Fritz, CP Sommerhoff, W Bode. Human β-tryptase is a ring-like tetramer with active sites facing a central pore. Nature 392:306–311, 1998.

90. SC Alter, JA Kramps, A Janoff, LB Schwartz. Interactions of human mast cell tryptase with biological protease inhibitors. Arch Biochem Biophys 276:26–31, 1990.

91. JS Miller, EH Westin, LB Schwartz. Cloning and characterization of complementary DNA for human tryptase. J Clin Invest 84:1188–1195, 1989.

92. JS Miller, G Moxley, LB Schwartz. Cloning and characterization of a second complementary DNA for human tryptase. J Clin Invest 86:864–870, 1990.

93. P Vanderslice, SM Ballinger, EK Tam, SM Goldstein, CS Craik, GH Caughey. Human mast cell tryptase: multiple cDNAs and genes reveal a multigene serine protease family. Proc Natl Acad Sci USA 87:3811–3815, 1990.

94. M Pallaoro, MS Fejzo, L Shayesteh, JL Blount, GH Caughey. Characterization of genes encoding known and novel human mast cell tryptases on chromosome 16p13.3. J Biol Chem 274:3355–3362, 1999.

95. HP McNeil, DS Reynolds, V Schiller, N Ghildyal, DS Gurley, KF Austen, RL Stevens. Isolation, characterization, and transcription of the gene encoding mouse mast cell protease 7. Proc Natl Acad Sci USA 89:11174–11178, 1992.

96. DS Reynolds, DS Gurley, KF Austen, WE Serafin. Cloning of the cDNA and gene of mouse mast cell protease-6. Transcription by progenitor mast cells and mast cells of the connective tissue subclass. J Biol Chem 266:3847–3853, 1991.

97. GH Caughey. Mast cell chymases and tryptases: phylogeny, family relations, and biogenesis. In: GH Caughey, ed. Mast Cell Proteases in Immunology and Biology. New York: Marcel Dekker, Inc., 1995, pp 305–329.

98. E Baker, TJ Sayers, GR Sutherland, MJ Smyth. The genes encoding NK cell granule serine proteases, human tryptase-2 (*TRYP2*) and human granzyme A (*HFSP*), both map to chromosome 5q11-q12 and define a new locus for cytotoxic lymphocyte granule tryptases. Immunogenetics 40:235–237, 1994.

99. D Hudig, NJ Allison, CM Kam, JC Powers. Selective isocoumarin serine protease inhibitors block RNK-16 lymphocyte granule-mediated cytolysis. Mol Immunol 26:793–798, 1989.

100. TJ Sayers, AR Lloyd, DW McVicar, MD O'Connor, JM Kelly, CRD Carter, TA Wiltrout, RH Wiltrout, MJ Smyth. Cloning and expression of a second human natural killer cell granule tryptase, HNK-Tryp-2/granzyme 3. J Leuk Biol 59:763–768, 1996.

101. H Kido, A Fukutomi, N Katunuma. A novel membrane-bound serine esterase in human T4+ lymphocytes immunologically reactive with antibody inhibiting syncytia induced by HIV-1. Purification and characterization. J Biol Chem 265:21979–21985, 1990.

102. H Kido, Y Yokogoshi, K Sakai, M Tashiro, Y Kishino, A Fukutomi, N Katunuma.

Isolation and characterization of a novel trypsin-like protease found in rat bronchiolar epithelial Clara cells. A possible activator of the viral fusion glycoprotein. J Biol Chem 267:13573–13579, 1992.

103. GW Wong, YZ Tang, RL Stevens. Cloning of the human homolog of mouse transmembrane tryptase. Int Arch Allergy Immunol 118:419–421, 1999.

104. K Sakai, S Ren, LB Schwartz. A novel heparin-dependent processing pathway for human tryptase: autocatalysis followed by activation with dipeptidyl peptidase I. J Clin Invest 97:988–995, 1996.

105. K Sakai, SD Long, DAD Pettit, GA Cabral, LB Schwartz. Expression and purification of recombinant human tryptase in a baculovirus system. Protein Expression Purif 7:67–73, 1996.

106. MA Sherman, VH Secor, SK Lee, RD Lopez, MA Brown. STAT6-independent production of IL-4 by mast cells. Eur J Immunol 29:1235–1242, 1999.

107. LB Schwartz, AMA Irani, K Roller, C Castells, NM Schechter. Quantitation of histamine, tryptase and chymase in dispersed human T and TC mast cells. J Immunol 138:2611–2615, 1987.

108. S Ren, AE Lawson, M Carr, CM Baumgarten, LB Schwartz. Human tryptase fibrinogenolysis is optimal at acidic pH and generates anticoagulant fragments in the presence of the anti-tryptase monoclonal antibody B12. J Immunol 159:3540–3548, 1997.

109. D Proud, ES Siekierski, GS Bailey. Identification of human lung mast cell kininogenase as tryptase and relevance of tryptase kininogenase activity. Biochem Pharmacol 37:1473–1480, 1988.

110. S Ren, K Sakai, LB Schwartz. Regulation of human mast cell β-tryptase: conversion of inactive monomer to active tetramer at acid pH. J Immunol 160:4561–4569, 1998.

111. NM Schechter, JE Fraki, JC Geesin, GS Lazarus. Human skin chymotryptic protease. Isolation and relation to cathepsin G and rat mast cell proteinase. J Biol Chem 258:2973–2978, 1983.

112. GH Caughey, EH Zerweck, P Vanderslice. Structure, chromosomal assignment, and deduced amino acid sequence of a human gene for mast cell chymase. J Biol Chem 266:12956–12963, 1991.

113. IA Osman, JR Garrett, RE Smith. Enzyme histochemical discrimination between tryptase and chymase in mast cells of human gut. J Histochem Cytochem 37:415–421, 1989.

114. R Huber, W Bode, NM Schechter, S Strobl. The 2.2 Å crystal structure of human chymase in complex with succinyl-Ala-Ala-Pro-Phe-chloromethylketone: structural explanation for its dipeptidyl carboxypeptidase specificity. J Mol Biol 286:163–173, 1999.

115. A Kinoshita, H Urata, FM Bumpus, A Husain. Multiple determinants for the high substrate specificity of an angiotensin II-forming chymase from the human heart. J Biol Chem 266:19192–19197, 1991.

116. M Murakami, SS Karnik, A Husain. Human prochymase activation. A novel role for heparin in zymogen processing. J Biol Chem 270:2218–2223, 1995.

117. G Pejler, JE Sadler. Mechanism by which heparin proteoglycan modulates mast cell chymase activity. Biochemistry 38:12187–12195, 1999.

118. M Walter, RM Sutton, NM Schechter. Highly efficient inhibition of human chymase by alpha(2)macroglobulin. Arch Biochem Biophys 368:276–284, 1999.

119. H-Z Xia, CL Kepley, K Sakai, J Chelliah, A-MA Irani, LB Schwartz. Quantitation of tryptase, chymase, FcεRIα, and FcεRIgamma mRNAs in human mast cells and basophils by competitive reverse transcription-polymerase chain reaction. J Immunol 154:5472–5480, 1995.

120. NM Schechter, LF Brass, RM Lavker, PJ Jensen. Reaction of mast cell proteases tryptase and chymase with protease activated receptors (PARs) on keratinocytes and fibroblasts. J Cell Physiol 176:365–373, 1998.

121. CP Sommerhoff, KC Fang, JA Nadel, GH Caughey. Classical second messengers are not involved in proteinase-induced degranulation of airway gland cells. Am J Physiol 271:L796–L803, 1996.

122. BJ Longley, L Tyrrell, YS Ma, DA Williams, R Halaban, K Langley, HS Lu, NM Schechter. Chymase cleavage of stem cell factor yields a bioactive, soluble product. Proc Natl Acad Sci USA 94:9017–9021, 1997.

123. MW Kofford, LB Schwartz, NM Schechter, DR Yager, RF Diegelmann, MF Graham. Cleavage of type I procollagen by human mast cell chymase initiates collagen fibril formation and generates a unique carboxyl-terminal propeptide. J Biol Chem 272:7127–7131, 1997.

124. I Gotis-Graham, HP McNeil. Mast cell responses in rheumatoid synovium—association of the MC_{TC} subset with matrix turnover and clinical progression. Arthritis Rheum 40:479–489, 1997.

125. NM Schechter, A-MA Irani, JL Sprows, J Abernethy, B Wintroub, LB Schwartz. Identification of a cathepsin G-like proteinase in the MC_{TC} type of human mast cell. J Immunol 145:2652–2661, 1990.

126. A-MA Irani, SM Goldstein, BU Wintroub, T Bradford, LB Schwartz. Human mast cell carboxypeptidase: selective localization to MC_{TC} cells. J Immunol 147:247–253, 1991.

127. SM Goldstein, CE Kaempfer, JT Kealey, BU Wintroub. Human mast cell carboxypeptidase: purification and characterization. J Clin Invest 83:1630–1636, 1989.

128. DS Reynolds, DS Gurley, RL Stevens, DJ Sugarbaker, KF Austen, WE Serafin. Cloning of cDNAs that encode human mast cell carboxypeptidase A, and comparison of the protein with mouse mast cell carboxypeptidase A and rat pancreatic carboxypeptidases. Proc Natl Acad Sci USA 86:9480–9484, 1989.

129. C Sillalber, M Baghestanian, D Bevec, M Willheim, H Agis, S Kapiotis, W Füreder, HC Bankl, HP Kiener, W Speiser, BR Binder, K Lechner, P Valent. The mast cell as site of tissue-type plasminogen activator expression and fibrinolysis. J Immunol 162:1032–1041, 1999.

130. N Kanbe, A Tanaka, M Kanbe, A Itakura, M Kurosawa, H Matsuda. Human mast cells produce matrix metalloproteinase 9. Eur J Immunol 29:2645–2649, 1999.

131. KC Fang, PJ Wolters, M Steinhoff, A Bidgol, JL Blount, GH Caughey. Mast cell expression of gelatinases A and B is regulated by *kit* ligand and TGF-β. J Immunol 162:5528–5535, 1999.

132. A Tanaka, K Arai, Y Kitamura, H Matsuda. Matrix metalloproteinase-9 production, a newly identified function of mast cell progenitors, is downregulated by c-kit receptor activation. Blood 94:2390–2395, 1999.

133. H Fujishima, ROS Mejia, CO Bingham, III, BK Lam, A Sapirstein, JV Bonventre, KF Austen, JP Arm. Cytosolic phospholipase A_2 is essential for both the immediate and the delayed phases of eicosanoid generation in mouse bone marrow-derived mast cells. Proc Natl Acad Sci USA 96:4803–4807, 1999.

134. KR Lynch, GP O'Neill, Q Liu, DS Im, N Sawyer, KM Metters, N Coulombe, M Abramovitz, DJ Figueroa, Z Zeng, BM Connolly, C Bai, CP Austin, A Chateauneuf, R Stocco, GM Greig, S Kargman, SB Hooks, E Hosfield, DL Williams, Jr., AW Ford-Hutchinson, CT Caskey, JF Evans. Characterization of the human cysteinyl leukotriene CysLT1 receptor. Nature 399:789–793, 1999.

135. T Colamorea, R Di Paola, F Macchia, MC Guerrese, A Tursi, JH Butterfield, MF Caiaffa, JZ Haeggstrom, L Macchia. 5-lipoxygenase upregulation by dexamethasone in human mast cells. Biochem Biophys Res Commun 265:617–624, 1999.

136. LJII Roberts, BJ Sweetman, RA Lewis, KF Austen, JA Oates. Increased production of prostaglandin D2 in patients with systemic mastocytosis. N Engl J Med 303:1400–1404, 1980.

137. M Murakami, CO Bingham, III, R Matsumoto, KF Austen, JP Arm. IgE-Dependent activation of cytokine-primed mouse cultured mast cells induces a delayed phase of prostaglandin D_2 generation via prostaglandin endoperoxide synthase-2. J Immunol 155:4445–4453, 1995.

138. DM Underhill, A Ozinsky, AM Hajjar, A Stevens, CB Wilson, M Bassetti, A Aderem. The Toll-like receptor 2 is recruited to macrophage phagosomes and discriminates between pathogens. Nature 401:811–815, 1999.

139. DG Raible, ES Schulman, J DiMuzio, R Cardillo, TJ Post. Mast cell mediators prostaglandin-D_2 and histamine activate human eosinophils. J Immunol 148:3536–3542, 1992.

140. T Matsuoka, M Hirata, H Tanaka, Y Takahashi, T Murata, K Kabashima, Y Sugimoto, T Kobayashi, F Ushikubi, Y Aze, N Eguchi, Y Urade, N Yoshida, K Kimura, A Mizoguchi, Y Honda, H Nagai, S Narumiya. Prostaglandin D(2) as a mediator of allergic asthma. Science 287:2013–2017, 2000.

141. M Wang, A Saxon, D Diaz-Sanchez. Early IL-4 production driving Th2 differentiation in a human *in vivo* allergic model is mast cell derived. Clin Immunol Immunopathol 90:47–54, 1999.

142. A-M Irani, KT Nouri-Aria, MR Jacobson, EM Varga, SJ Till, SR Durham, LB Schwartz. Basophil, eosinophil and IL-4 mRNA-positive cell numbers increase in the bronchial mucosa of atopic asthmatics 24 h after segmental bronchial allergen challenge. J Allergy Clin Immunol 105:827–2000.

143. G Devouassoux, B Foster, LM Scott, DD Metcalfe, C Prussin. Frequency and characterization of antigen-specific IL-4- and IL-13- producing basophils and T cells in peripheral blood of healthy and asthmatic subjects. J Allergy Clin Immunol 104:811–819, 1999.

144. CS Lantz, M Yamaguchi, HC Oettgen, IM Katona, I Miyajima, JP Kinet, SJ Galli. IgE regulates mouse basophil Fcε RI expression in vivo. J Immunol 158:2517–2521, 1997.

145. M Yamaguchi, CS Lantz, HC Oettgen, IM Katona, T Fleming, I Miyajima, JP Kinet, SJ Galli. IgE enhances mouse mast cell FcεRI expression in vitro and in

vivo: Evidence for a novel amplification mechanism in IgE-dependent reactions. J Exp Med 185:663–672, 1997.

146. D MacGlashan, JT Schroeder. Functional consequences of Fc epsilon RI alpha up-regulation by IgE in human basophils. J Leuk Biol 68:479–486, 2000.

147. M Yamaguchi, K Sayama, K Yano, CS Lantz, N Noben-Trauth, C Ra, JJ Costa, SJ Galli. IgE enhances Fcε receptor I expression and IgE-dependent release of histamine and lipid mediators from human umbilical cord blood-derived mast cells: synergistic effect of IL-4 and IgE on human mast cell Fcε receptor I expression and mediator release. J Immunol 162:5455–5465, 1999.

148. K Yano, M Yamaguchi, F De Mora, CS Lantz, JH Butterfield, JJ Costa, SJ Galli. Production of macrophage inflammatory protein-1α by human mast cells: increased anti-IgE-dependent secretion after IgE-dependent enhancement of mast cell IgE-binding ability. Lab Invest 77:185–193, 1997.

149. J-F Gauchat, S Henchoz, G Mazzei, J-P Aubry, T Brunner, H Blasey, P Life, D Talabot, L Flores-Romo, J Thompson, K Kishi, J Butterfield, C Dahinden, J-Y Bonnefoy. Induction of human IgE synthesis in B cells by mast cells and basophils. Nature 365:340–343, 1993.

150. B Baird, ED Sheets, D Holowka. How does the plasma membrane participate in cellular signaling by receptors for immunoglobulin E? Biophys Chem 82:109–119, 1999.

151. D Dombrowicz, SQ Lin, V Flamand, AT Brini, BH Koller, JP Kinet. Allergy-associated FcRβ is a molecular amplifier of IgE- and IgG-mediated in vivo responses. Immunity 8:517–529, 1998.

152. SQ Lin, C Cicala, AM Scharenberg, JP Kinet. The FcεRIβ subunit functions as an amplifier of FcεRIgamma-mediated cell activation signals. Cell 85:985–995, 1996.

153. JM Oliver, DL Burg, BS Wilson, JL McLaughlin, RL Geahlen. Inhibition of mast cell FcεR1-mediated signaling and effector function by the Syk-selective inhibitor, piceatannol. J Biol Chem 269:29697–29703, 1994.

154. VM Rivera, JS Brugge. Clustering of Syk is sufficient to induce tyrosine phosphorylation and release of allergic mediators from rat basophilic leukemia cells. Mol Cell Biol 15:1582–1590, 1995.

155. A Vallé, J-P Kinet. N-acetyl-L-cysteine inhibits antigen-mediated Syk, but not Lyn tyrosine kinase activation in mast cells. FEBS Lett 357:41–44, 1995.

156. CL Kepley, L Youssef, RP Andrews, BS Wilson, JM Oliver. Syk deficiency in nonreleaser basophils. J Allergy Clin Immunol 104:279–284, 1999.

157. CL Kepley, L Youssef, RP Andrews, BS Wilson, JM Oliver. Multiple defects in Fc epsilon RI signaling in Syk-deficient nonreleaser basophils and IL-3-Induced recovery of Syk expression and secretion. J Immunol 165:5913–5920, 2000.

158. H Lienard, P Bruhns, O Malbec, WH Fridman, M Daeron. Signal regulatory proteins negatively regulate immunoreceptor-dependent cell activation. J Biol Chem 274:32493–32499, 1999.

159. SA Berger, TW Mak, CJ Paige. Leukocyte common antigen (CD45) is required for immunoglobulin E-mediated degranulation of mast cells. J Exp Med 180:471–476, 1994.

160. H Suzuki, M Takei, M Yanagida, T Nakahata, T Kawakami, H Fukamachi. Early

and late events in FcεRI signal transduction in human cultured mast cells. J Immunol 159:5881–5888, 1997.

161. D Hata, Y Kawakami, N Inagaki, CS Lantz, T Kitamura, WN Khan, M Maeda-Yamamoto, T Miura, W Han, SE Hartman, L Yao, H Nagai, AE Goldfeld, FW Alt, SJ Galli, ON Witte, T Kawakami. Involvement of Bruton's tyrosine kinase in FcεRI-dependent mast cell degranulation and cytokine production. J Exp Med 187: 1235–1247, 1998.

162. R Setoguchi, T Kinashi, H Sagara, K Hirosawa, K Takatsu. Defective degranulation and calcium mobilization of bone-marrow derived mast cells from Xid and Btk-deficient mice. Immunol Lett 64:109–118, 1998.

163. VI Pivniouk, TR Martin, JM Lu-Kuo, HR Katz, HC Oettgen, RS Geha. SLP-76 deficiency impairs signaling via the high-affinity IgE receptor in mast cells. J Clin Invest 103:1737–1743, 1999.

164. L Frigeri, JR Apgar. The role of actin microfilaments in the down-regulation of the degranulation response in RBL-2H3 mast cells. J Immunol 162:2243–2250, 1999.

165. R Sullivan, LS Price, A Koffer. Rho controls cortical F-actin disassembly in addition to, but independently of, secretion in mast cells. J Biol Chem 274:38140–38146, 1999.

166. D Baram, R Adachi, O Medalia, M Tuvim, BF Dickey, YA Mekori, R Sagi-Eisenberg. Synaptotagmin II negatively regulates Ca^{2+}-triggered exocytosis of lysosomes in mast cells. J Exp Med 189:1649–1657, 1999.

167. WR Sperr, HC Bankl, G Mundigler, G Klappacher, K Grossschmidt, H Agis, P Simon, P Laufer, M Imhof, T Radaszkiewicz, D Glogar, K Lechner, P Valent. The human cardiac mast cell: localization, isolation, phenotype, and functional characterization. Blood 84:3876–3884, 1994.

168. M Mousli, TE Hugli, Y Landry, C Bronner. Peptidergic pathway in human skin and rat peritoneal mast cell activation. Immunopharmacology 27:1–11, 1994.

169. M Iikura, M Yamaguchi, M Miyamasu, Y Morita, T Iwase, I Moro, K Yamamoto, K Hirai. Secretory IgA-mediated basophil activation. Biochem Biophys Res Commun 264:575–579, 1999.

170. M Iikura, M Yamaguchi, T Fujisawa, M Miyamasu, T Takaishi, Y Morita, T Iwase, I Moro, K Yamamoto, K Hirai. Secretory IgA induces degranulation of IL-3-primed basophils. J Immunol 161:1510–1515, 1998.

171. V Patella, G Florio, A Petraroli, G Marone. HIV-1 gp120 induces IL-4 and IL-13 release from human Fc epsilon RI+ cells through interaction with the V(H)3 region of IgE. J Immunol 164:589–595, 2000.

172. PT Peachell, LM Lichtenstein, RP Schleimer. Differential regulation of human basophil and lung mast cell function by adenosine. J Pharmacol Exp Ther 256:717–726, 1991.

173. I Feoktistov, I Biaggioni. Pharmacological characterization of adenosine A_{2B} receptors—studies in human mast cells co-expressing A_{2A} and A_{2B} adenosine receptor subtypes. Biochem Pharmacol 55:627–633, 1998.

174. ES Schulman, MC Glaum, T Post, YH Wang, DG Raible, J Mohanty, JH Butterfield, A Pelleg. ATP modulates anti-IgE-induced release of histamine from human lung mast cells. Am J Respir Cell Mol Biol 20:530–537, 1999.

175. SM MacDonald, T Rafnar, J Langdon, LM Lichtenstein. Molecular identification of an IgE-dependend histamine-releasing factor. Science 269:688–690, 1995.

176. JT Schroeder, LM Lichtenstein, SM MacDonald. Recombinant histamine-releasing factor enhances IgE-dependent IL-4 and IL-13 secretion by human basophils. J Immunol 159:447–452, 1997.

177. M Baggiolini, M Uguccioni, P Loetscher. Chemokines and chemokine receptors in allergic inflammation. In: G Marone, LM Lichtenstein, KF Austen, ST Holgate, eds. Asthma and Allergic Diseases: Physiology, Immunopharmacology and Treatment. New York: Academic Press, 1998, pp 157–167.

178. M Uguccioni, CR Mackay, B Ochensberger, P Loetscher, S Rhis, GJ LaRosa, P Rao, PD Ponath, M Baggiolini, CA Dahinden. High expression of the chemokine receptor CCR3 in human blood basophils. Role in activation by eotaxin, MCP-4, and other chemokines. J Clin Invest 100:1137–1143, 1997.

179. K Hartmann, F Beiglböck, BM Czarnetzki, T Zuberbier. Effect of CC chemokines on mediator release from human skin mast cells and basophils. Int Arch Allergy Immunol 108:224–230, 1995.

180. MD Silverstein, CE Reed, EJ O'Connell, LJ Melton, III, WM O'Fallon, JW Yunginger. Long-term survival of a cohort of community residents with asthma. N Engl J Med 331:1537–1541, 1994.

181. M Baghestanian, R Hofbauer, HP Kiener, HC Bankl, F Wimazal, M Willheim, O Scheiner, W Füreder, MR Müller, D Bevec, K Lechner, P Valent. The c-kit ligand stem cell factor and anti-IgE promote expression of monocyte chemoattractant protein-1 in human lung mast cells. Blood 90:4438–4449, 1997.

182. S Imayama, Y Shibata, Y Hori. Epidermal mast cells in atopic dermatitis. Lancet 346:1559–1559, 1995.

183. K Rajakulasingam, SR Durham, F O'Brien, M Humbert, LT Barata, L Reece, AB Kay, JA Grant. Enhanced expression of high-affinity IgE receptor (FcεRI) a chain in human allergen-induced rhinitis with co-localization to mast cells, macrophages, eosinophils, and dendritic cells. J Allergy Clin Immunol 100:78–86, 1997.

184. CL Kepley, SS Craig, LB Schwartz. Identification and partial characterization of a unique marker for human basophils. J Immunol 154:6548–6555, 1995.

185. AR McEuen, MG Buckley, SJ Compton, AF Walls. Development and characterization of a monoclonal antibody specific for human basophils and the identification of a unique secretory product of basophil activation. Lab Invest 79:27–38, 1999.

186. AM Irani, C Huang, HZ Xia, C Kepley, A Nafie, ED Fouda, S Craig, B Zweiman, LB Schwartz. Immunohistochemical detection of human basophils in late-phase skin reactions. J Allergy Clin Immunol 101:354–362, 1998.

187. S Ying, DS Robinson, Q Meng, LT Barata, AR McEuen, MG Buckley, AF Walls, PW Askenase, AB Kay. C-C chemokines in allergen-induced late-phase cutaneous responses in atopic subjects: Association of eotaxin with early 6-hour eosinophils, and of eotaxin-2 and monocyte chemoattractant protein-4 with the later 24-hour tissue eosinophilia, and relationship to basophils and other C-C chemokines (Monocyte chemoattractant protein-3 and RANTES). J Immunol 163:3976–3984, 1999.

188. AJ Macfarlane, OM Kon, SJ Smith, K Zeibecoglou, LN Khan, LT Barata, AR McEuen, MG Buckley, AF Walls, Q Meng, M Humbert, NC Barnes, DS Robinson, S Ying, AB Kay. Basophils, eosinophils, and mast cells in atopic and nonatopic

asthma and in late- phase allergic reactions in the lung and skin. J Allergy Clin Immunol 105:99–107, 2000.

189. A KleinJan, AR McEuen, MD Dijkstra, MG Buckley, AF Walls, WJ Fokkens. Basophil and eosinophil accumulation and mast cell degranulation in the nasal mucosa of patients with hay fever after local allergen provocation. J Allergy Clin Immunol 106:677–686, 2000.

190. DR Wilson, A-M Irani, SM Walker, M Baran, MR Jacobson, LB Schwartz, SR Durham. Grass pollen immunotherapy reduces seasonal increases in epithelial basophils but not mast cells. J Allergy Clin Immunol 105:211–2000.

191. WD Travis, C-Y Li, EJ Bergstralh, LT Yam, RG Swee. Systemic mast cell disease. Analysis of 58 cases and literature review. Medicine (Baltimore) 67:345–368, 1988.

192. DD Metcalfe. Classification and diagnosis of mastocytosis: current status. J Invest Dermatol 96:2S–4S, 1991.

193. LB Schwartz, K Sakai, TR Bradford, SL Ren, B Zweiman, AS Worobec, DD Metcalfe. The α form of human tryptase is the predominant type present in blood at baseline in normal subjects and is elevated in those with systemic mastocytosis. J Clin Invest 96:2702–2710, 1995.

194. LB Schwartz, TR Bradford, C Rouse, A-M Irani, G Rasp, JK Van der Zwan, P-WG Van Der Linden. Development of a new, more sensitive immunoassay for human tryptase: use in systemic anaphylaxis. J Clin Immunol 14:190–204, 1994.

195. LB Schwartz, DD Metcalfe, JS Miller, H Earl, T Sullivan. Tryptase levels as an indicator of mast-cell activation in systemic anaphylaxis and mastocytosis. N Engl J Med 316:1622–1626, 1987.

196. LB Schwartz, JW Yunginger, JS Miller, R Bokhari, D Dull. The time course of appearance and disappearance of human mast cell tryptase in the circulation after anaphylaxis. J Clin Invest 83:1551–1555, 1989.

197. P-WG Van der Linden, CE Hack, J Poortman, YC Vivié-Kipp, A Struyvenberg, JK Van der Zwan. Insect-sting challenge in 138 patients: Relation between clinical severity of anaphylaxis and mast cell activation. J Allergy Clin Immunol 90:110–118, 1992.

198. MK Church, SP Skinner, LJ Burrows, AP Bewley. Microdialysis in human skin. Clin Exp Allergy 25:1027–1029, 1995.

199. H Behrendt, J Ring. Histamine, antihistamines and atopic eczema. Clin Exp Allergy 20 (suppl 4):25–30, 1990.

200. M Hannuksela, K Kalimo, K Lammintausta, T Mattila, K Turjanmaa, E Varjonen, PJ Coulie. Dose ranging study: cetirizine in the treatment of atopic dermatitis in adults. Ann Allergy 70:127–133, 1993.

201. T Langeland, HE Fagertun, S Larsen. Therapeutic effect of loratadine on pruritus in patients with atopic dermatitis. A multi-crossover-designed study. Allergy 49:22–26, 1994.

202. JM Hanifin. The role of antihistamines in atopic dermatitis. J Allergy Clin Immunol 86:666–669, 1990.

203. CF Wahlgren. Itch and atopic dermatitis: clinical and experimental studies. Acta Derm Venereol Suppl (Stockh) 165:1–53, 1991.

204. G Heyer, OP Hornstein, HO Handwerker. Skin reactions and itch sensation induced

by epicutaneous histamine application in atopic dermatitis and controls. J Invest Dermatol 93:492–496, 1989.

205. A Giannetti, G Girolomoni. Skin reactivity to neuropeptides in atopic dermatitis. Br J Dermatol 121:681–688, 1989.

206. R Rukwied, G Lischetzki, F McGlone, G Heyer, M Schmelz. Mast cell mediators other than histamine induce pruritus in atopic dermatitis patients: a dermal microdialysis study. Br J Dermatol 142:1114–1120, 2000.

207. AA Irani, G Nilsson, LK Ashman, LB Schwartz. Dexamethasone inhibits the development of mast cells from dispersed human fetal liver cells cultured in the presence of recombinant human stem cell factor. Immunology 84:72–78, 1995.

208. DG Malone, RL Wilder, AM Saavedra-Delgado, DD Metcalfe. Mast cell numbers in rheumatoid synovial tissues. Correlations with quantitative measures of lymphotic infiltration and modulation by anti-inflammatory therapy. Arthritis Rheum 30: 130–137, 1987.

209. RM Lavker, NM Schechter. Cutaneous mast cell depletion results from topical corticosteroid usage. J Immunol 135:2368–2373, 1985.

210. P Goldsmith, B McGarity, AF Walls, MK Church, GH Millward-Sadler, DAF Robertson. Corticosteroid treatment reduces mast cell numbers in inflammatory bowel disease. Digest Dis Sci 35:1409–1413, 1990.

211. AM Bentley, MR Jacobson, V Cumberworth, JR Barkans, R Moqbel, LB Schwartz, A- MA Irani, AB Kay, SR Durham. Immunohistology of the nasal mucosa in seasonal allergic rhinitis: Increases in activated eosinophils and epithelial mast cells. J Allergy Clin Immunol 89:877–883, 1992.

212. L Enerbäck, U Pipkorn, G Granerus. Intraepithelial migration of nasal mucosal mast cells in hay fever. Int Arch Allergy Appl Immunol 80:44–51, 1986.

213. C Stellato, A De Paulis, A Ciccarelli, R Cirillo, V Patella, V Casolaro, G Marone. Anti-inflammatory effect of cyclosporin A on human skin mast cells. J Invest Dermatol 98:800–804, 1992.

214. R Cirillo, M Triggiani, L Siri, A Ciccarelli, GR Pettit, M Condorelli, G Marone. Cyclosporin A rapidly inhibits mediator release from human basophils presumably by interacting with cyclophilin. J Immunol 144:3891–3897, 1990.

215. G Marone, M Triggiani, R Cirillo, A Giacummo, L Siri, M Condorelli. Cyclosporin A inhibits the release of histamine and peptide leukotriene C4 from human lung mast cells. Ric Clin Lab 18:53–59, 1988.

216. JM Naeyaert, JM Lachapelle, H Degreef, BM de la, M Heenen, J Lambert. Cyclosporin in atopic dermatitis: review of the literature and outline of a Belgian consensus. Dermatology 198:145–152, 1999.

217. T Ruzicka, T Bieber, E Schopf, A Rubins, A Dobozy, JD Bos, S Jablonska, I Ahmed, K Thestrup-Pedersen, F Daniel, A Finzi, S Reitamo. A short-term trial of tacrolimus ointment for atopic dermatitis. European Tacrolimus Multicenter Atopic Dermatitis Study Group. N Engl J Med 337:816–821, 1997.

16
Eosinophils and Atopic Dermatitis

Kristin M. Leiferman,* Douglas A. Plager, and Gerald J. Gleich*
Mayo Clinic and Mayo Foundation, Rochester, Minnesota

I. INTRODUCTION

Atopic dermatitis has been associated with allergies since its delineation as a disease entity (1). Eosinophils are prominently associated with allergic reactions, but a pathogenic role for eosinophils in atopic dermatitis has emerged only recently. Investigations have shown that eosinophils elaborate potent toxins and mediators of inflammation. Increased circulating eosinophils have been noted in patients with atopic dermatitis since early descriptions of the disease. Despite a paucity of eosinophils infiltrating affected skin, eosinophil granule proteins are prominently deposited in lesions of atopic dermatitis and eosinophil granule proteins are elevated in the peripheral blood of patients with atopic dermatitis (2,3). These studies indicate that eosinophil degranulation is occurring in atopic dermatitis. The recognition that the eosinophil and its granule proteins have potent inflammatory functions suggests a pathogenic role in diseases in which eosinophil infiltration and granule protein deposition are prominent. Observations demonstrating eosinophil involvement in atopic dermatitis are reviewed herein, summarized in Table 1, and schematically represented in Figure 1.

II. PHLOGISTIC PROPERTIES OF EOSINOPHILS

Studies over the past two decades have shown that the eosinophil has the potential for multiple inflammatory activities. The eosinophil contains several cationic

---

* *Current affiliation*: University of Utah, Salt Lake City, Utah.

Table 1   Evidence for Eosinophil Involvement in Atopic Dermatitis

Eosinophils and eosinophil granule proteins possess phlogistic activities and cytotoxic effects that are associated with allergic inflammation

Eosinophil granule proteins are extensively deposited in lesional skin with evidence of cytolytic eosinophil degeneration

Eosinophil granule proteins are increased in peripheral blood and correlate with disease activity

Peripheral blood eosinophils are increased in severe disease, decrease with therapeutic improvement; "activated" hypodense eosinophils with prolonged survival, i.e., delayed programmed cell death, correlate best with disease activity

Th2 immunological reactivity is present in atopic dermatitis associated with IL-5 expression; IL-5 has specific activities on eosinophils inducing eosinophilopoiesis, activation, and chemotaxis

Adhesion molecule expression needed for eosinophil transendothelial migration is present in atopic dermatitis

Eosinophil chemotaxins are expressed in atopic dermatitis

Eosinophil infiltration and extracellular eosinophil granule protein deposition occur in patch test allergen models of atopic dermatitis

---

granule proteins including major basic protein (MBP), eosinophil peroxidase (EPO), eosinophil cationic protein (ECP), and eosinophil-derived neurotoxin (EDN); MBP, EPO, and ECP are potent toxins to various targets including helminths, protozoa, bacteria, and normal mammalian cells (4) and are cytostimulants for basophil and mast cell mediator release (4,5) and for neutrophil (6) and platelet (7) activation. MBP, EPO, ECP, and EDN all increase microvascular permeability (8), and all four proteins induce wheal-and-flare reactions in human skin (9). Activated eosinophils not only release granule proteins but also generate lipid mediators such as leukotriene (LT)C_4 and platelet-activating factor (PAF), generate reactive oxygen species, and participate in antibody-dependent cytotoxicity reactions. The oxidative products of eosinophils including superoxide anions, hydroxyl radicals, and singlet oxygen (10,11) are, like the granule proteins, damaging to cells. The low molecular weight mediators produced by eosinophils, PAF, and LTC_4 (12,13) increase vascular permeability. PAF has several other activities including attraction and activation of leukocytes to areas of inflammation, and LTC_4 stimulates smooth muscle contraction. Eosinophils are also capable of synthesizing and secreting important inflammatory and regulatory cytokines (14–16); these include interleukin (IL)-1α, transforming growth factor (TGF)-α and -β_1, granulocyte-macrophage colony-stimulating factor (GM-CSF), IL-3, IL-4, IL-5, IL-6, IL-8, IL-12, tumor necrosis factor (TNF)-α, and macrophage inhibitory protein (MIP)-1α. The stimuli that trigger eosinophils to produce cytokines are only now being elucidated, but the chemotactic factors C5a and N-formyl-methionyl-leucyl-phenylalanine (FMLP) have been found to induce production of IL-8 and GM-CSF by eosinophils (17). Through expression of MHC class II molecules and IL-1a production, eosinophils may act as specialized antigen-presenting cells (16,18). Eosinophils may be involved in tissue repair by promoting collagen synthesis through release of TGF-α and -β_1 (19); they may also promote fibrosis by their ability to stimulate fibroblast DNA synthesis and extracellular matrix protein production (20). Therefore, the functional diversity of the eosinophil has manifold implications for its role in disease. Moreover, it is not currently known whether eosinophil-derived cytokines interact with other eosinophil mediators or other cell types to enhance inflammatory consequences (16, 21).

Eosinophil activation with deposition of toxic cationic proteins occurs in many diseases (22–24). Levels of blood eosinophil granule proteins are increased in patients with asthma (25) and other diseases, such as episodic angioedema with eosinophilia (9) and the eosinophilia-myalgia syndrome (26); levels of eosinophil granule proteins are also increased in the blood of patients receiving IL-2 in cancer protocols (27). In episodic angioedema with eosinophilia and in IL-2–treated patients, increased IL-5 concentrations temporally precede increases of blood eosinophils (27,28).

Granule proteins released from eosinophils are detected in tissues by immunohistological staining (29–36), and such staining methods are useful in determining the involvement of eosinophils in disease because extensive granule protein deposition is not detectable by routine histological studies such as hematoxylin and eosin or Giemsa staining. Using indirect immunofluorescence with polyclonal antibodies to purified eosinophil granule proteins injected in cadaver skin, the detectable concentrations in tissue are as follows: EPO, 0.05 μM; MBP, 0.1 μM; ECP, 0.25 μM; and EDN, 1.0 μM. These concentrations result in minimal detectable staining, and it is likely that much greater concentrations are deposited in diseased tissues showing extensive staining. Moreover, these concentrations of proteins are capable of inducing biologically damaging effects. The granule proteins appear to be deposited in some lesions, not through classical exocytotic degranulation, but by cytolytic degranulation. For example, by electron microscopy, disrupted eosinophils with free membrane-bound granules have been found in lesional tissues (9,33).

III. CLINICAL AND HISTOLOGICAL FEATURES OF ATOPIC DERMATITIS

Several schema of diagnostic criteria for atopic dermatitis have been used for clinical definition of the disease and for investigations of the disorder (37–39). The principal, basic features of the disease are pruritus and scratching, characteristic morphology and distribution of skin lesions, chronic or chronically relapsing course, and personal or family history of atopy. Other diagnostic features include

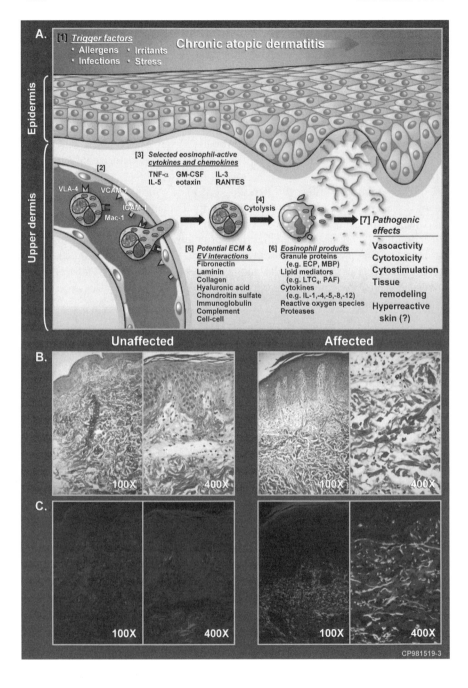

facial pallor and erythema, itch with sweating, white dermographism and delayed blanch to acetylcholine injection. No specific clinical feature or laboratory test is diagnostic for atopic dermatitis. Inclusion of the various additional features for diagnosis of atopic dermatitis emphasizes the importance of cutaneous inflammation in association with aberrant pharmacophysiological responses in the disease.

The histopathological changes in atopic dermatitis observable from examination of hematoxylin- and eosin-stained tissue sections are nonspecific and contribute little to understanding the immunopathogenesis of the disease (1). With Giemsa staining of epon-embedded tissues from atopic dermatitis lesions, more detail has been observed (40). Acute lesions show epidermal spongiosis and dermal perivascular inflammatory cell infiltration. Chronic lesions show thickening

---

Figure 1 Eosinophil involvement in atopic dermatitis. (A) As skin inflammation in atopic dermatitis is established, a variety of factors [1] can lead to extravasation of eosinophils [2] and other immune cells (e.g., CD4+ T cells and macrophages, not shown). Eosinophil extravasation is not fully understood, but the interaction of eosinophil CD49d/CD29 (i.e., VLA-4 or $\alpha4\beta1$ integrin) with endothelial cell VCAM-1 and eosinophil CD11b/CD18 (i.e., Mac-1, $\alpha M\beta2$ integrin) with endothelial cell ICAM-1 appears to be key to eosinophil extravasation and activation. Cytokines and chemokines [3] derived from various cellular sources also contribute to eosinophil chemotaxis and activation. Following allergen challenge, eosinophil extravasation can occur as early as 15 minutes postchallenge, peaking in the skin approximately 6–8 hours postchallenge. The timing and mechanism of eosinophil degranulation [4] following extravasation remains largely unknown. Deposition of granule proteins likely occurs by cytolysis of eosinophils in the upper dermis. Interaction with extracellular matrix (ECM) or extravascular (EV) immune molecules may mediate eosinophil activation [5]. Activation and subsequent degranulation results in mediator release and deposition of eosinophil granule proteins [6]. Release of eosinophil-derived IL-12 has recently been proposed to contribute to the Th2 to Th1 cytokine profile shift observed in chronic atopic dermatitis lesions. The potential for eosinophils to function as antigen-presenting cells (APC) has also recently been proposed. Cutaneous eosinophil activation and degranulation may contribute to disease pathology via several mechanisms [7]. (B) Hematoxylin and eosin staining of clinically unaffected (left two panels) and affected (right two panels) atopic dermatitis skin. Low-power (left) and high-power (right) (100X and 400X original magnification, respectively) images are shown for both unaffected and affected skin. Affected skin shows perivascular inflammation and upper dermal edema. The epidermis is thickened with elongated rete pegs, and the basement membrane is thickened. Unaffected skin shows minimal perivascular inflammation. (C) Indirect immunofluorescence staining for MBP in affected and unaffected atopic dermatitis skin serial sections as in B. Extensive fibrillar extracellular MBP staining is observed in the upper dermis of the affected skin. Minimal, but detectable, MBP is observed in the upper dermis of unaffected atopic dermatitis. Normal skin shows no MBP staining, and control sections of each stained with protein A purified rabbit IgG were negative (not shown).

of the epidermis with elongation of and fibrosis around the rete ridges. Langerhans cells and mast cells are increased in chronic lesions, and endothelial cells are enlarged (40). Eosinophils may be found in any lesional stage, but the majority of cells in biopsy specimens are T lymphocytes possessing the CD4 phenotype (41,42) and expressing activation and memory markers (43).

Several observations suggest that IgE and allergens contribute to the pathogenesis of atopic dermatitis in a large subset of patients with atopic dermatitis. Serum IgE levels are elevated in approximately 80% of patients with atopic dermatitis, and a correlation between serum IgE level and extent of skin involvement has been reported (44). Mast cell numbers are increased in chronic lesions (40). Cells infiltrating atopic dermatitis lesion, such as Langerhans cells and macrophages, as well as mast cells, bear IgE receptors, both FcεRI (high affinity) and FcεRII (low affinity) (45,46). IgE antibody present on cell surfaces is bound to these receptors (46–48). Allergen presentation in atopic dermatitis appears to be mediated by epidermal Langerhans cells bearing IgE (49), and allergens are capable of stimulating IgE-bearing macrophages to synthesize and secrete leukotrienes, PAF, IL-1, and TNF-α (50,51). Antigen-presenting cells then may regulate the local accumulation of inflammatory cells and/or preferentially influence the infiltration of T cells showing Th2-type activity. Atopic dermatitis patients also have circulating autoantibodies to IgE that may bind to and activate IgE-bearing cells (41,52).

Allergen studies in atopic dermatitis patients indicate that IgE antibodies are common and may contribute to disease exacerbations. When prick or intradermal skin tests are performed, patients with atopic dermatitis often show wheal-and-flare responses to multiple allergens, and they frequently have serum IgE antibodies to multiple allergens. Controlled studies have shown that ingestion of foods by children with atopic dermatitis sensitive to these foods provokes cutaneous pruritus and erythema leading to scratching and subsequent development of eczematous lesions (53). Furthermore, these cutaneous exacerbations after food challenges are associated with significant increases in plasma histamine concentrations (indicative of mast cell degranulation). These findings are consistent with the concept that repeated ingestion of food and the reactions that result from such exposure contribute to the development of chronic atopic dermatitis skin lesions in some patients.

The role of inhalant allergens in atopic dermatitis has been observed in numerous studies; exacerbations of atopic dermatitis have been reported after inhalational exposure to a variety of allergens including horse dander, ragweed pollen, and mold (54–56). Recent studies have focused on the role of direct skin contact by inhalant allergens in the development of atopic dermatitis lesions. Eczematoid lesions in atopic dermatitis patients have been provoked by application of allergens to superficially abraded skin (57). Subsequently, eczematous reactions have been demonstrated on nonabraded skin of atopic dermatitis patients to a variety of inhalant allergens (58). These reactions require the presence of epidermal cells coexpressing IgE and CD1a to develop (59). Avoidance of aeroallergens that elicit eczematous reactions at patch test sites or cause immediate hypersensitivity reactions has been reported to improve atopic dermatitis (58,60,61).

Approximately 50% of patients with chronic atopic dermatitis have circulating IgE directed to staphylococcal enterotoxins; these toxins have been identified on skin of atopic dermatitis patients colonized with *Staphylococcus aureus* (43,62); also, atopic dermatitis patients' own basophils release histamine on exposure to relevant staphylococcal enterotoxins. These findings indicate that local production of enterotoxin by *S. aureus* on the skin surface could induce IgE-mediated histamine release and trigger an inflammatory reaction that exacerbates atopic dermatitis (62). In addition, staphylococcal enterotoxin superantigens have recently been shown to augment allergen-specific IgE synthesis (63).

Although the exact role of IgE in atopic dermatitis remains to be clarified, the observations cited above along with studies showing that IgE-bearing Langerhans cells bind allergen, present it to T lymphocytes, and induce an allergen-specific Th2 response with IgE synthesis (49), suggest that IgE, as a product of Th2 immunological activity, which includes both IL-4 and IL-5 production, is important in atopic dermatitis.

IV. CYTOKINE EXPRESSION AND EOSINOPHILS IN ATOPIC DERMATITIS

Several lines of investigation indicate that eosinophils are recruited to and activated in tissue sites by Th2 cytokines; deposition of granule proteins occurs as a function of eosinophil activation and/or cytolytic degranulation (64). Mast cell cytokines may also contribute to eosinophil activation (65). IL-3, IL-5, and GM-CSF stimulate eosinophil growth, maturation, and differentiation. These cytokines along with TNF-α and interferon (IFN)-γ activate eosinophils and prime them for various functions. IL-5, for example, affects eosinophils by increasing their viability, decreasing their density, decreasing their granule content, and inducing release of their cytoplasmic granule proteins into the extracellular environment (66,67). In addition, IL-5 enhances eosinophilopoiesis in and eosinophil release from bone marrow (68) and is chemotactic for eosinophils (69). IL-5 likely accounts for the common presence of eosinophils in allergic inflammation. The presence of a functional IL-4 receptor has recently been identified on eosinophils, through which IL-4 can prime eosinophils to certain chemotactic stimuli (70). While several cytokines enhance eosinophil differentiation, survival, and activation, TGF-β_1, a multifunctional cell growth–regulating cytokine, counteracts the survival enhancing activities of IL-5, IL-3, GM-CSF, and IFN-γ on eosinophils (71). TGF-β_1 inhibits eosinophil survival in a dose-dependent manner and appears to act by inducing apoptosis of eosinophils (71). As noted above, eosinophils elaborate TGF-β_1 as well as IL-3 and GM-CSF (72), suggesting that activated eosinophils produce factors that both enhance and inhibit their own longevity in inflammatory conditions.

Evidence for various patterns of cytokine production in atopic dermatitis has been reported. Comparisons of typical or "atopic" atopic dermatitis (with evidence for IgE involvement) and "nonatopic" atopic dermatitis (atopic dermatitis without an identifiable IgE relationship) demonstrate Th2-type cytokine expression with increased spontaneously released IL-4 and IL-5 from peripheral blood lymphocytes in patients with "atopic" atopic dermatitis. In contrast, "nonatopic" atopic dermatitis patients displayed increased IL-5 but low IL-4 levels (73). Supernatants from lesional skin biopsies showed similar findings; increased IL-4 levels were present only in "atopic" atopic dermatitis biopsies, whereas IL-5 was increased in both "atopic" atopic dermatitis and "nonatopic" atopic dermatitis specimens. A subsequent study showed that the expression of IL-5 and IL-13 as well as the capacity to produce these cytokines by skin T cells is reduced in "nonatopic" atopic dermatitis patients compared to "atopic" atopic dermatitis (74). Cytokine mRNA expression in acute and chronic atopic dermatitis lesions (75) has also been studied and compared. Both acute and chronic lesions had significantly greater numbers of cells positive for IL-4 and IL-5 mRNA than uninvolved skin, but chronic atopic dermatitis lesions had significantly fewer IL-4 mRNA–expressing cells and significantly more IL-5 mRNA–expressing cells than acute lesions; the chronic lesions also showed greater eosinophil infiltration (75). In the peripheral blood and lesional skin of atopic dermatitis patients, both CD4+ and CD8+ T cells expressing the cutaneous lymphocyte-associated antigen (CLA), proliferate in response to superantigen stimulation and produce IL-5 and IL-13 (76). Considering the effects of IL-5 in promoting differentiation, adhesion, and enhanced survival of eosinophils, these studies emphasize that inductive factors are present for the important involvement of eosinophils in atopic dermatitis.

V. EOSINOPHIL INFILTRATION INTO ATOPIC DERMATITIS SKIN

The factors determining eosinophil infiltration into tissue have been under investigation in recent years and involve at least three interrelated signals: chemoattractants, adhesion molecules, and activating cytokines such as GM-CSF, IL-3, and IL-5. A combination of signals likely determines whether eosinophils infiltrate tissues and whether activation and degranulation occurs.

Several members of the C-C chemokine gene superfamily are chemotactic for eosinophils including eotaxin and regulated upon activation, normal T-cell–expressed and –secreted (RANTES) (77–80). Eotaxin, a recently cloned C-C chemokine, is specifically chemotactic for eosinophils (80–83). RANTES is potently chemotactic for eosinophils and is also chemotactic for monocytes, T lymphocytes, natural killer (NK) cells, and basophils, but not neutrophils. In addition to their chemotactic properties, eotaxin and RANTES stimulate production of reactive oxygen species by eosinophils, indicating that they have both chemotactic and functional activation effects on eosinophils (84). Eotaxin is similar in potency to RANTES as an eosinophil chemoattractant, but is a stronger stimulant for production of reactive oxygen species by eosinophils (85). Both eotaxin and RANTES are produced by dermal fibroblasts (79,86), and RANTES is also inducibly produced by keratinocytes (87,88). Enhanced production of RANTES has been found in both keratinocytes (88) and fibroblasts from atopic dermatitis patients (79). Intradermal injection of RANTES into both nonallergic and allergic subjects is attended with a concentration- and time-dependent recruitment of eosinophils (89). However, a difference in the kinetics of eosinophil recruitment and degranulation as detected by MBP staining is observed between nonallergic and allergic subjects; nonallergic subjects show virtually no eosinophil infiltration at 30 minutes and 6 hours, whereas significant eosinophil recruitment and degranulation are observed in allergic subjects by 30 minutes, reaching near maximum levels by 6 hours. However, by 24 hours, eosinophil infiltration and degranulation in both groups reaches a peak and is similar. RANTES injections resulted in E-selectin expression in both subject groups; however, RANTES had no effect on adhesion molecule expression by endothelial cells in vitro, suggesting that the in vivo effects may be indirect (89).

In order for eosinophils to migrate into tissues from the peripheral blood, the cells must transmigrate blood vessels; this information has been reviewed (90) and is briefly summarized here. Three gene superfamilies regulating expression of cell-surface proteins (91,92) contribute to the signaling needed for transmigration. First, selectins are involved in the early, high-sheer force stage of leukocyte adhesion to endothelium. Second, integrins, another gene superfamily of adhesion molecules, recognize counterreceptor members of the third gene superfamily, namely the immunoglobulin gene superfamily. Together, members of the integrin and immunoglobulin families interact to promote flattening and migration of cells onto and through the endothelium. Following migration through vessels, eosinophils are present in the extracellular matrix where integrins, expressed on the cell surfaces, recognize substances such as the fibrous proteins, fibronectin, laminin, and collagen and the glycosaminoglycans hyaluronic acid and chondroitin sulfate. These interactions may modulate eosinophil activity (93).

The importance of E-selectin expression by endothelial cells for tissue infiltration of lymphocytes in atopic dermatitis is supported by the observation that T cells in atopic dermatitis express the skin-specific homing receptor, CLA, a ligand for E-selectin. E-selectin expression is also associated with neutrophil adherence. Endothelial cell expression of vascular cell adhesion molecule-1 (VCAM-1) is also important in atopic dermatitis. Adherence of eosinophils expressing very late antigen (VLA)-4, a counterligand for VCAM-1, and VCAM-1, but not E-selectin expression, is found after IL-4 stimulation of endothelial cells (94). The number of eosinophils and deposits of MBP, EPO, and ECP are significantly and strongly correlated with the staining intensity of VCAM-1 (95). These findings implicate VCAM-1 expression in the mechanism of eosinophil recruitment in atopic dermatitis.

Evidence supports an important role for adhesion molecules, not only in leukocyte transmigration but also in leukocyte function. Simultaneous monitoring of eosinophil adhesion and degranulation has shown that degranulation is always preceded by cellular adhesion (96). Human eosinophils express the β_2-integrin CD11b/CD18 (Mac-1). Monoclonal antibodies to CD18 markedly inhibit eosinophil adhesion, degranulation, and superoxide production induced by PAF or GM-CSF; monoclonal antibodies to CD11b also inhibit eosinophil adhesion and degranulation (96). These findings indicate that CD11b/CD18-dependent cellular adhesion plays a crucial role in eosinophil degranulation and superoxide production. This mechanism may be important when eosinophils contact tissues after transmigrating vessels.

Migratory responses of eosinophils to C5a and TNF-α are the same in normals and in patients with atopic dermatitis. Following IL-5 exposure, eosinophils from normal donors show potentiation of migratory responses to PAF and platelet factor 4. (97,98). However, intracutaneous injection of PAF or allergen in patients with atopic dermatitis is associated with a much stronger skin eosinophilia at allergen-injected sites than at PAF-injected sites. This indicates that PAF alone does not account for eosinophil mobilization in atopic dermatitis. Taken together, these findings suggest in vivo priming of eosinophils in atopic dermatitis; however, this priming for migratory responses is apparently not maximal because it can be further potentiated by IL-5 (98).

VI. EOSINOPHIL DEGRANULATION IN ATOPIC DERMATITIS

Peripheral blood eosinophilia is found in many diseases and, specifically, has been associated with atopic dermatitis (1). Measurement of peripheral blood eosinophils and serum MBP levels in a group of subjects including 16 patients with atopic dermatitis showed that all normal control subjects had normal eosinophil numbers and low MBP levels in the peripheral blood; in contrast, over half of the patients with atopic dermatitis had elevated MBP levels in the peripheral blood, some with normal eosinophil counts and some with elevated eosinophil counts (99). These results suggested that the toxic eosinophil granule MBP was "escaping" from eosinophils through degranulation, secretion, or another process.

The common presence of peripheral blood eosinophilia in atopic dermatitis, the histological findings that show few infiltrating tissue eosinophils, and the prominent elevation of a granule protein from eosinophils in peripheral blood prompted studies to determine whether eosinophils were degranulating in the disease; these degranulated cells may not be recognizable morphologically, yet their granule proteins may be exerting biological effects. Immunohistological detection of eosinophil MBP was studied as a marker of eosinophil degranulation (31). Nineteen biopsy specimens of affected atopic dermatitis skin with chronic dermatitis and one of unaffected skin were obtained from 18 patients satisfying the diagnostic criteria for atopic dermatitis (37). Biopsy specimens were taken simultaneously from the affected and unaffected skin of one patient; two biopsy specimens from the affected skin of another patient were obtained 2 years apart. All 20 biopsy specimens from these patients showed extracellular MBP staining by indirect immunofluorescence using polyclonal affinity chromatography purified antibody to MBP (31). The dominant staining pattern was extracellular fibrillar fluorescence in the upper dermis, often with staining of scattered extracellular granules in the dermis. The specimen from unaffected skin showed minimal fluorescence with fine fibrillar extracellular MBP staining in the upper dermis; in contrast, a specimen of affected skin from the same patient showed marked upper dermal fibrillar MBP fluorescence (Fig. 1C). The two affected skin specimens obtained from the same patient 2 years apart both showed marked upper dermal fibrillar MBP fluorescence (31). The findings from these studies demonstrated eosinophil activity in atopic dermatitis through deposition of granule products.

A striking observation in the atopic dermatitis tissue specimens was extensive extracellular MBP staining with very few intact eosinophils. The identifiable eosinophils were located predominantly within perivascular foci of mononuclear cell infiltration. Yet in many of the biopsy specimens, extracellular MBP staining was prominent throughout the upper dermis. With increased MBP levels (99) and low-density eosinophils in the peripheral blood of patients with atopic dermatitis (100), the dermal MBP deposition in lesions of atopic dermatitis could have resulted from tissue deposition of eosinophil granule proteins from activated eosinophils in the circulation. However, the focal patchy localization of MBP principally in the upper dermis and the minimal staining of uninvolved skin argue against this possibility and suggest that eosinophils deposit granule proteins directly in the skin in this disease.

Following the initial demonstration of marked extracellular MBP deposition in lesions of atopic dermatitis (31), 22 additional patients with atopic dermatitis patients were studied (35). Skin biopsy specimens were obtained from each of these patients; blood and urine specimens were collected the same day as the biopsies from 19 and 14 of the patients, respectively. Specimens from 15 of the 22 patients showed prominent extracellular staining of at least one eosinophil granule protein in lesional skin specimens; tissue deposition of the eosinophil granule proteins was markedly out of proportion to the few infiltrating cells. Only 4 of 19 patients in whom blood differential counts were available exhibited peripheral blood eosinophilia of greater than 760 cells/μL. Yet serum levels of MBP, EDN, and ECP were elevated in more than half of the patients' sera (15 of 19, 14 of 19, and 10 of 19 specimens, respectively); mean MBP, EDN, and ECP serum levels in the group of 19 atopic dermatitis patients were elevated compared to 50 nonatopic normal subjects. Urine levels of MBP, EDN, and ECP were elevated in 3 of 14, 7 of 14, and 0 of 14 specimens, respectively (35).

Eight significant positive correlations were found from statistical comparisons (35). Serum levels of MBP and EDN were correlated ($r_s = 0.64$, $p < 0.007$) and serum levels of EDN and ECP were correlated ($r_s = 0.63$, $p < 0.008$). Tissue deposits of MBP and EDN were correlated ($r_s = 0.76$, $p < 0.0005$), as were tissue deposits of MBP and ECP ($r_s = 0.67$, $p < 0.003$), and tissue deposits of EDN and ECP ($r_s = 0.68$, $p < 0.002$). Urinary MBP levels correlated with serum EDN levels ($r_s = 0.60$, $p < 0.04$). Peripheral blood eosinophils correlated with MBP deposition in tissues ($r_s = 0.49$, $p < 0.04$). A relationship between body surface involvement and peripheral blood MBP levels ($r_s = 0.59$, $p < 0.02$) was also found (35).

Monoclonal antibodies to ECP and MBP are commercially available and have been used in studies to delineate eosinophil involvement in atopic dermatitis. With respect to staining with EG2 (Pharmacia & Upjohn, Uppsala, Sweden), a monoclonal antibody to ECP, studies have shown that EG2 stains not only ECP in and from eosinophils but ECP in and from neutrophils in tissues as well (101). Therefore, the detection of ECP may be from an eosinophil or a neutrophil source or both. With respect to staining with BMK13 (Biodesign International, Kennebunk, ME), a monoclonal antibody to MBP, the sensitivity in detecting extracellular MBP deposition is much less than with polyclonal antibodies. Figure 2 illustrates the prominent extracellular eosinophil granule MBP staining observed in chronic atopic dermatitis lesions by both indirect immunofluorescence and by immunoperoxidase staining methods. Figure 2 also comparatively demonstrates staining with monoclonal and polyclonal antibodies to MBP. Considerably less MBP is detected in tissues stained with monoclonal antibodies than with polyclonal antibodies using either method. This has been observed with other monoclonal antibodies to MBP as well (unpublished observations). Therefore, eosinophil involvement may be underestimated in tissue assays with monoclonal MBP antibodies.

Over the past several years, various studies have reported relationships between eosinophils and atopic dermatitis disease activity; they are reviewed elsewhere (102). For example, peripheral blood eosinophils are increased in severe

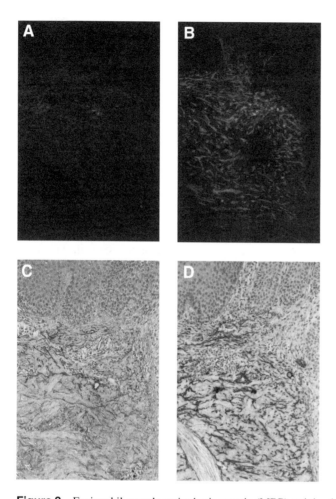

Figure 2 Eosinophil granule major basic protein (MBP) staining in an atopic dermatitis lesion as detected by different antibodies and indirect staining techniques; polyclonal MBP antibodies (panels B and D) revealed greater MBP staining than monoclonal antibodies (panels A and C) in tissue with both immunofluorescence and immunoperoxidase methods. Comparable fields were photographed from serial sections and show extensive extracellular MBP deposition in the dermis with few intact infiltrating cells. In addition, the features of chronic dermatitis are evident with elongation of the epidermal rete pegs, thickening of the basement membrane zone and perivascular mononuclear cell infiltration (160 × original magnification). Negative controls using protein A purified rabbit IgG and irrelevant monoclonal antibodies did not show staining. Lesional atopic dermatitis skin stained by: (A) indirect immunofluorescence with monoclonal MBP antibody (BMK13, Biodesign International, Kennebunk, ME); (B) indirect immunofluorescence with affinity-chromatography purified polyclonal MBP antibody; (C) immunoperoxidase with BMK13 monoclonal MBP antibody; (D) Immunoperoxidase with affinity-chromatography purified polyclonal MBP antibody.

disease, and peripheral blood eosinophils decrease with therapeutic improvement (61,103–109). These studies showed that blood eosinophil counts roughly correlate with disease severity, although many patients with severe disease show normal peripheral blood eosinophil counts. The patients with normal eosinophil counts were mainly those with atopic dermatitis alone; patients with severe atopic dermatitis and concomitant respiratory allergies commonly had increased peripheral blood eosinophils (106). Other studies have shown that serum ECP levels are increased in atopic dermatitis and correlate with disease activity (103,105,110–121). Similar results were found in both adults (115–117) and children (110,114), although children usually had lower ECP levels (102). Correlations between ECP levels and eosinophil counts in the peripheral blood were variable (110,114). Serum ECP levels did not correlate with serum IgE levels, and serum ECP levels were increased in patients with atopic dermatitis who did not have elevated IgE. None the less, the relationship between ECP levels in peripheral blood and the clinical activity of atopic dermatitis provides additional strong support for the eosinophil's role in the disease, although, as noted above, caution must be exercised in attributing ECP solely to eosinophil activity because ECP is present in neutrophils and, thus, may be derived from neutrophils as well (101).

VII. FATE OF EOSINOPHILS IN ATOPIC DERMATITIS

The striking extracellular deposition of eosinophil granule proteins in lesions of atopic dermatitis and the granule protein elevations in peripheral blood that correlate with disease activity suggest that these granule-associated proteins are released from the eosinophil in the disease process. In the IgE-mediated LPR, extracellular eosinophil granule protein deposition corresponds with electron microscopic observations showing obvious eosinophil disruption and free granules in the tissue (33). Electron microscopic studies of specimens from 10 patients with atopic dermatitis revealed disrupted eosinophils and/or free eosinophil granules in 7 patients' lesions. No normal eosinophils were found, and various degrees of eosinophil degeneration were observed in the dermis ranging from intact eosinophils with granule abnormalities, to intact eosinophils with granule abnormalities and prominent pseudopod-like extensions, to eosinophils with degenerating cell and/or nuclear membranes, to free eosinophil granules in proximity to or in the absence of nearby degenerating eosinophils. Free granules as well as cytoplasmic granules in degenerating eosinophils showed lucency and loss of core density (122). This electron microscopic study of lesional atopic dermatitis specimens showed a spectrum of disrupted eosinophils; no evidence of other forms of degranulation such as classical granule exocytosis (piecemeal degranulation) or vesicular transport was seen. On the basis of these findings, it appears that deposition of eosinophil granules and granule proteins in atopic dermatitis may be mainly the result of a cytolytic process.

Programmed cell death (PCD) of peripheral blood eosinophils is delayed in atopic dermatitis to an even greater extent than in inhalant allergy (123). Delayed PCD was the same in "atopic" and "nonatopic"atopic dermatitis subjects, indicating that it is not likely specifically related to sensitization and, based on studies of eosinophils in culture, may be due to autocrine production of growth factors by eosinophils (123). On the other hand, apoptosis in eosinophils from atopic dermatitis patients could be induced in a dose-dependent manner with glucocorticoids (124). At this time, it is difficult to reconcile the delayed eosinophil apoptosis, or PCD, observed in atopic dermatitis (123) with the prominence of cytolytic eosinophil degeneration also observed in the disease (122); however, delayed PCD may be an indicator of eosinophil activation that, once eosinophils infiltrate tissues, is associated with granule release and cytolytic cell death.

VIII. IGE-MEDIATED LATE PHASE REACTIONS AND ATOPIC DERMATITIS

Eosinophil degranulation occurs in several in vivo models of hypersensitivity including the IgE-mediated late phase reaction (LPR) (33). Intradermal allergen injection in allergic patients causes the LPR and release of eosinophil granule proteins into tissues (and into blister fluids bathing these lesions) (125,126) with marked disruption of eosinophils and extracellular deposition of eosinophil granule proteins (33). Eosinophil survival–enhancing cytokines are also present in LPR blister fluids (127), and increased mRNA expression of the cytokine gene cluster IL-3, IL-4, IL-5, and GM-CSF is found in the cutaneous LPR (128). Similarly, after nasal challenge with antigen, the LPR is accompanied by a dramatic increase of eosinophils along with eosinophil degranulation as indicated by increases in MBP and EDN in nasal lavage fluids (129), and eosinophil-active cytokines are present in nasal secretions (130). In studies of cytokine expression during allergen-induced late nasal responses, the expression of IL-4 and IL-5 mRNA was found predominantly in eosinophils early in the reaction at 6 hours (131). Analyses of eosinophil granule proteins in the pulmonary LPR induced by segmental challenge with ragweed extract have shown that MBP, EDN, EPO, and ECP are elevated in bronchoalveolar lavage (BAL) fluids (132) and IL-5 is the predominant eosinophil-active cytokine (133). Thus, allergen challenge of sensitized persons causes eosinophil infiltration and degranulation into the skin, nose, and lung.

The late phase of the IgE-mediated reaction has been proposed as a model for chronic allergic inflammation, including that seen in atopic dermatitis (134,135). Immediate hypersensitivity reactions in the skin are characterized by the development of a wheal and flare, which peaks in 10–20 minutes; the LPR is an inflammatory reaction developing hours later at the same site but over a much larger area with painful, pruritic edema. Pathological examination of the cutaneous LPR has shown infiltration with mononuclear cells, neutrophils, basophils, and eosinophils along with edema and mast cell degranulation (136–138). Eosinophil infiltration occurs quickly after antigen challenge with eosinophils marginating in blood vessels within 15 minutes of challenge (33). Extracellular deposition of eosinophil and neutrophil granule proteins in the LPR begins within one hour after antigen challenge and persists to 56 hours (33). Extracellular eosinophil and neutrophil granule protein deposition are prominent at the peak of the reaction, 6–8 hours after antigen challenge (33).

Both the IgE-mediated cutaneous LPR and atopic dermatitis lesions are associated with the induction of leukocyte adhesion molecules including E-selectin, VCAM-1, and intercellular adhesion molecule-1 (ICAM-1). In children with atopic dermatitis, increased circulating soluble ICAM-1 levels are found (139), and soluble E-selectin correlates with disease activity (140). The induction of these leukocyte adhesion molecules can be blocked by neutralizing antibodies to IL-1 and TNF-α (94), implicating these cytokines in the expression of leukocyte adhesion molecules. Therefore, the release of such cytokines likely is an important regulatory event in the local accumulation of inflammatory cells at the sites of allergic reactions.

Immunohistological studies comparing atopic dermatitis and the cutaneous LPR have shown differences. In the LPR, extracellular deposition of both eosinophil and neutrophil granule proteins is found (33). In contrast, in atopic dermatitis lesions, prominent extracellular eosinophil granule protein deposition is present but neutrophil granule protein deposition is not (35). Immunoassay of sera from atopic dermatitis patients for eosinophil granule proteins and neutrophil elastase showed similar findings; levels of eosinophil granule proteins were increased compared to normals studied in the same assay, whereas neutrophil elastase levels in sera from atopic dermatitis patients were within the normal range (35). Overall, the results indicate that eosinophils actively participate in the pathogenesis of atopic dermatitis, but, unlike the IgE-mediated LPR, neutrophils do not appear to play a role in established lesions of atopic dermatitis (35).

The differences that are observed in the inflammatory cell activity comparing atopic dermatitis to the LPR may have several explanations (Table 2). The mode of antigen exposure may be linked to the pathophysiological outcome. For example, in atopic dermatitis, antigens are likely ingested, inhaled, or contacted rather than intradermally injected as in the LPR. The inflammatory response may be modified depending on antigen presentation and processing in the different anatomical areas. Moreover, atopic dermatitis skin may differ from skin of patients who have respiratory allergies in whom LPRs are elicited; patients with respiratory allergies have essentially normal skin, whereas patients with atopic

Table 2 Possible Explanations for Differences in Inflammatory Cell Involvement Comparing Atopic Dermatitis to the IgE-Mediated Late Phase Reaction

Different mode of antigen exposure
    In atopic dermatitis likely ingested, inhaled or contacted rather than intradermal as in the LPR
    Disease expression may be modified depending on antigen processing and presentation
Atopic dermatitis skin may be constitutionally different than skin of patients with respiratory allergies
Repeated or continuous antigen exposure may show a different inflammatory response than single exposure

dermatitis show altered pharmacophysiological responsiveness and aberrant fatty acid composition. Finally, repeated or continuous antigen exposure may cause a different inflammatory response pattern than single exposure.

Allergen challenge models other than the LPR have been studied to delineate the pathogenesis of atopic dermatitis and further establish links between the eosinophil and the pathophysiology of atopic dermatitis. They suggest that a different mode of antigen exposure, namely the epicutaneous route, compares favorably to the intradermal route. Biopsies of aeroallergen patch test sites in atopic dermatitis patients showed that lymphocytes and eosinophils infiltrate the dermis 2–6 hours after allergen application. By 24–48 hours after patch test application, eosinophils had infiltrated the epidermis and released ECP (141). Activated eosinophils are also in the epidermis and dermis in contact with antigen-presenting (OKT6-positive) cells (142). Furthermore, eosinophil granules are present outside of intact cells, and ECP is present in macrophage-like dermal cells (142). In other studies of house dust mite patch test sites, tissue biopsies revealed that eosinophils localize in dermal postcapillary venules at 2 hours, followed by tissue infiltration at 6 hours, peaking at 24 and 48 hours with spongiosis in the epidermis at 48 hours. Endothelial cell expression of E-selectin and ICAM-1 was upregulated as infiltrating eosinophils increased (143). Increased expression of IL-4, IL-5, IL-6, IL-7, and TNF-α was also observed (144). Taken together, these studies demonstrate a relationship between eosinophil activity and eczematous dermatitis and indicate that cutaneous eosinophil infiltration and degranulation may be induced with epicutaneous allergen contact.

Emerging evidence also indicates that repeated or constant allergen exposure may be associated with a changing inflammatory pattern. In monkeys, for example, repeated allergen challenge by inhalation is attended with airway neutrophils early, followed by a prolonged inflammatory reaction and a marked increase of airway eosinophils. The airway eosinophilia is associated with an increase in airway responsiveness (145). It is likely that repeated or continual antigen challenge in skin is attended with further development of the IgE-mediated reaction (146) including eosinophil involvement. As mentioned previously, chronic lesions of atopic dermatitis that may result from chronic allergen exposure show significantly fewer IL-4 and more IL-5 mRNA-expressing cells than acute lesions, and chronic lesions also show more eosinophil infiltration (75). IL-12 mRNA-expressing cells are also greater in chronic lesions. Because eosinophils have recently been found to express IL-12 (147,148), these cells may be eosinophils. A corresponding increase in IL-12 may promote a Th0 to Th1 switch in chronic lesions, resulting in IFN-γ production as is also found in chronic atopic dermatitis lesions (43). The evolution of the chronic IgE response toward Th1 activity may help explain why the histopathology of chronic atopic dermatitis is similar to delayed-type hypersensitivity. Although the role of eosinophils in delayed-type hypersensitivity has not been well characterized, IFN-γ is a prominent cytokine in delayed-type hypersensitivity reactions and IL-4 mRNA is expressed in contact dermatitis (149); because eosinophils possess both functional IFN-γ and IL-4 receptors, they may be involved in Type IV, delayed and contact, hypersensitivity as well as Type I, IgE-mediated and immediate hypersensitivity. Results from recent studies indicate that Th2 cells require signals in addition to antigen for maximal inflammatory cell recruitment and that Th1 and Th2 cells together promote a robust eosinophil-predominant inflammatory response (150).

IX. THERAPEUTIC POTENTIALS

Many pathogenic pathways involved in inducing atopic dermatitis have been and continue to be investigated. IgE-bearing antigen-presenting cells, IgE-bearing mast cells and basophils, Th2 lymphocytes, and monocytes evidently are important in the pathogenic process. Eosinophils also appear to be intricately involved, although they may not be central cells for initiating the immunological response but rather for perpetrating the response. As such, interference with eosinophil activity as a therapeutic approach may ameliorate the end results of the inflammatory process and will likely not have such potentially grave consequences as interference with other, more centrally acting immunoresponsive cells. Glucocorticoids are the mainstay of treatment for eosinophil-related diseases, and they are widely used to treat atopic dermatitis especially in topical form. Lidocaine mimics certain activities of glucocorticoids in blocking IL-5 activity on eosinophils in vitro. Two recent studies have shown beneficial effects in using nebulized lidocaine for asthma (151,152); studies in atopic dermatitis remain to be initiated. IFN-γ effectively reduces total leukocyte and eosinophil counts in patients with the hypereosinophilic syndrome (153), and studies in atopic dermatitis have shown that improvement with IFN-γ treatment correlates with decreased eosinophil counts (108). Humanized monoclonal anti IL-5 is currently in clinical trials of asthma (154), and it will be interesting to learn whether it is effective in atopic dermatitis. IL-4 is important in Th2 development and eosinophil infiltration, therefore, soluble IL-4 is being investigated as treatment for eosinophil-associated diseases. Agents that block eosinophil chemotaxins, including eotaxin, and chemotaxin receptor blockers are under development as are agents that block eosinophil adhesion and, hence, activation. Leukotriene antagonists have also been studied, and the leukotriene receptor antagonist zafirlukast has been found to be beneficial in treating atopic dermatitis (155). Finally, polyanions, such as heparin and polyglutamic acid, can neutralize the toxicity of the intensely cationic eosinophil granule proteins, and they have been shown to block bronchial hyperreactivity caused by MBP (156). Thus, analyses of the therapeutic effects of neutralizing acidic substances is warranted.

X. CONCLUSION

Strong evidence supports a role for eosinophils in the pathogenesis of atopic dermatitis. The cutaneous inflammatory reaction in atopic dermatitis includes recruitment, activation, and cytolytic degranulation of eosinophils with release of cytotoxic granule proteins and other mediators from eosinophils, which contributes to the disease expression. The IgE-mediated reaction, as currently understood, is an incomplete or inadequate model for atopic dermatitis; however, repeated or continuous allergen challenge may show a multiphasic response beyond the classical dual phase IgE response with persistent inflammation and eosinophil involvement (Fig. 1). What initiates the disease, why only certain individuals are afflicted, and whether blocking the effects of eosinophil activity will modify the manifestations of atopic dermatitis are important questions for continuing investigations.

ACKNOWLEDGMENTS

Supported in part by grants from the National Institutes of Health AR36008, AI34577, AI15231, AI09728, AI31155, the Kieckhefer Foundation, Prescott, AZ, and the Mayo Foundation.

REFERENCES

1. Rajka G. Atopic dermatitis. Major Prob Dermatol 1975; 3:42.
2. Leiferman KM. The role of eosinophils in atopic dermatitis. In: DYM Leung, ed.

The Atopic Dermatitis: From Pathogenesis to Treatment. Austin, TX: R. G. Landes Company, 1996.

3. Leiferman KM. Eosinophils in atopic dermatitis. J Allergy Clin Immunol 1994; 94:1310–1317.

4. Gleich GJ, Adolphson CR, Leiferman KM. Eosinophils. In: Gallin JI, Goldstein IM, Snyderman R, eds. Inflammation, Basic Principles and Clinical Correlates. New York: Raven Press, 1992:663–700.

5. Zheutlin LM, Ackerman SJ, Gleich GJ, Thomas GJ, Thomas LL. Stimulation of basophil and rat mast cell histamine release by eosinophil granule-derived cationic proteins. J Immunol 1984; 133:2180–2185.

6. Moy JN, Gleich GJ, Thomas LL. Noncytotoxic activation of neutrophils by eosinophil granule major basic protein: effect on superoxide anion generation and lysosomal enzyme release. J Immunol 1990; 145:2626–2632.

7. Rohrbach MS, Wheatley CL, Slifman NR, Gleich GJ. Activation of platelets by eosinophil granule proteins. J Exp Med 1990; 172:1271–1274.

8. Minnicozzi M, Duran WN, Gleich GJ, Egan RW. Eosinophil granule proteins increase microvascular macromolecular transport in the hamster cheek pouch. J Immunol 1994; 153:2664–2670.

9. Gleich GJ, Schroeter AL, Marcoux JP, Sachs MI, O'Connell EJ, Kohler PF. Episodic angioedema associated with eosinophilia. N Engl J Med 1984; 310:1621–1626.

10. Kanofsky JR, Hoogland H, Wever R, Weiss SJ. Singlet oxygen production by human eosinophils. J Biol Chem 1988; 263:9692–9696.

11. Petreccia DC, Nauseef WM, Clark RA. Respiratory burst of normal human eosinophils. J Leukocyte Biol 1987; 41:283–288.

12. Lee T, Lenihan DJ, Malone B, Roddy LL, Wasserman SI. Increased biosynthesis of platelet activating factor in activated human eosinophils. J Biol Chem 1984; 259:5526–5530.

13. Shaw RJ, Walsh GM, Cromwell O, Moqbel R, Spry CJF, Kay AB. Activated human eosinophils generate SRS-A leukotrienes following physiological (IgG-dependent) stimulation. Nature 1985; 316:150–152.

14. Hansel TT, Braun RK, DeVries IJ, Boer C, Boer L, Rihs S, Walker C. Eosinophils and cytokines. Agents Actions 1993; 43(suppl):197–208.

15. Moqbel R. Eosinophils, cytokines, and allergic inflammation (review). Ann NY Acad Sci 1994; 725:223–233.

16. Moqbel R, Levi-Schaffer F, Kay AB. Cytokine generation by eosinophils. J Allergy Clin Immunol 1994; 94:1183–1188.

17. Miyamasu M, Hirai K, Takahashi Y, Lida M, Yamaguchi M, Koshino T, Takaishi T, Morita YO. Chemotactic agonists induce cytokine generation in eosinophils. J Immunol 1995; 154:1339–1349.

18. Shi HZ, Humbles A, Gerard C, Jin Z, Weller PF. Lymph node trafficking and antigen presentation by endobronchial eosinophils. J Clin Invest 2000; 105:945–953.

19. Elovic A, Wong DT, Weller PF, Matossian K, Galli SJ. Expression of transforming growth factors-alpha and beta 1 messenger RNA and product by eosinophils in nasal polyps. J Allergy Clin Immunol 1994; 93:864–869.

20. Birkland TP, Cheavens MD, Pincus SH. Human eosinophils stimulate DNA synthesis and matrix production in dermal fibroblasts. Arch Dermatol Res 1994; 286: 312–318.

21. Ochi H, De Jesus NH, Hsieh FH, Austen KF, Boyce JA. IL-4 and -5 prime human mast cells for different profiles of IgE-dependent cytokine production. Proc Natl Acad Sci USA 2000; 97:10509–10512.

22. Butterfield JH, Leiferman KM. Eosinophil-associated diseases. In: Page CP, ed. The Handbook of Immunopharmacology, Immunopharmacology of Eosinophils. New York: Academic Press, 1993:151–192.

23. Leiferman KM. Current perspective on the role of eosinophils in dermatologic diseases. J Am Acad Dermatol 1991; 24:1101–1112.

24. Leiferman KM. Eosinophil granule proteins in cutaneous disease. In: Gleich GJ, Kay AB, ed. Eosinophils in Allergy and Inflammation. New York: Marcel Dekker, Inc., 1994:455–469.

25. Gleich GJ. The eosinophil and bronchial asthma: Current understanding. J Allergy Clin Immunol 1990; 85:422–436.

26. Hertzman PA, Blevins WL, Mayer J, Greenfield B, Ting M, Gleich GJ. Association of the eosinophilia-myalgia syndrome with the ingestion of tryptophan. N Engl J Med 1990; 322:869–873.

27. van Haelst Pisani C, Kovach JS, Leiferman KM, Gleich GJ, Silver JE, Dennin R, Abrams JS. Administration of interleukin-2 (IL-2) results in increased plasma concentrations of IL-5 and eosinophilia in patients with cancer. Blood. 1991; 78: 1538–1544.

28. Butterfield JH, Leiferman KM, Abrams J, Silver JE, Bower J, Gonchoroff N, Gleich GJ. Elevated serum levels of interleukin-5 in patients with the syndrome of episodic angioedema and eosinophilia. Blood 1992; 79:688–692.

29. Filley WV, Ackerman SJ, Gleich GJ. An immunofluorescent method for specific staining of eosinophil granule major basic protein. J Immunol Meth 1981; 47:227–238.

30. Filley WV, Holley KE, Kephart GM, Gleich GJ. Identification by immunofluorescence of eosinophil granule major basic protein in lung tissues of patients with bronchial asthma. Lancet 1982; 2:11–16.

31. Leiferman KM, Ackerman SJ, Sampson HA, Haugen HS, Venencie PY, Gleich GJ. Dermal deposition of eosinophil-granule major basic protein in atopic dermatitis: comparison with onchocerciasis. N Engl J Med 1985; 313:282–285.

32. Leiferman KM, Peters MS, Gleich GJ. The eosinophil and cutaneous edema. J Am Acad Dermatol 1986; 15:513–517.

33. Leiferman KM, Fujisawa T, Gray BH, Gleich GJ. Extracellular deposition of eosinophil and neutrophil granule proteins in the IgE-mediated cutaneous late phase reaction. Lab Invest 1990; 62:579–589.

34. Peters MS, Schroeter AL, Kephart GM, Gleich GJ. Localization of eosinophil granule major basic protein in chronic urticaria. J Invest Dermatol 1983; 81:39–43.

35. Ott NL, Gleich GJ, Peterson EA, Fujisawa T, Sur S, Leiferman KM. Assessment of eosinophil and neutrophil participation in atopic dermatitis: comparison with the IgE-mediated late phase reaction. J Allergy Clin Immunol 1994; 94:120–128.

36. Perez GL, Peters MS, Reda AM, Butterfield JH, Peterson EA, Leiferman KM. Mast

cells, neutrophils and eosinophils in prurigo nodularis. Arch Dermatol 1993; 129: 861–866.

37. Hanifin JM, Rajka G. Diagnostic features of atopic dermatitis. Acta Derm Venereol (Stockh) 1980; 92(suppl):44–47.

38. Williams HC. What is atopic dermatitis and how should it be defined in epidemiological studies? In: Williams HC, ed. Atopic Dermatitis: The Epidemiology, Causes and Prevention of Atopic Eczema. Cambridge, UK: Cambridge University Press, 2000:3–24.

39. Archer CB. The pathophysiology and clinical features of atopic dermatitis. In: Williams, HC, ed. Atopic Dermatitis: The Epidemiology, Causes and Prevention of Atopic Eczema. Cambridge, UK: Cambridge University Press, 2000:25–40.

40. Mihm MC, Soter NA, Dvorak HF, Austen KF. The structure of normal skin and the morphology of atopic eczema. J Invest Dermatol 1976; 67:305–312.

41. Leung DYM. Immunopathology of atopic dermatitis. Springer Semin Immunopathol 1992; 13:427–440.

42. Lever R, Turbitt M, Sanderson A, MacKie R. Immunophenotyping of the cutaneous infiltrate and of the mononuclear cells in the peripheral blood in patients with atopic dermatitis. J Invest Dermatol 1987; 89:4–7.

43. Leung DYM. Pathogenesis of atopic dermatitis. J Allergy Clin Immunol 1999; 104: S99–108.

44. Stone SP, Muller SA, Gleich GJ. IgE levels in atopic dermatitis. Arch Dermatol 1973; 108:806–811.

45. Vercelli D, Jabara HH, Lee BW, Woodland N, Geha RS, Leung DYM. Human recombinant interleukin-4 induces FcεRII/CD23 on normal human monocytes. J Exp Med 1988; 167:1406–1416.

46. Wang B, Rieger A, Kilgus O, Ochiai K, Maurer D, Fodinger D, Kinet JP, Stingl G. Epidermal Langerhans cells from normal human skin bind monomeric IgE via FcεRI. J Exp Med 1992; 175:1353.

47. Bruijnzeel-Koomen C, van Wichen DF, Toonstra J, Berrens L, Bruijnzeel PL. The presence of IgE molecules on epidermal Langerhans' cells in patients with atopic dermatitis. Arch Dermatol Res 1986; 278:199–205.

48. Barker JN, Alegre VA, MacDonald DM. Surface-bound immunoglobulin E on antigen-presenting cells in cutaneous tissue of atopic dermatitis. J Invest Dermatol 1988; 90:117–121.

49. Mudde GC, VanReijsen FC, Boland GJ, DeGast GC, Bruijnzeel PL, Bruijnzeel-Koomen C. Allergen presentation by epidermal Langerhans' cells from patients with atopic dermatitis is mediated by IgE. Immunology 1990; 69:335–341.

50. Fuller RW, Morris PK, Richmond R, Sykes P, Varndell IM, Kemeny DM, Cole PJ, Dollery CT, MacDermot J. Immunoglobulin E-dependent stimulation of human alveolar macrophages: significance in Type 1 hypersensitivity. Clin Exp Immunol 1986; 65:416–426.

51. Rouzer CA, Scott WA, Hamill AL, Liu F-T, Katz DH, Cohn ZA. Secretion of leukotriene C and other arachidonic acid metabolites by macrophages challenged with immunoglobulin E immune complexes. J Exp Med 1982; 156:1077–1086.

52. Quinti I, Brozek C, Wood N, Geha RS, Leung DYM. Circulating IgG antibodies to IgE in atopic syndromes. J Allergy Clin Immunol 1986; 77:586–594.

53. Sampson HA. The immunopathogenic role of food hypersensitivity in atopic dermatitis. Acta Derm Venereol (Stockh). 1992; 176(suppl):34–37.

54. Tuft L, Heck VM. Studies in atopic Dermatitis. IV. Importance of seasonal inhalant allergens, especially ragweed. J Allergy 1952; 23:528–540.

55. Tuft L, Tuft HS, Heck VM. Atopic dermatitis. I. An experimental clinical study of the role of inhalant allergens. J Allergy 1950; 21:181–186.

56. Walker IC. Causation of eczema, urticaria, and angioneurotic edema by proteins other than those derived from foods. JAMA 1918; 70:897–900.

57. Mitchell EB, Crow J, Chapman MD, Jouhal SS, Pope FM, Platts-Mills TAE. Basophils in allergen-induced patch test sites in atopic dermatitis. Lancet 1982; 1:127–130.

58. Clark RA, Adinoff AD. The relationship between positive aeroallergen patch test reactions and aeroallergen exacerbations of atopic dermatitis. Clin Immunol Immunopathol 1989; 53:S132–S140.

59. Langeveld-Wildschut EG, Bruijnzeel PL, Mudde GC, Versluis C, Van Ieperen-Van Dijk AG, Bihari IC, Knol EF, Thepen T, Bruijnzeel-Koomen CA, van Reijsen FC. Clinical and immunologic variables in skin of patients with atopic eczema and either positive or negative atopy patch test reactions. J Allergy Clin Immunol 2000; 105:1008–1016.

60. Platts-Mills TAE, Chapman MD, Mitchell B, Heymann PW, Deuell B. Role of inhalant allergens in atopic eczema. In: Ruzicka T, Ring J, Przybilla B, ed. Handbook of Allergens in Atopic Eczema. Heidelberg: Springer-Verlag, 1991:192–203.

61. Sanda T, Yasue T, Oohashi M, Yasue A. Effectiveness of house dust-mite allergen avoidance through clean room therapy in patients with atopic dermatitis. J Allergy Clin Immunol 1992; 89:653–657.

62. Leung DYM, Harbeck R, Bina P, Reiser RF, Yang E, Norris DA, Hanifin JM. Presence of IgE antibodies to staphylococcal exotoxins on the skin of patients with atopic dermatitis. Evidence for a new group of allergens. J Allergy Clin Immunol 1993; 92:1374–1380.

63. Hofer MF, Harbeck RJ, Schlievert PM, Leung DYM. Staphylococcal toxins augment specific IgE responses by atopic patients exposed to allergen. J Invest Dermatol 1999; 112:171–176.

64. Abu-Ghazaleh RI, Kita H, Gleich GJ. Eosinophil activation and function in health and disease. Immunology Series 1992; 57:137–167.

65. Bradding P, Roberts JA, Britten KM, Montefort S, Djukanovic R, Mueller R, Heusser CH. Interleukin-4, -5, and -6 and tumor necrosis factor-alpha in normal and asthmatic airways: evidence for the human mast cell as a source of these cytokines. Am J Respir Cell Mol Biol 1994; 10:471–480.

66. Kita H, Weiler DA, Abu-Ghazaleh R, Sanderson CJ, Gleich GJ. Release of granule proteins from eosinophils cultured with IL-5. J Immunol 1992; 149:629–635.

67. Rothenberg ME, Petersen J, Stevens RL, Silberstein DS, McKenzie DT, Austen KF, Owen W. IL-5 dependent conversion of normodense human eosinophils to the hypodense phenotype use 3T3 fibroblasts for enhanced viability, accelerated hypodensity, and sustained antibody dependent cytotoxicity. J Immunol 1989; 143:2311–2316.

68. Silberstein DS, Austen KF, Owen WF, Jr. Hemopoietins for eosinophils; glycopro-

tein hormones that regulate the development of inflammation in eosinophilia-associated diseases. Hematol Oncol Clin North Am 1989; 3:511–533.

69. Yamaguchi Y, Hayashi Y, Sugama Y, Miura Y, Kasahara T, Kitamuras TM, Mita S, Tominag A, Takatsu K. Highly purified murine interleukin 5 (IL-5) stimulates eosinophil function and prolongs in vitro survival. IL-5 as an eosinophil chemotactic factor. J Exp Med 1988; 167:1737–1742.

70. Dubois GR, Schweizer RC, Versluis C, Bruijnzeel-Koomen CAFM, Bruijnzeel PLB. Human eosinophils constitutively express a functional interleukin-4 receptor: Interleukin-4-induced priming of chemotactic responses and induction of PI-3 kinase activity. Am J Respir Cell Mol Biol 1998; 19:691–699.

71. Atsuta J, Fujisawa T, Iguchi K, Terada A. Inhibitory effect of TGF-beta 1 on cytokine-enhanced eosinophil survival. Jpn J Allergol 1994; 43:1194–1200.

72. Kita H, Ohnishi T, Okubo Y, Weiler D, Abrams JS, Gleich GJ. Granulocyte/macrophage colony-stimulating factor and interleukin 3 release from human peripheral blood eosinophils and neutrophils. J Exp Med 1991; 174:745–781.

73. Kagi MK, Wüthrich B, Montano E, Barandun J, Blaser K, Walker C. Differential cytokine profiles in peripheral blood lymphocyte supernatants and skin biopsies from patients with different forms of atopic dermatitis, psoriasis and normal individuals. Int Arch Allergy Immunol 1994; 103:332–340.

74. Akdis CA, Akdis M, Simon D, Dibbert B, Weber M, Gratzl S, Kreyden O, Disch R, Wüthrich B, Blaser K, Simon H-U. T cells and T cell-derived cytokines as pathogenic factors in the nonallergic form of atopic dermatitis. J Invest Dermatol 1999; 113:628–634.

75. Hamid Q, Boguniewicz M, Leung DYM. Differential in situ cytokine gene expression in acute versus chronic atopic dermatitis. J Clin Invest 1994; 94:870–876.

76. Akdis M, Simon H-U, Weigl L, Kreyden O, Blaser K, Akdis CA. Skin homing (cutaneous lymphocyte-associated antigen-positive) CD8+ T cells respond to superantigen and contribute to eosinophilia and IgE production in atopic dermatitis. J Immunol 1999; 163:466–475.

77. Kaplan AP, Kuna P, Reddigari SR. Chemokines and the allergic response. Exp Dermatol 1995; 4:260–265.

78. Schröder JM. Cytokine networks in the skin. J Invest Dermatol 1995; 105(1 suppl): 20S–24S.

79. Schröder J-M, Noso N, Sticherling M, Christophers E. Role of eosinophil-chemotactic C-C chemokines in cutaneous inflammation. J Leukocyte Biol 1996; 59:1–5.

80. Ponath PD, Qin S, Ringler DJ, Clark-Lewis I, Wang J, Kassam N, Smith H, Shi X, Gonzalo JA, Newman W, Gutierrez-Ramos JC, Mackay CR. Cloning of the human eosinophil chemoattractant, eotaxin. Expression, receptor binding, and functional properties suggest a mechanism for the selective recruitment of eosinophils. J Clin Invest 1996; 97:604–612.

81. Hein H, Schluter C, Kulke R, Christophers E, Schröder JM, Bartels J. Genomic organization, sequence, and transcriptional regulation of the human eotaxin gene. Biomed Biophys Res Com 1997; 237:537–542.

82. Jose PJ, Griffiths-Johnson DA, Collins PD, Walsh DT, Moqbel R, Totty NF, Truong O, Hsuan JJ, Williams TJ. Eotaxin: A potent eosinophil chemoattractant cytok-

ine detected in a guinea pig model of allergic airways inflammation. J Exp Med 1994; 179:881–887.

83.   Ganzalo JA, Jia GQ, Aguirre V, Friend D, Coyle AJ, Jenkins NA, Lin GS, Katz H, Lichtman A, Copeland N, Kopf M, Gutierrez-Ramos JC. Mouse eotaxin expression parallels eosinophil accumulation during lung allergic inflammation but it is not restricted to a Th2-type response. Immunity 1996; 4:1–14.

84.   Kapp A, Zeck-Kapp G, Czech W, Schopf E. The chemokine RANTES is more than a chemoattractant: characterization of its effect on human eosinophil oxidative metabolism and morphology in comparison with IL-5 and GM-CSF. J Invest Dermatol 1994; 102:906–914.

85.   Elsner J, Hochstetter R, Kimmig D, Kapp A. Human eotaxin represents a potent activator of the respiratory burst of human eosinophils. Eur J Immunol 1996; 26: 1919–1925.

86.   Bartels J, Schluter C, Richter E, Noso N, Kulke R, Christophers E, Schröder JM. Human dermal fibroblasts express eotaxin: Molecular cloning, mRNA expression, and identification of eotaxin sequence variants. Biochem Biophys Res Commun 1996; 225:1045–1051.

87.   Li J, Ireland GW, Farthing PM, Thornhill MH. Epidermal and oral keratinocytes are induced to produce RANTES and IL-8 by cytokine stimulation. J Invest Dermatol 1996; 106:661–666.

88.   Yamada H, Matsukura M, Yudate T, Chihara J, Stingl G, Tezuka T. Enhanced production of RANTES, an eosinophil chemoattractant factor, by cytokine-stimulated epidermal keratinocytes. Int Arch Allergy Immunol 1997; 114:28–32.

89.   Beck LA, Dalke S, Leiferman KM, Bickel CA, Hamilton R, Rosen H, Bochner BS, Schleimer RP. Cutaneous injection of RANTES causes eosinophil recruitment: comparison of nonallergic and allergic subjects. J Immunol 1997; 159:2962–2972.

90.   Gleich GJ. Mechanisms of eosinophil-associated inflammation. J Allergy Clin Immunol 2000; 105:651–663.

91.   Springer TA. Adhesion receptors of the immune system. Nature 1990; 346:425–434.

92.   Bochner BS, Schleimer RP. The role of adhesion molecules in human eosinophil and basophil recruitment. J Allergy Clin Immunol 1994; 94:427–438.

93.   Teti A. Regulation of cellular functions by extracellular matrix. J Am Soc Nephrol 1992; 2(suppl 10):S83–S87.

94.   Schleimer RP, Ebisawa M, Georas SN, Bochner BS. The role of adhesion molecules and cytokines in eosinophil recruitment. In: Gleich GJ, Kay AB, eds. Eosinophils in Allergy and Inflammation. New York: Marcel Dekker, Inc., 1994:99–112.

95.   Wakita H, Sakamoto T, Tokura Y, Takigawa M. E-selectin and vascular cell adhesion molecule-1 as critical adhesion molecules for infiltration of T lymphocytes and eosinophils in atopic dermatitis. J Cutan Pathol 1994; 21:33–39.

96.   Horie S, Kita H. CD11b/CD18 (Mac-1) is required for degranulation of human eosinophils induced by human recombinant granulocyte-macrophage colony-stimulating factor and platelet-activating factor. J Immunol 1994; 152:5457–5467.

97.   Morita E, Schröder J-M, Christophers E. Chemotactic responsiveness of eosinophils isolated from patients with inflammatory skin diseases. J Dermatol 1989; 16: 348–351.

98. Bruijnzeel PL, Kuijper PH, Rihs S, Betz S, Warringa RA, Koenderman L. Eosinophil migration in atopic dermatitis. I: Increased migratory responses to N-formyl-methionyl-leucyl-phenylalanine, neutrophil-activating factor, platelet-activating factor, and platelet factor 4. J Invest Dermatol 1993; 100:137–142.

99. Wassom DL, Loegering DA, Solley GO, Moore SB, Schooley RJ, Fauci AS, Gleich GJ. Elevated serum levels of the eosinophil granule major basic protein in patients with eosinophilia. J Clin Invest 1981; 67:651–661.

100. Miyasato M, Iryo K, Kasada M, Tsuda S. Varied density of eosinophils in patients with atopic dermatitis reflecting treatment with anti-allergic drug (abstr). J Invest Dermatol 1988; 90:589.

101. Sur S, Glitz DG, Kita H, Kujawa SM, Peterson EA, Weiler DA, Kephart GM, Wagner JM, George TJ, Gleich GJ, Leiferman KM. Localization of eosinophil-derived neurotoxin and eosinophil cationic protein in neutrophilic leukocytes. J Leukocyte Biol 1998; 63:715–722.

102. Kapp A. The role of eosinophils in the pathogenesis of atopic dermatitis—eosinophil granule proteins as markers of disease activity. Allergy 1993; 48:1–5.

103. Kagi MK, Joller-Jemelka H, Wüthrich B. Correlation of eosinophils, eosinophil cationic protein and soluble interleukin-2 receptor with the clinical activity of atopic dermatitis. Dermatologica 1992; 185:88–92.

104. Mukai H, Noguchi T, Kamimura K, Nishioka K, Nishiyama S. Significance of elevated serum LDH (lactate dehydrogenase) activity in atopic dermatitis. J Dermatol 1990; 17:477–481.

105. Suagai T, Shoji A, Nagareda T. Changes of ECP values, number of eosinophils and EG2 eosinophils in the peripheral blood following oral ketotifen in patients with atopic dermatitis. Skin Res 1992; 34:368–386.

106. Uehara M, Izukura R, Sawai T. Blood eosinophilia in atopic dermatitis. Clin Exp Dermatol 1990; 15:264–266.

107. Businco L, Meglio P, Ferrara M. The role of food allergy and eosinophils in atopic dermatitis. Pediatr Allergy Immunol 1993; 4:33–37.

108. Stevens SR, Hanifin JM, Hamilton T, Tofte SJ, Cooper KD. Long-term effectiveness and safety of recombinant human interferon gamma therapy for atopic dermatitis despite unchanged serum IgE levels. Arch Dermatol 1998; 134:799–804.

109. Schneider LC, Baz Z, Zarcone C, Zurakowski D. Long-term therapy with recombinant interferon-gamma (rIFN-gamma) for atopic dermatitis. Ann Allergy Asthma Immunol 1998; 80:263–268.

110. Paganelli R, Fanales-Belasio E, Carmini D, Scala E, Meglio P, Businco L, Aiuti F. Serum eosinophil cationic protein in patients with atopic dermatitis. Int Arch Allergy Appl Immunol 1991; 96:175–178.

111. Czech W, Krutmann J, Schopf E, Kapp A. Serum eosinophil cationic protein (ECP) is a sensitive measure for disease activity in atopic dermatitis. Br J Dermatol 1992; 126:351–355.

112. Juhlin L, Venge P. Eosinophilic cationic protein (ECP) in skin disorders. Acta Derm Venereol (Stockh) 1991; 71:495–501.

113. Krutmann J, Czech W, Diepgen T, Niedner R, Kapp A, Schopf E. High-dose UVA1 therapy in the treatment of patients with atopic dermatitis. J Am Acad Dermatol 1992; 26:225–230.

114. Sugai T, Sakiyama Y, Matumoto S. Eosinophil cationic protein in peripheral blood of pediatric patients with allergic diseases. Clin Exp Allergy 1992; 22:275–281.

115. Tsuda S, Kato K, Miyasato M, Sasai Y. Eosinophil involvement in atopic dermatitis as reflected by elevated serum levels of eosinophil cationic protein. J Dermatol 1992; 19:208–213.

116. Kapp A, Czech W, Krutmann J, Schoepf E. Eosinophil cationic protein in sera of patients with atopic dermatitis. J Am Acad Dermatol 1991; 24:555–558.

117. Jakob T, Hermann K, Ring J. Eosinophil cationic protein in atopic eczema. Arch Dermatol Res 1991; 283:5–6.

118. Miyasato M, Tsuda S, Nakama T, Kato K, Kitamura N, Nagaji J, Sasai Y. Serum levels of eosinophil cationic protein reflect the state of in vitro degranulation of blood hypodense eosinophils in atopic dermatitis. J Dermatol 1996; 23:382–388.

119. Caproni M, Agata AD', Cappelli G, Fabbri P. Modulation of serum eosinophil cationic protein levels by cyclosporin in severe atopic dermatitis. Br J Dermatol 1996; 135:336.

120. Halmerbauer G, Frischer T, Koller DY. Monitoring of disease activity by measurement of inflammatory markers in atopic dermatitis in childhood. Allergy 1997; 52: 765–769.

121. Krutmann J, Diepgen TL, Luger TA, Grabbe S, Meffert H, Sonnichsen N, Czech W, Kapp A, Stege H, Grewe M, Schopf E. High-dose UVA1 therapy for atopic dermatitis: results of a multicenter trial. J Am Acad Dermatol 1998; 38:589–593.

122. Cheng JF, Ott NL, Peterson EA, George TJ, Hukee M, Gleich GJ, Leiferman KM. Dermal eosinophils in atopic dermatitis undergo cytolytic degeneration. J Allergy Clin Immunol 1997; 99:683–692.

123. Wedi B, Raap U, Lewrick H, Kapp A. Delayed eosinophil programmed cell death in vitro: a common feature of inhalant allergy and extrinsic and intrinsic atopic dermatitis. J Allergy Clin Immunol 1997; 100:536–543.

124. Matsukura M, Yamada H, Yudate T, Tezuka T, Chihara J. Corticosteroid-induced apoptosis of eosinophils in atopic dermatitis patients. J Clin Lab Immunol 1996; 48:109–122.

125. Zweiman B, Atkins PC, von Allmen C, Gleich GJ. Release of eosinophil granule proteins during IgE-mediated allergic skin reactions. J Allergy Clin Immunol 1991; 87:984–992.

126. Nish WA, Charlesworth EN, Davis TL, Whisman BA, Valtier S, Charlesworth MG, Leiferman KM. The effect of immunotherapy on the cutaneous late phase response to antigen. J Allergy Clin Immunol 1994; 93:484–493.

127. Charlesworth EN, Nish WA, Charlesworth MG, Valtier S, George T, Leiferman KM. Standard high dose immunotherapy decreases the production of IL-3, IL-5 and GM-CSF during the cutaneous late-phase response (LPR) to antigen (abstr). J Allergy Clin Immunol 1993; 91:252.

128. Kay AB, Ying S, Varney V, Gaga M, Durham SR, Moqbel R, Wardlaw AJ, Hamid Q. Messenger RNA expression of cytokine gene cluster, interleukin 3 (IL-3), IL-4, IL-5, and granulocyte/macrophage colony stimulating factor, in allergen-induced late-phase cutaneous reactions in atopic subjects. J Exp Med 1991; 173:775–778.

129. Bascom R, Pipkorn U, Proud D, Dunnette S, Gleich GJ, Lichtenstein LM, Naclerio RM. Major basic protein and eosinophil-derived neurotoxin concentrations in nasal-

lavage fluid after antigen challenge: effect of systemic corticosteroids and relationship to eosinophil influx. J Allergy Clin Immunol 1989; 84:338–346.

130. Sim TC, Grant JA, Hilsmeier KA, Fukuda Y, Alam R. Proinflammatory cytokines in nasal secretions of allergic subjects after antigen challenge. Am J Respir Crit Care Med 1994; 149:339–344.

131. Nouri-Aria KT, O'Brien F, Noble W, Jabcobson MR, Rajakulasingam K, Durham SR. Cytokine expression during allergen-induced late nasal responses: IL-4 and IL-5 mRNA is expressed early (at 6 h) predominantly by eosinophils. Clin Exp Allergy 2000; 30:1709–1716.

132. Sedgwick JB, Calhoun WJ, Gleich GJ, Kita H, Abrams JS, Schwartz LB, Volovitz B, Ben-Yaakov M, Busse WW. Immediate and late airway response of allergic rhinitis patients to segmental antigen challenge. Characterization of eosinophil and mast cell mediators. Am Rev Respir Dis 1991; 144:1274–1281.

133. Ohnishi T, Kita H, Weiler D, Sur S, Sedgwick JB, Calhoun WJ, Busse WW, Abrams JS, Gleich GJ. IL-5 is the predominant eosinophil-active cytokine in the antigen-induced pulmonary late-phase reaction. Am Rev Respir Dis 1993; 147:901–907.

134. Gleich GJ. The late phase of the immunoglobulin-E mediated reaction: a link between anaphylaxis and common allergic disease? J Allergy Clin Immunol 1982; 70:160–169.

135. Sampson HA. Late-phase response to food in atopic dermatitis. Hosp Pract (Off) 1987; 22:111–128.

136. Charlesworth EN, Hood AF, Soter NA, Kagey-Sobotka A, Norman PS, Lichtenstein LM. Cutaneous late-phase response to allergen: mediator release and inflammatory cell infiltration. J Clin Invest 1989; 83:1519–1526.

137. Dolovich J, Hargreave FE, Chalmers R, Shier KJ, Gauldie J, Bienenstock J. Late cutaneous allergic responses in isolated IgE-dependent reactions. J Allergy Clin Immunol. 1973; 52:38–46.

138. Solley GO, Gleich GJ, Jordon RE, Schroeter AL. The late phase of the immediate wheal and flare skin reaction. Its dependence upon IgE antibodies. J Clin Invest 1976; 58:408–420.

139. Kojima T, Ono A, Aoki T, Kameda-Hayashi N, Kobayashi Y. Circulating ICAM-1 levels in children with atopic dermatitis. Ann Allergy 1994; 73:351–355.

140. Wolkerstorfer A, Plaan M, Savelkoul HFJ, Neijens HJ, Mulder PGH, Oudesluys-Murphy AM, Sukhai RN, Oranje AP. Soluble E-selectin, other markers of inflammation and disease severity in children with atopic dermatitis. Br J Dermatol 1998; 138:431–435.

141. Bruijnzeel PL, Kuijper PH, Kapp A, Warringa RA, Betz S, Bruijnzeel-Koomen CA. The involvement of eosinophils in the patch test reaction to aeroallergens in atopic dermatitis: its relevance for the pathogenesis of atopic dermatitis. Clin Exp Allergy 1993; 23:97–109.

142. Maeda K, Yamamoto K, Tanaka Y, Anan S, Yoshida H. The relationship between eosinophils, OKT6-positive cells and house dust mite (HDM) antigens in naturally occurring lesions of atopic lesions. J Dermatol Sci 1992; 3:151–156.

143. Wakugawa M, Nakagawa H, Yamada N, Tamaki K. Chronologic analysis of eosinophil granule protein deposition and cell adhesion molecule expression in mite al-

lergen-induced dermatitis in atopic subjects. Int Arch Allergy Immunol 1996; 111 (suppl 1):5–11.

144. Yamada N, Wakugawa M, Kuwata S, Nakagawa H, Tamaki K. Changes in eosinophil and leukocyte infiltration and expression of IL-6 and IL-7 messenger RNA in mite allergen patch test reactions in atopic dermatitis. J Allergy Clin Immunol 1996; 98:S201–206.

145. Gundel RH, Gerritsen ME, Gleich GJ, Wegner CD. Repeated antigen inhalation results in a prolonged airway eosinophilia and airway hyperresponsiveness in primates. J Appl Physiol 1990; 68:779–786.

146. Bruin-Weller MS, Weller FR, De Monchy JGR. Repeated allergen challenge as a new research model for studying allergic reactions. Clin Exp Allergy 1999; 29: 159–165.

147. Grewe M, Czech W, Morita A, Klammer M, Kapp A, Ruzicki T, Schopf E, Krutmann J. Human eosinophils produce biologically active IL-12: implications for control of T cell responses. J Immunol 1998; 161:415–420.

148. Nutku E, Gounni AS, Olivenstein R, Hamid Q. Evidence for expression of eosinophil-associated IL-12 messenger RNA and immunoreactivity in bronchial asthma. J Allergy Clin Immunol 2000; 106:288–292.

149. Ohmen JD, Hanifin JM, Nickoloff BJ, Rea TH, Wyzykowski R, Kim J, Jullien D, McHugh T, Nassif AS, Chan SC. Overexpression of IL-10 in atopic dermatitis. Contrasting cytokine patterns with delayed-type hypersensitivity reactions. J Immunol 1995; 154:1956–1963.

150. Randolph DA, Stephens R, Carruthers CJL, Chaplin DD. Cooperation between TH1 and TH2 cells in a murine model of eosinophilic airway inflammation. J Clin Invest 1999; 104:1021–1029.

151. Hunt LW, Swedlund HA, Gleich GJ. Effect of nebulized lidocaine on severe glucocorticoid-dependent asthma. Mayo Clin Proc 1996; 71:361–368.

152. Hunt LW, Frigas EF, Butterfield JH, Li JT, Patel A, Kita H, Offord KP, Gleich GJ. Nebulized lidocaine prevents deterioration of pulmonary function following withdrawal of inhaled glucocorticoids. Am J Respir Crit Care Med 1999; 159:A644.

153. Butterfield JH, Gleich GJ. Interferon-γ treatment of six patients with the idiopathic hypereosinophilic syndrome. Ann Intern Med 1994; 121:648–653.

154. Milgrom H, Fick RB Jr, Su JQ, Reimann JD, Bush RK, Watrous ML, Metzger WJ. Treatment of allergic asthma with monoclonal anti-IgE antibody. N Engl J Med 1999; 341:1966–1973.

155. Carucci JA, Washenik K, Weinstein A, Shupack J, Cohen DE. The leukotriene antagonist zafirlukast as a therapeutic agent for atopic dermatitis. Arch Dermatol 1998; 134:785–786.

156. Barker RL, Gundel RH, Gleich GJ, Checkel JL, Loegering DA, Pease LR, Hamann KJ. Acidic polyamino acids inhibit human eosinophil granule major basic protein toxicity: evidence of a functional role for proMBP. J Clin Invest 1991; 88:798–805.

17

Aeroallergens

Elizabeth A. Erwin and Thomas A. E. Platts-Mills
University of Virginia, Charlottesville, Virginia

I. INTRODUCTION

In 1892 Besnier was the first to describe a familial pruritic skin disorder that begins during infancy, fluctuates with seasonal variations, and often occurs with asthma and hay fever. As such, the condition was called prurigo Besnier or infantile eczema. In 1902 Brocq used the term diffuse neurodermatitis, implying that the nervous system played an important role in its pruritus. The concept of allergic causation developed in conjunction with skin test studies in the 1920s, and the term atopic dermatitis (AD) was introduced by Wise and Sulzberger in 1933 due to the association with atopy (1). Acceptance of this new name reflected not only the growing awareness of an association between the disease and asthma or allergic rhinitis, but also the view that exposure to allergens played a significant role in the disease (2–4). In 1949 Tuft reported that most adult patients with AD had positive skin tests to "autologous" house dust, i.e., dust from their own homes (5). He went on to demonstrate both exacerbations of eczema with inhaled dust as well as improvement of skin symptoms when houses were "cleaned."

In spite of such evidence that allergens played a role in the disease, objections remained, largely based on the failure of allergens to produce delayed or eczematous skin lesions during skin testing and the observation that immunotherapy with suspected allergens was not effective. These arguments blocked further understanding and investigation of the allergic etiology of eczema for many years. Today, with the development of techniques to better define specific allergens and a clearer understanding of the pathogenesis of eczema, the role of allergens can be studied in detail. Still, it is important to remember that AD is multifactorial and needs to be approached in this way if successful management is to be achieved. Recently, it has been proposed that AD can be classified as extrinsic or intrinsic. The extrinsic cases ($\sim$70%) have a total immunoglobulin E (IgE) $\geq$ 300 IU/mL and positive IgE antibodies. In addition, these cases have FcεR1 expressed on skin Langerhans cells. The comments in this chapter apply to extrinsic cases and probably not to the minority (<30%) of cases with IgE < 200 IU/mL.

To further understand the relevance of allergens in AD, we will review the relationship between IgE levels and AD, results of patch tests in atopic individuals, and the more recent findings regarding T cells in AD lesions and genetic linkage analyses. We will then discuss in more detail the specific inhalant allergens implicated in the disease, and finally, evaluate the evidence about their role in the development of AD.

II. IMMUNOPATHOLOGY

A. IgE and IgE Antibodies

With the discovery of IgE by Ishizaka in 1967 and the development of the radioallergosorbent test (RAST) in 1971 by Wide and Johannson, it became clear that at least 80% of patients with AD had elevated levels of these antibodies. Ogawa et al. reported an association between IgE levels and severity of disease, which has been supported in subsequent studies (6). Furthermore, early studies established that the patients had specific IgE antibodies to a range of allergens that are present in the air both outdoors and indoors. Recently the quantity of specific IgE to various allergens was compared in serum assays of patients with atopic dermatitis. The greatest concentration of IgE was specific for dust mite. In fact concentrations of IgE to dust mite allergens in patients with AD were in general at least 20-fold higher than those found in sera from patients with asthma (7) (Fig. 1). Nevertheless, there are some confounding issues in the association of high IgE levels and AD. In AD with associated respiratory symptoms, the relationship between exposure and the disease may be easier to recognize. However, patients with "pure" AD can be considered separately (20–40% of all patients with AD) (6). These patients can be further divided by IgE levels. In our own studies we have identified patients who have no respiratory tract symptoms but who have very high total and specific IgE (8). We do not think that the absence of respiratory symptoms argues against the relevance of IgE antibody to the skin disease (6). Elevated IgE levels are also found in other dermatoses, such as cutaneous T-cell lymphoma and scabies, as well as helminthic infestations (9). The elevated total and specific IgE in scabies reflects immediate hypersensitivity to the mite *Sarcoptes scabeii*, which is a close relative of Dermatophagoides and has considerable antigenic cross-reactivity (10).

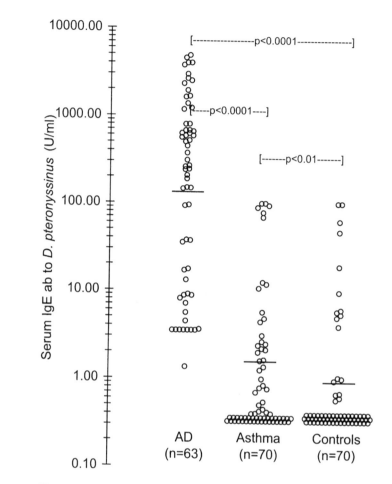

Figure 1 IgE antibodies to dust mite among patients with AD compared to a random group of patients with asthma and controls. Odds ratio for AD for IgE antibody ≥ Class 4; 46 (CI 15–151) compared to control group. (Data from Ref. 7.)

Using biopsies from patients with eczema, Bruijnzeel-Koomen et al. demonstrated IgE bound to Langerhans cells in epidermal cell suspensions (11). This suggests a linkage between type I and cellular hypersensitivity mechanisms. Their group went on to suggest a role for IgE-bearing Langerhans cells. They hypothesized that aeroallergens could penetrate the skin and bind to IgE on Langerhans cells contributing to a local T-lymphocyte response. T lymphocytes could be involved in induction of the eczematous response as well as being responsible for production of IL-4. In addition to its role in the production of IgE by B cells, IL-4 may be involved in induction of FcεRI. This can be expressed on monocytes, which differentiate into dendritic cells, or directly on dendritic cells, thus amplifying the response to allergens (12). Some authors continue to argue that it is possible that elevated IgE levels in AD patients are simply an incidental finding or are a consequence of altered B cell regulation. However the strength of the association with IgE antibodies to common inhalant allergens strongly argues that they are directly relevant to the pathogenesis of the disease (Fig. 2).

B. Results of Patch Tests with Inhalant Allergens

Exacerbation of skin rash in AD patients has been reported following allergen challenge by nasal provocation, bronchial provocation, and conventional skin testing. None of these approaches, however, provided a consistent model in which the response of the skin to allergen exposure could be studied. Indeed, it was often argued that allergens were not relevant to AD because they only produced an ''urticarial'' response in the skin. Perhaps the best technique reported so far for studying the role of inhalant allergens in AD has been the patch test. Mitchell et al., using a technique of ''stripping'' the skin (to remove the lipid barrier that would normally prevent penetration of proteins of MW ≥5000) followed by the application of a patch containing 5 µg of purified mite allergen, found a consistent eczematous response in AD patients at 48 hours as manifested by confluent papular erythema in mild cases and edema and exudation in those with stronger response (13). This finding was limited to AD patients who gave a positive immediate skin reaction to the same allergen. Subsequent studies have confirmed the finding of positive patch test results in AD patients and coined the term ''atopy patch test'' (see Ref. 14). It has been suggested that abrasion (which is similar to scratching) and prolonged exposure simulate naturally occurring conditions of AD. One study, performed in pediatric patients with AD using patch tests of house dust mite, cockroach, mold mix, and grass mix, induced an eczematous response in 90% of the children tested with AD. The control group, atopic children without AD, developed an eczematous response in only 10% of the cases, yielding an impressive p-value of $<10^{-6}$ (15). Others have performed patch testing without abrasion and have still identified allergens that were demonstrated to be clinically significant by resolution of symptoms when the exposure was removed (16).

C. Eosinophils and Basophils in Natural and Induced Eczema

Biopsy of patch test responses has shown cellular infiltrates of eosinophils and mononuclear cells (13,17,18). Mitchell et al. also reported the finding of basophils

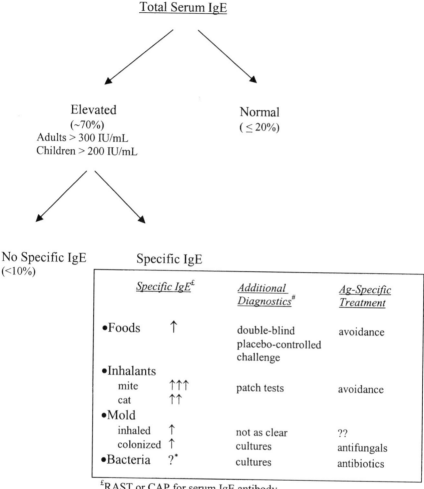

Figure 2 Relevance of inhalant allergy as part of the evaluation and management of atopic dermatitis.

in biopsies from patch reactions (13), although this finding has not been reproduced in all subsequent studies (17,18). Recently Irani et al. reported positive staining in AD using a basophil-specific monoclonal antibody (19). The finding of eosinophils in patch tests was surprising since eosinophils are not obvious in biopsies of naturally occurring eczematous skin lesions. In fact, eosinophils were predominant in the cellular infiltrate. When the patch test was extended by reapplying allergen every two days, the biopsies showed a progressive increase in eosinophils up to the sixth day but showed a dramatic decrease at 10 days (20) (Table 1). This finding could be interpreted as showing that continued exposure to antigen leads to degranulation of eosinophils with release of their toxic contents, substances that go on to perpetuate the eczematous lesions. This view is strongly supported by studies investigating eosinophil major basic protein (MBP) in lesions of patients with AD. Gleich and colleagues found strong staining in skin biopsies using anti-MBP even though the skin did not have identifiable eosinophils (21). Similarly, Kapp et al. found increased levels of eosinophil cationic protein (ECP) in sera of patients with atopic dermatitis (22).

Further research was undertaken to examine the relevance of serum ECP to atopic dermatitis. As there was very little correlation between blood eosinophil count and ECP, it was not simply a reflection of eosinophilia. Additionally, some patients with low serum IgE levels and without specific IgE also had increased serum ECP levels. It has been suggested that increased ECP reflects the activation state of eosinophils or the release of eosinophil granules in eczematous skin (23). Czech et al. showed that serum ECP level significantly correlated with disease activity in AD by clinical scores. Clinical improvement was also associated with a decrease in serum ECP level, suggesting that it could be used as an objective measure of response to treatment (24).

The complexity of the AD lesion was further emphasized by the finding of basophils in biopsies from patch tests. Basophils are typically found in a form

Table 1   Accumulation of Inflammatory Cells in Atopy Patch Tests over 10 Days

Patch applied	Time of bx	Basophils	Mast	Eosinophils	Monocytes	Neutrophils	Total
Saline	2 days	2	46	0	303	16	367
Der p I	2 days	26	56	337	795	37	1251
Der p I	6 days	22	77	1249	833	13	2194
Der p I	10 days	21	113	96	932	9	1171

Note: 5 μg Der p I was applied on a patch of gauze to three separate sites and was reapplied every 2 days. Biopsies carried out with a 4 mm patch biopsy were sized with Karnovsky embedded in plastic and stained with Giemsa.
Source: Adapted from Ref. 20.

of delayed hypersensitivity termed cutaneous basophil hypersensitivity. Using systemically administered plasma or locally administered antibody from patients with AD, it was possible to demonstrate that the eosinophil response could be passively transferred with IgE antibody, suggesting that eosinophil infiltration could be explained by release of mediators from passively sensitized mast cells in the skin. The local basophil response could only be transferred with whole serum injected intradermally, which suggests that T cells in the recipient were playing an active role in their recruitment (25). Presently, there is no general agreement about the existence of T-cell–derived factors that could sensitize the skin to produce a local basophil infiltrate (26,27).

E. T Lymphocytes

While the role of T cells has not been completely elucidated, patients with AD have circulating T cells that respond in vitro to dust mite and other allergens. Furthermore, the number of T cells in the skin is dramatically increased in patients with lesions of atopic dermatitis. This can also be demonstrated over the course of an atopy patch test. Thepen et al. observed different cytokine-producing sub-populations of lymphocytes by double staining for IL-4 and IFN-γ. They showed a shift in balance between different T-helper-cell populations during patch testing. At 24 hours, an increase in Th2 occurs with predominant IL-4 production. Between 24 and 48 hours, an increase in the percentage of CD4 cells with a Th1 phenotype occurs associated with a decrease in Th2 resulting in IFN-γ production prevailing over IL-4 (28). In addition, investigators have reported increased soluble IL-2 receptor levels in patients with AD suggesting T-cell activation (29). The circulating T-cells in patients with AD that respond in vitro to mite antigens are predominantly CD45RO+. In addition, they carry the skin homing marker, cutaneous lymphocyte antigen (CLA+), strongly suggesting that the cells were primed in the skin and can preferentially localize to the skin (30).

F. Genetic Analyses

In the search for the genetic basis of IgE levels and allergic diseases, associations between total serum IgE concentration and polymorphism in several candidate genes have been reported. The region in 5q31-q33 is full of candidate genes, including clustered cytokine genes such as IL-4 and IL-13, which are known to be important in class switching to IgE and in the differentiation of naïve T cells into Th2/Th0 cells. Liu et al. reported a novel sequence variant in the IL-13–coding region and demonstrated a significant association of the allele with both high total serum IgE level and AD (31). Although it is likely that there is a genetic component to AD, it remains unclear whether this reflects a factor controlling

IgE production, specific IgE responses to a dominant antigen such as dust mite, or some more nonspecific control over the activation of helper T cells.

Clearly, there is evidence to support a role for inhalant allergens in the exacerbation and pathophysiology of AD. While it has been shown that eosinophils play a role in this response, the role of mast cells, basophils, and T cells is less clear. The issue of whether inhalant allergen induced inflammation of the skin involves a direct role for T cells remains undecided.

III. INHALANT ALLERGENS

A. Dust Mites

As early as 1932, Rost reported that patients with eczema improved when living in a dust-free environment (4). Later, Tuft confirmed that patients improved when taken out of their homes (5). However, true placebo-controlled trials are difficult. First, it is difficult to standardize avoidance measures, and the degree to which avoidance is carried out by one individual is hard to quantitate. Second, it is difficult to control for each avoidance measure allowing for an overlap in responses. Finally, the presence of complicating factors such as food allergy, bacterial infection, and possibly even fungal colonization of the skin might result in failure to improve in spite of decreased dust mite exposure. Kolmer et al. reported several patients with positive fungal cultures, immediate hypersensitivity to the species of fungi grown, and clinical improvement when treated with extended courses of antifungals (32). These patients had failed to improve with environmental allergen avoidance, and cases of this kind would confound controlled trials.

As a result, only a few controlled trials have been published to add support to anecdotal reports. In 1984, Roberts noted improvement in 15 out of 18 patients with severe atopic dermatitis after a 6-week period of efforts to decrease house dust mite exposure (33). Tan et al. (34) reported a controlled trial of dust mite avoidance measures in which they compared levels of house dust mite to improvement in clinical symptoms. They found that anti–house dust mite measures produced significant improvements in eczema severity. As with avoidance studies for asthma, there was also improvement in the patients in the control group, but part of this reflects reduced exposure secondary to increased cleaning (i.e., a Hawthorne effect in the placebo group).

Specific avoidance measures addressed in the studies described include covering the pillow, mattress, and box springs with allergen-impermeable covers, washing bedding in hot water, and cleaning carpets with an efficient vacuum cleaner on a weekly basis. Additional helpful measures include replacing carpets with polished flooring, keeping humidity at <50% in the house, and reducing the temperature to <70^{0}F. In general, the measures proposed for AD are not different from the mite-avoidance measures that are well established in the treatment of asthma in mite-allergic patients (35).

There is conflicting evidence regarding whether dust mite allergens have their primary role through direct contact with the skin, or whether inhalation and absorption through the respiratory tract is equally important. Some researchers have shown that patients with AD have increased sensitivity to irritants and that irritant reactions occur during patch testing. Specifically, house dust mite allergen, which is a cystein proteinase with catalytic sites distinct from the allergenic epitopes, may function not only as an allergen but also because it is an enzyme (36). Carswell and Thompson (37) addressed the mechanism of sensitization when they found that serum concentrations of IgE Ab specific for allergens in the dust mite body were greater in children with eczema than in children with asthma. They suggested that increased exposure to mite body allergens was a consequence of skin inflammation and thus the pattern of antibodies provided evidence for sensitization through the skin. On the other hand, Tupker et al. later demonstrated the induction of skin symptoms consisting of new lesions as well as exacerbation of existing lesions by inhalation of house dust mite in a double-blind, randomized, placebo-controlled trial (38).

B. Other Inhalants

If dust mite can induce AD through inhalation or topical exposure as described above, logically there should be a role for other inhalant allergens. In fact, earlier investigators published anecdotal reports involving pollens, animal dander, and molds. In 1918 Walker (39) reported two patients who experienced significant clearing of their skin following pollen avoidance. He noted that these patients had previously suffered seasonal exacerbations. In a horse-allergic patient, he observed worsening of rash following inhalation of horse dander (39). Hopkins suggested a possible role for molds in 1930 when he observed worsening of a patient's skin lesions following the inhalation of *Alternaria* (40), and Tuft reported immediate pruritus in two ragweed-allergic AD patients upon inhalation of ragweed allergen (41).

It has been difficult to obtain controlled evidence for allergens other than dust mite. Patch test results have supported a role for other inhalant allergens, but not as frequently as dust mite. Adinoff et al. (42) published a collection of case reports on a subset of AD patients who displayed positive patch tests to animal dander, molds, grasses, trees, and ragweed. They found that in their 10 patients positive patch tests could be predicted by history and thus correlated with aeroallergens identified in their patients' environments. In 1989, Clark and Adinoff (43) expanded on their previous findings, detailing that patients were able to associate contact with specific allergens and exacerbations or experience seasonal variability in their disease severity. They also observed that removal of patients from their homes or local environments resulted in marked improvement in skin symptoms. In their experience they found that approximately 30% of positive skin prick tests resulted in positive patch tests. When Ring et al. (14) investigated whether the patch test could be used to evaluate the role of aeroallergens in AD, they found that their patients could be divided into two groups according to the clinical distribution of their AD lesions. Group I exhibited an air-exposed pattern with lesions on skin that was not covered by clothing, including head, neck, forearms, ankles, and hands. In this group, 69% had positive atopy patch tests. In Group II, which did not show such a pattern of lesions, 39% had positive atopy patch tests. Despite these reports, it would seem that the role of pollen exposure is modest in patients with AD because their symptoms are not markedly influenced by pollen seasons. In fact, most AD patients actually improve during the spring and summer at the time when pollen levels are elevated.

In view of the recent attention to the role of cockroach allergen in asthma in inner city children, it is not surprising that its contribution to AD has begun to be investigated. Wananukul et al. (15) demonstrated positive intradermal reactions to cockroach in 86% of pediatric patients studied. Additionally, 70% of these children had positive patch test results to cockroach. Purification of the allergens has been fairly recent, and further studies dealing solely with cockroach allergy and AD have yet to be done. Given its fairly impressive role in asthma and the information described above, one might predict that cockroach allergen will come to be seen as playing an important role in AD.

A few studies have looked at specific IgE to other aeroallergens. Haatela and Jaakonmaki reported elevated specific IgE to cat and dog (44), and Scalabrin et al. found correlations between serum total IgE levels and specific IgE levels to fungi in their patients with AD (7) (Fig. 3). However, it is important to remember that some fungi can also colonize the skin and play a role in disease. Our experience is that most, but not all patients with fungal infection of the skin have high levels of total IgE and specific IgE to dust mite. Thus it is likely that there is a role for both colonizing fungi and inhaled fungi and inhaled or topical mite exposure.

In contrast to the increased sensitization to dust mite that is seen with increased exposure, we have recently published data that show that high exposure to cat allergen Fel d 1 induces production of IgG and IgG4 antibodies but not IgE antibodies in otherwise allergic children (45). This tolerant response has the features of a modified Th2 response rather than a Th1 response. Preliminary data from measurement of serum IgE and IgG in AD patients by RIA and CAP demonstrated only one patient with IgG to Fel d 1 without evidence of hypersensitivity. This raises the possibility that patients with AD may be unable to develop a similar "tolerance" to Fel d 1, suggesting that their T cells respond differently to high-dose antigen.

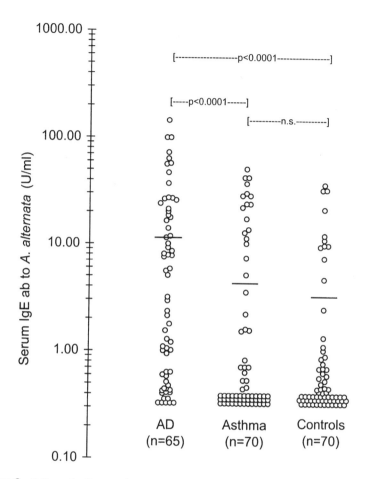

Figure 3 IgE antibodies to alternaria in patients with atopic dermatitis, asthma and controls. Odds ratio for AD among patients with IgE antibody ≥ 4.9 compared to controls (CI 2.8–8.6). (From Ref. 7.)

IV. THE DEVELOPMENT OF ATOPIC DERMATITIS

Exposure to allergens starts before birth since it is quite clear that food allergens can be absorbed and can be transferred across the placenta. After birth, food antigen exposure occurs through eating or through breast milk. Given the quantities inhaled per day, i.e., ~5–50 ng of the mite allergen Der p 1, it seems very unlikely that the fetus is exposed to sufficient mite allergen to produce an immune response to the antigen before birth. The T-cell proliferative responses that have been reported in cord blood have not convincingly been shown to relate to exposure or to a subsequent allergic response (46). Exposure to dust mite and other indoor allergens is generally low in the first few months. Furthermore, very few children develop IgG antibodies to mite allergens before 2 years of age. Obviously, the great majority of children do not go on to develop allergic disease, and only a small minority, i.e., <1%, have persistent trouble with atopic dermatitis. For food antigens it is clear that the infant, and subsequently the child, is exposed to sufficient allergen to produce an immune response. Thus, the nonallergic state to foods must indeed be some form of tolerance. By contrast, for inhalant allergens, including dust mites, exposure is low or very low. In addition, studies to find a correlation between dust mite exposure and eczema have been unsuccessful. Henderson et al. were unable to find a relationship between Der p1 exposure (as measured in mattress dust) and either eczema severity or immediate hypersensitivity to Der p1 (47). Gutgesell et al. (48) went one step further to say that an antigen load greater than 25 μg/g of dust was usually associated with a negative patch test. They suggested that high antigen exposure may cause induction of anergy. Specific T cells are present in allergic children, but in vitro proliferative responses do not distinguish between groups of children with different types of allergic disease (49). At present it is not clear whether severe atopic dermatitis develops because of excessive environmental exposure, failure to develop tolerance, infection of the skin, or some other event that leads to an exaggerated immune response and the associated excessive inflammatory response in the skin.

V. SUMMARY AND CONCLUSIONS

A. Mechanisms

If we consider dust mite allergens as the primary example of an "inhaled" foreign antigen related to AD, there are many questions about how these proteins contribute to the disease. Our data about the quantity of IgE antibody to mite allergens (Fig. 1) raise the possibility that these antigens play a significant role in the increase in total serum IgE. Given the remarkable contrast in the levels of total IgE found in AD compared to other allergic disease, it seems likely that immunopathological events occurring in the skin or its draining lymph nodes are central to the development of the serum IgE. In turn, this could be explained if chronic topical exposure of the inflamed skin to a foreign antigen was the stimulus for IgE production. Whether bacteria in the skin or the enzymatic activity of mite allergens is necessary as adjuvant in this process is not clear. However, priming of CLA+ T cells in the skin may be central to the continuation of the inflammation. In addition, inflammatory events in the skin will lead to upregulation of receptors on the endothelial lining of the small blood vessels in the skin. These changes in the blood vessels must be important in the localization of T cells or circulating allergens. Some of the evidence also suggests that allergen inhaled and absorbed through the respiratory tract can exacerbate the disease and may be particularly important in pruritus. Thus it seems likely that the allergens of dust mite play two distinct roles: (1) contributing to the inflammation, priming of T cells, and production of IgE by direct contact with the skin; and (2) as a trigger for acute exacerbations and itching either from inhalation or direct contact.

B. Relevance to Treatment

Many different specific and nonspecific treatments have been proposed for AD. The primary specific treatment is allergen avoidance, which is very effective in some cases and should be considered as an essential part of treatment in all severe cases. There are some very interesting treatments being developed, including humanized monoclonal antibodies to IgE and IL-5. In addition, there are at least two approaches to blocking the actions of IL-4: (1) soluble IL-4 receptor that has been used successfully as an inhaled drug in the treatment of moderately severe asthma and (2) the inactive mutants of IL-4, which can block both IL-4 and IL-13. These treatments focus on IgE, eosinophils, or T cells, i.e., different parts of the immune response. However, these proposed treatments are not antigen specific. Traditionally, it has been considered that immunotherapy was contraindicated in AD. Indeed, immunotherapy can cause severe exacerbations of the skin disease. However, logically changing or modifying the immune response to allergens should be the correct approach to treatment. The question is whether this would best be achieved safely by using peptides (50,51), modified recombinant proteins (52), antigens combined with the CpG motif of bacterial DNA (53), or a different route of exposure, e.g., oral.

C. Evidence for a Causal Role of Inhalant Allergens

In 1949, Louis Tuft concluded that sensitization to foods was the major factor in AD in young children but that by age 7 years most patients were sensitive to inhalants (5). Since the discovery of IgE many of his observations have been confirmed and explained, in particular, the high prevalence of IgE antibodies to inhalants and clinical efficacy of reducing exposure to house dust (8,43). The case that inhalants contribute to AD is best considered in relation to several different observations (Table 2):

Table 2 Evidence Favoring a Causal Relationship Between Atopic Dermatitis and Dust Mite Allergy

1. Prevalence of sensitization and the quantity of IgE Ab to *D. pteronyssinus* is higher in AD than in any other condition (odds ratio > 20).
2. Patch tests with purified mite allergens can induce the histological and cellular infiltrate typical of the disease.
3. Experimental studies:
   In anecdotal cases, hospital studies, and controlled trials of avoidance, reduced exposure can decrease disease.
   Nasal challenge leads to an exacerbation of AD.

1. Patients with AD have very high titer IgE antibodies to dust mites and other inhalants. In keeping with this they have specific T cells of the Th2 type and specific IgG_4 antibodies.
2. Application of dust mite allergens to the skin (the atopy patch test) can produce a macroscopic, eczematous response and a marked infiltrate including eosinophils, basophils, and T cells. In uncontrolled experiments, inhaling allergens can also exacerbate the skin rash.
3. Reducing exposure to dust mite allergens produces improvement in the rash. This has been demonstrated both with hospital admission and in controlled trials of avoidance measures in the patients' houses.

Atopic dermatitis, like all allergic diseases, ranges from mild (or very mild) to severe and sometimes debilitating. In mild cases a change in the environment or modest doses of topical steroids may provide adequate treatment. Among cases with moderate disease careful avoidance of dust mite allergens has been proven to be effective treatment (34), and it is safe to assume that avoidance measures can help with other inhalants. However, as cases become more severe, they also become more complex with multiple factors contributing to the disease. It is well recognized that skin infection with *Staphylococcus aureus* can exacerbate the skin rash. However, it is less well recognized that colonization of the skin with so-called nonpathogenic bacteria or a wide range of fungi can contribute. Thus managing the most severe cases may require attention to dietary factors, control of environmental exposure, antibiotics, and even antifungal treatment (32). Establishing the specific sensitization of patients with AD to inhalants using skin testing or in vitro assays is essential in order to define appropriate avoidance measures and should be a routine part of treatment.

ACKNOWLEDGMENT

Research supported by NIH grants AI-20565 and AI-34607.

REFERENCES

1. Hanifin J. Atopic dermatitis. J Allergy Clin Immunol 73:211–222, 1984.
2. Atherton DJ. Allergy and atopic eczema, I and II. Clinical Exp Dermatol 6:191, 317–326, 1981.
3. Sulzberger MB, Vaughan WT. Experiments in silk hypersensitivity and inhalation of allergen in atopic dermatitis (neurodermatitis disseminatus) J allergy 5:544–560, 1934.
4. Rost GA. Über Erfahrungen mit der allergenfreien Kammer nach Storm von Leeuwen: insbesondere in der Spätperiode der exsudaten diathese. Arch Dermatol Syphilol 155:297–308, 1932.
5. Tuft LA. Importance of inhalant allergen in atopic dermatitis. J Invest Dermatol 12: 211–219, 1949.
6. Wuthrich B. Atopic dermatitis flare provoked by inhalant allergens. Dermatologica 178:51–53, 1989.
7. Scalabrin DMF, Baubek S, Perzanowski MS, Wilson BB, Platts-Mills TAE, Wheatley LM. Use of specific IgE in assessing the relevance of fungal and dust mite allergens to atopic dermatitis: a comparison with asthmatic and nonasthmatic control subjects. J Allergy Clin Immunol 104:1273–1279, 1999.
8. Chapman MD, Rowntree S, Mitchell EB, Di Priso de Fuenmajor MC, Platts-Mills TAE. Quantitative assessments of IgG and IgE antibodies to inhalant allergens in patients with atopic dermatitis. J Allergy Clin Immunol 72:27–33, 1983.
9. Guerevitch A, Heiner D, Reiner R. IgE in atopic dermatitis and other common dermatoses. Arch Dermatol Forsch 2:712–715, 1973.
10. Arlian LG, Geis DP, Vyszenski-Moher DL, Bernstein IL, Gallagher JS. Crossed antigenic and allergenic properties of the house dust mite *Dermatophagoides farinae* and the storage mite *Tyrophagus putrescentiae*. J Allergy Clin Immunol 74:172–179, 1984.
11. Bruijnzeel-Koomen C, van Wichen D, Toonstra J, Berrens L, Bruijnzeel-Koomen P. The presence of IgE molecules on epidermal Langerhans cells in patients with atopic dermatitis. Arch Dermatol Res 278:199–205, 1986.
12. Bruijnzeel-Koomen CAFM, Mudde GC, Bruijnzeel PLB. New aspects in the pathogenesis of atopic dermatitis. Acta Derm Venereol 144:558–563, 1989.
13. Mitchell EB, Crow J, Chapman MD, Jouhal SS, Pope FM, Platts-Mills TAE. Basophils in allergen-induced patch test sites in atopic dermatitis. Lancet I:127–301, 1982.
14. Ring J, Darsow U, Gfessor M, Vieluf D. The 'atopy patch test' in evaluating the role of aeroallergens in atopic eczema. Int Arch Allergy Immunol 113:379–383, 1997.

15. Wananukul S, Huiprasert P, Pongprasit P. Eczematous skin reaction from patch test-ing with aeroallergens in atopic children with and without atopic dermatitis. Pediatric Dermatol 10:209–213, 1993.

16. Clark R, Adinoff A. The relationship between positive aeroallergen patch reactions and aeroallergen exacerbations of atopic dermatitis. Clin Immunol Immunopath 53: S132–140, 1989.

17. Bruijnzeel-Koomen CAFM, van Wichesn DF, Spry CJF, Venge P, Bruijnzeel PLB. Active participation of eosinophils in patch test reactions to inhalant allergens in patients with atopic dermatitis. Br J Dermatol 118:229–238, 1988.

18. Henoque E, Vargaftig BB. Skin eosinophilia in atopic dermatitis. J Allergy Clin Immunol 81:691–695, 1988.

19. Irani AA, Leung DYM, Boguniewicz M, Strickland I, Baran ML, Schwartz LB. Acute atopic dermatitis is associated with increased infiltration of basophils. J Al-lergy Clin Immunol 107:S237, 2001.

20. Mitchell EB, Crow J, Williams G, Platts-Mills TAE. Increase in skin mast cells following chronic house dust mite exposure. Br J Dermatol 114:65–73, 1986.

21. Leiferman KM, Ackerman SJ, Sampson HA, Haugen HS, Venencie PY, Gleich GJ. Dermal deposition of eosinophil granule major basic protein in atopic dermatitis. N Engl J Med 313:282–285, 1985.

22. Kapp A, et al. Eosinophil cationic protein in sera of patients with atopic dermatitis. J Am Acad Dermatol 24:555–558, 1991.

23. Kapp A. The role of eosinophils in the pathogenesis of atopic dermatitis- eosinophil granule proteins as markers of disease activity. Allergy 48:1–5, 1993.

24. Czech W, Krutmann J, Schopf E, Kapp A. Serum eosinophilic cationic protein (ECP) is a sensitive measure for disease activity in atopic dermatitis. Br J Dermatol 126: 351–355, 1992.

25. Mitchell EB, Crow J, Rowntree S, Webster AD, Platts-Mills TAE. Cutaneous baso-phil hypersensitivity to inhalant allergens: local transfer of basophil accumulation with immune serum but not IgE antibody. J Invest Dermatol 83:290–295, 1984.

26. Borish L, Rosenwasser L. T_{H1}/T_{H2} lymphocytes: doubt some more. J Allergy Clin Immunol 99:161–164, 1997.

27. Mitchell EB, Askenase PW. Suppression of T cell mediated cutaneous basophil hy-persensitivity by serum from guinea pigs immunized with mycobacterial adjuvant. J Exp Med 156:159–172, 1982.

28. Thepen T, Langeveld-Wildschut EG, Bihari IC, van Wichen DF, van Reijsen FC, Mudde GC, Bruijnzeel-Koomen CAFM. Biphasic response against aeroallergen in atopic dermatitis showing a switch from an initial TH2 response to a TH1 response in situ: An immunocytochemical study. J Allergy Clin Immunol 97:828–837, 1996.

29. Wuthrich B, Joller-Jemelka H, Helfenstein U, Grob PJ. Levels of soluble IL-2 recep-tor correlate with severity of atopic dermatitis. Dermatologica 181:92–97, 1990.

30. Santamaria LF, Picker LJ, Perez Soler MT, Drzimalla K, Flohr P, Blaser K, Hauser C. Circulating allergen-reactive T cells from patients with atopic dermatitis and aller-gic contact dermatitis express the skin-selective homing receptor the cutaneous lym-phocyte-associated antigen (CLA). J Exp Med 181:1935–1940, 1995.

31. Liu X, Nickel R, Beyer K, Wahn U, Ehrlich E, Freidhoff LR, Bjorksten B, Beaty TH, Huang S, MAS-Study Group. An IL-13 coding region variant is associated with

a high total serum IgE level and atopic dermatitis in the German Multicenter Atopy Study (MAS-90). J Allergy Clin Immunol 106:167–170, 2000.

32. Kolmer HL, Taketomi EA, Hazen KC, Hughs E, Wilson BB, Platts-Mills TAE. Effect of combined antibacterial and antifungal treatment in severe atopic dermatitis. J Allergy Clin Immunol 98:702–707, 1996.

33. Roberts DL. House dust mite avoidance and atopic dermatitis. Br J Dermatol 110: 735–736, 1994.

34. Tan BB, Weald D, Strickland I and Friedman PS. Double blind controlled trial of effect of house dust mite allergen avoidance on atopic dermaitis. Lancet 347:15–18, 1996.

35. Platts-Mills TAE, Vaughan JW, Carter MC, Woodfolk JA. The role of intervention in established allergy: avoidance of indoor allergens in the treatment of chronic allergic disease. J Allergy Clin Immunol 106: 787–804, 2000.

36. Deleuran M, et al. Purified Der p1 and p2 patch tests in patients with atopic dermatitis: evidence for both allergenicity and proteolytic irritancy. Acta Derm Venereol 798: 241–243, 1998.

37. Carswell F, Thompson S. Does natural sensitization in eczema occur through the skin? Lancet 2:13–15, 1986.

38. Tupker RA, De Monchy JGR, Coenraads PJ, Homan A, Van De Meer J. Induction of atopic dermatitis by inhalation of house dust mite. J Allergy Clin Immunol 97: 1064–70, 1996.

39. Walker C. Causation of eczema, urticaria and angioneurotic edema. JAMA 70:897–900, 1918.

40. Hopkins J, Kesten B, Benham R. Sensitization to saprophytic fungi in a case of eczema. Proc Soc Exp Biol Med 27:342–344, 1930.

41. Tuft L, Heck V. Studies in atopic dermatitis. IV. Importance of seasonal inhalant allergens, especially ragweed. J Allergy 23:528–540, 1952.

42. Adinoff AD, Tellez P, Clark RAF. Atopic dermatitis and aeroallergen contact sensitivity. J Allergy Clin Immunol 81:736–742, 1988.

43. Adinoff AD, Clark RAE. The allergic nature of atopic dermatitis. Immunol Allergy Prac xi:17–28, 1989.

44. Haatela T, Jaakonmaki I. Relationship of allergen-specific IgE antibodies, skin prick tests and allergic disorders in unselected adolescents. Allergy 36:251–256, 1981.

45. Platts-Mills TAE, Vaughan J, Squillace S, Woodfolk J, Sporik R. Sensitisation, asthma, and a modified Th2 response in children exposed to cat allergen: a population based cross-sectional study. Lancet 356:752–756, 2001.

46. Platts-Mills TAE, Woodfolk JA. Cord blood proliferative responses to inhaled allergens: Is there a phenomenon? J Allergy Clin Immunol 106:441–443, 2000.

47. Henderson AJW, Kennedy CTC, Thompson SJ, Carswell F. Temporal association between Der p1 exposure, immediate hypersensitivity and clinical severity of eczema. Allergy 45:445–450, 1990.

48. Gutgesell C, Seubert A, Junghans V, Neumann CH. Inverse correlations of domestic exposure to *Dermatophagoides pteronyssinus* antigen patch test reactivity in patients with atopic dermatitis. Clin Exp Allergy 29:920–925, 1999.

49. Rawle FC, Mitchell EB, Platts-Mills, TAE. T cell responses to the major allergen from the house dust mite *Dermatophagoides pteronyssinus* antigen P1: comparison

of patients with asthma, atopic dermatitis, and perennial rhinitis. J Immunol 133: 195–201, 1984.

50. Marcotte GV, Braun CM, Norman PS, Nicodemus CF, Kagey-Sobotka A, Lichtenstein LM, Essayan DM. Effects of peptide therapy on ex vivo T-cell responses. J Allergy Clin Immunol 101:506–513, 1998.

51. Haselden BM, Kay AB, Larch M. Immunoglobulin E-independent major histocompatibility complex-restricted T cell peptide epitope-induced late asthmatic reactions. J Exp Med 189:1885–1894, 1999.

52. Mueller GA, Smith AM, Chapman MD, Rule GS Benjamin DC. Hydrogen exchange nuclear magnetic resonance spectroscopy mapping of antibody epitopes on the house dust mite allergen Der p 2. J Biol Chem 276:9359–9365, 2001.

53. Tighe H, Takabayashi K, Schwartz D, Ban Nest G, Tuck S , Eiden JJ, Kagey-Sobotka A, Creticos PS, Lichtenstein LM, Speigelberg HL, Raz E. Conjugation of immunostimulatory DNA to the short ragweed allergen Amb a 1 enhances its immunogenicity and reduces its allergenicity. J Allergy Clin Immunol 106:124–134, 2000.

18
Atopic Dermatitis and Foods

Lisa Ellman-Grunther and Hugh A. Sampson
Mount Sinai School of Medicine, New York, New York

Atopic dermatitis (AD) is a chronically relapsing skin disorder that is associated with severe pruritis and a "classic" distribution. There are international standards for diagnosis based upon the criteria recommended by Hanifin and Rajka (1) and a standardized method for gauging severity based on the SCORAD Index (2) adapted by the European Task Force on Atopic Dermatitis. Symptoms present in the first year of life in about 50% of patients, and in 80% by 5 years. Depending upon a patient's age, the distribution of lesions will vary. The cheeks and extensor surfaces of the arms and legs are typically affected in infants, the flexor surfaces of the arms and legs in the young child, and the flexor surfaces, hands, and feet in the teenage patient and young adult (3). Lesions are erythematous, papulovesicular eruptions, which are sometimes associated with weeping and crusting in early life, and progress to a scaly lichenified eruption with age (4). Most patients have a significant elevation in total serum IgE as well as environmental- and food-specific IgE antibody concentrations (5). A large number of cell types are involved in the pathogenesis of AD, including B cells, T cells, monocytes, macrophages, dendritic cells, eosinophils, platelets, and Langerhans cells (6–8). Early (9) studies showed that the intense pruritus and resultant scratching that develops in patients following exposure to irritants and relevant allergens is an important cause of the physical signs and typical distribution of this disorder.

The importance of IgE-mediated mechanisms in atopic dermatitis has been debated since the first comprehensive description of this disorder made by Besnier in 1892 (10). He observed the hereditary nature, chronically relapsing course, and association of eczematous rash with asthma and hay fever. Since that time, certain observations have supported the idea that IgE-mediated mechanisms play a significant role in AD: other atopic disorders such as allergic rhinitis and asthma develop in 50–80% of children with AD (11,12); a positive family history of atopy is present in 65–85% of patients with AD (13), serum IgE levels are elevated in 80–90% of AD children (14), and positive immediate skin tests and RASTS to various dietary and environmental allergens are present in approximately 80% of children with AD (15,16). Identification and strict avoidance of relevant allergens has been of significant therapeutic benefit.

Food hypersensitivity has been shown to cause worsening of skin symptoms in 33–40% of children with moderate to severe disease (17,18). In 1988, Burks et al. studied 46 patients with mild to severe atopic dermatitis who were evaluated in a pediatric allergy or dermatology clinic (17). Thirty-three percent of patients had positive double-blind, placebo-controlled food challenges (DBPCFC) to at least one food, with the onset of symptoms occurring within 2 hours in all patients. Skin symptoms were present in 96% of positive challenges and were the sole symptom in 30%. In 1998, Eigenmann et al. (18) found a similar prevalence of 35–40% among children with moderate to severe atopic dermatitis referred to a pediatric dermatologist. Most recently, Eigenmann et al. (19) reported that out of 74 Swiss children referred to a pediatric allergist or dermatologist for atopic dermatitis, 34% had food hypersensitivity.

Over the past two decades, a large number of studies have been conducted that would fulfill Koch's postulates and therefore support a causal role for food hypersensitivity in children with atopic dermatitis. In other words, studies have shown that elimination of the causal factor leads to clearing of the disorder, introduction of the causal factor brings on the disorder, and avoidance of the causal factor prevents the development of the disorder. Children with AD and food hypersensitivity who follow diets strictly eliminating suspected food allergens have shown significant improvement in their skin symptoms (20–22). Conversely, children with AD and food allergy who have been eliminating certain food allergens have been shown to develop worsening of their chronic dermatitis when given the food in blinded oral food challenges (23,24). Because many of the studies in this area have been performed by physicians in the field of allergy and immunology, it has been somewhat difficult to convince physicians in other specialties of the importance of the immunopathogenic association between food hypersensitivity and atopic dermatitis. However, in recent years the increasing number of clinical and laboratory studies supporting this association has led to more widespread acceptance (25,26). In addition, we recently developed a murine model of a food-induced atopic dermatitis–like syndrome (27). In this chapter we will review the abundance of laboratory and clinical investigations that have provided convincing evidence that food allergy plays a significant causative role in a subgroup of children with atopic dermatitis. The studies done in adults are very limited and less conclusive, but these data will be discussed as well.

I. EVIDENCE FOR IGE-MEDIATED CUTANEOUS RESPONSE IN ATOPIC DERMATITIS

Through the examination of skin biopsy specimens, the typical histological features of both acute and chronic AD have been described. The clinical and histological phenotype of AD depends on the acuity of the skin lesions (28–31). However, even clinically normal-appearing skin of AD patients is histologically abnormal with mild hyperkeratosis and a slight perivascular cellular infiltrate consisting primarily of T cells. Acute AD lesions are marked by spongiosis of the epidermis and a marked perivenular infiltrate consisting predominantly of lymphocytes with occasional monocytes in the dermis. Lymphocytes are primarily CD4+, CD45RO+, CLA+ lymphocytes, suggesting that cells have had a previous encounter with an inciting antigen. Mast cell numbers are normal or slightly increased and rare eosinophils may be seen, although immunohistochemical staining with anti-MBP antibodies has revealed diffuse deposition of eosinophil major basic protein (MBP), an activated eosinophil product (32). In chronic lesions, the epidermis is hyperplastic with elongation of the rete pegs and hyperkeratosis, increased numbers of IgE-bearing Langerhans cells (professional antigen-presenting cells) in the epidermis and dermis, increased numbers of mast cells, especially of the T type (33), and increased numbers of eosinophils. Eosinophil major basic protein, eosinophil cationic protein, and eosinophil-derived neurotoxin are elevated in the sera of AD patients and correlate with disease severity (34).

In situ hybridization studies suggest that the acute lesion of AD is the result of a Th2-induced (allergic) inflammatory response, whereas the chronic lesion is the result of a Th1/Th0 ("mixed") response. Although various disease states may have a combination of cytokine profiles, IL-4, IL-5, and IL-13 classically are considered Th2 cytokines, whereas IL-2, IL-12, and IFN-γ are Th1 cytokines. Compared to the skin of healthy controls, normal-appearing skin of AD patients has increased numbers of cells expressing IL-4 and IL-13 mRNA, but not IL-5, IL-12, or IFN-γ (27,28). In acute AD lesions, there are increased numbers of cells expressing mRNA for IL-4, IL-5, and IL-13 compared to healthy-appearing skin, but not IL-12 or IFN-γ. Eosinophils as well as MBP (35) have been isolated from biopsy specimens of acute AD lesions, and the cytokine mileu as described above is likely to play a role in their recruitment to this area. This is in contrast to classic Type IV cellular responses, such as PPD (purified protein derivative) or rhus dermatitis (poison ivy), where cells express primarily mRNA for IFN-γ and IL-2, but not IL-4 and IL-5 (36). Chronic AD skin lesions have fewer IL-4 and IL-13 mRNA–expressing cells but increased numbers of IL-5–, IL-12–, GM-CSF–, and IFN-γ–expressing cells than in the acute skin lesions. It is felt that the expression of IL-12 by eosinophils or macrophages plays a key role in the switch to Th1 cells, which are prominent in chronic AD (28). Many of the histological features of chronic AD described are consistent with the terminal stages of allergen-induced IgE-mediated hypersensitivity reactions (37). The elevated numbers of IgE-bearing mast cells and Langerhans cells (38,39) within these lesions further suggest atopic mechanisms.

A recent study utilizing a murine model of AD induced by cutaneous sensitization with ovalbumin examined the consequences of IL-4, IL-5, or IFN-γ knockout (40). These investigators showed that IL-5 knockout mice had no detectable eosinophils in the skin and exhibited decreased epidermal and dermal thickening, IL-4 knockouts displayed normal thickening of the skin but had drastically reduced numbers of eosinophils, and IFN-γ knockouts had reduced dermal thickening. The systemic Th2-skewing in patients with AD is supported by the propensity of patients' PBMCs to produce increased levels of IL-4, IL-5, and IL-13 and decreased levels of IFN-γ in response to various allergens and mitogens in vitro (41–43).

II. MURINE MODEL OF ATOPIC DERMATITIS INDUCED BY ORAL SENSITIZATION

Recently several investigators have reported murine models that may prove useful in the elucidation of underlying immunopathogenic mechanisms of atopic dermatitis (44,45). Recently we have been evaluating the development of an eczematous rash that occurs in a subset of mice orally sensitized to food proteins (27). Oral sensitization with milk protein and cholera toxin led to IgE-mediated anaphylaxis (46). Interestingly, a number of the mice developed a dry, apparently pruritic rash resulting in scratching and hair loss. A review of potential causes revealed that the new mouse chow was contaminated with low levels of milk protein. Subsequent attempts to reproduce the dermatitis resulted in approximately one third of mice similarly sensitized with milk or peanut proteins developing a dry, erythematous, scaly, pruritic rash involving 15–100% of their body surface within 9–14 weeks of initiating the sensitization protocol (27). As with human AD, treatment of the skin lesions with topical corticosteroids led to decreased pruritus and erythema, with return of hair growth. In addition, episodic dermatitis was noted in untreated mice, with recurrences and remissions occurring over an 8-month observation period. Histological examination of the skin lesions in the sensitized mice revealed findings similar to those reported in humans with atopic dermatitis (29,30). We believe that this is the first murine model of an AD-like disorder induced by oral sensitization with a food protein.

III. FOOD HYPERSENSITIVITY AND ATOPIC DERMATITIS

A. Clinical Studies in Children

Many studies done in the early part of the twentieth century clearly showed that ingested food allergens were readily accessible to cutaneous mast cells and the "skin-associated lymphoid tissue." After studying the absorption of food antigens from various locations in the gastrointestinal tract and other sites, Walzer and colleagues concluded that "the absorption of unaltered protein into the circulation is a normal, physiologic process occurring in nonatopic as well as atopic individuals at all ages with many allergens" (47). Some of the same investigators (48,49) also demonstrated unequivocally that these ingested food antigens readily penetrate the gastrointestinal barrier and are transported in the circulation to mast cells in the skin. To demonstrate this process, 65 normal adults were passively sensitized by intracutaneous injection of serum (i.e., P-K test) from a patient with severe fish allergy and a normal control (48). The following day the volunteers were fed fish, and 61 of 65 subjects developed a wheal-and-flare reaction within 90 minutes at the sensitized site but not at the control site. Similar results were found in a series of experiments conducted in 66 normal children with serum from an egg-allergic subject (49). In addition, intravenous injection of the protein nitrogen equivalent of 1/44,000 of one peanut kernel was sufficient to induce wheal and flare at a passively sensitized skin site.

Other early studies showed that food allergens could produce intense pruritus and subsequent scratching and rubbing that lead to typical eczematous lesions in the sensitized host. In 1936, Engman et al. (9) performed a provocation study in a child with atopic dermatitis and wheat allergy. Within 2 hours of being challenged with two wheat crackers, the child complained of itching and began scratching. The following morning he had typical eczematous lesions, except under the areas where bandages had been placed on his left arm and leg in order to prevent scratching. Patients with similar findings have been described in several other case reports.

A number of large studies included children who either underwent unblinded food challenges or were placed on food-exclusion diets. Although most of these studies failed to control for other "trigger" (or inciting) factors of AD, placebo effect or observer bias, many of them supported a role for food intolerance in the exacerbation of atopic dermatitis (50–52). In the late 1970s Hammar reported the induction of eczematous skin lesions in 15 of 81 hospitalized children less than 5 years of age after 2–3 days of ingesting 100 mL of milk daily (51). These challenges were done openly. When challenges were repeated 18 months later, symptoms recurred in about 25% of patients (4 of 15) reflecting the high rate of "outgrowing" milk allergy in this age group. Juto et al. (52) reported that out of 20 infants with eczema who followed a highly restricted elimination diet, 7 had complete resolution and 12 had at least some improvement. Unblinded challenges to cow's milk reportedly resulted in increased pruritus and rash in 12 of 20 infants. Atherton et al. (53) reported that two thirds of children with atopic dermatitis between 2 and 8 years of age showed marked improvement of skin during a double-blind crossover trial of egg and milk exclusion that was conducted over a 12-week period in the patients' homes. The results of this study could only be taken in the context of several confounders (high dropout/exclusion rate, failure to control for other trigger factors for AD).

Neild et al. (54) demonstrated improvement in an older group of patients during a milk and egg exclusion phase, but overall no statistically significant difference was seen in 40 patients completing a crossover trial. Businco et al. (55) found that dietary exclusion of milk and/or egg from the diets of 59 children with severe AD resulted in clinical improvement in 80% of cases. Younger children were more likely to have a good response to the diet. Other factors, such as the severity of eczema, family history of atopy, and total and/or specific IgE levels, were not predictive of clinical response. Hill and Lynch (56) treated 8 children with severe atopic dermatitis with Vivonex followed by the addition of two vegetables and two fruits for 3 months. All patients experienced marked improvement in their eczematous rash while maintaining the diet, but relapsed within weeks of discontinuing it.

In a more recent prospective, randomized controlled dietary trial, Lever et al. (57) initiated a trial of egg exclusion in children with suspected egg hypersensitivity (based upon clinical history and or RAST test results) who presented to a pediatric dermatology clinic for evaluation of atopic dermatitis. After undergoing a "washout" period of optimized skin care, 55 children were randomized to one of two groups: a dietary group, which was instructed on the maintenance of strict egg exclusion from the diet and general skin care, or a control group, where only general skin care recommendations were made. The group that received dietary advice had a significantly greater mean reduction in body surface area affected by eczematous rash (19.6 to 10.9%) in comparison to the control group (21.9 to 18.9%) and also had a significant improvement in severity score (33.9 to 24 SCORAD units) compared with only a slight decrease in the control group (36.7 to 33.5 units). At the end of the dietary phase, egg hypersensitivity was confirmed by positive DBPCFC in 42 of 49 patients who completed the study (22/26 patients who underwent food challenges in the egg exclusion group and 20/23 patients who underwent food challenges in the control group).

In 1978, May and Bock performed double-blind, placebo-controlled oral food challenges on 68 children whose parents and/or physicians suspected an adverse food reaction (24). The population studied included ambulatory patients, as well as patients who were hospitalized for poorly controlled asthma. Of the 29 patients who had positive challenges, 10 developed a pruritic, erythematous rash within 2 hours of the challenge. For 5 of these patients, this was the only manifestation of their clinical reactivity. Using similar challenge protocols, Burks et al. (17) performed similar studies as previously described.

In the past 20 years, many of our studies have addressed the etiological role of IgE-mediated food hypersensitivity in atopic dermatitis (15,58–60), and we have several ongoing studies as well. The current approach to diagnosing food hypersensitivity in a child with atopic dermatitis has been developed through these protocols. Using predominantly double-blind placebo-controlled food challenges (at times single blind and open challenges have been performed as well), 578 patients with atopic dermatitis have been evaluated for food hypersensitivity. Subjects ranged in age from 3 months to 25 years, with a median age of 3.4 years. For a subset of these patients (470), more detailed analysis revealed that family history was positive for atopic disease in 91%. One hundred and fifty-seven patients (~40%) had allergic rhinitis and asthma at the time of initial evaluation, and only 94 (20%) had neither allergic rhinitis nor asthma. In 376 (~80%) of patients, serum total IgE concentration was elevated with a median of 3410 IU/mL and a range of 1.5–45,000 IU/mL.

Any patient with chronic moderate to severe eczema fulfilling the criteria of Hanifin and Rajka (1) for the diagnosis of atopic dermatitis was eligible for the study, regardless of whether clinical history or previous allergy tests suggested a diagnosis of food hypersensitivity. All patients were admitted to the Clinical Research Center to provide a stable, low-allergen environment. Foods administered during DBPCFC were selected on the basis of skin test (and RAST) results or a strongly suggestive history of food hypersensitivity. Foods selected for the challenge protocol were excluded from the patient's diet for 7–10 days prior to admission. In addition, the following medications were withheld: oral corticosteroids for at least one month prior to admission, antihistamines for at least 7–10 days, and inhaled and oral β-adrenergic drugs for 8 hours prior to the challenge. Subjects were allowed to continue on inhaled cromolyn sodium and oral theophylline.

To determine which foods each individual patient would ingest during his or her food challenge, prick skin testing with a battery of 20 food antigens was performed. In order to achieve control of erythema and pruritus prior to the challenges, patients were treated with an aggressive skin care regimen for 3 days preceding challenges, which included two to three soaking baths (or wet wraps) per day, followed by the application of a lubricating cream to the entire body and topical corticosteroid (1% hydrocortisone cream for the face and 0.025% or 0.1% triamcinolone ointment for the trunk and extremities) to active eczematous areas. Antistaphylococcal antibiotics were generally administered if infection was suspected. Chloral hydrate was used for sedation. Once a stable baseline was established, a venous line was placed prior to initiating challenges to provide an ''open line'' in case of a major anaphylactic reaction and to provide access for atraumatic serial blood sampling.

Over 20 years, a total of 2907 diagnostic food challenges were conducted in 578 children. In instances where clinical history indicated a convincing account of a major anaphylactic reaction, (mostly to peanuts and nuts) challenges were not performed. Of the 2907 challenges performed, 1348 had positive results and 1559 were interpreted as negative. Intense pruritus and scratching frequently resulted in superficial excoriations and occasionally bleeding. Gastrointestinal and/ or respiratory symptoms were present in close to 50% of the reactors in a subset of these patients.

Virtually all symptoms developing during the blinded food challenges occurred between 5 minutes and 2 hours of initiating the food challenge. Symptoms associated with the immediate response were generally abrupt in onset, beginning with marked pruritus, followed by the development of an erythematous, macular eruption that lasted 1–2 hours. Several patients experienced a recurrence of symptoms that consisted of increased cutaneous pruritus and a transient morbilliform eruption 6–10 hours after the initial positive challenge. Symptoms associated with the later response were less pronounced than the immediate symptoms and tended to last for several hours. Less than 1% of the placebo challenges were interpreted as positive, i.e., false positive. To confirm negative food challenges, all patients were fed the food openly in a meal form under observation prior to discharge. Less than 3% of food challenges concluded to be negative were found to be false-negative studies.

Although many reports have suggested that children with atopic dermatitis are sensitive to a large number of foods, analysis of data from a subset of these patients revealed that most patients (80%) developed symptoms to only one to three foods by DBPCFC. Most children in this subset of patients had positive prick skin tests to several foods (mean: 3.5; range: 0–10), although only about one third of positive skin tests correlated with positive food challenges. Five foods (egg, peanut, milk, wheat, and soy) accounted for approximately 60% of the positive clinical responses. In a previous analysis of a subset of these patients, these foods accounted for 80% of positive food challenges in this patient population. This decrease is due to the fact that fewer patients have been challenged to these foods in the past several years, since use of the 95% predictive "decision points" for major food allergens have eliminated the need for food challenges in patients whose food-specific IgE levels exceed these values (i.e., ~40–50% of patients) (61). A summary of the challenge data from these patients is depicted in Tables 1 and 2.

In a second study we compared patterns of food hypersensitivity in children with atopic dermatitis in two different decades (unpublished data). We found that the major food allergens (milk, egg, wheat, soy peanut, tree nut, and seafood) accounted for 87% of positive food challenges in the one year between 1988 and 1989 and 91% of positive food challenges in the period between 1998 and 1999. In an earlier study by Burks (17), all positive challenges were accounted for by

Table 1 21 Years of Oral Food Challenges in 578 Patients with Atopic Dermatitis

Challenges	Positive	Negative	Total
All foods	1348	1559	2907
Major food allergens	777	766	1543
Egg	351	160	511
Milk	202	185	387
Peanut	40	56	96
Wheat	79	164	243
Soy	105	201	306

seven foods—peanut, egg, milk, wheat, fish, soy, and chicken. Eigenmann et al. (18) recently found that egg, milk, and peanuts were most frequently responsible for positive food challenges in 74 Swiss children with atopic dermatitis.

B. Laboratory Investigations in Children

Since many atopic dermatitis patients develop pruritic, morbilliform rashes instead of classic urticarial lesions, the senior author and colleagues have sought markers of mast cell activation in patients undergoing DBPCFC in order to demonstrate that the ingestion of food antigens led to IgE-mediated reactions (62).

Table 2 Hypersensitivity Rates to Major Food Allergens in Children with Atopic Dermatitis[a]

Food	Percent positive food challenges (positive challenges total challenges per food)	Percent of patients with IgE $\geq$ 95% predictive range[b] (# pts with positive values/ # patients tested)
Milk	52 (202/387)	60 (52/87)
Egg	69 (351/511)	66 (57/87)
Peanut	42 (40/96)	82 (71/87)
Wheat	33 (79/243)	
Soy	34 (105/306)	

[a] All data obtained from 578 children with atopic dermatitis who had at least one oral food challenge between 1979 and 2000.

[b] IgE data analyzed for milk, egg, and peanut in children NOT challenged to any of these three foods (due to IgE level above 95% predictive value) but challenged to at least one other food between 1998 and 2000.

Thirty-three patients undergoing DBPCFC were monitored for changes in circulating plasma histamine. Histamine concentration was measured prior to initiating the challenge and following the ingestion of the test antigen. Following the blinded challenge, patients experiencing clinical symptoms developed a rise in their plasma histamine (mean: 296 ± 80 pg/mL to 1055 ± 356 pg/mL; $p <$ 0.001). Subjects ingesting placebo or a food that did not provoke clinical symptoms (i.e., had a negative DBPCFC) had no demonstrable rise in their plasma histamine concentration. Figure 1 illustrates these results. In order to determine whether this phenomenon could be accounted for by circulating basophils, blood samples were obtained prior to, immediately following, and 30 minutes after the challenge. No difference was observed in circulating basophil number or total histamine content of the circulating basophils at any time point.

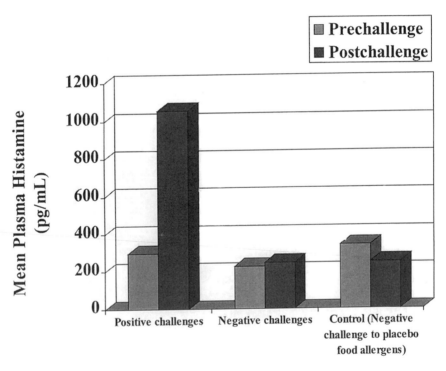

Figure 1 Mean plasma histamine levels in atopic dermatitis patients. Mean histamine levels in patients with positive food challenges were significantly higher after DBPCFC compared to levels prior to challenges. Patients with negative challenges had no significant change in levels before and after challenge. (Data adapted from Ref. 62.)

Children with AD and newly diagnosed food hypersensitivity have been found to have high "spontaneous" basophil histamine release (SBHR) from peripheral blood basophils in vitro compared to patients with atopic dermatitis and no food allergy or normal control subjects (mean: 35.1% ± 3.9% vs. 2.3% ± 0.2%; $p < 0.001$) (63). When food-allergic patients were placed on appropriate elimination diets for at least one year, they experienced good clearing of their atopic dermatitis and normalization of SBHR. Unstimulated peripheral blood mononuclear cells from food-allergic subjects with high SBHR were found to produce a histamine-releasing factor (HRF) in vitro that could activate basophils from other food-sensitive individuals, but not basophils from non–food-sensitive subjects. The specificity of the HRF was found to lie with food-allergic patient IgE molecules, possibly specific isoforms of IgE. Food-allergic patient's IgE antibodies placed on "stripped" basophils from food-nonallergic individuals could be activated by HRF, whereas food-allergic patient "stripped" basophils coated with food-nonallergic patient IgE were unresponsive to HRF. It was postulated that ingestion of food allergens leads to the production of HRF in vivo, which can then activate, or lower the threshold of activation, of basophils and possibly mast cells. The loss of spontaneously generated HRF appeared to correlate with the loss of cutaneous hyperreactivity and inversely with improvement in the patient's skin.

T cells from children with milk-induced eczema have been found to express homing receptors, cutaneous lymphocyte antigens (CLA), which are thought to be responsible for the skin-seeking behavior of these T cells (64). Blood samples from three patient populations were studied: a group of children with atopic dermatitis and milk-induced eczema (milk hypersensitivity defined by the presence of milk-specific IgE as well as a positive DBPCFC to milk), patients with milk-induced allergic eosinophilic gastroenteritis (AEG) or enterocolitis syndrome, and a group of normal adult subjects. More recently a group of patients with milk-induced wheezing was also studied. When exposed to the milk protein casein in vitro, PBMCs from all four study groups proliferated equally well. After 6 days of incubation with casein, children with AD and milk-induced eczema had a significantly greater numbers of CLA+ T cells in culture than the other three groups (see Fig. 2). There was no significant difference in CLA expression on T cells in the different patient populations after incubation with *Candida albicans*. Previous investigations (65,66) have demonstrated that the vascular counter receptor for CLA (E-selectin) has increased expression on cutaneous venules in patients with chronic AD and provides a mechanism for the selective homing of CLA+ T cells to the skin. Similar studies evaluating the expression of the lymph node homing receptor, L-selectin, in these patient populations found no significant differences in the four patient populations, thereby supporting the theory that the chronic skin symptoms in patients with AD and food hypersensitivity

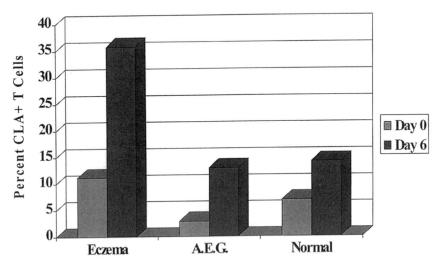

Figure 2 Casein stimulation of CLA expression on T cells. T cells from milk-allergic patients with atopic dermatitis had a significant increase in expression of cutaneous lymphocyte antigen (CLA), as kin homing receptor, after 6 days of incubation with casein. T cells from patients with milk-induced gastrointestinal disease (AEG) and normal controls did not have similar expression. (Data adapted from Ref. 64.)

may be a result of an organ-specific immunological response. In a similar study, PBMCs from AD patients with and without dust mite allergy were separated into CLA+ and CLA− cells and then stimulated with dust mite antigen in vitro. Activated CLA+ cells were found to be Th2+, whereas activated CLA− were found to be Th1+ (67).

Table 3 summarizes the findings from many of the studies discussed thus far.

C. Diagnosis and Management in Children

1. Diagnosis

Food hypersensitivity should be considered in any child with moderate to severe atopic dermatitis whose symptoms persist despite standard therapy, or who requires high-potency topical steroids in order to be controlled. The more severe the atopic dermatitis, the more likely that food allergy is involved in the pathogenesis (25). In addition, a personal and/or family history of atopy should raise the suspicion that food allergy is contributing to the patient's overall skin symptoms. Although many patients report a history of specific foods exacerbating their skin

Table 3 Studies Supporting the Role of Food Hypersensitivity in Children with Atopic Dermatitis

Clinical studies
1. Dietary elimination of food allergens results in resolution of eczema
   a. Children on restricted diets
   b. Breastfeeding mothers on restricted diets
2. Food challenges result in worsening of eczema
3. Delayed introduction of food allergens in infants delays development of eczema

Laboratory studies
1. Elevated plasma histamine levels in AD patients following positive food challenges
2. Elevated spontaneous histamine release in patients with atopic dermatitis ingesting food allergens
3. Casein stimulated elevated expression of cutaneous lymphocyte antigen on T cells from AD patients with milk allergy
4. Elevated total and food-specific IgE levels in AD patients
5. Elevated levels of activated eosinophils and eosinophil products in AD patients with positive food challenges
6. Murine model of food-induced atopic dermatitis

symptoms, less than 40% of foods implicated by the patient can be shown to provoke skin symptoms by blinded food challenge. Regular ingestion of food allergens leads to "downregulation" of immediate responses, thereby making it difficult to determine by history alone if a particular food antigen is causing worsening of eczema. Therefore, the standard approach in diagnosing food allergy in these patients begins with obtaining a detailed dietary history in order to determine which of the most common food antigens are in the child's diet. After that has been done, prick skin and/or in vitro (RAST) testing is performed in order to detect any food-specific IgE antibody that may be present. If prick skin tests are positive, the quantitative level of IgE present to each individual food antigen should be tested. For some of the most common food antigens, 90 and 95% positive predictive values have been determined, as listed in Table 4 (61). Any patient with a food-specific IgE level greater than these values (decision points) to a specific food should be considered clinically reactive and is instructed to follow a diet that strictly eliminates that food antigen. If the food-specific IgE level is below the known predictive value and there is no recent history of a severe, life-threatening reaction, DBPCFC are performed in order to confirm or rule out clinical reactivity to the food. This is done with any food antigen that is suspected to be contributing to eczema symptoms, and therefore one child may need to undergo a number of challenges. See Table 5 for a review of this diagnostic approach.

When food challenges are performed, symptoms that develop are usually abrupt in onset and generally resolve within 1–2 hours. Children with mild AD

Table 4 Positive Predictive Values for Common Food Antigens

Food	>95%	>90%
Egg	6	2
Milk	32	23
Peanut	15	9
Fish	20	9.5
Wheat	Best PPV = 75% at 100 kU/L	
Soy	Best PPV = 50% at 65 kU/L	

IgE values determined by the Pharmacia CAP-RAST system FEIA.
Source: Adapted from Ref. 61.

symptoms at the time of challenge may develop urticarial lesions as their cutaneous manifestation at the time of challenge, whereas those with more extensive, poorly controlled disease usually develop a markedly pruritic, erythematous morbilliform eruption. For children who are admitted to our clinical research center for multiple food challenges on consecutive days, their skin condition at the time of discharge often has deteriorated compared to baseline if more than one of their challenges are positive.

There has been increasing interest in the use of the atopy patch test (APT) to detect the late-onset skin symptoms following the ingestion of food allergens (68–70). Kekki et al. found that 54 of 113 children with AD and suspected milk

Table 5 Diagnosing Food Hypersensitivity in Children with Atopic Dermatitis

History—factors that increase suspicion for food hypersensitivity
  Moderate to severe disease
  Requirement for medium- to high-potency topical corticosteroids for symptom
    control
  Atopic history
  Known history of food hypersensitivity
  Detailed dietary history which identifies common food allergens in diet
Diagnostic tools
  Skin prick tests—highly sensitive
  RAST testing—quantitative values may identify 95% predictive values for certain
    food antigens
  Double-blind, placebo-controlled food challenges

allergy had positive milk challenges (68). Reactions were reportedly immediate in 36 of 54 and delayed in 18 of 54 children. The immediate reactions were associated with positive prick skin tests and the delayed reactions with positive APTs. In 26% of the cases, only the atopy patch test was positive. More recently, Niggemann et al. reported that prick skin tests were a highly sensitive, but moderately specific indicator of immediate food reactions while the APT was a moderately sensitive but highly specific indicator of late reactions (70). Studies examining the immunohistology of skin lesions induced by atopy patch tests have been confined to IgE-associated allergens. The immunohistology of APT-generated lesions is very similar to AD lesions, but the cellular composition of non–IgE-mediated patch test–induced lesions has not been studied and remains to be elucidated.

2. Management

a. Allergen Avoidance Diets. When positive food challenges confirm the diagnosis of food hypersensitivity, allergen-avoidance diets are recommended. The importance of educating patients' families about hidden sources of food antigens is critical. It is imperative that the patient and/or family members realize that food labels may use a variety of terms to connote the presence of a specific food antigen. Once the proper food-elimination diet is instituted, patients typically experience significant improvement in their symptoms compared to patients without food allergy or those who fail to comply with the allergen-elimination diet (71). If no significant clinical improvement is seen with the restricted diet within 2–3 weeks (in addition to the child following the hydrating skin care regimen discussed earlier), food challenges with less common food allergens may be indicated in order to determine if other foods still in the patient's diet may be provoking the persistent symptoms.

b. Immunological Changes Associated with Allergen-Elimination Diets. Several investigators have identified changes in a number of immunological parameters after allergen avoidance diets have been instituted. In a previously described study by Sampson et al., (63) 38 patients with AD and food hypersensitivity who followed an allergen-elimination diet for at least one year had significantly lower SBHR levels (mean $3.7 \pm 0.5\%$) compared to that of 25 patients with AD who had not yet begun an allergen elimination diet (mean $35.1 \pm 3.9\%$). However, this SBHR level was still significantly higher than that in AD patients without food hypersensitivity. In 10 patients with food hypersensitivity and AD who followed an allergen elimination diet, levels of SBHR were measured prior to and one year after starting the elimination diet (63). All patients had a significant decrease in the rate of spontaneous histamine release ($38 \pm 9.6\%$ before vs. $4.3 \pm 2.1\%$ after). In addition, allergen avoidance resulted in the loss of spontaneous production of the histamine-releasing factor, which was found to be produced by the mononuclear cells of patients with newly diagnosed food hypersensitivity who had not followed an allergen elimination diet.

We found that an allergen-elimination diet resulted in a change in the activation profile of peripheral eosinophils (72). After 2 weeks of a specific elimination diet in 23 children with AD and food hypersensitivity, eosinophil density shifted from an activated/hypodense profile (before allergen elimination) to an unactivated/normodense profile. In addition, positive DBPCFCs in 4 of these patients resulted in a shift in eosinophil density back toward the activated profile, a finding that had been demonstrated previously (73). Patients with more severe AD demonstrated a transient fall in serum ECP levels within 4 hours of a positive DBPCFC compared to baseline levels, with a return to baseline within 24 hours. The proposed mechanism for this decrease was the migration of eosinophils from the periphery into target organs with the onset of acute symptoms. Several other investigators, however, have reported a rise in serum ECP levels in children with positive DBPCFC, particularly those with cutaneous reactions (74,75). In one of these studies (75), the challenges were performed after a period of dietary restriction, illustrating the fact that reintroduction of the inciting food allergen will cause immunological abnormalities similar to those that were likely to be present prior to allergen avoidance.

In another study, James and Sampson (76) found that out of 29 cow's milk–allergic children who had returned for three annual milk challenges, 11 became clinically tolerant (median age 7 years; median time to clinical tolerance 3 years). Initial (at the time of diagnosis) and final (at the time of DBPCFC) milk-, casein-, and β-lactoglobulin–specific IgE and IgG antibody concentrations of the patients who became clinically tolerant were compared to those of 18 children who retained their clinical reactivity. For the patients who had developed clinical tolerance, casein- and β-lactoglobulin–specific IgE concentrations were significantly lower, and decreased significantly from the initial to the final evaluation. There were slight but significant decreases from the initial to final IgG1 and IgG4 casein-specific antibody concentrations. IgE/IgG ratios for casein and β-lactoglobulin were lower in comparison to that of the patients who remained clinically reactive at both points in time. These levels decreased significantly from the initial evaluation to the time they had developed clinical tolerance. IgE/IgG1 ratios for β-lactoglobulin and IgE/IgG4 ratios for casein and β-lactoglobulin were significantly lower for the clinically tolerant patients at initial evaluation and final evaluation compared to those who had persistent cow's milk allergy.

D. Natural History of Food Hypersensitivity in Children with Atopic Dermatitis

A number of investigators have followed patients for many years in order to determine the natural history of food hypersensitivity in children. In 1982 Bock

(77) performed an interview follow-up study of 79 children with food hypersensitivity diagnosed 1–7 years earlier. For 30 children diagnosed with food allergy under 3 years of age, 44% of the foods that had previously caused clinical reactivity were well tolerated, whereas only 19% of foods previously associated with reactivity in 49 children older than 3 years of age at diagnosis were tolerated. After 3–9 years of follow-up of nine children diagnosed with severe food allergic reactions within the first 2 years of life, Bock (78) found that three could tolerate normal quantities of the food, four could tolerate small amounts, and two patients remained highly reactive. In 25 egg-allergic patients, 24 of whom had AD, Ford and Taylor (79) found that after 2–2.5 years, 44% of the children had lost their clinical reactivity.

In some of the senior author's studies that have addressed the natural history of food hypersensitivity in children with atopic dermatitis, three factors have appeared to have the greatest importance in determining the probability of patients losing their clinical reactivity: the food to which the patient was allergic (71) (i.e., patients allergic to peanuts, nuts, fish, and shellfish were unlikely to lose their clinical reactivity, whereas those allergic to soy, wheat, milk, and egg were much more likely to develop clinical tolerance), the level of specific IgE antibody to a particular food (i.e., the higher the level of food antigen-specific IgE, the less likely that clinical tolerance would develop in the subsequent few years) (76), and the degree to which the patient adhered to the elimination diet (i.e., patients ingesting small amounts of allergen or having frequent accidental ingestions were less likely to develop clinical tolerance). Prick skin tests did not correlate with the loss of clinical reactivity and remained positive for 5 or more years after the food had been reintroduced into the diet. Therefore, it is recommended that patients be rechallenged intermittently (e.g., egg: every 2–3 years; milk, soy, wheat: every 1–2 years; foods other than peanut, nuts, fish, and shellfish: every 1–2 years) to determine whether their food allergies persist. Determination of food-specific IgE antibody concentration may be useful in determining when to rechallenge patients allergic to egg or milk. Specific IgE antibody levels < 1.5 kU_A/L to egg or 7.5 kU_A/L to milk appear to be associated with < 50% chance of clinical reactivity in a patient known to be reactive to the food (20). Once patients are able to tolerate a food, i.e., "outgrown" food allergy, no patient has had a recurrence of allergic symptoms or worsening of eczema.

E. Prevention of Atopic Dermatitis in Children with Food Hypersensitivity

Many investigators have attempted to determine the effect of prophylactic food allergen avoidance in newborns and infants predisposed to atopic dermatitis, as well as other atopic diseases. The role of breast-feeding in the prevention of food allergy and atopic dermatitis has been evaluated as well. In the 1930s, Grulee and Sanford (80) reported a decreased incidence of atopic dermatitis in breast-fed infants. Since children are exposed to maternal dietary food antigens passed in breast milk (81), maternal dietary restriction of common food allergens may be necessary in order to guarantee that any protective effect of breast-feeding is not counteracted by the infant's exposure to dietary antigens in the maternal milk. In evaluating six breast-fed infants (age 2.5–6 months), all of whom had classic infantile AD as well as positive prick skin tests to egg, we found that all of these infants had complete clearing of eczematous lesions when their mothers totally eliminated egg-containing foods from their diets. Four of the six infants were challenged in a research unit by first feeding eggs to their mothers and then having their mothers breast-feed their babies. Each child developed an erythematous morbilliform rash within 4–36 hours after feeding. Based upon these findings it is apparent that if the maternal diet is not evaluated and limited as necessary, breast-feeding may result in an atopic infant's early exposure to dietary food antigens and possibly a worse outcome.

A number of investigators have evaluated the effect of breast-feeding on the incidence of AD in high-risk infants when the maternal diet is restricted of major food allergens. In two series, mothers eliminated milk, egg, and fish from their diets during the first 3 months of breast-feeding and delayed introduction of cow's milk until 6 months and egg and fish until 9 months. Their children had a lower incidence of atopic dermatitis during the first 6 months of life, compared to controls whose mothers followed no dietary restrictions while breast-feeding (82,83). There was no significant difference in the incidence of atopic dermatitis in the children at 9, 12, or 18 months of age, but there was a trend toward lower AD rates in the prophylaxis group until 18 months of age. At 4 years of age, the prophylaxis group had less atopic dermatitis, but no differences were detected in food or respiratory allergies (83).

Zeiger and colleagues (84,85) designed a double-blind, randomized, prospective controlled study of infants from atopic families whose mothers were assigned to one of two dietary regimens: (group 1) a prophylactic dietary group, which restricted all cow's milk, egg, and peanut during the last trimester of pregnancy and while breast-feeding (12 months), and delayed introduction of solid foods as follows: nonlegume vegetables, rice cereal, meats, and noncitrus fruits between 6 and 12 months; cow's milk, wheat, soy, corn, and citrus fruits between 12 and 18 months; eggs at 24 months; and peanut and fish at 36 months. When supplemented, a casein hydrolysate formula (Nutramigen) was used. In the control group (group 2), mothers and infants followed the dietary recommendations of the Academy of Obstetrics and Gynecology during pregnancy and the Academy of Pediatrics during the duration of breast-feeding. When supplemented, a cow's milk–based formula was used (Enfamil). The prevalence of food allergy, cow's milk sensitization, and atopic dermatitis in the prophylaxis group were reduced significantly during the first 2 years of life. There was no significant difference in the period prevalence of atopic dermatitis after that time. When followed up at 4 and 7 years, the cumulative prevalence of food allergy remained lower in the prophylaxis group.

Consistent with the above findings, delayed introduction of solid foods has also been found to play a role in the prevention of atopic dermatitis. A prospective, nonrandomized study of 1265 unselected neonates evaluated the effect of the introduction of solid foods over a 10-year period (86,87). A significant linear relationship was found between the number of solid foods introduced into the diet by 4 months of age and the subsequent development of atopic dermatitis. There was a threefold increase in recurrent eczema noted at 10 years of age in infants receiving four or more solid foods in the first 4 months compared to infants receiving no solid foods in that time. No relationship was found between asthma and the introduction of solid foods. A similar study compared breast-fed infants who had received solid foods at 3–6 months of age (88). A reduction in AD at 1 year of age was seen in the patients with later introduction of solid foods, but this difference was no longer present at 5 years of age (89).

F. Clinical and Laboratory Investigation in Adults

Although there has been a wealth of information supporting the role of food hypersensitivity in children with atopic dermatitis, there are fewer data supporting the role of food allergy in adult patients. Many adult patients do, however, observe food-related worsening of their disease. There has been evidence that birch pollen–related fruits can cause worsening of eczema symptoms in a subpopulation of adults with atopic dermatitis who have no obvious clinical reactivity to these foods (90). In a recent study, adult patients with atopic dermatitis and evidence of sensitization to birch pollen were instructed to avoid birch pollen–associated foods (carrot, celery, hazelnut, apple etc.) for a 4-week time period. When patients underwent DBPCFC with these foods after this elimination period, 17 of 37 patients had worsening of eczema symptoms (with a median increase of 21 SCORAD points) within 48 hours of the challenge. In addition, when sera from the patients who had responded to challenges were compared to sera of those who did not, a significantly higher proportion of their lymphocytes expressed cutaneous lymphocyte antigen (CLA+) after incubation with birch pollen antigens than those of nonresponders. Skin-derived T-cell lines also showed significantly greater degrees of stimulation after exposure to birch pollen antigen. Additional studies are being done by these investigators in order to confirm and expand upon these findings.

Some of the same investigators (91) also demonstrated that 22 out of 88 adolescent and adult atopic dermatitis patients who reported worsening of skin symptoms after ingestion of milk products showed confirmation of these findings by double-blind, placebo-controlled food challenges. The lymphocytes of these patients showed significantly higher proliferative responses to casein compared to those of atopic dermatitis patients whose milk sensitivity was not confirmed by food challenge and normal controls. Casein-specific IgE was elevated in only 41% of these patients, suggesting that the mechanism for food hypersensitivity in these patients may be IgE independent.

Worm et al. (92) evaluated the effect of food additives on clinical symptoms in adult patients with atopic dermatitis. They proposed that these substances may act as "pseudoallergens," resulting in direct mast cell release. Out of 41 adult patients with atopic dermatitis recruited from a dermatology clinic (mean age 28 years), 63% had improvement in their eczema symptoms after 6 weeks on a low-pseudoallergen diet. These patients also had a significant reduction in their serum ECP levels (previously shown to correlate with clinical skin assessment (74,93–95) compared to patients who had no clinical improvement ($p < 0.05$). Although the majority of adult patients on the avoidance diet in this study had clinical improvement, the broad dietary restrictions make it difficult to identify the mechanism by which any of the foods avoided would cause worsening of AD symptoms if ingested.

It has been our clinical experience that many adult patients with atopic dermatitis describe worsening of skin symptoms after ingestion of spicy foods and/or alcohol. The vasodilatation that can occur secondary to the chemical properties of these substances is most likely to be responsible for this effect. These patients may therefore benefit from a trial of dietary elimination of these substances if clinical history is suggestive.

G. Conclusions

There are clear and convincing data that food hypersensitivity plays a significant role in the symptomatology of atopic dermatitis in a subgroup of children with moderate to severe disease. Evaluations of skin biopsy and serological specimens from children with atopic dermatitis, as well as skin biopsy specimens from a murine model of food-induced atopic dermatitis, have demonstrated the importance of IgE-mediated mechanisms. The clinical trials using double-blind, placebo-controlled food challenges and of food-elimination diets in these patients have proven that clinical symptomatology is directly affected by the ingestion or avoidance of certain food antigens in this subpopulation of patients. As the number of referrals for food hypersensitivity evaluation in children with atopic dermatitis appears to have increased in recent years, it seems that this association is becoming better recognized among physicians. For adult patients with atopic dermatitis, more studies need to be performed in order to further determine the role of food allergens as triggers.

REFERENCES

1. Hanifin JM, Rajka G. Diagnostic features of atopic dermatitis. Acta Derm Venereol Suppl (Stockh) 1980; 92:44–47.
2. European Task Force on Atopic Dermatitis. Severity scoring of atopic dermatitis: the SCORAD index. Dermatology 1993; 186:23–31.
3. Hill LSM. Evaluation of atopic dermatitis. Arch Dermatol Syph 1935; 32:451–463.
4. Blaylock WK. Atopic dermatitis: diagnosis and pathobiology. J Allergy Clin Immunol 1976; 57:62–79.
5. Sampson HA. Food sensitivity and the pathogenesis of atopic dermatitis. J Roy Soc Med 1997; 90:3–9.
6. Capron M, Capron A, Joseph M. IgE receptors on phagocytic cells and immune response to Schistosome infection. Monograph Allergy 1983; 18:33–44.
7. Joseph M, Capron A, Ameisen J-C. The receptors for IgE on blood platelets. Eur J Immunol 1986; 16:306–312.
8. Spiegelberg H. Structure and function of Fc receptors for IgE on lymphocytes, monocytes and macrophages. Adv Immunol 1984; 35:61–88.
9. Engman WF, Weiss RS, Engman MF. Eczema and environment. Med Clin North Am 1936; 20:651–663.
10. Besnier E. Premiere ntoe et observations preliminaries pour sevir d'introduction a l'etude des pruripos diathesiques. Ann Dermatol Syphil 1892; 23:634–637.
11. Pasternack B. The prediction of asthma in infantile eczema. J Pediatrics 1965; 66:166–167.
12. Stifler W. A twenty-one year follow-up of infantile eczema. J Pediatrics 1965; 66:164–165.
13. National Institute of Allergy and Infectious Disease Task Force Report. Dermatologic allergy, asthma and the other allergic diseases. 1979.
14. Johnson E, Irons J, Pattereon R, Roberts M. Serum IgE concentration in atopic dermatitis. J Allergy Clin Immunol 1974; 59:94–99.
15. Sampson HA. Atopic dermatitis [review]. Ann Allergy 1992; 69:469–479.
16. Hoffman DR. Diagnosis of IgE mediated reactions to food antigens by radioimmunoassay. Clin Immunol 1975; 55:256–267.
17. Burks AW, Mallory SB, Williams LW, Shirrell MA. Atopic dermatitis: clinical relevance of food hypersensitivity reactions. J Pediatr 1988; 113:447–451.
18. Eigenmann PA, Sicherer SH, Borkowski TA, Cohen BD, Sampson HA. Prevalence of IgE-mediated food allergy among children with atopic dermatitis. Pediatrics 1998; 101:e8.
19. Eigenmann PA CA. Diagnosis of IgE mediated food allergy among swiss children witha atopic dermatitis. Pediatr Allergy Immunol 2000; 11:95–100.
20. Sampson HA. Utility of food-specific IgE concentrations in predicting symptomatic food allergy. J Allergy Clin Immunol 2001; 107:891–896.
21. Schloss OM. Allergy to common foods. Trans Am Pediatr Soc 1915; 27:62–68.
22. Talbot FB. Eczema in childhood. Med Clin North Am 1918; 1:985–996.
23. Sampson HA. Role of immediate food hypersensitivity in the pathogenesis of atopic dermatitis. J Allergy Clin Immunol 1983; 71:473–480.

24. Bock S, Lee W, Remigio L, May C. Studies of hypersensitivity reactions to food in infants and children. J Allergy Clin Immunol 1978; 62:3327–3334.

25. Guillet MH, Guillet G. Allergologic survey in 251 patients with moderate or severe dermatitis: incidence and value of the detection of contact eczema and food allergy sensitization to airborne allergens. Ann Dermatol Venereol 1996; 123:157–164.

26. Patriza AGVRGNISFMM. The Natural history of sensitization to food and aeroallergens in atopic dermatitis: a 4 year follow-up. Pediatr Dermatol 2000; 17:261–265.

27. Li XM, Kleiner G, Huang CK, Lee SY, Schofield B, Soter N, Sampson HA. Murine model of atopic dermatitis associated with food hypersensitivity. J Allergy Clin Immunol 2001; 107(4):693–702.

28. Grewe M, Bruijnzeel-Koomen C, Schopf E, Thepen T, Langeveld-Wildshut EG, Ruzicka T, et al. A role for Th1 and Th2 cells in the immunopathogenesis of atopic dermatitis. Immunol Today 1998; 19:359–361.

29. Hamid Q, Naseer T, Minshall EM, Song YL, Boguniewicz M, Leung DYM. In vivo expression of IL-12 and IL-13 in atopic dermatitis. J Allergy Clin Immunol 1996; 98:225–231.

30. Hamid Q, Boguniewicz M, Leung DYM. Differential in situ cytokine gene expression in acute versus chronic atopic dermatitis. J Clin Invest 1994; 94:870–876.

31. Mihm MC, Soter NA, Dvorak HF, Austen KJ. The structure of normal skin and the morphology of atopic eczema. J Invest Dermatol 1976; 67:305–312.

32. Leiferman K, Ackerman S, Sampson H, Haugen H, Venencie P, Gleich G. Dermal deposition of eosinophil-granule major basic protein in atopic dermatitis. Comparison with onchocerciasis. N Engl J Med 1985; 313:282–285.

33. Irani AM, Sampson HA, Schwartz LB. Mast cells in atopic dermatitis. Allergy 1989; 44 (suppl 9):31–34.

34. Pucci N, Lombardi E, Novembre E, Farina S, Bernardini R, Rossi E, et al. Urinary eosinophil protein X and serum eosinophil cationic protein in infants and young children with atopic dermatitis: correlation with disease activity. J Allergy Clin Immunol 2000; 105:353–357.

35. Tong AKF, Mihm MC. The pathology of atopic dermatitis. Clin Rev Allergy 1986; 4:27–42.

36. Tsicopoulos A, Hamid Q, Varney V, Ying S, Moqbel R, Durham S, Kay A. Preferential messenger RNA expression of Th-1-type cells [IFN-gamma, IL-2] in classical delayed-type [tuberculin] hypersensitivity reactions in human skin. J Immunol 1992; 148:2058–2061.

37. Lemanske R, Kaliner M. Late-phase allergic reactions. In: Middleton E, Reed C, Ellis E, Adkinson N, Yuninger J, eds. Allergy: Principles and Practice. St. Louis: CV Mosby Company, 1988:12–30.

38. Mudde G, van Reijsen F, Boland G, de Gast G, Bruijnzeel P, Bruijnzeel-Koomen C. Allergen presentation by epidermal Langerhan's cells from patients with atopic dermatitis is mediated by IgE. Immunology 1990; 69:335–341.

39. Mudde G, Bheekha R, Bruijnzeel-Koomen C. Consequences of IgE/CD23-mediated antigen presentation in allergy. Immunol Today 1995; 16:380–383.

40. Spergel JM, Mizoguchi E, Oettgen HC, Bhan AK, Geha RS. Role of Th1 and Th2 cytokines in a murine model of allergic dermatitis. J Clin Invest 1999; 103:1103–1111.

41. Kimura M, Tsuruta S, Yoshida T. Unique profile of IL-4 and IFN-gamma production by peripheral blood mononuclear cells in infants with atopic dermatitis. J Allergy Clin Immunol 1998; 102:238–244.

42. Kimura M, Tsuruta S, Yoshida T. Correlation of house dust mite-specific lymphocyte proliferation with IL-5 production, eosinophilia, and the severity of symptoms in infants with atopic dermatitis. J Allergy Clin Immunol 1998; 101:84–89.

43. Schade RP. Differences in Antigen-specific T-cell responses between infants with atopic dermatitis with and without cow's milk allergy. Relevance of Th-2 cytokines. J Allergy Clin Immunol 2000; 106:1155–1162.

44. Spergel JM, Mizoguchi E, Brewer JP, Martin TR, Bhan AK, Geha RS. Epicutaneous sensitization with protein antigen induces localized allergic dermatitis and hyperresponsiveness to methacholine after single exposure to aerosolized antigen in mice. J Clin Invest 1998; 101:1614–1622.

45. Vestergaard C, Yoneyama H, Murai M, Nakamura K, Temaki K, Terrashima Y, Imai T, Yoshie O, Irimura T, Mizutani H, Matsushima K. Overproduction of Th2-specific chemokines in NC/Nga mice exhibiting atopic dermatitis-like lesions. J Clin Invest 1999; 104:1097–1105.

46. Li XM, Schofield B, Huang MS, Kleiner GA, Sampson HA. A murine model of IgE-mediated cow's milk hypersensitivity. J Allergy Clin Immun 1999; 103:206–214.

47. Walzer M. Absorption of allergens. J Allergy 1942; 13:554–562.

48. Brunner M, Walzer M. Absorption of undigested proteins in human beings: The absorption of unaltered fish protein in adults. Arch Intern Med 1928; 42:173–179.

49. Wilson SJ, Walzer M. Absorption of undigested proteins in human beings. IV. Absorption of unaltered egg protein in infants. Am J Dis Child 1935; 50:49–54.

50. David TJ, Waddington E, Stanton RHJ. Nutritional hazards of elimination diets in children with atopic dermatitis. Arch Dis Child 1984; 59:323–325.

51. Hammar H. Provocation with cow's milk and cereals in atopic dermatitis. Acta Derm Veneorol (Stockh) 1977; 7:159–163.

52. Juto P, Engberg S, Winberg J. Treatment of infantile atopic dermatitis with a strict elimination diet. Clin Allergy 1978; 8:493–500.

53. Atherton DJ, Soothill JF, Sewell M, Wells RS, Chilvers CED. A double-blind controlled crossover trial of an antigen-avoidance diet in atoic eczema. Lancet 1978; 1:401–403.

54. Neild VS, marsden RA, Bailes JA, Bland JM. Egg and milk exclusion diets in atopic eczema. Br J Dermatol 1986; 114:117–123.

55. Businco L, Businco E, Cantani A, Galli E, Infussi R, Benincori N. Results of a milk and/or egg free diet in children with atopic dermatitis. Allergol Immunopathol (Madr) 1982; 10:283–288.

56. Hill DJ, Lynch BC. Elemental diet in the management of severe eczema in childhood. Clin Allergy 1982; 12:313–315.

57. Lever R, MacDonald C, Waugh P, Aitchison T. Randomized controlled trial of advice on an egg exclusion diet in young children with atopic eczema and sensitivity to eggs. Pediatr Allergy Immunol 1998; 9:13–19.

58. Jones SM, Sampson HA. The role of allergens in atopic dermatitis. In: Leung DYM,

ed. Atopic Dermatitis: From Pathogenesis to Treatment. Georgetown, TX: R.G. Landes Company, 1996:41–65.

59. Sampson HA, McCaskill CC. Food hypersensitivity and atopic dermatitis: evaluation of 113 patients. J Pediatr 1985; 107:669–675.

60. Sampson HA. Role of immediate hypersensitivity in the pathogenesis of atopic dermatitis [review]. Allergy 1989; 44 (suppl 9):52–58.

61. Sampson H, Ho D. Relationship between food-specific IgE concentration and the risk of positive food challenges in children and adolescents. J Allergy Clin Immun 1997; 100:444–451.

62. Sampson HA, Jolie PL. Increased plasma histamine concentrations after food challenges in children with atopic dermatitis. N Engl J Med 1984; 311:372–376.

63. Sampson HA, Broadbent KR, Bernhisel-Broadbent J. Spontaneous release of histamine from basophils and histamine-releasing factor in patients with atopic dermatitis and food hypersensitivity. N Engl J Med 1989; 321:228–232.

64. Abernathy-Carver K, Sampson H, Picker L, Leung D. Milk-induced eczema is associated with the expansion of T cells expressing cutaneous lymphocyte antigen. J Clin Invest 1995; 95:913–918.

65. Berg EL, Yoshino LS, Rott MK, Robinson RA, Warnock TK, Kishimoto LJ, Picker LJ, Butcher EC. The cutaneous lymphocyte antigen, CLA, is a skin lymphocyte homing receptor for the vascular lectin ELAM-1. J Exp Med 1991; 174:1461–1466.

66. Groves RW, Allen MH, Barker JN, Haskard DO, Macdonald DM. Endothelial leukocyte adhesion molecule-1 (ELAM-1) expression in cutaneous inflammation. Br J Dermatol 1991; 124:117–123.

67. Santamaria BLF, Picker LJ, Perez Soler MT, Drzimalla K, Flohr P, Blaser K, Hauser C. Circulating allergen-reactive T cells from patients with atopic dermatitis and allergic contact dermatitis express the skin-selective homing receptor, the cutaneous lymphocyte-associated antigen. J Exp Med 1995; 18:1935–1940.

68. Kekki OM, Turjanman K, Isolauri E. Differences in skin-prick and patch-test reactivity are related to the heterogeneity of atopic eczema in infants. Allergy 1997; 52: 755–759.

69. Majamaa H, Moisio P, Holm K, Turjanmaa K. Wheat allergy: diagnostic accuracy of skin prick and patch tests and specific IgE. Allergy 1999; 54:851–856.

70. Niggemann B, Reibel S, Wahn U. The atopy patch test (APT)–a useful tool for the diagnosis of food allergy in children with atopic dermatitis. Allergy 2000; 55:281–285.

71. Sampson HA, Scanlon SM. Natural history of food hypersensitivity in children with atopic dermatitis. J Pediatr 1989; 115:23–27.

72. Sampson HA. Food sensitivity and pathogenesis of atopic dermatitis. J Roy Soc Med 1997; 90(Supp 30):2–8.

73. Magnarin M, Knowles A, Ventura A, Vita F, Fanti L, Zabucchi G. A role for eosinophils in the pathogenesis of skin lesions in patients with food-sensitive atopic dermatitis. J Allergy Clin Immunol 1995; 96:200–208.

74. Niggemann B, Beyer K, Wahn U. The role of eosinophils and eosinophil cationic protein in monitoring oral challenge tests in children with food-sensitive atopic dermatitis. J Allergy Clin Immunol 1994; 94:963–971.

75. Suomalainen. Evidence for eosinophil activation in cow's milk allergy. Pediatr Allergy Immunol 1993; 4:1–5.
76. James JM, Sampson HA. Immunologic changes associated with the development of tolerance in children with cow milk allergy. J Pediatr 1992; 121:371–377.
77. Bock SA. The natural history of food sensitivity. J Allergy Clin Immunol 1982; 69: 173–177.
78. Bock SA. Natural history of severe reactions to food in young children. J Pediatr 1985; 107:676–680.
79. Ford RPK, Taylor B. Natural history of egg hypersensitivity. Arch Dis Child 1982; 57:649–652.
80. Grulee CG, Sanford HN. The influence of breast feeding and artificial feeding in infantile eczema. J Pediatr 1936; 9:223–225.
81. Jakobsson I, Lindberg T, Benediktsson B, et al. Dietary bovine B-lactoglobulin is transferred to human milk. Acta Pediatr Scand 1985; 74:342–345.
82. Hattevig G, Kjellman B, Bjorksten B, Kjellman N. Effect of maternal avoidance of eggs, cow's milk and fish during lactation upon allergic manifestations in infants. Clin Exp Allergy 1989; 19:27–32.
83. Sigurs N, Hattevig G, Kjellman B. Maternal avoidance of eggs, cow's milk, and fish during lactation: Effect on allergic manifestation, skin-prick tests, and specific IgE antibodies in children at age 4 years. Pediatrics 1992; 89:735–739.
84. Zeiger R, Heller S, Mellon M, Forsythe A, O'Connor R, Hamburger R. Effect of combined maternal and infant food-allergen avoidance on development of atopy in early infancy: a randomized study. J Allergy Clin Immunol 1989; 84:72–89.
85. Zeiger R, Heller S. The development and prediction of atopy in high-risk children: follow-up at seven years in a prospective randomized study of combined maternal and infant food allergen avoidance. J Allergy Clin Immunol 1995; 95:1179–1190.
86. Fergusson DM, Horwood LJ, Shannon FT. Early solid feeding and recurrent eczema: a 10-year longitudinal study. Pediatrics 1990; 86:541–546.
87. Fergusson D, Horwood L, Shannon F. Asthma and infant diet. Arch Dis Child 1983; 58:48–51.
88. Kajosaari M, Saarinen UM. Prophylaxis of atopic disease by six months; total solid food elimination. Arch Paediatr Scand 1983; 72:411–414.
89. Kajosaari M. Atopy prophylaxis in high-risk infants: prospective 5-year follow-up study of children with six months exclusive breastfeeding and solid food elimination. Adv Exp Med Biol 1991; 310:453–458.
90. Reekers R, Busche M, Wittman M, Kapp A, Werfel T. Birch pollen-related foods trigger atopic dermatitis in patients with specific cutaneous T-cell responses to birch pollen antigens. J Allergy Clin Immunol 1999; 104:466–472.
91. Werfel T, Ahlers G, Schmidt P, Boeker M, Kapp A, Neumann C. Milk-responsive atopic dermatitis is associated with a casein-specific lymphocyte response in adolescent and adult patients. J Allergy Clin Immunol 1997; 99:124–133.
92. Worm M, Ehlers I, Sterry W, Zuberbier T. Clinical relevance of food additives in adult patients with atopic dermatitis. Clin Exp Allergy 2000; 30:407–414.
93. Czeck W, Krutmann J, Schopf E, Kapp A. Serum Eosinophil cationic protein is a sensitive measure for disease activity in atopic dermatitis. Br J Dermatol 1992; 126: 351–355.

94. Jakob T, Hermann K, Ring J. Eosinophil cationic protein in atopic eczema. Arch Dermatol Resources 1991; 283:5–6.

95. Walker C. Atopic dermatitis. Correlation of peripheral blood T cell activation, eosinophilia and serum factors with clinical severity. Clin Exp Allergy 1993; 1993:145–153.

19

Role of *Staphylococcus aureus* in Atopic Dermatitis

Donald Y. M. Leung
National Jewish Medical and Research Center, Denver, Colorado

I. INTRODUCTION

Atopic dermatitis (AD) is a chronic relapsing, pruritic skin disease frequently seen in patients with a history of respiratory allergy (1). Skin lesions evolve as the result of complex interactions between IgE-bearing antigen-presenting cells, T-cell activation, mast cell degranulation, keratinocytes, eosinophils, and a combination of immediate and cellular immune responses (see Chapters 8–16 for further discussion). Population studies indicate that the prevalence of AD in children has been steadily increasing since World War II and that it now affects more than 10% of children in most parts of the world (2). The rapid rise in prevalence of AD is thought to be primarily related to changes in our environment. A number of factors can trigger AD, including irritants, foods, aeroallergens, and infection. The relative contribution of allergens to the course of this illness is reviewed in Chapters 17, 18, and 20.

The current review examines the evidence that *Staphylococcus aureus* plays an important role in the pathogenesis of AD, acting not only as a trigger but having disease-sustaining effects as well. These effects appear to be related to the potent toxins they produce. An understanding of the mechanisms underlying enhanced *S. aureus* colonization in AD and identification of the molecules involved in triggering atopic skin inflammation has important implications in our approach to the management of AD and the development of new therapies for patients with this common illness.

II. PREVALENCE OF *S. AUREUS* IN ATOPIC DERMATITIS

S. aureus is found on the skin of over 90% of patients with AD (3). Using electron microscopy, Morishita et al. (4) found *S. aureus* distributed on the surface of the epidermis as well as growing between layers of keratinocytes. Interestingly, staphylococcal toxins (superantigens, see below) could be identified by immuno-fluorescence as deeply into the skin as on the inflammatory cells infiltrating into the dermis. In contrast, only 5% of normal subjects harbor this bacterium on their skin, and its localization is mainly in the nose and intertriginous areas. The density of *S. aureus* on acutely inflamed AD lesions is frequently more than 1000 times higher than on nonlesional atopic skin. Clinical superinfection with *S. aureus* can reach 10^7 organisms per cm^2 on acute lesional skin. Honey-colored crusting, extensive serous weeping, folliculitis, and pyoderma indicate bacterial infection usually secondary to *S. aureus* in patients with AD. These patients can have a sudden exacerbation of skin disease and respond rapidly to antibiotic therapy. However, even AD patients without overt *S. aureus* infection show greater clinical improvement to combined treatment with antistaphylococcal antibiotics and topical corticosteroids, as compared to topical corticosteroids alone, supporting the concept that *S. aureus* contributes to atopic skin inflammation in AD (5,6).

III. MECHANISM(S) FOR ENHANCED *S. AUREUS* COLONIZATION IN AD

The mechanism(s) leading to increased *S. aureus* colonization in AD are poorly understood. It is likely to result from a combination of processes, including disruption of skin barrier function from scratching, loss of certain innate antibacterial activities from changes in β-defensin levels or reduced immune responses necessary for eradication and defense against bacteria, as well as changes in skin surface pH values toward alkalinity (7). There has also been much interest in the potential role of lipid deficiencies in atopic skin since lipids have antimicrobial effects and an altered lipid content in the skin may lead to increased transepidermal water loss contributing to the dryness and cracked, brittle skin that predisposes to *S. aureus* colonization (8,9). None of these factors are mutually exclusive. Indeed, all are likely to play a role in *S. aureus* colonization of AD skin, varying according to the patient's genetic predisposition and environmental exposure.

The initial event in colonization requires "adherence" of *S. aureus* to the skin, and if it results in firm attachment of *S. aureus* to skin surfaces, there is an increased risk for subsequent infection or immunoreaction. Studies have demonstrated increased adherence of *S. aureus* to keratinocytes from atopic skin (10). The reason for increased binding of *S. aureus* to AD skin is not completely understood but is likely to be driven by atopic inflammation. This concept is supported by several observations.

First, it has been found that treatment with topical corticosteroids or tacrolimus significantly reduces the numbers of *S. aureus* found on atopic skin (11,12). In vitro studies from our lab indicate that corticosteroids have no direct antibiotic effects on the growth of cultured *S. aureus*. Thus, it is very likely that atopic skin inflammation leads to the expression of attachment sites, which promote colonization of *S. aureus*.

Second, acute inflammatory skin lesions have more *S. aureus* than chronic skin lesions or unaffected atopic skin (3). Scratching likely enhances *S. aureus* binding by disturbing the skin barrier, releasing proinflammatory cytokines, which upregulate extracellular matrix molecules known to act as adhesins for *S. aureus* (13). Alternatively breaks in the epidermal layer from scratching or skin dryness can expose underlying extracellular matrix molecules, which can serve as an anchor for adherence of *S. aureus* to the skin.

Third, we have directly examined *S. aureus* binding to skin lesions in mice undergoing allergen-driven Th1 vs. Th2 inflammatory responses using a novel in vitro bacterial binding assay (14). Bacterial binding to frozen skin sections was found to be significantly greater at skin sites with Th2-mediated inflammation than skin sites with Th1-mediated inflammation. Importantly, this increased bacterial binding did not occur in IL-4 gene knockout mice. Conversely when normal mouse skin was incubated in vitro with IL-4, as compared to interferon-γ, increased *S. aureus* binding occurred in skin explants treated with IL-4. These data indicate that IL-4 plays a crucial role in the enhancement of *S. aureus* binding to skin.

The microbial components responsible for adherence are termed "adhesins." During the past few years, a number of important staphylococcal adhesins (aside from protein A) have been identified, which are responsible for the initial interactions between *S. aureus* and matrix proteins in different tissues. These include fibronectin-binding proteins A and B; clumping factor A and B, which are fibrinogen-binding proteins; and collagen adhesins (13). Importantly, it is well established that the tissue ligands for some of these staphylococcal adhesins, e.g., fibronectin, are modulated by proinflammatory cytokines. Of interest, IL-4, but not interferon-γ, is known to induce fibronectin production by skin fibroblasts (15).

Recently, we demonstrated that fibronectin and fibrinogen, but not collagen, are the key proteins used in the binding of *S. aureus* to Th2-induced skin inflammatory reactions. This is supported by the following observations: first, isogenic mutants of *S. aureus* that were selectively deficient in fibronectin- or fibrinogen-binding proteins, as compared to their corresponding wild-type parent strains, demonstrated reduced binding to allergen-sensitized/challenged Th2, but not Th1, skin reactions in mice (14). Consistent with these studies, *S. aureus* mutants deficient in fibronectin- or fibrinogen-binding proteins demonstrated reduced binding to human AD skin but not psoriatic skin or normal skin (16). In contrast, a collagen adhesin–negative mutant did not show decreased binding to Th2-mediated inflamed skin. Second, when *S. aureus* were preincubated with either saline, human serum albumin, fibronectin, collagen, or fibrinogen in an attempt to block the *S. aureus*–binding proteins, only fibronectin and fibrinogen, but not saline, collagen, or human serum albumin, significantly reduced the level of *S. aureus* binding to Th2-induced skin inflammation sites. Of note, the bacterial binding sites were mainly confined to the stratum corneum. This was shown in both mouse models of Th1 vs. Th2 skin inflammation as well as a comparison of human AD vs. psoriasis skin (14–16).

While fibronectin and fibrinogen are plasma proteins that can exudate from the blood at sites of skin inflammation, it is unlikely that this represents the exclusive process by which *S. aureus* binding is increased to atopic skin. As discussed above, in vitro incubation of skin explants with recombinant IL-4 increases *S. aureus* binding to a level significantly greater than incubation of skin from the same skin sites with either media control or interferon-γ. Furthermore, we have found that IL-4 but not interferon-γ also increases supra-basal epidermal fibronectin deposition (14). This suggests a selective mechanism by which Th2, as compared to Th1, responses can enhance *S. aureus* binding to the skin. Thus, IL-4–induced fibronectin synthesis, in combination with plasma exudation of fibrinogen, could provide a mechanism by which the atopic/inflammatory environment mediates enhanced *S. aureus* attachment to the skin. Interestingly, a recent study by Wann et al. (17) demonstrated that the *S. aureus* fibronectin-binding MSCRAMM FnbpA is a bifunctional protein that also binds to fibrinogen. This observation is consistent with our observations suggesting that blocking the binding of *S. aureus* to fibrinogen and fibronectin may be an important therapeutic target for reduction of *S. aureus* colonization in atopic skin.

IV. STAPHYLOCOCCAL VIRULENCE FACTORS

A. Superantigens

Recent studies suggest that one strategy by which *S. aureus* exacerbates or maintains skin inflammation in AD is by secreting a group of toxins known to act as superantigens (Fig. 1). These potent toxins bind directly without antigen processing to constitutively expressed HLA-DR molecules on professional antigen-presenting cells such as macrophages or dendritic cells and to cytokine-induced HLA-DR molecules on nonprofessional APC such as keratinocytes (18). This can have profound biological consequences due to the local or massive systemic release of cytokines and mediators of inflammation by these HLA-DR+ cells or via the subsequent activation of T cells. The stimulation of T cells by superanti-

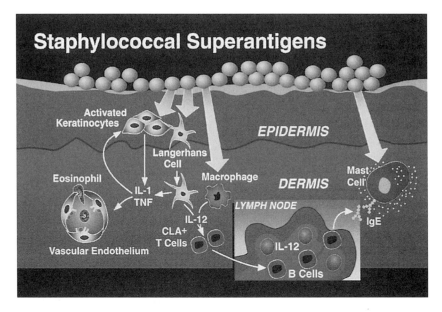

Figure 1   Immune mechanisms of staphylococcal superantigen action. (From Ref. 1.)

gens results in the activation and expansion of lymphocytes expressing specific T-cell receptor Vβ regions. Such T cells may include autoreactive T cells that migrate to the target tissue containing the autoantigen recognized by that T cell and mediate damage via cytotoxic mechanisms or the secretion of proinflammatory cytokines. While all bacterial superantigens can cause marked stimulation of T cells, they frequently cause the expansion of different portions of the T-cell repertoire. Identification of specific T-cell receptor Vβ expansions can be useful in supporting the concept that tissue inflammation is mediated by superantigens (19).

A variety of observations support a role for superantigens in the pathogenesis of AD (Table 1). First, over half of AD patients have *S. aureus* cultured from their skin that secrete superantigens such as enterotoxins A, B, and toxic shock syndrome toxin-1 (TSST-1) (20–22). An analysis of the peripheral blood skin homing CLA+ T cells from these patients as well as their skin lesions reveals that they have undergone a T-cell receptor Vβ expansion within both their CD4+ T cells and their CD8+ T cells consistent with superantigenic stimulation (Fig. 2) (23,24). TCR Vβ skewing was not present within the CLA+ T-cell subsets of patients with plaque psoriasis or normal controls. TCR BV genes from the presumptively superantigen-expanded populations of skin-homing T cells were cloned and sequenced from three AD subjects and, consistent with a superanti-

Table 1 Evidence for Role of Staphylococcal Superantigens in Atopic Dermatitis

AD severity correlates with presence of IgE antibodies to superantigens.
Superantigens augment allergen-induced skin inflammation by activating infiltrating
  mononuclear cells and inducing mast cell degranulation.
Superantigens induce dermatitis on application to skin by patch testing.
Patients recovering from toxic shock syndrome develop chronic eczema.
Superantigens induce the skin-homing receptor on T cells.
Peripheral blood mononuclear cells from AD, as compared to normal controls, have
  higher proliferative responses to superantigens.

gen-driven effect, were found to be polyclonal. These data suggest that superantigens can contribute to AD pathogenesis by increasing the frequency of memory T cells able to migrate to and be activated within AD lesions.

Second, most AD patients make specific IgE antibodies directed against the staphylococcal superantigens found on their skin (Fig. 3) (20–22). Basophils from patients with IgE to superantigens release histamine on exposure to the relevant superantigen, but not in response to superantigens to which they make no specific IgE (20). These findings raise the intriguing possibility that superantigens induce specific IgE in AD patients and chronic mast cell degranulation in vivo when the superantigens penetrate their disrupted epidermal barrier. This promotes the itch-scratch cycle contributing to the evolution of skin rashes in AD.

Third, a correlation has been found between the presence of IgE to superantigens and severity of AD (21,22). Furthermore, colonization with superantigen-producing *S. aureus* is at greatest density in patients with IgE to staphylococcal

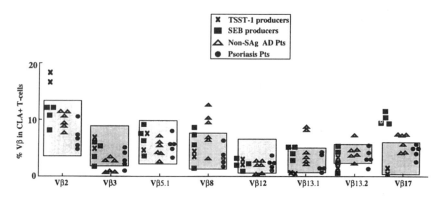

Figure 2 Increased superantigen-reactive skin-homing T cells in AD patients with superantigen-producing *S. aureus*. (From Ref. 23.)

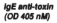

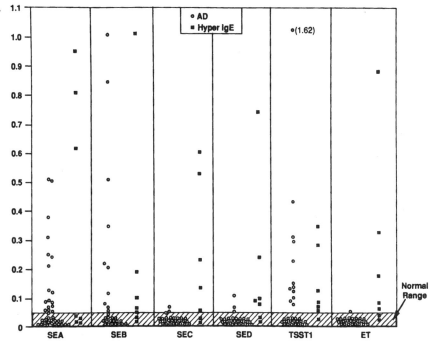

Figure 3 Atopic dermatitis and hyper IgE syndrome are associated with increased serum IgE anti-*S. aureus* toxin. (From Ref. 20.)

superantigens. Of note, in one study there was no difference in skin severity between patients with or without superantigen-producing *S. aureus* unless patients made an IgE response to the superantigen present on their skin (22). Patients with superantigens on their skin generally have increased IgE levels to specific allergens. This is consistent with in vitro studies demonstrating superantigens augment allergen-specific IgE synthesis by binding to HLA-DR on B cells (25). Utilizing a humanized murine model of skin inflammation, *S. aureus* superantigen plus allergen was found to have an additive effect in inducing cutaneous inflammation (26). Skin-homing CLA+ T cells have also been shown to respond to superantigen and contribute to eosinophilia and IgE production in AD (27,28).

Fourth, epicutaneous application of SEB to normal skin or unaffected AD skin has also been found to induce skin erythema and induration (29). In one study, three of the six AD subjects studied experienced a flare of their skin disease in the elbow flexure ipsilaterally to where the SEB was applied. These observations provide direct evidence that superantigens can exacerbate and sustain skin inflammation with AD. More recently, it was found that the infiltrating T cells into SEB patch test sites are selectively expanded with a T-cell repertoire (T-cell receptor Vβ 3, 12, and 17) reflecting SEB stimulation (30). Furthermore, in a prospective study of patients recovering from toxic shock syndrome, 14 of 68 patients developed chronic eczematoid dermatitis, whereas no patients recovering from gram-negative sepsis developed eczema (31). These investigators concluded that superantigens may induce an atopic eczematoid process in the skin. Kawasaki syndrome, a multisystem vasculitis of childhood thought to be caused by superantigens, has also been associated with a 10-fold higher prevalence of atopic dermatitis than disease controls (32).

A number of factors likely contribute to the induction of skin inflammation by superantigens. In this regard, superantigens can cause marked activation of Th2 cells. Mouse Th2 cells expanded in vitro by superantigen induce IL-4– dependent skin inflammation when injected into the skin of mice (33). Saloga et al. (34,35). also found that epicutaneous application and intracutaneous injection of SEB elicits a strong inflammatory skin response in wild-type BALB/c mice, but not T-cell–deficient SCID mice. These results suggest that superantigen-induced skin inflammation is T-cell–dependent.

Importantly superantigens have been demonstrated to induce T-cell expression of the skin homing receptor, cutaneous lymphoid antigen (CLA) via stimulation of IL-12 production (36). As shown in Figure 1, staphylococcal superantigens secreted at the skin surface can penetrate the skin to stimulate epidermal macrophages or Langerhans cells to produce IL-1, tumor necrosis factor-α (TNF-α) and IL-12. Local production of IL-1 and TNF induces the expression of E-selectin on vascular endothelium (37), allowing an initial influx of CLA+ Th2 memory/effector cells. IL-12 secreted by superantigen-stimulated Langerhans cells which migrate to skin-associated lymph nodes can upregulate the expression of CLA on T cells and influence the functional profile of virgin T cells activated by the superantigens. These actions result in the formation of additional skin-homing memory T cells, which can contribute to ongoing skin inflammation.

The environmental triggers that contribute to chronicity of AD are unknown. However, chronic AD is frequently associated with colonization by superantigen-producing S. aureus and increased infiltration of monocyte/macrophages (1). To examine a potential role for microbial superantigens in the prolongation of monocyte-macrophage survival, Bratton et al. (38) incubated peripheral blood monocytes from AD subjects with various concentrations of TSST-1, a prototypic superantigen, and examined their effects on monocyte apoptosis. TSST-1, in a concentration-dependent manner, significantly inhibited monocyte apoptosis and stimulated production of the prosurvival cytokines GM-CSF, IL-1, and TNF-α. Their data also showed GM-CSF was the primary cytokine responsible for inhibition of apoptosis, creating conditions favoring persistent tissue inflammation and skin colonization with *S. aureus*.

B. Nonsuperantigenic Toxins

Aside from superantigens, staphylococci can express other molecules that contribute to skin inflammation. Ezepchuk et al. (39) found that AD *S. aureus* isolates that failed to secrete superantigenic toxins produced α-toxin. All of these staphylococcal strains also expressed staphylococcal protein A. There were significant differences in the action of these molecules on keratinocytes. The superantigens TSST-1, SEA, SEB, and exfoliative toxin as well as protein A did not induce significant cytotoxic damage on keratinocytes. In contrast, α-toxin induced profound keratinocyte cytotoxicity that was time and dose dependent. The morphological and functional characteristics of cell death induced by α-toxin was consistent with cell necrosis, but not apoptosis. Additionally, α-toxin induced the release of TNF-α release from keratinocytes within 30 minutes of addition to cultures. In contrast, protein A and staphylococcal superantigens stimulated TNF-α secretion from keratinocytes over a 6- to 12-hour period. Lipoteichoic acid found in all *S. aureus* strains are also potent inducers of proinflammatory cytokine production by mononuclear cells (40). Thus, a wide variety of staphylococcal products can have proinflammatory effects on the skin.

V. THERAPEUTIC IMPLICATIONS

A. Antibiotic/Steroid Combinations

The growing evidence that infection with *S. aureus* can exacerbate acute AD and colonization promotes the chronic inflammatory process of AD provides a rationale for use of anti staphylococcal therapy in patients with poorly controlled AD (Table 2). Systemic antistaphylococcal antibiotics are particularly helpful in the

Table 2 Therapeutic Approach to Reducing *S. aureus*

Restore skin barrier
Topical antibiotic/corticosteroid combinations
Topical corticosteroids
Topical macrolide immunomodulators
Anti-infectives
Phototherapy

treatment of acute exacerbations of AD due to diffuse *S. aureus* infection (41–43). Erythromycin and the newer macrolide antibiotics (azithromycin and clarithromycin) are usually beneficial for patients who are not colonized with a macrolide-resistant *S. aureus* strain. However, for macrolide-resistant *S. aureus*, a penicillinase-resistant penicillin (e.g., dicloxacillin) may be needed. First-generation cephalosporins and oral fusidic acid (Fucidin) also offer effective coverage for *staphylococci*. Topical fusidic acid or mupirocin is useful in the treatment of localized impetiginized skin lesions (44). However, in patients with extensive superinfection, topical antibiotics can be very expensive. In this situation, a course of systemic antibiotics is most practical.

Due to the increased risk of bacterial resistance accompanying frequent use of antibiotics, it is important to combine antimicrobial therapy with effective skin care since it is well established that the excoriated inflamed skin of AD predisposes to *S. aureus* colonization. Therefore use of antibiotic therapy must be carried out with good skin hydration to restore skin barrier function and effective anti-inflammatory therapy to reduce overall skin inflammation and *S. aureus* colonization (11,12). Exacerbating factors such as food allergens, inhalant allergens, irritants, and emotional triggers should be identified and eliminated because they can alter response to therapy. Since the major reservoir for *S. aureus* is in the nose, intranasal antibiotics may be needed to reduce overall skin carriage of *S. aureus* (45).

Several studies have now demonstrated that the combination of topical corticosteroids with an antibiotic is significantly more effective at reducing skin inflammation due to AD than using the topical corticosteroid or topical antibiotic alone (46–48). Topical fusidic acid (Fucidin) combined with corticosteroid has been particularly effective because fusidic acid inhibits growth of even methicillin-resistant *S. aureus* (49). In contrast, topical neomycin can be a problem since it frequently leads to the development of allergic contact dermatitis (50).

The observation that combined treatment of AD with antibiotics and corticosteroids is more effective than corticosteroids alone suggests that *S. aureus* secretes products that can induce GC insensitivity. This may contribute to the spectrum of corticosteroid responsiveness that exists in clinical treatment of AD (51). Thus, an understanding of the mechanism of corticosteroid insensitivity in this clinical setting is important and may lead to improved therapy for patients with AD. Recently, we made the interesting observation that when T cells are stimulated with superantigens, as compared to other stimuli, they become insensitive to the immunosuppressive effects of corticosteroids (Fig. 4) (52). This may be clinically important because use of antibiotics, even at concentrations that do not suppress their growth, are known to reduce superantigen production by *S. aureus* (53).

At a cellular level, GCs exert their biological effects by binding to a specific intracellular receptor, i.e., the GC receptor (GR). Cloning of the human GR gene has revealed that alternative splicing of the GR pre-mRNA generates two homolo-

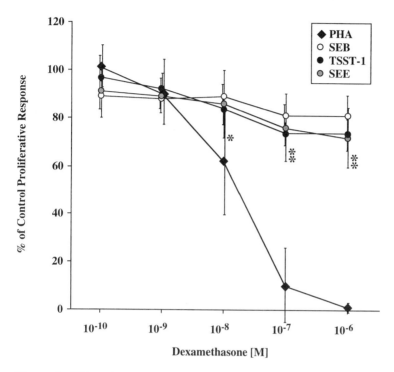

Figure 4 Effect of dexamethasone (DEX) on T-cell proliferation response to superantigens in comparison to PHA. (From Ref. 51.)

gous isoforms: GRα and GRβ (54). GRα is the steroid-activated transcription factor that, in the hormone-bound state, modulates the expression of steroid-sensitive genes. GRβ differs from GRα only in its COOH terminus with replacement of the last 50 amino acids of the latter with a unique 15-amino-acid sequence. This difference renders GRβ unable to bind GC hormones and antagonizes the activity of GRα. Interestingly, superantigens are a potent inducer of GRβ expression in T cells and may account for their ability to induce GC insensitivity (55).

By eliminating superantigens and augmenting corticosteroid sensitivity, combination antibiotic-topical corticosteroid therapy can potentially allow clinicians to use low- to medium-potency topical corticosteroids to achieve the same clinical effects as high-potency corticosteroids when used alone. Since prolonged use of high-potency corticosteroids can lead to marked side effects, this concept is worth pursuing further. Taken together, these data indicate the importance of combining anti-inflammatory therapy with the eradication of bacteria secreting superantigens to effectively treat inflammatory skin diseases such as AD.

B. Nonantibiotic Approaches for Control of *S. aureus*

1. Anti-infectives

In patients who cannot wean off antibiotic therapy, alternative topical approaches should be considered for control of *S. aureus* (see Chapter 22). This would include antibacterial cleansers, which have been shown to be effective in reducing bacterial skin flora (55). The antiseptic gentian violet has been shown to significantly decrease *S. aureus* on AD skin accompanied by a reduction in the clinical severity of skin disease (56,57). Use of 10% povidone iodine solution has been reported to result in a 10-to 100-fold decrease in the density of *S. aureus* in AD patients (58). Finally, daily bathing with an antibacterial soap, as compared to placebo soap, has been found to significantly reduce the number of *S. aureus* on the skin and result in clinical improvement of AD (59). Of note, all these anti-infective strategies may be limiting as they can be too irritating for the inflamed skin of some patients with AD.

2. Phototherapy

It is generally accepted that phototherapy or photochemotherapy is effective in the treatment of atopic dermatitis (see Chapter 25). Although its mechanisms of action are not completely understood, it is thought that this may be due to immunosuppressive and anti-inflammatory effects of phototherapy. Interestingly, it has also been shown that UV-B irradiation or psoralen plus UVA (PUVA) inhibits growth of *S. aureus* via a direct bactericidal effect (60). In addition, in vitro treatment of *S. aureus* with UV-B irradiation or PUVA has been found to inhibit superantigen production in an ultraviolent dose-dependent manner (61). These bacteriostatic effects of UV radiation along with its suppressive effects on superantigen production may contribute to the therapeutic efficacy of phototherapy in AD.

3. Topical Tacrolimus

Several multicenter controlled studies have demonstrated that FK506 in ointment form (tacrolimus) can effectively reduce the clinical symptoms of AD (see Chapter 27) with markedly diminished pruritus within 3–5 days of initiating therapy (62,63). Tacrolimus does not act on glucocorticoid receptors but instead interacts with a cyclophilin-like cytoplasmic protein, FK506-binding protein, and this complex in turn inhibits calcineurin, interfering with gene transcription of multiple Th1- and Th2-like cytokines including IL-2, IL-4, and IL-5 (64). In a 1-year study, Remitz et al. (12) found that application of 0.1% tacrolimus ointment markedly decreased the number of *S. aureus* on the skin of AD patients within the first week of treatment. Tacrolimus has no direct inhibitory effect on bacterial growth. Since the reduction in number of *S. aureus* followed the clinical improve-

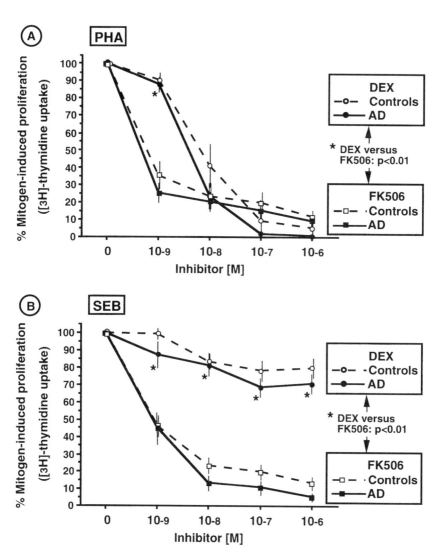

Figure 5 Effect of dexamethasone (DEX) and FK506 on PHA (A) vs. SEB (B) stimulated T-cell proliferation response to superantigens vs. PHA. (From Ref. 65.)

ment of AD following tacrolimus treatment, it is likely that the healing of skin lesions due to the anti-inflammatory actions of tacrolimus is the mechanism for the observed reduction in *S. aureus* counts on AD skin. As shown in Figure 5, superantigen-induced T-cell activation is resistant to the anti proliferation effects of dexamethasone, a prototypic corticosteroid. However, FK506 was highly effective at inhibiting superantigen-induced T-cell activation (65). Thus, tacrolimus ointment may be an effective new treatment option for steroid-insensitive diseases such as AD colonized with *S. aureus*–secreting superantigens. However, it should be noted that there is currently no data supporting the use of topical tacrolimus as first line therapy in the treatment of AD flares that result from *S. aureus* infections. In those situations, oral antibiotics or topical antibiotic/steroid combinations such as fusidic acid/hydrocortisone (Fucidin H) with fusidic acid/betamethasone (Fucicort) would be most useful.

VI. CONCLUSIONS

Colonization and infection with *S. aureus* contributes to the severity of atopic dermatitis. Recent studies demonstrating that bacterial toxins produced by *S. aureus* act as superantigens provide mechanism(s) by which *S. aureus* could mediate an inflammatory skin lesion. The inflamed skin of atopic patients avidly bind *S. aureus*. Once attached to the skin, staphylococcal superantigens can augment allergic skin inflammation and reduce corticosteroid sensitivity. Reduction in *S. aureus* colonization requires effective skin care to control skin inflammation, which predisposes *to S. aureus* colonization/infection. These observations suggest a role for antibiotic/corticosteroid combinations or topical macrolide immunosuppressive ointments in the treatment of atopic dermatitis.

REFERENCES

1. Leung DYM. Atopic dermatitis: new insights and opportunities for therapeutic intervention. J Allergy Clin Immunol 105:860–876, 2000.
2. Williams H, Robertson C, Stewart A, Ait-Khaled N, Anabwani G, Anderson R, Asher I, Beasley R, Bjorksten B, Burr M, Clayton T, Crane J, Ellwood P, Keil U, Lai C, Mallol J, Martinez F, Mitchell E, Montefort S, Pearce N, Shah J, Sibbald B, Strachan D, von Mutius E, Weiland SK. Worldwide variations in the prevalence of symptoms of atopic eczema in the International Study of Asthma and Allergies in Childhood. J Allergy Clin Immunol 103:125–138, 1999.
3. Leyden JJ, Marples RR, Kligman AM. *Staphylococcus aureus* in the lesions of atopic dermatitis. Br J Dermatol 90:525–530, 1974.
4. Morishita Y, Tada J, Sato A, Toi Y, Kanzaki H, Akiyama H, Arata J. Possible influ-

ences of *Staphylococcus aureus* on atopic dermatitis—the colonizing features and the effects of staphylococcal enterotoxins. Clin Exp Allergy 29:1110–1117, 1999.

5. Lever R, Hadley K, Downey D, Mackie R. Staphylococcal colonization in atopic dermatitis and the effect of topical mupirocin therapy. Br J Dermatol 119:189–198, 1988.

6. Nilsson EJ, Henning CG, Magnusson J. Topical corticosteroids and *Staphylococcus aureus* in atopic dermatitis. J Am Acad Dermatol 27:29–34, 1992.

7. Mempel M, Schmidt T, Weidinger S, Schnopp C, Foster T, Ring J, Abeck D. Role of *Staphylococcus aureus* surface-associated proteins in the attachment to cultured HaCaT keratinocytes in a new adhesion assay. J Invest Dermatol 111:452–456, 1998.

8. Miller SJ, Aly R, Shinefeld HR, Elias PM. *In vitro* and *in vivo* antistaphylococcal activity of human stratum corneum lipids. Arch Dermatol 124:209–215, 1988.

9. Imokawa G, Abe A, Jin K, Higaki Y, Kawashima M, Hidano A. Decreased level of ceramides in stratum corneum of atopic dermatitis: an etiologic factor in atopic dry skin? J Invest Dermatol 96:523–526, 1991.

10. Cole GW, Silverberg NL. The adherence of *Staphylococcus aureus* to human corneocytes. Arch Dermatol 122:166–169, 1986.

11. Stalder JF, Fleury M, Sourisse M, Rostin M, Pheline F, Litoux P. Local steroid therapy and bacterial skin flora in atopic dermatitis. Br J Dermatol 131:536–540, 1994.

12. Remitz A, Kyllonen H, Granlund H, Reitamo S. Tacrolimus ointment reduces staphylococcal colonization of atopic dermatitis lesions. J Allergy Clin Immunol 107: 196–197, 2001.

13. Foster TJ, Höök M. Surface protein adhesins of *Staphylococcus aureus*. Trends Microbiol 6:484–488, 1998.

14. Cho SH, Strickland I, Tomkinson A, Fehringer AP, Gelfand EW, Leung DYM. Preferential binding of *Staphylococcus aureus* to skin sites of Th2-mediated inflammation in a murine model. J Invest Dermatol 116:658–663, 2001.

15. Postlethwaite AE, Holness MA, Katai H, Raghow R. Human fibroblasts synthesize elevated levels of extracellular matrix proteins in response to interleukin 4. J Clin Invest 90:1479–1485, 1992.

16. Strickland I, Cho SH, Boguniewicz M, Leung DYM. Fibronectin contributes to the enhanced binding of *Staphylococcus aureus* to atopic skin. J Allergy Clin Immunol 107:778A, 2001.

17. Wann ER, Gurusiddappa S, Höök M. The fibronectin-binding MSCRAMM FnbpA of *Staphylococcus aureus* is a bifunctional protein that also binds to fibrinogen. J Biol Chem 275:13863–13871, 2000.

18. Kotzin BL, Leung DYM, Kappler J, Marrack P. Superantigens and their potential role in human disease. Adv Immunol 54:99–166, 1993.

19. Leung DYM, Schlievert PM. Superantigens in human disease: Future directions in therapy and elucidation of disease pathogenesis. In: Leung DYM, Huber B Schlievert PM. Superantigens: Molecular Biology, Immunology and Relevance to Human Disease. New York, Marcel Dekker, Inc, 581–602, 1997.

20. Leung DYM, Harbeck R, Bina P, Reiser RF, Yang E, Norris DA, Hanifin JM, Sampson HA. Presence of IgE antibodies to staphylococcal exotoxins on the skin of pa-

tients with atopic dermatitis. Evidence for a new group of allergens. J Clin Invest 92:1374–1380, 1993.

21. Bunikowski R, Mielke M, Skarabis H, Herz U, Bergmann RL, Wahn U, Renz H. Prevalence and role of serum IgE antibodies to the *Staphylococcus aureus*-derived superantigens SEA and SEB in children with atopic dermatitis. J Allergy Clin Immunol 103:119–124, 1999.

22. Nomura I, Tanaka K, Tomita H, Katsunuma T, Ohya Y, Ikeda N, Takeda T, Saito H, Akasawa A. Evaluation of the staphylococcal exotoxins and their specific IgE in childhood atopic dermatitis. J Allergy Clin Immunol 104:441–446, 1999.

23. Strickland I, Hauk PJ, Trumble AE, Picker LJ, Leung DYM. Evidence for superantigen involvement in skin homing of T cells in atopic dermatitis. J Invest Dermatol 112:249–253, 1999.

24. Bunikowski R, Mielke ME, Skarabis H, Worm M, Anagnostopoulos I, Kolde G, Wahn U, Renz H. Evidence for a disease-promoting effect of *Staphylococcus aureus*–derived exotoxins in atopic dermatitis. J Allergy Clin Immunol 105:814–819, 2000.

25. Hofer MF, Harbeck RJ, Schlievert PM, Leung DYM. Staphylococcal toxins augment specific IgE responses by atopic patients exposed to allergen. J Invest Dermatol 112: 171–176, 1999.

26. Herz U, Schnoy N, Borelli S, Weigl L, Kasbohrer U, Daser A, Wahn U, Kottgen E, Renz H. A human-SCID mouse model for allergic immune response bacterial superantigen enhances skin inflammation and suppresses IgE production. J Invest Dermatol 110:224–231, 1998.

27. Akdis M, Akdis CA, Weigl L, Disch R, Blaser K. Skin-homing, CLA+ memory T cells are activated in atopic dermatitis and regulate IgE by an IL-13-dominated cytokine pattern: IgG4 counter-regulation by CLA-memory T cells. J Immunol 159: 4611–4619, 1997.

28. Akdis M, Simon HU, Weigl L, Kreyden O, Blaser K, Akdis CA. Skin homing (cutaneous lymphocyte-associated antigen-positive) CD8+ T cells respond to superantigen and contribute to eosinophilia and IgE production in atopic dermatitis. J Immunol 163:466–475, 1999.

29. Strange P, Skov L, Lisby S, Nielsen PL, Baadsgaard O. Staphylococcal enterotoxin B applied on intact normal and intact atopic skin induces dermatitis. Arch Dermatol 132:27-33, 1996.

30. Skov L, Olsen JV, Giorno R, Schlievert PM, Baadsgaard O, Leung DYM. Application of Staphylococcal enterotoxin B on normal and atopic skin induces up-regulation of T cells by a superantigen-mediated mechanism. J Allergy Clin Immunol 105: 820–826, 2000.

31. Michie CA, Davis T. Atopic dermatitis and staphylococcal superantigens. Lancet 347:324, 1996.

32. Brosius CL, Newburger JW, Burns JC, Hojnowski-Diaz P, Zierler S, Leung DYM. Increased prevalence of atopic dermatitis in Kawasaki disease. Pediatr Infect Dis J 7:863–866, 1988.

33. Müller KM, Jaunin F, Masouye I, Saurat JH, Hauser C. Th2 cells mediate IL-4-dependent local tissue inflammation. J Immunol 150:5576–5584, 1993.

34. Saloga J, Enk AH, Becker D, Mohamadzadeh M, Spieles S, Bellinghausen I, Leung

DYM, Gelfand EW, Knop J. Modulation of contact sensitivity responses by bacterial superantigen. J Invest Dermatol 105:220–224, 1995.

35. Saloga J, Leung DYM, Reardon C, Giorno RC, Born W, Gelfand EW. Cutaneous exposure to the superantigen staphylococcal enterotoxin B elicits a T-cell-dependent inflammatory response. J Invest Dermatol 106:982–988, 1996.

36. Leung DYM, Gately M, Trumble A, Ferguson-Darnell B, Schlievert PM, Picker LJ. Bacterial superantigens induce T cell expression of the skin-selective homing receptor, the cutaneous lymphocyte-associated antigen, via stimulation of interleukin 12 production. J Exp Med 181:747–753, 1995.

37. de Vries IJ, Langeveld-Wildschut EG, van Reijsen FC, Dubois GR, van den Hoek JA, Bihari IC, van Wichen D, de Weger RA, Knol EF, Thepen T, Bruijnzeel-Koomen CA. Adhesion molecule expression on skin endothelia in atopic dermatitis: effects of TNF-alpha and IL-4. J Allergy Clin Immunol 102:461–468, 1998.

38. Bratton DL, Hamid Q, Boguniewicz M, Doherty DE, Kailey JM, Leung DYM. Granulocyte macrophage colony-stimulating factor contributes to enhanced monocyte survival in chronic atopic dermatitis. J Clin Invest 95:211–218, 1995.

39. Ezepchuk YV, Leung DYM, Middleton MH, Bina P, Reiser R, Norris DA. Staphylococcal toxins and protein A differentially induce cytotoxicity and release of tumor necrosis factor-alpha from human keratinocytes. J Invest Dermatol 107:603–609, 1996.

40. Morath S, Geyer A, Hartung T. Structure-function relationship of cytokine induction by lipoteichoic acid from *Staphylococcus aureus*. J Exp Med 193:393–398, 2001.

41. Abeck D, Mempel M. *Staphylococcus aureus* colonization in atopic dermatitis and its therapeutic implications. Br J Dermatol 139 Suppl 53:13–16, 1998.

42. Boguniewicz M, Sampson HA, Bina P, Reiser R, McCormick D, Harbeck R, Leung DYM. Effects of antibiotic treatment on *S. aureus* colonization in atopic dermatitis (AD). J Allergy Clin Immunol 103:S178 (#684A), 1999.

43. Skov L, Baadsgaard O. Role of infection in atopic dermatitis. In: Leung DYM, Greaves MW. Allergic Skin Diseases: A Multidisciplinary Approach. New York: Marcel Dekker, 2000:449–462.

44. Lever R, Hadley K, Downey D, Mackie R. Staphylococcal colonization in atopic dermatitis and the effect of topical mupirocin therapy. Br J Dermatol 119:189–198, 1988.

45. Ramsay CA, Savoie LM, Gilbert M. The treatment of atopic dermatitis with topical fusidic acid and hydrocortisone acetate. J Eur Acad Dermatol Venereol 7:S15–22, 1996.

46. Wachs GN, Maibach HI. Co-operative double-blind trial of an antibiotic/corticoid combination in impetiginized atopic dermatitis. Br J Dermatol 95:323–328, 1976.

47. Leyden JJ, Kligman AM. The case for steroid–antibiotic combinations. Br J Dermatol 96:179–187, 1977.

48. Verbist L. The antimicrobial activity of fusidic acid. J Antimicrob Chemother 25 Suppl B:1–5, 1990.

49. Albert MR, Gonzalez S, Gonzalez E. Patch testing reactions to a standard series in 608 patients tested from 1990 to 1997 at Massachusetts General Hospital. Am J Contact Dermat 9:207–211, 1998.

50. Clayton MH, Leung DY, Surs W, Szefler SJ. Altered glucocorticoid receptor binding in atopic dermatitis. J Allergy Clin Immunol 96:421–423, 1995.
51. Hauk PJ, Hamid QA, Chrousos GP, Leung DYM. Induction of corticosteroid insensitivity in human PBMCs by microbial superantigens. J Allergy Clin Immunol 105: 782–787, 2000.
52. Herbert S, Barry P, Novick RP. Subinhibitory Clindamycin Differentially Inhibits Transcription of Exoprotein Genes in *Staphylococcus aureus*. Infect Immun 69: 2996–3003, 2001.
53. Bamberger CM, Bamberger AM, de Castro M, Chrousos GP. Glucocorticoid receptor beta, a potential endogenous inhibitor of glucocorticoid action in humans. J Clin Invest 95:2435–2441, 1995.
54. Doebbeling BN, Reagan DR, Pfaller MA, Houston AK, Hollis RJ, Wenzel RP. Long-term efficacy of intranasal mupirocin ointment. A prospective cohort study of *Staphylococcus aureus* carriage. Arch Intern Med 154:1505–1508, 1994.
55. Stalder JF, Fleury M, Sourisse M, Allavoine T, Chalamet C, Brosset P, Litoux P. Comparative effects of two topical antiseptics (chlorhexidine vs KMn04) on bacterial skin flora in atopic dermatitis. Acta Derm Venereol Suppl 176:132–134, 1992.
56. Brockow K, Grabenhorst P, Abeck D, Traupe B, Ring J, Hoppe U, Wolf F. Effect of gentian violet, corticosteroid and tar preparations in Staphylococcus-aureus-colonized atopic eczema. Dermatology 199:231–236, 1999.
57. Brockow K, Grabenhorst P, Traupe B. Gentian violet for the treatment of atopic eczema antibacterial and clinical efficacy. J Invest Dermatol 109:463, 1997.
58. Akiyama H, Tada J, Toi J, Kanzaki H, Arata J. Changes in *Staphylococcus aureus* density and lesion severity after topical application of povidone-iodine in cases of atopic dermatitis. J Dermatol Sci 16:23–30, 1997.
59. Breneman DL, Hanifin JM, Berge CA, Keswick BH, Neumann PB. The effect of antibacterial soap with 1.5% triclocarban on *Staphylococcus aureus* in patients with atopic dermatitis. Cutis 66:296–300, 2000.
60. Yoshimura M, Namura S, Akamatsu H, Horio T. Antimicrobial effects of phototherapy and photochemotherapy *in vivo* and *in vitro*. Br J Dermatol 135:528–532, 1996.
61. Yoshimura-Mishima M, Akamatsu H, Namura S, Horio T. Suppressive effect of ultraviolet (UVB and PUVA) radiation on superantigen production by *Staphylococcus aureus*. J Dermatol Sci 19:31–36, 1999.
62. Ruzicka T, Bieber T, Schopf E, Rubins A, Dobozy A, Bos JD, Jablonska S, Ahmed I, Thestrup-Pedersen K, Daniel F, Finzi A, Reitamo S. A short-term trial of tacrolimus ointment for atopic dermatitis. European Tacrolimus Multicenter Atopic Dermatitis Study Group. N Engl J Med 337:816–821, 1997.
63. Boguniewicz M, Fiedler VC, Raimer S, Lawrence ID, Leung DYM, Hanifin JM. A randomized, vehicle-controlled trial of tacrolimus ointment for treatment of atopic dermatitis in children. Pediatric Tacrolimus Study Group. J Allergy Clin Immunol 102:637–644, 1998.
64. Fleischer AB, Jr.. Treatment of atopic dermatitis: role of tacrolimus ointment as a topical noncorticosteroidal therapy. J Allergy Clin Immunol 104:S126–130, 1999.
65. Hauk PJ, Leung DYM. Tacrolimus (FK506): new treatment approach in superantigen-associated diseases like atopic dermatitis? J Allergy Clin Immunol 107:391–392, 2001.

20

Fungal Allergens

Hachiro Tagami, Hiroaki Aoyama, Mikiko Okada,* and Tadashi Terui
Tohoku University School of Medicine, Sendai, Japan

The skin protects our body not only physicochemically by covering its surface with the stratum corneum (SC) but also immunologically with the unique skin immune system (1). However, immunological reactivity against environmental substances may induce so-called allergic skin reactions. Individuals with atopic histories tend to develop IgE-mediated immediate hypersensitivity reactions against various aeroallergens, which are mostly derived from other living organisms such as animals, plants, and microorganisms including fungi. Patients with atopic dermatitis (AD) display not only delayed contact sensitivity but also immediate reactions to allergens (2). Unlike small molecular haptens that can penetrate even normal SC to induce allergic skin reactions, large molecular aeroallergens cannot penetrate through the intact SC of normal skin. For their percutaneous penetration, barrier function of the SC must be compromised.

I. STRATUM CORNEUM AS A PHYSICOCHEMICAL BARRIER

The primary defense mechanism of the skin depends on the production of a physicochemical barrier, the SC, by the epidermis. The SC is a thin biological membrane less than 20 μm in thickness but is nevertheless efficient as a barrier. The SC is composed of about 15 tightly stacked layers of corneocytes, except for at certain bodily locations such as the genitals or the palmoplantar skin, where it is extremely thin or thick (3).

The SC prevents invasion from the environment of injurious agents with

---

* *Current affiliation*: Sendai Shakaihoken Hospital, Sendai, Japan.

a molecular mass larger than 500 daltons. It is basically comprised of a two-compartment system of corneocytes, flattened dead cell bodies of keratinocytes covered by a tough, highly cross-linked proteinaceous cornified envelope, and extracellular lipid lamellae (4). The latter, which play a crucial role in the barrier function of the SC, fill the continuous extracellular matrix consisting of roughly equimolar concentrations of ceramides, long-chain free fatty acids and cholesterol released from lamellar granules of differentiated granular cells. It is so efficient as a barrier that it hardly allows easy passage of a small molecule like water. Thus, the SC protects our body from desiccation even in a dry environment. Accordingly, large molecular components of fungi cannot penetrate the skin through intact SC but only through injured sites caused by scratching or through fissures observed in dry skin or the lesional skin of dermatitis.

Epidermal appendages such as hair follicles and sweat ducts are not well equipped with an intact SC barrier (4). In fact, they provide an alternative permeation pathway even for large molecules like protein allergens, although in a restricted fashion. Thus, in AD patients with sensitivity to environmental protein antigens, we can induce positive reactions with atopy patch test even when conducted on the unabraded skin of the back that is dotted with large hair follicular orifices (5). In such patch testing, antigenic substances are applied under occlusion for 48 hours, which produces an extremely wet condition that is not experienced in daily life. In contrast, it is not easy to produce similar positive reactions on the flexor surface of the forearms, where the orifices of hair follicles are much smaller than those on the back. On the flexor surface of the forearms, partial stripping of the SC with adhesive tape or scarification using a needle is required to obtain definite positive reactions (6,7).

The SC also plays another important role at the skin surface by binding water to keep the skin smooth and flexible even in an extremely dry environment (1,4). Water renders these dry stacked layers of corneocytes supple enough to allow free movement of the body without producing cracks or fissures in the skin surface. There is always a water supply from the underlying hydrated living tissue at the deeper portion of the SC. Therefore, it is the water content at the upper portion of the SC that determines the skin surface properties, keeping the skin smooth and soft, as long as the water-holding capacity is intact. The presence of intercellular lipids in the SC between each corneocyte, together with skin surface lipids derived from sebum and water-soluble amino acids (natural moisturizing factor) produced by the enzymatic degradation of filaggrin, gives the SC a water-holding capacity as well as a barrier function. However, the SC produced in pathological skin conditions is deficient in water-holding capacity, being firm and brittle and producing fissures and scales even under normal ambient conditions. These changes in the SC, which are always observed in the lesional skin of dermatitis, enable permeation of even large molecules such as protein allergens.

II. ATOPIC XEROSIS

Clinically observable erythema reflects one facet of inflammation occurring in the skin. Invisible but microscopically observable inflammatory changes persist far longer than the clinically observable erythematous changes. For example, mildly functionally deficient SC is always observed in the clinically noninflamed, dry nonlesional skin of patients with atopic xerosis (8), much like the scaly skin lesions caused by the physical insult of tape-stripping (9). In such skin, mild residual inflammation is accompanied by hyperproliferation of the epidermis with rapid turnover of the SC, which leads to the production of functionally defective SC. Thus, atopic xerosis skin shows higher transepidermal water loss (TEWL) and lower skin surface hydration levels than does normal control skin.

The contents of ceramides and water-soluble amino acids in the SC of atopic xerosis are reduced, which is responsible for its compromised barrier function as well as the deficient water-holding capacity (8,10). The corneocytes in atopic xerosis tend to desquamate in clumps of cell aggregates instead of as individual cells. Although the number of stratum corneum cell layers in atopic xerosis (21 ± 4) was substantially larger than that in controls (15 ± 1), its turnover time (7 ± 2 days) was appreciably shorter than that for controls (14 ± 2 days) when studied on the volar forearms. As noted in the skin with increased epidermal proliferation, the size of superficial corneocytes in patients with atopic xerosis is substantially smaller than in controls. In fact, histopathological examination reveals acanthotic epidermis, mild perivascular mononuclear cell infiltrate, and pigment incontinence. All these changes seem to reflect the increased epidermal proliferation due to the low-level ongoing dermatitis. This SC dysfunction as well as the reduced ceramide and amino acid contents are no longer observable when the xerotic changes eventually disappear from the skin surface (11,12).

Patch testing with detergents such as 1% sodium lauryl sulfate (SLS) in petrolatum for 24 hours on atopic xerosis induces much more severe damage in the SC barrier function (>1 week) than in normal individuals (13). It also makes a sharp contrast with the finding that in atopic xerosis the barrier recovery is not impaired after infliction of a physical insult such as scratching (12,14). The effects on the skin of chemical insults such as those caused by detergents that induce inflammation may be more prominent than those resulting from physical traumas.

The mild barrier dysfunction of the SC as noted in atopic xerosis does not seem to be a prerequisite for the development of dermatitis. Even the skin of the face and genitals of normal individuals shows high TEWL values, almost comparable to those noted in scaly dermatitis skin, which far exceed those of atopic xerosis (3). In the case of skin tests for various environmental allergens, scarification or pricking with a needle is required to produce a compromised state in the SC barrier. Likewise, fissuring or cracking that develops even in the intact

SC due to the decreased water content of the SC opens a new penetration pathway for aeroallergens through the SC. Thus, nummular eczema can occur even in elderly individuals with senile xerosis who show immediate skin hypersensitivity as well as contact hypersensitivity reactions to aeroallergens as in young patients with AD (15). These patients tend to show more severe xerotic changes than similarly aged normal people.

III. SKIN TESTS WITH FUNGAL ANTIGENS

All the subjects are prohibited from taking antihistamines and systemic steroids and from applying topical steroids on the volar aspects of the forearms for one week before the skin testing.

Various test agents containing fungal allergens are commercially available. However, a modern allergen tray should integrate relevant aeroallergens prepared from adequate aerial as well as cutaneous fungal flora.

Because these agents are too large to penetrate normal skin, we must prepare the test skin area by compromising the barrier function of the SC to assure definite permeation of the antigen. For prick testing to check immediate hypersensitivity, after placing a droplet of each test extract reagent, a commercially available disposable prick test needle that is equipped with a guard to prevent deeper piercing is passed though the drop and inserted 1 mm deep into the skin. Alternatively, a disposable hypodermic needle (27 gauge) is passed through the droplet and inserted into the epidermal surface at a low angle, with the bevel of the needle facing away from the skin surface. Then the needle tip is gently lifted upward to raise a small portion of the skin without causing bleeding. A whealing reaction is evaluated after 15 minutes. A wheal with a diameter of more than 5 mm is regarded as positive. When the subject shows a reaction to the solvent (control solution), the reaction to allergen is recorded as positive if the diameter of the reaction is two times larger than the reaction to the solvent. A high correlation is observed between the prick test in the skin and RAST with the serum (2).

The site should be examined 6–8 hours later to check for the late phase reaction, which is characterized by tissue infiltration with Th2 lymphocytes and eosinophils. When the tests are done in outpatient clinics, we ask the patient to trace the outline of the erythematous reaction at 8 hours at home with a ball point pen. The size of the reaction area can be kept as a record on transparent adhesive tape, which is later applied to the site to strip the skin surface with the tracing line. From our experience, the late phase reaction tends to develop in those who have high levels of IL-5.

Aeroallergens can induce positive reactions with atopy patch tests conducted even on the unabraded skin of the back, which has large hair follicular orifices (5). However, for patch testing on the flexor aspect of the forearm, the skin should be pretreated to assure penetration of large molecular substances through the SC. To avoid missing a positive response, the skin is lightly abraded four times with a 27-gauge needle in a crisscross fashion (1,7). Another way to compromise the barrier function of the SC is partial tape stripping. Ten strippings with adhesive cellophane tape is sufficient to obtain a response positive in reactive subjects without causing any skin damage that lasts more than 48 hours (6). Furthermore, to assure sufficient penetration of antigenic substances into the skin, the test solutions should be concentrated. Concentrations of at least 100 times those used for intradermal skin tests are desirable as long as the agent is not an irritant. To prevent bacterial proliferation, phenol can be added at a final concentration of 0.1%.

Twenty μL of the test solution in a Finn chamber is applied to the site for 48 hours. A control vehicle solution is applied in the same way. The patch test reaction is read at 48 and 72 hours and 1 week after the application of the patches and evaluated according to the International Contact Dermatitis Research Group criteria for patch tests (16).

IV. CUTANEOUS IMMUNE REACTIVITY INDUCED BY ARTIFICIAL EXPOSURE TO FUNGAL ALLERGENS

It is difficult to induce a skin immune response by simply applying fungal allergens on normal skin. However, from the observations in artificial exposure to fungal components by inducing experimental cutaneous infections with pathogenic fungi such as dermatophytes and *Candida albicans*, which can invade the SC, we can study the development of immune responses that lead to regression of the lesions (7,17,18). When spores of *Trichophytin mentagrophytes* are inoculated on the normal skin of guinea pigs under occlusion for 24 hours, the inoculated sites first become erythematous at 1–2 days after infection (17). This is simply a sign of irritant dermatitis induced by substances released from the proliferating fungus in the SC. The intensity of erythema increases gradually. After 7 days, almost concurrently with the demonstrability of delayed contact sensititivity reactions to the dermatophyte allergen trichophytin, the lesions become infiltrated and covered by silvery scales. Climax inflammatory changes are observed between 9 and 14 days. Thereafter the crusty scales are sloughed off and healing begins to take place. By week 4 the lesions are replaced by smooth alopecic scars. By reinfecting such recovered animals in the same way with *T. mentagrophytes*, a much more rapid onset of inflammatory change is produced, reaching a peak within 2 days. Because a similar reaction can be induced even with heat-killed spore suspensions, the inflammation is thought to depend on contact sensitivity to dermatophyte. Subsequently, the inflammation begins to subside and completely regresses within 10 days. Thus, contact sensitivity to fungal antigen is crucial to eliminate the fungus from the skin surface by inducing prominent inflammation that enhances epidermal proliferation associated with rapid desquamation of the SC infected by the fungus (18).

The development of delayed contact hypersensitivity to fungal allergens is also observable 4–5 days after application of the spore suspensions in guinea pig skin experimentally infected with *C. albicans* (7).

We cannot study the development of immune reactivity induced by experimental innoculation of *Candida* in human subjects because most individuals have been exposed since birth (7). *C. albicans* is a common commensal of human oral and vaginal mucosae and the intestinal tract, existing as part of the normal flora (19). Thus, whenever possible it readily colonizes or infects the moist skin area under diapers or intertriginous areas such as the interdigital spaces, inframammary folds, and perianal skin. Therefore, in humans we can utilize only experimental dermatophytosis for the study of the development of skin immune reactivity after exposure to fungal allergens.

There is a difference between the uniform experimental dermatophyte infections of guinea pigs and dermatophytosis in humans, the infection patterns of which are rich in variety. Jones et al. (20) found that, as noted in guinea pigs, healthy human volunteers also develop delayed hypersensitivity at first, which enhances the inflammatory changes of the skin lesions to induce spontaneous regression. However, they found that in certain subjects the infected lesions became chronic and widespread. This phenomenon occurred in those having an atopic history. Their group also found that patients who were extensively and chronically infected with dermtophytes were atopic by demonstrating multiple immediate skin test sensitivity and elevated levels of serum IgE (21). They obtained evidence that type I hypersensitivity in atopic subjects antagonizes the effect of cellular immunity locally that induces prominent inflammation to eliminate the invading fungus from the skin. In parallel with these in vivo observations, in vitro assays of T-lymphocyte functions also demonstrated a deficiency of cellular immunity as well as a high incidence of atopy in individuals with chronic dermatophytosis (22,23). Thus, it is reasonable to presume that the exposure to fungal allergens induces at first Th1-lymphocyte–dependent, delayed-type hypersensitivity in every individual and that those with an atopic background tend to develop Th2-cell–dependent IgE antibody production later.

In fact, the incidence of positive patch testing with trichophytin, the dermatophyte allergen, on the skin partially stripped with tape was demonstrated to be statistically marginally low ($p < 0.1$) in dermatophytosis patients with evidence of atopy compared with nonatopic patients (6). In various types of dermatophytosis, a high frequency of this response is observed in patients with the vesiculobullous type of tinea pedis, whereas a very low incidence is observed in tinea corporis and the squamous hyperkeratotic type of tinea pedis. Recently, we have found that IgE antibodies against dermatophyte allergen are significantly higher in adult AD patients than in nonatopic patients with dermatophytosis or than normal individuals, when measured with RAST (CAP system, Pharmacia, Uppsala, Sweden) (Fig. 1). Most of them had no past history of dermatophytosis. These patients have a compromised barrier function in the SC, allowing a exposure to various environmental fungi including dermatophytes for a long period of time. Also, we cannot rule out the possibility of a cross-reaction to allergens of other fungi.

Recent experimental evidence indicates that the shift from Th1 to Th2 immune reactivity seems to occur with any antigen under a situation where persistent skin contact to it is maintained. Kitagaki et al. (24) found that repeated epicutaneous application of hapten, a small molecular contact-sensitizing agent, on the original sensitized site for 24–48 days could induce a shift from a delayed-type hypersensitivity to an immediate-type response followed by a late reaction when skin reactions were repeatedly elicited. There were epidermal hyperplasia, the accumulation of large numbers of mast cells and CD4+ T cells beneath the epidermis, and elevated serum levels of antigen-specific IgE. We have observed that murine Th2 lymphocytes that release IL-4, IL-5 and IL-13 upon exposure to allergens produce an inflammatory skin response with a peak at 24 hours. In contrast, Th1 lymphocytes that release IL-1, IL-2 and IFN-γ produce skin inflammation that has a peak at 48 hours after stimulation with allergen (25). Partic-

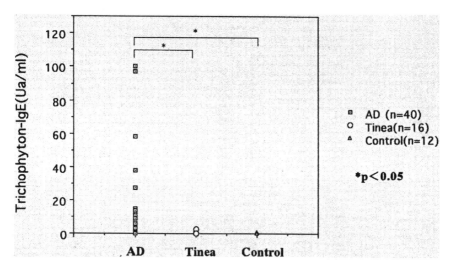

Figure 1 IgE antibody level against dermatophyte antigen in patients with atopic dermatitis (AD), those with tinea, and normal controls measured with RAST. Far higher IgE levels were noted in AD patients.

ularly, such circumstances can easily occur in AD patients, because their skin shows extensive xerotic changes with cracks and fissures in addition to many scratch marks. Moreover, they have a propensity to develop Th2-dependent immune reactions to various substances more readily than normal individuals.

IV. SKIN REACTIVITY TO *CANDIDA ALBICANS* ANTIGEN

Delayed contact sensitivity to dermatophyte occurs only after the inflammatory changes of dermatophytosis. By contrast, although neonates do not show any skin reactions to *C. albicans* allergen, most healthy adults show positive, delayed-type patch test reactions to *C. albicans* allergen without any history of cutaneous candidiasis (1,7,26,27). These findings indicate that everybody has been infected at least once by *C. albicans* early in life, with a skin change being overlooked as a mild diaper dermatitis or nonspecific intertrigo. Because it is such a potent contact sensitizer, the patch test with *C. albicans* allergen can be used as a prospective measure to evaluate patients' immune function. Its contact sensitivity is reduced in patients with autoimmune diseases or elderly patients with skin malignancies who have a deficiency in cellular immunity (7). Moreover, it is remarkable that adult AD patients tend to show decreased contact sensitivity to *C. albicans* together with enhanced immediate hypersensitivity to this antigen, showing also high RAST scores (Fig. 2). Namely, many of them show a shift from Th1 to Th2 reactivity. This shift is observed against no other aeroallergens

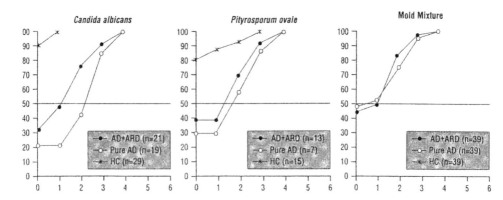

Figure 2 Cumulative frequency distribution of the radioallergosorbent test (RAST). Fifty percent corresponds to the median of RAST scores. They are much higher in patients with AD than in healthy controls. AD, Atopic dermatitis; ARD, atopic respiratory disease; HC, healthy age-matched control subjects. (Modified from Ref. 2.)

to such a degree (2). AD patients who have contact sensitivity to a certain allergen such as dust mite or cedar pollen usually show higher levels of specific IgE antibodies against the same allergen than healthy controls (2,26). Thus, a definite shift from Th1 to Th2 reactivity is observable only for *C. albicans* allergen in AD patients. Moreover, when we studied the immune reactivity of adult patients with atopic respiratory diseases (allergic rhinitis and atopic asthma), their reactivity profile was unchanged from that of normal adults. Namely, they showed a high incidence of contact sensitivity with a low RAST score against *C. albicans* antigen (26). Thus, the altered reactivity against *C. albicans* antigen is quite unique to AD patients. It is further demonstrable with their peripheral blood lymphocytes (PBL). PBL from AD patients showed a significantly lower response to *C. albicans* antigen, although their responses to staphylococcal superantigens did not differ from those of healthy controls (28). All of these findings suggest that the specific shift from Th1- to Th2-type immune reactivity against *C. albicans* allergen takes place only in the presence of the chronic dermatititis of AD (Fig. 3).

As mentioned above, because neonates do not show skin reactions to *C. albicans* allergen, delayed-type contact sensitivity to this allergen is acquired later in life (7). According to Munoz and Limbert (29), who examined immune reactivity with an intradermal test against *C. albicans* allergen, after the first 3 months of life when the skin reactivity is quite low there is a progressive increase in the frequency of positive delayed skin reactions. About one third of infants under 1 year of age and four fifths of 1- to 5-year-old children showed positive test reactions.

Our own data indicate that infantile AD patients begin to show delayed contact sensitivity to *C. albicans* allergen like normal infants (Table 1). With the persistence of the AD skin lesions, however, they tend to show a shift from Th1- to Th2-type immunoreactivity later in life. Kimura et al. (30) found higher *Candida*-specific proliferation of peripheral blood lymphocytes in children with AD, which was not related to the levels of *Candida*-specific IgE antibodies. They

Table 1 Incidence of Reactors to *Candida* Prick Test and Scarification Patch Test

	Prick test	Scarification patch test
Healthy infants (1–2 years)	0/7 (0%)	8/9 (89%)
Healthy adults (19–38 years)	1/36 (3%)	27/32 (84%)
Patients with infantile atopic dermatitis (1–12 years)	1/8 (13%)	7/8 (83%)
Adult patients with atopic dermatitis (17–36 years)	18/43 (42%)	14/46 (30%)

further demonstrated that IL-5 production by PBL was significantly lower in children with AD than in those with bronchial asthma (31). Thus, immune reactivity against a commensal like *C. albicans* can be used as a parameter for the chronicity of the skin disease; infants with a short history of AD show Th1-dependent immune reactivity to it, whereas adults with a long history of AD tend to display Th2-dependent immune reactivity. In many adult AD patients, however, there still seems to be coexistence of Th1 and Th2 immunoreactivity. Our recent analysis in adult AD patients with increased levels of IgE antibodies against *C. albicans*, based on the difference in the dependency on CD80 or CD86 costimulation between T-helper type 1 and T-helper type 2 immune responses, indicates that they are not completely shifted to a Th2 subset (32).

There is no agreement in the reported data about mucosal colonization of *C. albicans* in AD patients. Although there is one report showing no difference (33), others indicate a higher incidence of *C. albicans* colonization in AD patients (34), particularly in recalcitrant cases (35,36). Thus, there is not only a possibility of mucosal absorption but also a possibility of continuous exposure of the skin to *C. albicans* allergen in severe AD patients.

There are many antigenic components including proteins and polysaccharides in *C. albicans* allergen. Akiyama et al. (37) demonstrated that acid proteases secreted by *C. albicans* constitute the major antigenic materials in crude *C. albicans* extract. In contrast, antibodies to the cell-wall polysaccharide mannan of *C. albicans* show cross-reaction with that of other fungi (38), especially the lipophilic yeast *Malassezia* in the IgE response (39). However, despite their presence, IgE antibodies directed to such cross-reactive carbohydrate determinants of fungal glycoprotein may have only poor biological activity to induce the skin immune response (40). By contrast, *C. albicans* mannan has the ability to induce the production of Th1 cytokines such as IL-2 and IFN-γ in AD patients (38, 41).

V. SKIN REACTIVITY TO *MALASSEZIA*

The genus *Malassezia* (*Pityrosporum*) consists of lipophilic dimorphic yeasts existing as a commensal on seborrheic skin regions, i.e., the head, neck, and face. It is etiologically implicated in tinea versicolor, pityrosporum folliculitis, and seborrheic dermatitis in humans. Formerly denoted as *P. ovale* and *P. orbiculare*, which are differentiated by their morphology, there are now seven species identified by means of their phenotypic and biochemical characteristics as well as their ability to assimilate polyethylene (20)-sorbitan esters: *M. furfur*, *M. sympodialis*, *M. slooffiae*, *M. globosa*, *M. obtsusa*, *M. restricta*, and *M. pachydermatis*. Mixed strains are usually isolated from normal skin and lesional skin of seborrheic dermatitis or AD. *M. pachydermatis* can usually be isolated from warm-blooded animal skin but only rarely from human skin.

Unlike dermatophytes or *C. albicans*, however, it is difficult to produce an experimental infection with the spores of *Malassezia* in either humans or guinea pigs. Because its cellular components can be shown to have a proinflammatory property that activates the complement system (42), skin inflammation can be easily produced by repeated applications of even heat-killed spore suspensions on the skin of experimental animals (43). The induced inflammation is similar to that of seborrheic dermatitis. We found that contact sensitivity to *Malassezia* allergen becomes demonstrable in 5 days in hairless guinea pigs in which experimental inflammation was induced by the repeated applications of heat-killed spore suspensions (unpublished data). However, it does not seems to be a potent contact sensitizer as compared with *C. albicans* allergen, because the incidence of its positive patch test reactions is much lower than that observed with the latter in both AD patients and normal controls.

Findings that the incidence of contact sensitivity to *Malassezia* tends to be higher in AD patients suggest again that they have more chances to be exposed to the fungus allergen (44–46). As compared with *C. albcians* allergen, *Malassezia* allergen seems to stimulate Th1-type and Th2-type lymphocytes equally, and low levels of IgE antibodies are demonstrable even in normal individuals (2). However, adult patients with AD (Fig. 2), particularly those with head and neck involvement, show a higher incidence of IgE antibodies and positive prick tests against *Malassezia* allergen (2,45). Moreover, patch test–positive AD patients are reported to show significantly higher serum levels of *Malassezia*-specific IgE (46).

Malassezia is also a skin commensal of infants (19,47). Both contact sensitivity and IgE-mediated immediate hypersensitivity are also demonstrable in children with AD. IgE antibodies against *Malassezia* are reported to occur more frequently in children with AD than in those with other types of atopic diseases (47). The sensitization to *Malassezia* appears to be of little importance in early childhood AD. However, it is likely to carry a poor prognosis because severe itch that disturbs sleep is a characteristic clinical feature of anti-*Malassezia*-positive cases (48).

Malassezia allergen consists of proteins and polysaccharides (39,49). At least four protein antigens that are reactive with IgE antibodies of AD patients have been cloned and sequenced (50). Mannan antigen is the main cross-reacting component. There is a highly significant correlation between the levels of anti-*Malassezia* IgE and IgE reacting with *C. albicans* (51). The higher avidity of the former suggests that these anti-yeast IgE antibodies in AD result from sensitization to *Malassezia* and cross-react with *C. albicans*. Taken together, the presence of inflammatory skin lesions that allow a continuous exposure to these allergens

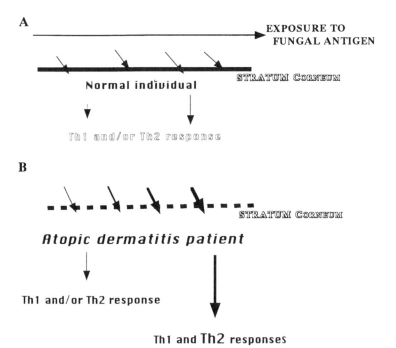

Figure 3 Immune responses to fungal allergens. (A) A normal healthy individual whose skin is covered with intact stratum corneum has little chance of being exposed to fungal allergen. Thus, he or she develops a weak Th1 and/or Th2 response according to the property of the antigenic components. (B) The skin of a patient with atopic dermatitis is covered by compromised stratum corneum, which allows easy penetration of fungal allergen. With such repeated exposure, the patient begins to show a more prominent Th2-dependent immune response than Th1-dependent reaction.

through the skin is important for the development of these types of immune reactivity.

VI. MOLD HYPERSENSITIVITY

Molds are the main components of aeroallergens. However, they seem to play a much less important role as a triggering factor in AD than *C. albicans* and *Malassezia*. In the outdoor air, *Cladosporium* and *Alternaria* are the most common in Japan. However, unlike skin microflora, their number greatly changes in the indoor air according to the environment; e.g., *Cladosporium*, *Trichoderma*, *Al-*

ternaria, and *Rhizopus* proliferate only in a humid air, whereas *Aspergillus restrictus*, *Penicillium*, and *Eruroticum* can tolerate a dry environment and thus exist as components of house dust. Moreover, they show a conspicuous seasonal change in number, being rather high in hot and humid summers and remarkably low in cold and dry winters. The pattern of seasonal change is just the opposite of AD, which, in most cases, shows exacerbation in winter rather than in summer. Moreover, their density in the air seems to greatly vary according to the distance from the floor i.e., the lower the relative humidity, the smaller, the number of organisms. This means that their number is very low in the air surrounding the face and neck, where AD is most severe.

Airborne molds such as *Alternaria*, *Aspergillus*, and *Penicillium*, to which adult patients with bronchial asthma show relatively high immediate hypersensitivity, can be a cause in some of nonatopic adult individuals of eczematous dermatitis with recurrence or aggravation every summer (52). However, aeroallergen patch testing is of little use in the evaluation of patients with suspected nonaeroallergen allergic contact dermatitis, because the prevalence of positive patch test reactions (2%) is significantly lower in them than in AD and respiratory allergy (19%) (53). Even in AD patients, the incidence of positive patch tests is much lower than that against *C. albicans* or *Malassezia* (2).

IgE antibodies are detectable with a higher incidence in AD patients than in asthmatic or nonasthmatic control subjects. However, the difference in the prevalence as compared with that in respiratory allergy patients is not as great as demonstrated with IgE against *Malassezia* (54), probably reflecting a smaller chance of skin exposure to them than to *Malassezia*, which is part of the normal skin microflora.

Children with AD also show a higher frequency of positive patch tests to mold mix than those with mucosal allergy, but in such cases no difference is noted in immediate hypersensitivity (55).

VII. TREATMENT OF AD PATIENTS WITH FUNGUS ALLERGY

The ultimate proof of whether certain allergens contribute to the lesions of AD must be by demonstrating that their removal from the skin surface improves the skin condition. So far there is no definite evidence indicating that fungus avoidance and appropriate intervention for fungus allergy improve all AD lesions. There is controversy about the effectiveness of topical antimycotic treatment (56). However, some patients with chronic head and neck lesions definitely show improvement with systemic therapy targeting *Malassezia* or *C. albicans* (57–59). It is reasonable to try antifungal therapy, either systemic or topical, in those who have recalcitrant chronic lesions, particularly on the face and neck. In a similar fashion, fungal allergen avoidance may afford some patients greater comfort than they have achieved previously.

VIII. CONCLUDING REMARKS

Fungi, both those constituting microflora of a human body like *C. albicans* and *Malassezia* and airborne molds, contain various antigenic components such as polysaccharides (mannan) and proteins. They induce Th1- and/or Th2-dependent immune responses if they penetrate the skin. The highest incidence of cutaneous immune responses is observed against *C. albicans*, being followed by *Malassezia*. *C. albicans* allergen is a potent contact sensitizer to which most normal healthy individuals react only with delayed contact sensitivity. Such exposure through the skin easily occurs in patients with AD, whose persistently xerotic skin has cracks and many scratch wounds that provide openings even to large molecular fungal allergens. Individuals with atopic histories tend to develop IgE-mediated immune reactions against various aeroallergens, which are mostly derived from other living organisms, including fungi. However, when tested with *C. albicans* antigen, most children with AD demonstrate only delayed hypersensitivity in a fashion similar to normal individuals or those with allergic respiratory diseases. In contrast, adult patients with AD show a markedly high incidence of immediate hypersensitivity with reduced contact sensitivity. Therefore, after continual exposure to fungal allergens for a prolonged period, AD patients seem to show a shift from a Th1 to Th2 dominance of the immune response even to an allergen that will normally stimulate Th1 lymphocytes to induce contact sensitivity in most individuals (Fig. 3). Although fungal allergy in AD patients may not be the primary cause for their skin disease, it can be an aggravating factor. Thus, it is worthwhile to try antifungal therapy, either systemic or topical, in patients who have recalcitrant chronic lesions, particularly on the face and neck.

ACKNOWLEDGMENT

This study was supported by Special Coordination Funds for Promoting Science and Technology from the Science and Technology Agency, Japan.

REFERENCES

1. Tagami H, Hashimoto-Kumasaka K, Terui T. The stratum corneum as a protective biological membrane of the skin. In: Tagami H, Parrish JA, Ozawa T, eds. Skin.

Interface of a Living Tissue. Perspective for Skin Care System in the Future. Amsterdam: Elsevier, 1998, pp. 23–37.

2. Tanaka M, Aiba S, Matsumura N, Aoyama H, Tabata N, Sekita Y, Tagami H. IgE-mediated hypersensitivity and contact sensitivity to multiple environmental allergens in atopic dermatitis. Arch Dermatol 1994; 130:1393–1401.

3. Ya-Xian Z, Suetake T, Tagami H. Number of cell layers of the stratum corneum in normal skin—relationship to the anatomical location on the body, age, sex and physical parameters. Arch Dermatol Res 1999; 291:555–559.

4. Schaefer H, Redelmeier TE. Skin Barrier. Principles of Percutaneous Absorption. Basel: Karger, 1996.

5. Ring J, Darsow U, Gfesser M, Vieluf D. The 'atopy patch test' in evaluating the role of aeroallergens in atopic eczema. Int Arch Allergy Immunol 1997; 113:379–383.

6. Tagami H, Watanabe S, Ofuji S, Minami K. Trichophytin contact sensitivity in patients with dermatophytosis. Arch Dermatol 1977; 113:1409–1414.

7. Tagami H, Urano-Suehisa S, Hatchome N. Contact sensitivity to *Candida albicans*—comparative studies in man and animal (guinea-pig). Br J Dermatol 1985; 113:415–424.

8. Watanabe M, Tagami H, Horii I, Takahashi M, Kligman AM. Functional analyses of the superficial stratum corneum in atopic xerosis. Arch Dermatol 1991; 137:1689–1692.

9. Tagami H, Yoshikuni K. Interrelationship between water-barrier and reservoir functions of pathologic stratum corneum. Arch Dermatol 1985; 121:642–645.

10. Imokawa G, Abe A, Jin K, Higaki Y, Kawashima M, Hidano A. Decreased level of ceramides in stratum corneum of atopic dermatitis: an etiologic factor in atopic dry skin? J Invest Dermatol 1991; 96:523–526.

11. Matsumoto M, Umemoto N, Sugiura H, Uehara M. Difference in ceramide composition between "dry" and "normal" skin in patients with atopic dermatitis. Acta Derm Venereol 1999; 79:246–247.

12. Tanaka M, Zhen YX, Tagami H. Normal recovery of the stratum corneum barrier function following damage induced by tape stripping in patients with atopic dermatitis. Br J Dermatol 1997; 136:966–967.

13. Tabata N, Tagami H, Kligman AM. A twenty-four-hour occlusive exposure to 1% sodium lauryl sulfate induces a unique histopathologicinflammatory response in the xerotis skin of atopic dermatitis patients. Acta Derm Venereol (Stockh) 1998; 78:244–247.

14. Gfesser M, Abeck D, Rugemer J, Schreiner V, Stab F, Disch R, Ring J. The early phase of epidermal barrier regeneration is faster in patients with atopic eczema. Dermatology 1997; 195:332–336.

15. Aoyama H, Tanaka M, Hara M, Tabata N, Tagami H. Nummular eczema: An addition of senile xerosis and unique cutaneous reactivities to environmental aeroallergens. Dermatology 1999; 199(2):135–139.

16. Fisher AA. Contact Dermatitis. Philadelphia: Lea & Febinger, 1986.

17. Tagami H, Watanabe S, Ofuji S. Trichophytin contact sensitivity in guinea pigs with experimental dermatophytosis induced by a new inoculation method. J Invest Dermatol 1973; 61:237–241.

18. Tagami H. Epidermal cell proliferation in guinea pigs with experimental dermato-
     phytosis. J Invest Dermatol 1985; 85:153–155.
19. Marples MJ. The Ecology of the Human Skin. Springfield, IL: Charles C Thomas,
     1965.
20. Jones HE, Reinhardt JH, Rinaldi MG. Immunologic susceptibility to chronic derma-
     tophytosis. Arch Dermatol 1974; 110:213–220.
21. Jones HE, Reinhardt JH, Rinaldi MG. A clinical, mycological, and immunological
     survey for dermatophytosis. Arch Dermatol 1973; 108:61–65.
22. Hanifin JM, Ray LF, Lobitz WC Jr. immunologicalreactivity in dermatophysosis.
     Br J Dermatol 1974; 110:213–220.
23. Hay RJ, Brostoff J. Immune responses in patients with chronic *Trichophyton rubrum*
     infections. Clin Exp Dermatol 1977; 2:373–380.
24. Kitagaki H, Fujisawa S, Watanabe K, Hayakawa K, Shiohara T. Immediate-type
     hypersensitivity response followed by a late reaction is induced by repeated epicuta-
     neous application of contact sensitizing agents in mice. J Invest Dermatol 1995; 105:
     749–755.
25. Terui T, Sano K, Okada M, Shirota H, Honda M, Ozawa M, Hirasawa N, Tamura G,
     Tagami H. Production and pharmacologic modulation of the granulocyte-associated
     allergic responses to ovalbumin in murine skin models induced by injecting
     ovalbumin-specific Th1 or Th2 cells. J Invest Dermatol 2001; 117:236–243.
26. Matsumura N, Aiba S, Tanaka M, Aoyama H, Tabata N, Tamura G, Tagami H.
     Comparison of immune reactivity profiles against various environmental allergens
     between adult patients with atopic dermatitis and patients with allergic respiratory
     diseases. Acta Derm Venereol (Stockh) 1997; 77:388–391.
27. Morita E, Hide M, Yoneya Y, Kannbe M, Tanaka A, Yamamoto S. An assessment
     of the role of *Candida albicans* antigen in atopic dermatitis. J Dermatol 1999; 26:
     282–287.
28. Tanaka M, Aiba S, Takahashi K, Tagami H. Reduced proliferative responses of
     peripheral blood mononuclear cells specifically to *Candida albicans* antigen in pa-
     tients with atopic dermatitis—comparison with their normal reactivity to bacterial
     superantigens. Arch Dermatol Res 1996; 288:495–459.
29. Munoz AI, Limbert D. Skin reactivity to *Candida* and streptokinase-streptodornase
     antigens in normal pediatric subjects: influence of age and acutte illness. J Pediatr
     1977; 91:565–568.
30. Kimura M, Tsuruta S, Yoshida T. Measurement of *Candida*-specific lymphocyte
     proliferation by flow cytometry in children with atopic dermatitis. Jpn J Allergol
     1998; 47:449–456 (in Japanese).
31. Kimura M, Tsuruta S, Yoshida T. Differences in cytokine production by peripheral
     blood mononuclear cells (PBMC) between patients with atopic dermatitis and bron-
     chial asthma. Clin Exp Immunol 1999; 118:192–196.
32. Kawamura MS, Aiba S, Tagami H: The importance of CD54 and CD86 costimula-
     tion in T cells stimulated with *Candida albicans* and *Dermatophagoides farinae*
     antigens in patients with atopic dermatitis. Arch Dermatol Res 1998; 290:603–609.
33. Henseler T, Tausch I. Mykosen bei Patienten mit Psoriasis oder atopischer Derma-
     titis. Mycosen 1997; 40(suppl 1):22–28.
34. Seebacher Cl. *Candida* in der Dermatologie. Mycoses 1999; 42(suppl 1):63–67.

35. Savolainen J, Lammintausta K, Kalimo K, Viander M. *Candida albicans* and atopic dermatitis. Clin Exp Allergy. 1993; 23:332–339.

36. Schempp CM, Effinger T, Czech W, Krutmann J, Simon JC, Schopf E. Charakterisierung von Non-Respondern bei der hochdosierten UVA1-Therapie der akut exazerbierten Atopischen Dermatitis. Hautarzt 1997; 48:94–99.

37. Akiyama K, Shida T, Yasueda H, Mita H, Yanagihara Y, Hasegawa M, Maeda Y, Yamamoto T, Takesako K, Yamaguchi H. Allergenicity of acid protease secreted by *Candida albicans*. Allergy 1996; 51:887–892.

38. Akiyama K, Shida T, Yasueda H, Saito A, Hasegawa M, Maeda Y, Takesako K, Yamaguchi H, Kato H. Assay for detecting IgE and IgG antigodies against *Candida albicans* cell-wall mannan. Allergy 1998; 153:173–179.

39. Lintu P, Savolainen J, Kalimo K, Kortekangas-Savolainen O, Nermes M, Terho EO. Cross-reacting IgE and IgG antibodies to *Pityrosporum ovale* mannan and other yeasts in atopic dermatitis. Allergy 1999; 54:1067–1073.

40. Nissen D, Petersen LJ, Esch R, Svejgaard E, Skov PS, Poulsen LK, Nolte H. IgE-sensitization to cellular and culture filtrates of fungal extracts in patients with atopic dermatitis. Ann Allergy Asthma Immunol 1998; 81:247–255.

41. Savolainen J, Kosonen J, Lintu P, Viander M, Pene J, Kalimo K, Terho EO, Bousquet J. *Candida albicans* mannan- and protein-induced humoral, cellular and cytokine responses in atopic dermatitis patients. Clin Exp Allergy 1999; 29:824–831.

42. Terui T, Rokugo M, Kato T, Tagami H. Analysis of the proinflammatory property of epidermal cyst contents: chemotactic C5a anaphylatoxin generation. Arch Dermatol Res 1989; 281:31–34.

43. Yoshimura T, Kudoh K, Aiba S, Tagami H. Antiinflammatory effects of topical ketoconazole for the inflammation induced on the skin of hairless guinea-pigs by repeated applications of heat-killed spores of *Malassezia furfur*. A comparative study with hydrocortisone 17-butyrate. J Dermatol Treatment 1995; 6:113–116.

44. Rokugo M, Tagami H, Usuba Y, Tomita Y. Contact sensitivity to *Pityrosporum ovale* in patients with atopic dermatitis. Arch Dermatol 1990; 126:627–632.

45. Kieffer M, Bergbrant IM, Faergemann J, Jemec GB, Ottevanger V, Stahl Skov P, Svejgaard E. Immune reactions to *Pityrosporum ovale* in adult patients with atopic and seborrheic dermatitis. J Am Acad Dermatol 1990; 22:739–742.

46. Tengvall-Linder M, Johansson C, Scheynius A, Wahlgren C. Positive atopy patch test reactions to Pityrosporum orbiculare in atopic dermatitis patients. Clin Exp Allergy 2000; 30:122–131.

47. Broberg A: Pityrosporum ovale in healthy children, infantile seborrhoeic dermatitis and atopic dermatitis. Acta Derm Venereol (Stockh) 1995; Suppl 191:1–47.

48. Lindgren L, Wahlgren CF, Johansson SG, Wklund I, Nordvall SI. Occurrence and clinical features of sensitization to *Pityrosporum orbiculare* and other allergens in children with atopic dermatitis. Acta Derm Venereol (Stockh) 1995; 75:300–304.

49. Lintu P, Savolainen J, Kalimo K. IgE antibodies to protein and mannan antigens of *Pityrosporum ovale* in atopic dermatitis patients. Clin Exp Allergy 1997; 27: 87–95.

50. Onishi Y, Kuroda M, Yasueda H, Saito A, Sono-Koyama E, Tunasawa S, Hashida-Okada T, Yagihara T, Uchida K, Yamaguchi H, Akiyama K, Kato I, Takesako K. Two-dimensional electrophoresis of *Malassezia allergens* for atopic dermatitis and

isolation of Maal f 4 homologs with mitochondrial malate dehydrogenase. Eur J Biochem 1999; 261:148–154.

51. Doekes G, van leperen van Dijk AG. Allergens of *Pityrosporum ovale* and *Candida albicans*. I. Cross- reacivity of IgE-binding components. Allergy 1993; 48:391–393.

52. Fujisawa S, So Y, Ofuji S. Eczematous dermatitis produced by airborne molds. Arch Dermatol 1966; 94:413–420.

53. Whitmore SE, Shererts EF, Belsito DV, Maibach HI, Nethrcott JR. Aeroallergen patch testing for patients presenting to contact dermatitis clinics. J Am Acad Dermatol 1996; 35:700–704.

54. Scalabrin DM, Bavbek S, Perzanowski MS, Wilson BB, Platts-Mills TA, Wheatley LM. Use of specific IgE in assessing the relevance of fungal and dust mite allergens to atopic dermatitis: a comparison with asthmatic and nonasthmatic control subjects. J Allergy Clin Immunol 1999; 104:1273–1279.

55. Wananukul S, Huiprasert P, Pongprasit P. Eczematous skin reaction from patch testing with aeroallergens in atopic children with and without atopic dermatitis. Pediatr Dermatol 1993; 10:209–213.

56. Broberg A, Faergemann J: Topical antimycotic treatment of atopic dermatitis in the head/neck area. A double-blind randomised study. Acta Derm Venereol (Stockh) 1995; 75:46–49.

57. Back O, Scheynius A, Johansson SG: Ketoconazolein atopic dermatitis: therapeutic response is correlated with decrease in serum IgE. Arch Dermatol Res 1995; 287: 448–451.

58. Adachi A, Horikawa T, Ichihashi M, Takashima T, Komura A. Role of *Candida* allergen in atopic dermatitis and efficacy of oral therapy with various antifungal agents. Jpn J Allergol 1999; 48:719–725 (in Japanese).

59. Hiruma M, Maeng DJ, Kobayashi M, Suto H, Ogawa H. Fungi and atopic dermatitis. Jpn J Med Mycol 1999; 40:79–83 (in Japanese).

21

Allergy Diagnosis in Atopic Eczema with the Atopy Patch Test

Ulf G. Darsow and Johannes Ring
Technical University Munich, Munich, Germany

I. INTRODUCTION

Atopic eczema (AE), or atopic dermatitis, is an inflammatory, chronically relapsing skin disease with a high prevalence of 2–5% (in children and young adults about 10%) (1–3). The discussion on the pathophysiology of AE is mirrored by the different names it has been given, such as prurigo Besnier, neurodermatitis, endogenous eczema, and *neurodermitis constitutionalis siva atopica*. Atopy is a very common finding in patients with this disease and their families (3–5). Atopy is defined as a familial tendency towards the development of certain diseases (extrinsic bronchial asthma, allergic rhinoconjunctivitis, and/or atopic eczema) based on a hypersensitivity of skin and mucous membranes against environmental substances. This is associated with elevated IgE production and/or altered unspecific reactivity (6,7). AE is also clinically defined by a typically age-related distribution and morphology (1,4,8,9).

The increased production of IgE is a result of an impaired balance of the CD4-positive T-helper-cell populations Th1 and Th2 with a predominance of interleukin (IL)-4 and IL-13 producing Th2 cells (10–14). IL-4 induces IgE synthesis (13,15) and inhibits the production of interferon (IFN)-γ on the level of transcription (15). The inflammatory infiltrate of AE lesions consists to a large proportion of T-helper cells. This concept is described elsewhere in this volume in more detail. AE is a multifactorial disease with a large number of individually different trigger factors (16–19). With regard to the Th2-driven immunopathophysiology in AE and other atopic diseases and the known epidermal barrier function disturbance in AE (20), a clinical fact seems to be of special interest: some patients with AE report exacerbations of their skin lesions after contact with certain aeroallergens like house dust mite, pollen, or animal dander. Appropriate avoidance strategies, on the other hand, often improve the course of AE (21–25). Aeroallergens, among other environmental influences, can play an important role as a trigger factor of AE (26,27). Thus, the identification of an allergic flare caused by aeroallergen contact is not only of theoretical, but also of essential practical significance for the patient. In such a case, a full remission of AE can only be expected when the *relevant* allergen is avoided. As in classical contact eczema diagnosis, in which the patch test is established to evaluate the specific cellular reaction of a contact allergy (28–30), it should be possible to obtain such a diagnostic tool for aeroallergen-triggered AE.

II. PROBLEMS OF DIAGNOSIS OF ALLERGIES IN ATOPIC ECZEMA

IgE-mediated sensitizations are usually diagnosed by determination of specific serum IgE and skin tests, which are read after 20 minutes: skin prick test or intracutaneous injections of allergen solutions (6,29). However, the mostly multiple sensitizations in AE remain often unclear with regard to their clinical relevance. Also, wheal-and-flare skin test reactions are neither intended to simulate the clinical picture of eczema, nor do they depict the appropriate dimension of skin immune system. In 1937 Rostenberg und Sulzberger (31) described a total of 12,000 patch tests with a wide variety of allergens, including aeroallergens in different patient groups. A patch test with aeroallergens especially for AE patients was first published 1982 by Mitchell et al. (32). Some groups tried to reproduce their results with different methodological approaches (27,33–41). Stratum corneum abrasion (32,42,43), tape stripping of the uppermost skin layer (44–46), and addition of sodiumlaurylsulfate (47) were used to enhance allergen penetration. Studies of aeroallergen patch testing on untreated, nonabraded skin were an exception (48). Accordingly, the number of positive reactions in these experimental systems varied (15–100%). This was also due to differences in allergen content of the used allergen preparations. Moreover, the physical measures to enhance allergen penetration may have irritative effects and hamper the reading of the test reactions. An atopy patch test (APT) study from our group with aqueous skin prick test preparations showed 30% positive reactions but no clear correlation with history or the classical tests of IgE-mediated hypersensitivity (skin prick test and specific IgE in the CAP-RAST) (48). Thus, controversy remained about the clinical utility of the APT.

Due to the position of the epicutaneous patch testing of immediate-type allergens between the classical reaction type I and type IV (Coombs and Gell), the term ''atopy patch test'' was proposed with the following definition: an epicutaneous patch test with allergens known to elicit IgE-mediated reactions, and the evaluation of eczematous skin lesions (49,50).

The aim of the atopy patch test is the identification of the patient group suffering from aeroallergen-induced AE flares. Due to the high molecular structure of used allergens, clear test results require an optimized galenic preparation. Irritation of the atopic skin should be avoided. If an allergen can elicit eczema exacerbations locally by direct skin penetration, the penetration enhancers formerly used should theoretically be not necessary. The allergen panel has to be fitted to the most common sensitizations in AE patients. Finally, for practical purposes the APT methods should resemble those of the patch test for classical (type IV) contact allergy. We investigated methodological aspects and clinical covariates of the APT in order to obtain a test for clinical use.

III. APT MATERIALS AND METHODS

We performed APT studies with allergen lyophilisates from house dust mite (*Dermatophagoides pteronyssinus*), cat dander, and grass pollen. Later, birch and mugwort pollen were also included. Lyophilisates were provided by Allergopharma (Reinbek, Germany) and preparations for testing according to our study plans were made by Hermal (Reinbek, Germany). Petrolatum and hydrogel (methylcellulose) vehicles were compared. Allergen dose varied between 500 and 10,000 protein nitrogen units (PNU) per gram in different trials. The studies with PNU-based preparations were sustained by a trial using biologically standardized (200 IR/g) extracts by Stallergénes (Antony, France), (Fig. 1).

The test substances were applied in large Finn chambers (12 mm diameter) on clinically uninvolved, nonabraded, and untreated back skin. In control areas, vehicles without allergens were tested. A 0.5% solution of sodium lauryl sulfate was simultaneously tested as an irritative model. Results were evaluated after 48 and 72 hours. Grading of positive APT reactions resembled the criteria used in conventional contact allergy patch testing (ICDRG rules, 28–30). All APT studies were performed after discontinuation of antihistamines and systemic and topical (test area) steroids for at least 7 days.

APT with 1,000 and 10,000 PNU/g of the most common allergens in petrolatum and hydrogel were compared in 36 patients with atopic eczema in a pilot method trial (51). After 48 hours the reactions of 17 patients were graded as clear-cut positive. Allergens in petrolatum elicited twice as many APT reactions as allergens in hydrogel vehicle. Also, the higher allergen concentration increased the reactivity to APT significantly, as previously shown by others (46). Thirty-six percent of patients reacted to house dust mite (*D. pter.*), 22% to cat dander, and 16% to grass pollen. Ten nonatopic controls and 4 patients suffering from allergic rhinoconjunctivitis only were also tested and showed no positive APT reactions. Irritant sodium lauryl sulfate reactions (33% of patients), clinically distinguishable from APT by their clear-cut limitation to the Finn chambers, were not correlated with APT reactivity. Thus, allergen penetration without previous alteration of the skin barrier was shown to occur in patients with AE, but not in controls. The use of lipophilic petrolatum vehicles, initially not expected to give better results, is now widely accepted for APT systems and has since been standard in our further investigations.

Suitable allergen concentrations for the APT were obtained in a dose-response double-blind multicenter study involving 253 adult patients and 30 children with atopic eczema (52,53) (Table 1). This study investigated the important allergen concentration range from 5,000 to 10,000 PNU/g. The allergen dose with the most clear-cut results (positive or negative) could be determined for the most frequent aeroallergens—house dust mite, cat dander, and grass pollen—by means of a two-step McNemar-statistics. For *D. pter.* and cat dander, 5000–7000 PNU/g gave the best results. Grass pollen may be tested with 5000 PNU/g. For children, lower allergen doses seem possible (53). The allergen doses of 7000 PNU/g and 200 IR/g (biological unit) showed comparable concordance with the patients clinical history as a substitute for clinical relevance (Table 2).

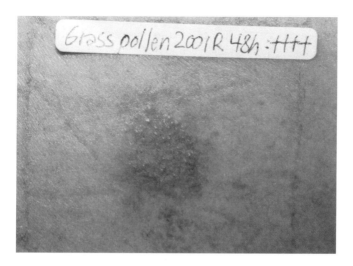

Figure 1 APT with grass pollen in a patient with atopic eczema: eczematous reaction after 48 hours.

Table 1 Clinical Covariates of the APT in a Randomized, Double-Blind Multicenter Trial

	Skin prick		sIgE		APT		History	
	C	A	C	A	C	A	C	A
D. pter.	67%	59%	40%	56%	41%	34%	30%	52%
Cat dander	43%	54%	43%	49%	17%	12%	23%	23%
Grass pollen	57%	65%	57%	75%	15%	18%	20%	33%
Birch pollen (*n* = 88)	n.d.	65%	n.d.	65%	n.d.	11%	n.d.	13%

A: Adults 15–63 y; *n* = 253, 3,000–10,000 PNU/g.
C: Children 5–14 y; *n* = 30, 300–5,000 PNU/g.
sIgE, Specific IgE; APT, atopy patch test; history, aeroallergen-specific history of eczema flares after allergen contact; *D. pter.*, *Dermatophagoides pteronyssinus* (house dust mite); PNU, protein nitrogen units.
Source: Data from Refs. 52, 53.

Table 2 Comparison of Biological and PNU-Based Standardization of APT Preparations

Standardization:	7000 PNU/g		200 IR/g	
Corresponding history:	yes	no	yes	no
D. pter., n	25	25	31	19
Cat dander, n	36	14	37	13
Grass pollen, n	39	11	39	11
Birch pollen, n	41	9	38	12
Total, %	71	29	73	27

400 APT in $n = 50$ patients with atopic eczema.
PNU, Protein nitrogen units; IR, reactivity index (biological unit: skin prick test with 100 IR elicits mean 7 mm wheal diameter in sensitized patients). Both standardizations show comparable concordance of APT with clinical allergen-specific history.

IV. PATIENTS WITH HIGHER APT REACTIVITY

A clinical picture resembling airborne contact dermatitis may also be predictive in patients with AE. According to their eczema pattern, 57 patients were divided into two subgroups (54). Group I ($n = 26$) patients had eczematous skin lesions predominantly on air-exposed areas: hands, lower arms, head and neck area, and ankles. In group II, 31 patients were compared as a control group without a conspicuous distribution of skin lesions. APT were applied in four concentrations from 500 to 10,000 PNU/g. In 53% of patients, at least one APT reaction was graded as clear-cut positive. The percentage of patients with clear-cut positive reactions was significantly higher in group I patients with eczematous skin lesions predominantly in air-exposed areas (69%) compared with group II (39%; $p = 0.02$). A clear dose-response relationship between allergen concentration and number of patients with a positive APT result was obtained in both groups. Also, in the same patient exposed to an allergen, the strength of reaction typically increased with the allergen concentration in a dose-dependent manner. However, the mode of this dose-dependent increase in positive results in group I differed significantly from group II ($p = 0.03$). Both groups were best differentiated with 5000 PNU/g. In group I, the last concentration step doubling allergen concentration to 10,000 PNU/g increased APT reactivity only in 11%. The effect was independent from reaction intensity or kind of allergen. It was corroborated for grass pollen and cat dander in other studies (52,55). The results of this study confirmed that aeroallergens are able to elicit eczematous skin lesions in a dose-dependent way in different groups of patients with atopic eczema when applied epicutaneously. Patients with a predictive history of eczema flares after contact with a specific allergen also show significantly more often positive APT reactions to this allergen (see below).

V. APT AND CLASSICAL TESTS OF IgE-MEDIATED SENSITIZATION

In all studies, the frequency of positive APT was lower than the numbers of positive skin prick tests or radioallergosorbent tests in the investigated patient group, but the individually positive APT allergen pattern of the patients varied with their skin prick test and specific IgE results. Of patients with *D. pter.*-positive APT, 62% showed a corresponding positive skin prick test and 77% a corresponding elevated specific IgE. This results in allergen-specific concordance of 0.53 (skin prick) and 0.69 (specific IgE). For APT with cat allergen the concordance is 0.5 for skin prick and 0.67 for specific IgE; in grass pollen APT concordances of 0.39 (skin prick) and 0.42 (specific IgE) were observed (51).

The results of the larger German multicenter study are shown in Table 1 (percentages calculated with regard to *n*, including patients with questionable results and 10 dropouts). Patients were tested with *D. pter.*, cat dander, grass pollen, and in two study centers ($n = 88$) with birch pollen and mugwort pollen (data not shown) in petrolatum. APT reading was done 48 and 72 hours after application and after obtaining skin prick tests and specific serum IgE determination and a detailed history on aeroallergen-induced eczema flares. Cross-table analysis and logistic regression revealed significant concordances of APT results with history, skin prick test, and specific corresponding IgE for *D. pter.*, cat dander, and grass pollen ($p < 0.001$). However, the results also showed that high allergen-specific IgE in serum is not mandatory for a positive atopy patch test,

Table 3 Cross-Tabulation of Atopy Patch Test and Specific IgE (CAP) Results in a Multicenter Study

	CAP 0	CAP pos.	Total
APT neg.	49	29	78
APT pos.	13	60	73
Total	62	89	151

Fisher's exact test, $p < 0.00001$.
APT 48 h results in adult patients: house dust mite *D. pter.*
APT and specific IgE are significantly associated. In 18% of patients with clear-cut positive APT, no specific IgE to the corresponding aeroallergen was detected.
Source: Data from Ref. 52.

and the same holds true for the correlation with skin prick tests. An example is given in Table 3. One may conclude that the APT may give further diagnostic information in addition to a patient's history and classical tests of IgE-mediated hypersensitivity. On the other hand, a role for IgE in the reaction mechanism of APT is suggested, since in most APT-positive patients elevated specific IgE was found compared to those with negative APT.

VI. CLINICAL RELEVANCE AND ALLERGEN-SPECIFICITY OF APT

A prospectively obtained history of allergen-induced eczema exacerbation can be used as proof of clinical relevance of an allergy test result. The phenomenon of "summer eruption" of AE is well known. About one third of AE patients report eczema flares during spring and summer, the pollen seasons of birch and grass (5). Also, according to our results, one third of patients with specific IgE to grass pollen develop a positive APT result to this allergen (52). We tested 79 patients with an APT with 10,000 PNU/g grass pollen allergen mixture (*Holcus lanatus*, *Dactylis glomerata*, *Lolium perenne*, *Phleum pratense*, *Poa pratensis*, and *Festuca pratensis*) in petrolatum and simultaneously with 10 mg dry unprocessed pollen of *Dactylis glomerata* grass (55). Again, the APT results were compared with history, skin prick tests, specific corresponding IgE, and the eczema pattern. In this study, significantly higher frequencies of positive APT with both methods were seen in patients with corresponding history of exacerbation of their eczema in the summer months of the previous year and/or in direct contact with grass (12 of 79 patients; 75% had positive APT) compared to patients without this history (67 of 79; 16% had positive APT; $p < 0.001$). There was also a significant concordance of standardized and unprocessed grass pollen APT. The standardized allergen mixture also correlated with eczema pattern, skin prick, and specific IgE ($p < 0.01$). The fact that unprocessed pollen elicited eczematous skin reactions on nonpretreated skin of atopic eczema patients (in healthy and rhinoconjunctivitis controls, no positive reactions were observed) with good correlation to history suggests that pollen are involved in eczema flares in some patients. When comparing such calculations for seasonal pollen allergens with the most frequent allergen eliciting APT reactions, house dust mite, one has to keep in mind that a history on "house dust–elicited eczema flares" is by far more difficult to obtain.

In the German multicenter study, 13–52% of the 253 adult patients reported previous eczema flares after contact with specific allergen (Table 1). APT results of *D. pter.*, cat dander, and grass pollen were statistically significantly associated with clinical history in chi^2- and logistic regression analysis ($p < 0.001$; birch pollen, $p = 0.1$). The association of clinical history and APT was a starting point to calculate comparative sensitivity and specificity of the classical and new tests.

Table 4 Sensitivity and Specificity of Different Diagnostic Methods with Regard to Patient History in Two Studies with AE Patients

Test	Sensitivity[a] (%)	Specificity[a] (%)
Multicenter study $n = 253$, 3 allergens		
Skin prick	69–82	44–53
RAST	65–94	42–64
APT	42–56	69–92
Single center study $n = 79$; allergen: grass pollen		
Skin prick	100	33
RAST	92	33
APT	75	84

APT shows a higher specificity but lower sensitivity compared to skin prick test and measurement of specific IgE. For the APT, better results are obtained with a seasonal allergen.
[a] Referring to predictive history of eczema exacerbations in pollen season or in direct contact with allergen, excluding questionable cases, depending on allergen.
Source: Data from Refs. 52, 55.

The APT showed a higher specificity (depending on allergen) with regard to clinical relevance of an allergen as compared to skin prick test and specific IgE, but also under certain conditions lower sensitivity (sensitivity and specificity from both studies are given in Table 4).

Evidence for the allergen-specificity of APT reactions also comes from the association with specific IgE and the patients individual skin prick test results. As shown above, this association is significant, but far from 100% (Table 3). In a subgroup of our patients in the multicenter trial, specific activation of T cells in peripheral blood was compared with the patient's APT result. Also, specific lymphocyte proliferation was investigated in these patients (56). Positive APT reactions were significantly more frequent in patients with elevated CD 54+ or CD 30+ T cells after in vitro stimulation with the corresponding allergen. In addition, positive APT were associated with an allergen-specific lymphocyte proliferation ($p < 0.001$). These findings argue against the interpretation of APT results as irritative or nonspecific. There was no correlation of APT reactivity and eczema severity (SCORAD) (57) in these AE patients (56).

VII. IgE AND LANGERHANS CELLS IN AE AND APT

Langerhans cells bind and present allergens, which penetrate the impaired epidermal barrier in atopic eczema patients. The role of IgE in antigen presentation was shown by the group of Stingl (58). This concept, described elsewhere in this volume in more detail, is derived from studies showing IgE and IgE-binding structures on the surface of epidermal Langerhans cells (59–62) together with mite allergen (63). From APT biopsies, allergen-specific T cells have been cloned. These T cells showed a characteristic Th2 secretion pattern initially, whereas after 48 hours a Th1 pattern as seen in chronic AE lesions was predominant (64–66). Within the APT lesions, the inflammatory infiltrate is dominated by T lymphocytes with a T4:T8 ratio of 2–6:1 and, to a lesser degree, of Langerhans and indeterminate T6+ cells, when immunostaining is performed (37). A similar situation is found in natural lesions of atopic eczema characterized also by a predominance of CD4+ T cells (11). Other cell populations may also be involved in the initiation and perpetuation of APT reactions. Among these are basophils, present in the infiltrate after 48 hours (32), and activated eosinophils (44).

VIII. ROLE OF APT IN DIAGNOSIS IN AE PATIENTS

The described APT methodology was evaluated in a large group of patients with AE. For patients with aeroallergen-triggered disease, this test may provide an important diagnostic tool. At least in a subgroup of patients with AE, IgE-dependent allergic reactions elicited by the transdermal route play a pathophysiological role. This underscores the importance of appropriate allergy diagnosis in AE. As for bronchial asthma and rhinoconjunctivitis, the results of our studies sustain Wüthrich's concept of extrinsic/allergic versus intrinsic/cryptogenic atopic eczema with a heterogeneity of disease subgroups. From this point of view, the APT is a provocation test of the skin in analogy to the specific provocation methods in respiratory atopy. Some evidence for the practical relevance of positive APT reactions may be drawn from an early report on 18 patients by Clark and Adinoff (27,33). These authors described a positive experimental APT reaction in combination with a detection of specific IgE antibodies in skin prick tests associated with aeroallergens they identified in the patients' environment.

Questions remain concerning the clinical relevance of positive APT results in patients with a negative history and negative skin prick tests or RAST, since no gold standard exists for the provocation of eczematous skin lesions in aeroallergen-triggered atopic eczema. These questions may only be answered by controlled studies using specific provocation and elimination procedures in patients with positive and negative APT results. The final scientific proof for the relevance of aeroallergens identified by positive APT reactions for the management of the atopic eczema in the identified patients is still missing, but appropriate allergen specific avoidance strategies (21,22,24,67,68) are recommended in patients showing positive APT reactions. The diagnostic validity of APT in routine diagnosis of aeroallergen-triggered atopic eczema is investigated in ongoing controlled studies. We are currently coordinating a European multicenter study with biologically standardized APT extracts of the European Task Force on Atopic Dermatitis (ETFAD). Standardization of major allergen content is an important goal for the future. Meetings of most groups performing APT for clinical use in Europe were held on April 11, 1997, and June 30, 1998, in Munich. One result of these meetings is a consensus APT reading key for describing the intensity of APT reactions, which will be further evaluated. The European multicenter trial also deals with the investigation of food allergen patch testing. Further aeroallergens of regional significance are to be standardized. With the ongoing studies, a test for the clinical relevance of an aeroallergen sensitization that can be applied in the allergist's practice may evolve. The identified subgroup of patients may profit extraordinarily from allergen avoidance. More controversially, the APT may also prove valuable in selecting patients for specific immunotherapy.

IX. SUMMARY AND CONCLUSIONS

Aeroallergens are relevant eliciting factors of atopic eczema. The atopy patch test is an epicutaneous patch test with allergens known to elicit IgE-mediated reactions used to evaluate eczematous skin lesions. It can be used for the diagnosis in atopic eczema patients with suspected allergy to aeroallergens like house dust mite, cat dander, or pollen. The atopy patch test gave the most specific results with regard to clinical history as compared to the classical skin prick and radioallergosorbent tests.

REFERENCES

1. Hanifin JM, Rajka G. Diagnostic features of atopic dermatitis. Acta Derm Venereol (Stockh) 1980; 114:146–148.
2. Hanifin JM. Clinical and basic aspects of atopic dermatitis. Semin Dermatol 1983; 2:5.
3. Leung DYM, Rhodes AR, Geha RS, Schneider LC, Ring J. Atopic dermatitis (atopic eczema). In: Fitzpatrick TB, Eisen AZ, Wolff K, Freedberg IM, Austen KF, eds. Dermatology in General Medicine, 4th ed. New York: McGraw-Hill, 1993, pp. 1543–1563.
4. Jones HE, Inouye JC, McGerity JL, Lewis CW. Atopic disease and serum immunoglobulin-E. Br J Dermatol 1975; 92:17–25.
5. Rajka G. Essential Aspects of Atopic Dermatitis. Berlin: Springer, 1989.
6. Ring J. Angewandte Allergologie, 2d ed. München: MMV Medizin Verlag, 1995.
7. Ring J. Atopy: condition, disease, or syndrome? In: Ruzicka T, Ring J, Przybilla B, eds. Handbook of Atopic Eczema. Berlin: Springer, 1991, pp. 3–8.

8. Meneghini CL, Bonifazi E. Correlation between clinical and immunological findings in atopic dermatitis. Acta Derm Venereol (Stockh) 1985; 114:140–142.

9. Wüthrich B. Minimal forms of atopic eczema. In: Ruzicka T, Ring J, Przybilla B, eds. Handbook of Atopic Eczema. Berlin: Springer, 1991, pp. 46–53.

10. Grewe M, Gyufko K, Schöpf E, Krutmann J. Lesional expression of interferon-gamma in atopic eczema. Lancet 1994; I:25–26.

11. Leung DYM, Ghan AK, Schneeberger EE, Geha RS. Characterization of the mononuclear cell infiltrate in atopic dermatitis using mononuclear antibodies. J Allergy Clin Immunol 1983; 71:47–56.

12. Ohmen JD, Hanifin JM, Nickoloff BJ, Rea TH, Wyzykowski R, Kim J, Jullien D, McHugh T, Nassif AS, Chan SC. Overexpression of IL-10 in atopic dermatitis. Contrasting cytokine patterns with delayed-type hypersensitivity reactions. J Immunol 1995; 154:1956–1963.

13. Renz H, Jujo K, Bradley K, et al. Enhanced IL-4 production and IL-4 receptor expression in atopic dermatitis and their modulation by interferon-gamma. J Invest Dermatol 1992; 99:403–408.

14. Sowden J, Powell R, Allen B. Selective activation of circulating CD4+ lymphocytes in severe adult atopic dermatitis. Br J Dermatol 1992; 127:228–232.

15. Vercelli D, Jabara H, Lauener R, Geha R. IL-4 inhibits the synthesis of INF-gamma and induces the synthesis of IgE in human mixed lymphocyte cultures. J Immunol 1990; 144:570–573.

16. Morren MA, Przybilla B, Bamelis M, et al. Atopic dermatitis: triggering factors. J Am Acad Dermatol 1994; 31:467–473.

17. Przybilla B, Ring J. Food allergy and atopic eczema. Semin Dermatol 1990; 9:220–225.

18. Skov L, Baadsgaard O. Ultraviolet B-exposed major histocompatibility complex class II positive keratinocytes and antigen-presenting cells demonstrate a differential capacity to activate T cells in the presence of staphylococcal superantigens. Br J Dermatol 1996; 134:824–830.

19. Van Bever HP, Docx M, Stevens WJ. Food and food additives in severe atopic dermatitis. Allergy 1989; 44:588–594.

20. Schäfer L, Kragballe K. Abnormalities in epidermal lipid metabolism in patients with atopic dermatitis. J Invest Dermatol 1991; 96:10–15.

21. Fukuda H, Imayama S, Okada T. Mite-free room (MFR) for the management of atopic dermatitis. Jpn J Allergol 1991; 40:626–632.

22. Ring J, Brockow K, Abeck D. The therapeutic concept of "patient management" in atopic eczema. Allergy 1996; 51:206–215.

23. Sanda T, Yasue T, Oohashi M, Yasue A. Effectiveness of house dust-mite allergen avoidance with atopic dermatitis. J Allergy Clin Immunol 1992; 89:653–657.

24. Tan B, Weald D, Strickland I, Friedman P. Double-blind controlled trial of effect of housedust-mite allergen avoidance on atopic dermatitis. Lancet 1996; 347:15–18.

25. Tupker R, DeMonchy J, Coenraads P, Homan A, van der Meer J. Induction of atopic dermatitis by inhalation of house dust mite. J Allergy Clin Immunol 1996; 97:1064–1070.

26. Barnetson RSTC, MacFarlane HAF, Benton EC. House dust mite allergy and atopic eczema: a case report. Br J Dermatol 1987; 116:857–860.

27. Clark R, Adinoff A. Aeroallergen contact can exacerbate atopic dermatitis: patch test as a diagnostic tool. J Am Acad Dermatol 1989; 21:863–869.

28. Andersen KE, Benezra C, Burrows D, et al. The European environmental and contact dermatitis research group: contact dermatitis a review. Contact Dermatitis 1987; 16: 55–78.

29. Darsow U. Etablierte Diagnostikverfahren. In: Ring J, ed. Neurodermitis. Landsberg: Ecomed, 1998, pp. 61–73.

30. Fisher AA. Contact Dermatitis. 3rd ed. Philadelphia: Lea & Febiger, 1986, pp. 686–691.

31. Rostenberg A, Sulzberger MD. Some results of patch tests. Arch Dermatol 1937; 35:433–454.

32. Mitchell E, Chapman M, Pope F, Crow J, Jouhal S, Platts-Mills T. Basophils in allergen-induced patch test sites in atopic dermatitis. Lancet 1982; I:127–130.

33. Adinoff A, Tellez P, Clark R. Atopic dermatitis and aeroallergen contact sensitivity. J Allergy Clin Immunol 1988; 81:736–742.

34. Imayama S, Hashizuma T, Miyahara H, Tanahashi T, Takeishi M, Kubota Y, Koga T, Hori Y, Fukuda H. Combination of patch test and IgE for dust mite antigens differentiates 130 patients with atopic dermatitis into four groups. J Am Acad Dermatol 1992; 27:531–538.

35. Platts-Mills T, Mitchell E, Rowntree S, Chapman M, Wilkins S. The role of dust mite allergens in atopic dermatitis. Clin Exp Dermatol 1983; 8:233–247.

36. Reitamo S, Visa K, Kaehoenen K, Käykhö A, Lauerna I, Stubb S, Salo OP. Patch test reactions to inhalant allergens in atopic dermatitis. Acta Derm Venereol (Stockh) 1989; 144:119–121.

37. Reitamo S, Visa K, Kähönen K, Stubb S, Salo OP. Eczematous reactions in atopic patients caused by epicutaneous testing with inhalant allergens. Br J Dermatol 1986; 114:303–309.

38. Seidenari S, Manzini BM, Danese P, Giannetti A. Positive patch tests to whole mite culture and purified mite extracts in patients with atopic dermatitis, asthma and rhinitis. Ann Allergy 1992; 69:201–206.

39. Seidenari B, Manzini M, Danese P. Patch testing with pollens of Gramineae in patients with atopic dermatitis and mucosal atopy. Contact Dermatitis 1992; 27:125–126.

40. Seifert H, Wollemann G, Seifert B, Borelli S. Neurodermitis: Eine Protein-Kontaktdermatitis? Dtsch Derm 1987; 35:1204–1214.

41. Vocks E, Seifert H, Seifert B, Drosner M. Patch test with immediate type allergens in patients with atopic dermatitis. In: Ring J, Przybilla B, eds. New Trends in Allergy III. Berlin: Springer, 1991, pp. 230–233.

42. Gondo A, Saeki N, Tokuda Y. Challenge reactions in atopic dermatitis after percutaneous entry of mite antigen. Br J Dermatol 1986; 115:485–493.

43. Norris P, Schofield O, Camp R. A study of the role of house dust mite in atopic dermatitis. Br J Dermatol 1988; 118:435–440.

44. Bruijnzeel-Koomen C, van Wichen D, Spry C, Venge P, Bruynzeel P. Active participation of eosinophils in patch test reactions to inhalant allergens in patients with atopic dermatitis. Br J Dermatol 1988; 118:229–238.

45. Langeland T, Braathen L, Borch M. Studies of atopic patch tests. Acta Derm Venereol (Stockh) 1989; 144:105–109.

46. van Voorst Vader PC, Lier JG, Woest TE, Coenraads PJ, Nater JP. Patch tests with house dust mite antigens in atopic dermatitis patients: methodological problems. Acta Derm Venereol (Stockh) 1991; 71(4):301–305.

47. Tanaka Y, Anan S, Yoshida H. Immunohistochemical studies in mite antigen-induced path test sites in atopic dermatitis. J Derm Sci 1990; 1:361–368.

48. Vieluf D, Kunz B, Bieber T, Przybilla B, Ring J. "Atopy patch test" with aeroallergens in patients with atopic eczema. Allergo J 1993; 2:9–12.

49. Ring J, Bieber T, Vieluf D, Kunz B, Przybilla B. Atopic eczema, Langerhans cells and allergy. Int Arch Allergy Appl Immunol 1991; 94:194–201.

50. Ring J, Kunz B, Bieber T, Vieluf D, Przybilla B. The "atopy patch test" with aeroallergens in atopic eczema (abstr). J Allergy Clin Immunol 1989; 82:195.

51. Darsow U, Vieluf D, Ring J. Atopy patch test with different vehicles and allergen concentrations—an approach to standardization. J Allergy Clin Immunol 1995; 95: 677–684.

52. Darsow U, Vieluf D, Ring J for the APT study group. Evaluating the relevance of aeroallergen sensitization in atopic eczema with the "atopy patch test": a randomized, double-blind multicenter study. J Am Acad Dermatol 1999; 40:187–193.

53. Darsow U, Vieluf D, Berg B, Berger J, Busse A, Czech W, Heese A, Heidelbach U, Peters KP, Przybilla B, Richter G, Rueff F, Werfel T, Wistokat-Wülfing A, Ring J. Dose response study of atopy patch test in children with atopic eczema. Pediatr Asthma Allergy Immunol 1999; 13:115–122.

54. Darsow U, Vieluf D, Ring J. The atopy patch test: an increased rate of reactivity in patients who have an air-exposed pattern of atopic eczema. Br J Dermatol 1996; 135:182–186.

55. Darsow U, Behrendt H, Ring J. Gramineae pollen as trigger factors of atopic eczema: evaluation of diagnostic measures using the atopy patch test. Br J Dermatol 1997; 137:201–207.

56. Wistokat-Wülfing A, Schmidt P, Darsow U, Ring J, Kapp A, Werfel T. Atopy patch test reactions are associated with T lymphocyte-mediated allergen-specific immune responses in atopic dermatitis. Clin Exp Allergy 1999; 29:513–521.

57. European Task Force on Atopic Dermatitis. Severity scoring of atopic dermatitis: the SCORAD index. Dermatology 1993; 186:23–31.

58. Maurer D, Ebner C, Reininger B, Fiebiger E, Kraft D, Kinet JP, Stingl G. The high affinity IgE receptor mediates IgE-dependent allergen presentation. J Immunol 1995; 154:6285–6290.

59. Bieber T, de la Salle C, Wollenberg A, Hakimi J, Chizzonite R, Ring J. Constitutive expression of the high affinity receptor for IgE (FCeR1) on human Langerhans-cells. J Exp Med 1992; 175:1285–1290.

60. Bieber T, Rieger A, Neuchrist C, Prinz JC, Rieber EP, Boltz-Nitulescu G, Scheiner O, Kraft D, Ring J, Stingl G. Induction of FCeR2/CD23 on human epidermal Langerhans-cells by human recombinant IL4 and IFN. J Exp Med 1989; 170:309–314.

61. Bieber T. FCeRI on human Langerhans cells: a receptor in seach of new functions. Immunol Today 1994; 15:52–53.

62. Bruijnzeel-Koomen C, van Wichen DF, Toonstra J, Berrens L, Bruijnzeel PLB. The presence of IgE molecules on epidermal Langerhans-cells in patients with atopic dermatitis. Arch Dermatol Res 1986; 278:199–205.

63. Maeda K, Yamamoto K, Tanaka Y, Anan S, Yoshida H. House dust mite (HDM) antigen in naturally occurring lesions of atopic dermatitis (AD): the relationship between HDM antigen in the skin and HDM antigen-specific IgE antibody. J Derm Sci 1992; 3:73–77.

64. Ramb-Lindhauer CH, Feldmann A, Rotte M, Neumann CH. Characterization of grass pollen reactive T-cell lines derived from lesional atopic skin. Arch Dermatol Res 1991; 283:71–76.

65. Sager N, Feldmann A, Schilling G, Kreitsch P, Neumann C. House dust mite-specific T cells in the skin of subjects with atopic dermatitis: frequency and lymphokine profile in the allergen patch test. J Allergy Clin Immunol 1992; 89:801–810.

66. van Reijsen FC, Bruijnzeel-Koomen CAFM, Kalthoff FS, Maggi E, Romagnani S, Westland JKT, Mudde GC. Skin-derived aeroallergen-specific T-cell clones of TH2 phenotype in patients with atopic dermatitis. J Allergy Clin Immunol 1992; 90:184–192.

67. Darsow U, Abeck D, Ring J. Allergie und atopisches Ekzem: Zur Bedeutung des "Atopie-Patch-Tests." Hautarzt 1997; 48:528–535.

68. Lau S, Ehnert B, Cremer B, Nasert S, Büttner P, Czarnetzki BM, Wahn U. Häusliche Milbenallergenreduktion bei spezifisch sensibilisierten Patienten mit atopischem Ekzem. Allergo J 1995; 4:432–435.

22

Conventional Topical Treatment of Atopic Dermatitis

Mark Boguniewicz
National Jewish Medical and Research Center, and University of Colorado School of Medicine, Denver, Colorado

I. GENERAL MEASURES

Education of patients and their families is a critical component of successful management of atopic dermatitis (AD) (1). Learning about the course of AD along with exacerbating factors is important in dealing with a chronic illness. Adequate time and teaching materials are necessary to provide effective education. Most patients or parents will forget or confuse the skin care recommendations given them without written instructions. For many patients, a written step-care treatment plan will lead to improved outcomes. Patients or parents should demonstrate an appropriate level of understanding of the recommendations, and these should be adjusted and reviewed on follow-up visits. Educational brochures and videos can be obtained from the Eczema Association for Science and Education (800-818-7546 or *www.eczema-assn.org*) or the Lung Line (800 222-LUNG or *www.njc.org*). Patient-oriented support groups and updates on progress in AD research may also benefit patients.

II. IDENTIFICATION AND ELIMINATION OF EXACERBATING FACTORS

A. Irritants

Patients with AD have a lowered threshold of irritant responsiveness (2). Tabata et al. (3) showed that an abnormal stratum corneum is present even in noninvolved AD skin and is associated with increased diffusional water loss 7 days after application of a topical irritant, confirming a functional abnormality. Furthermore, the irritant was shown to induce inflammatory changes including spongiosis, perivenular mononuclear infiltrate, along with activated eosinophils. Thus, in AD, similarly to the other atopic diseases, both specific and nonspecific triggers may contribute to chronic inflammation. These studies also support the important concept that normal-appearing skin in AD is in fact abnormal. Identifying and avoiding irritants is integral to the successful management of this disease. Soaps should be used sparingly and have minimal defatting activity and a neutral pH. In one comparative study, 18 soaps and cleansers were rated for irritancy using a chamber test (4). The study rated erythema, scaling, and fissuring and found Dove® to be the mildest. Other mild cleansers available in sensitive skin formulation include Oil of Olay®. Of note, a recent double-blind study looked at whether daily bathing with an antibacterial soap would reduce the number of *Staphylococcus aureus* on the skin and result in clinical improvement of AD (5). Over a period of 9 weeks, 50 patients with moderately severe AD bathed daily with either an antimicrobial soap containing 1.5% triclocarban or a placebo soap. The antimicrobial soap regimen caused significantly greater improvement in the severity and extent of skin lesions than the placebo soap regimen, which correlated with reductions both in *S. aureus* in patients with positive cultures at baseline. Overall, daily bathing with an antibacterial soap was well tolerated, provided clinical improvement, and reduced levels of skin microorganisms. While antibacterial cleansers may reduce staphylococcal colonization, they may be too irritating for some patients with AD. Alcohol and astringents found in skin care products can be drying, and exposure to them should be minimized. New clothing should be laundered prior to wearing to remove formaldehyde and other chemicals. Residual laundry detergent in clothing may be irritating, and using a liquid rather than powder detergent and adding a second rinse cycle to facilitate removal of the detergent may be helpful. Occlusive clothing should be avoided, and open-weave, loose-fitting cotton or cotton blend garments substituted.

Temperature in the home and work environments should be temperate with moderate humidity to minimize sweating. Patients generally do better in an air-conditioned environment. Swimming is usually well tolerated; however, since pools typically are treated with chlorine or bromine, patients should shower and use a cleanser to help remove these drying chemicals afterwards, then apply a moisturizer. Sun exposure can lead to evaporation or overheating and sweating, both of which can be irritating. While ultraviolet rays in sunlight may be beneficial to some patients, photodamage can occur. Sunscreens should be used to protect the skin, and preparations made specifically for use on the face are often best tolerated by patients with AD.

B. Allergens

Clinical studies support the role of contact with aeroallergens causing exacerbations of AD (discussed in Chapter 17). Epicutaneous application of aeroallergens to uninvolved skin by patch test techniques results in eczematoid reactions in approximately 50% of aeroallergen-sensitized patients with AD (6,7). Positive reactions have been described with a number of allergens including house dust mite, pollens, animal danders, and molds. Corroborating laboratory data include the finding of specific IgE antibodies to inhalant allergens in most patients with AD. Ninety-five percent of sera from AD patients had IgE to house dust mite allergen compared with 42% of asthmatic subjects (8). The degree of sensitization to aeroallergens is directly associated with the severity of AD (9). The isolation from AD skin lesions and allergen patch test sites of T cells that recognize *Dermatophagoides pteronyssimus* (Der p 1) and other aeroallergens provides further evidence that the inflammatory response in AD can be elicited by inhalant allergens (10).

Environmental control measures aimed at decreasing dust mite load have also been shown in a double-blind controlled trial to improve AD in those patients who demonstrate specific IgE to dust mite allergen (11). Recently, the use of polyurethane-coated cotton encasings was compared to cotton encasings in a 12-month study of adults with AD (12). Eczema severity decreased in both groups but was more pronounced in patients using the treated covers. House dust mite exposure and specific IgE both decreased significantly in the active treatment group. Of note, patients not sensitized to house dust mite benefited from use of the allergy-proof covers as much as the sensitized patients. The authors speculate that impermeable covers may reduce exposure to other allergens (such as furred animals or yeast), irritants, or possibly superantigens. Dust mite control measures include use of dust mite–proof encasings on pillows, mattresses, and box springs; washing bedding in hot water weekly; removal of bedroom carpeting; and decreasing indoor humidity levels with air conditioning. HEPA filters are not particularly effective in reducing dust mite allergen levels and in addition have not been shown to improve clinical signs in pet-associated asthma and allergic rhinitis (13).

III. HYDRATION

Atopic dry skin shows an enhanced transepidermal water loss denoting an impaired water permeability barrier function (14,15). The water permeability barrier is formed by intercellular lipid lamellae located between the horny cells of stratum corneum (16). The stratum corneum has been shown to have reduced water-binding capacity when measured with an in vitro microbalance technique (17). In addition, transepidermal water loss measured with an evaporimeter is increased from both involved and normal-appearing atopic skin, and water content is decreased when measured with a corneometer. There have also been some reports that patients have decreased ceramide levels in their skin, which may contribute to reduced water-binding capacity, higher transepidermal water loss, and decreased water content (18).

In addition, bathing may also remove allergens from the skin surface and reduce colonization by *S. aureus*. Despite a drying or irritating effect, swimming in chlorinated pools results in clinical improvement in some patients with AD. Of interest, balneotherapy in acidic hot springs has been shown to help some patients with refractory AD (19). More recently, manganese and iodide ions in the latter have been shown to have a bactericidal effect on *S. aureus* (20).

Hydration, therefore, is an important component of successful therapy in AD. This can be accomplished by bathing or soaking the affected area for 15–20 minutes in warm water. Hydration of the face or neck can be achieved by applying a wet washcloth or towel to the involved area. A wet washcloth may be better tolerated when eye and mouth holes are cut out, allowing the patient to watch TV or engage in other activities. Isolated hand or foot dermatitis can be treated with soaks in basins. Baths may need to be taken on a long-term daily basis and may even need to be increased to two or three times daily during flares of AD. On the other hand, showers may be appropriate for patients with mild disease. Addition of substances such as oatmeal or baking soda to the bath water may be soothing to certain patients but does not promote increased water absorption. Bath oils, on the other hand, may give the patient a false sense of lubrication and can make the bathtub slippery.

After hydrating the skin, patients should gently pat away excess water with a soft towel and *immediately* apply an occlusive preparation. Since wet skin is more permeable to water, it is essential that the skin be covered within the first few minutes to prevent evaporation. Appropriate use of hydration and occlusives will help to reestablish the skin's barrier function. It is critical for patients and their families to understand the concept of proper hydration in order to achieve optimal control of their disease.

IV. MOISTURIZERS AND OCCLUSIVES

Use of an effective emollient, especially when combined with hydration therapy, will help restore and preserve the stratum corneum barrier (21). Emollients may also decrease the need for topical corticosteroids (22). Moisturizers are available in the form of lotions, oils, creams, and ointments. In general, ointments have the fewest additives and are the most occlusive, although in a hot, humid environment their use may lead to trapping of sweat with associated irritation of the skin. Lotions and creams may be irritating due to added preservatives, solubilizers, and fragrances. Lotions contain more water than creams and may be drying due to an evaporative effect. Oils are also less effective moisturizers. Recently, the effects of daily moisturizer therapy, while not inducing any change in the water barrier function of the stratum corneum or in the size of desquamating corneocytes (a parameter for turnover rate of the stratum corneum), were shown to substantially increase high-frequency conductance (a parameter for the hydration state of the skin surface) (23). This approach allows for ranking the efficacy of moisturizers according to either the duration of the lasting effects or the magnitude of an increase in the hydration levels of the stratum corneum.

Moisturizers should be obtained in the largest size available since they usually need to be applied several times each day on a long-term basis. Crisco® shortening can be used as an inexpensive moisturizer. An occlusive such as petroleum jelly (Vaseline®) can be used as a sealer after hydrating the skin; however, it should be noted that petroleum jelly is not a moisturizer and is most effective when used in conjunction with hydration. Urea-containing preparations have been used in AD primarily to treat the associated xerosis, as application on open, excoriated areas results in burning and discomfort. A recent study investigated the influence of treatment with a urea-containing moisturizer on the barrier properties of atopic skin with a twice-daily protocol (24). Skin capacitance and transepidermal water loss (TEWL) were measured at the start of the study and after 10 and 20 days. On day 21 the skin was exposed to sodium lauryl sulfate (SLS), and on day 22 the irritant reaction was measured noninvasively. Skin capacitance was significantly increased by the treatment, indicating increased skin hydration. The water barrier function, as reflected by TEWL values, tended to improve ($p = 0.07$), and the skin susceptibility to SLS was significantly reduced, as measured by TEWL and superficial skin blood flow ($p < 0.05$). This suggests that certain moisturizers could improve skin barrier function in AD and reduce skin susceptibility to irritants. In a recent double-blind, randomized study in AD, the combination of urea and sodium chloride applied in a topical moisturizing cream was found to be superior to the identical cream with urea alone with respect to ability to reverse impedance indices of atopic skin towards normal, an effect ascribed mainly to changes in hydration of the stratum corneum (25).

Alpha-hydroxy acids impact keratinization at the lowest levels of the stratum corneum, where they affect corneocyte cohesion and new stratum corneum formation. In addition, they increase dermal mucopolysaccharides and collagen formation. The efficacy and safety of 12% ammonium lactate emulsion has been assessed by clinical criteria and by noninvasive methods including electrical capacitance of stratum corneum, skin surface lipids, TEWL, skin surface topography, as well as the biomechanical properties of the skin (26). All patients tested showed a significant increase in electrical capacitance, skin surface lipids, extensibility and firmness of the skin, and an improvement in the skin barrier function and skin surface topography. Of potential clinical imortance in AD, Lavker et al. (27) reported that 12% ammonium lactate mitigates epidermal and dermal atrophy from a topically applied potent corticosteroid.

There has also been increased interest in the role of ceramides in atopic skin (28,29). Recently, an abnormal expression of sphingomyelin (SM) deacylase–like enzyme in the epidermis of patients with AD has been described, which results in decreased levels of ceramides in both involved and uninvolved stratum corneum (30). In this study, direct enzymatic measurements demonstrated that stratum corneum from lesional skin of AD patients has an extremely high SM deacylase activity that is at least five times higher than in the stratum corneum of normal controls. In stratum corneum from nonlesional AD skin, SM deacylase activity was still at least three times higher than in normal controls. Of interest, stratum corneum from contact dermatitis patients showed levels of SM deacylase similar to normal controls. In extracts of whole epidermis biopsies from AD patients, SM deacylase activities are significantly (threefold) increased over normal controls in the particulate fraction, whereas there is no significant difference in the activity of sphingomyelinase between AD and normal controls. In peripheral blood lymphocytes of AD patients, there is no increase in activity compared to normal controls, indicating a possibility that the high expression of SM deacylase is highly associated with the skin of AD patients. These findings suggest that, in contrast to changes in sphingolipid metabolism due to aging, the hitherto undiscovered enzyme SM deacylase is highly expressed in the epidermis of AD patients and competes with sphingomyelinase or beta-glucocerebrosidase for the common substrate SM or glucosylceramide, which leads to the ceramide deficiency of the stratum corneum in AD. Of potential practical significance, whereas an equimolar ratio of ceramides, cholesterol, and either the essential fatty acid linoleic acid or the nonessential fatty acids palmitic and stearic acids allows normal repair of damaged human skin, further acceleration of barrier repair occurs as the ratio of any of these ingredients is increased up to threefold (31).

V. CORTICOSTEROIDS

Topical corticosteroids have been the mainstay of treatment for AD. They reduce inflammation and pruritus and are useful for both the acute and chronic phases of the disease. Their mechanism of action is both broad and complex, impacting on multiple resident and infiltrating cells primarily through suppression of inflammatory genes (32). The complexity of the response is demonstrated in a recent study in AD that showed that expression of IL-12 p40 mRNA, which was significantly enhanced in lesional skin, was strongly downregulated after treatment with topical corticosteroids for 9–10 days (33). However, IL-12 p35 transcript levels were not affected by this treatment. Thus, the specific targets of corticosteroids in AD remain to be fully elucidated.

A large number of topical corticosteroids are available, ranging from extremely high- to low-potency preparations (Table 1). The vasoconstrictor assay, which measures the ability of a steroid to produce blanching when applied to normal human skin under controlled conditions, remains the gold standard for determining the potency of a topical corticosteroids. Most authors rank topical corticosteroids into seven potency groups (34). The vehicle the product is formulated in can alter the potency of the steroid and move it up or down in this classification. Generic formulations of topical steroids are required to have the same active ingredient and the same concentration as the original product. However, many generics do not have the same formulation of the vehicle, and the bioequivalence of the product can vary significantly (35). In general the same steroid will be most potent in an ointment base, followed by emollient, gel, cream, and lotion. An exception is Halog® cream, which because of added penetration enhancers, is a class II potency corticosteroid, while Halog® ointment is rated class III.

Use of a particular drug should depend on the severity and distribution of the skin lesions. Patients should be informed of the strength of topical corticosteroid they are given and the potential side effects. Patients often make the mistake of assuming that the potency of their prescribed corticosteroid is based solely on the percent noted after the compound name (e.g., believing that hydrocortisone 2.5% is more potent than fluticasone 0.005%) and may thus apply the preparations incorrectly. As a general rule, the lowest-potency corticosteroid that is effective should be used. However, using a topical corticosteroid that is too low in potency may result in persistence or worsening of AD. In such cases, a step-care approach with a mid- or high-potency preparation (although usually not to the face, axillae, or groin) followed by low-potency preparations may be more successful. In addition, patients are often given a high-potency corticosteroid and told to discontinue it after a period of time without being given a lower-potency corticosteroid to step down to, which can result in rebound flaring of the AD, similar to that often seen with oral corticosteroid therapy. Occasionally, therapy-resistant lesions may respond to a potent topical corticosteroid under occlusion, although this approach should be used with caution and reserved primarily for eczema of the hands or feet (36). Of note, the combination product Lotrisone® contains beclomethasone dipropionate, a high-potency corticosteroid, and should rarely be used in AD and never in the diaper area, face, or axillae.

Despite their widespread use, side effects are infrequent with appropriately used low- to medium-potency topical corticosteroids, even when applied over extended periods of time (37). With use of potent topical steroids, thinning of the skin is the most common side effect. After many weeks of topical use, collagen and elastin synthesis are decreased, which can result in skin fragility, dermal

Table 1 Representative Topical Corticosteroid Preparations

Group[a]	Generic name	Brand name	Vehicle
I	Clobetasol propionate	Temovate 0.05%	Ointment/Cream/ Emollient
		Cormax Scalp Application 0.05%	Solution
	Flurandrenolide	Cordan	Tape
	Halobetasol propionate	Ultravate 0.05%	Ointment/Cream
	Betamethasone dipropionate	Diprolene 0.05%	Ointment/Cream
	Diflorasone diacetate	Psorcon 0.05%	Ointment
II	Amcinonide	Cyclocort 0.1%	Ointment
	Betamethasone dipropionate	Diprosone 0.05%	Ointment
	Mometasone furoate	Elocon 0.1%	Ointment
	Halcinonide	Halog 0.1%	Cream
	Fluocinonide	Lidex 0.05%	Ointment/Cream/Gel/ Solution
	Desoximetasone	Topicort 0.25%	Ointment/Cream/Gel
III	Fluticasone propionate	Cutivate 0.005%	Ointment
	Amcinonide	Cyclocort 0.1%	Cream/Lotion
	Betamethasone diproprionate	Diprosone 0.05%	Cream
	Halcinonide	Halog 0.1%	Ointment/Solution
	Betamethasone valerate	Luxiq 0.12%	Foam
IV	Mometasone furoate	Elocon 0.1%	Cream/Lotion
	Triamcinolone acetonide	Kenalog 0.1%	Ointment/Cream
	Fluocinolone acetonide	Synalar 0.025%	Ointment
V	Fluticasone propionate	Cutivate 0.05%	Cream
	Triamcinolone acetonide	Kenalog 0.1%	Lotion
	Fluocinolone acetonide	Synalar 0.025%	Cream
	Betamethasone valerate	Valisone 0.1%	Cream
	Hydrocortisone valerate	Westcort 0.2%	Ointment
VI	Desonide	DesOwen 0.05%	Ointment/Cream/ Lotion
	Alclometasone dipropionate	Aclovate 0.05%	Ointment/Cream
	Triamcinolone acetonide	Kenalog 0.025%	Cream/Lotion
	Fluocinolone acetonide	Synalar 0.01%	Cream/Solution
		Derma-Smoothe/FS	Oil/Shampoo
VII	Hydrocortisone	Hytone 2.5%, 1.0%	Ointment/Cream/ Lotion

[a] Group I (superpotent) through group VII (least potent).
Source: Adapted from Ref. 34.

atrophy, striae, telangiectasia, purpura, and poor wound healing. In addition, hypopigmentation, secondary infections, and acneiform eruptions may occur. Local side effects are most likely to occur on the face and in the intertriginous areas, and only a low-potency corticosteroid should be used in these areas on a routine basis. Perioral dermatitis is often associated with use of topical steroids on the face. It is characterized by erythema, scaling, and follicular papules and pustules that occur around the mouth, alar creases, and sometimes on the upper lateral eyelids. "Steroid addiction" describes an adverse effect primarily of the face of adult women treated with topical steroids who complain of a burning sensation (38). In a large retrospective review of eyelid dermatitis seen over an 18-year period, a subgroup of 100 patients was identified who had, as the basis for their ongoing problem, an "addiction" to the use of topical or systemic corticosteroids (39). Their recalcitrant eyelid or facial dermatitis often resulted in the use of increasing amounts of corticosteroids for longer periods of time, creating a vicious cycle leading to the steroid "addiction." These patients improved with total discontinuation of the corticosteroid therapy. High- and super-high-potency topical corticosteroids, especially if used under occlusion, may cause systemic side effects along with local atrophic changes and should be used cautiously (40).

Topical steroids are available in a variety of bases including ointments, creams, lotions, solutions, gels, sprays, foam, oil, and even tape (Table 1). There is, therefore, no need for the pharmacist or patient to compound these medications. In addition, applying an emollient immediately prior to or over a topical corticosteroid preparation may decrease the effectiveness of the latter. Ointments are most occlusive, providing better delivery of the medication and decreasing water loss from the skin with fewest additives. During periods of excessive heat or humidity, creams may be better tolerated than ointments since the increase in occlusion may result in itching or even folliculitis. In general, however, creams and lotions, while easier to spread, may be less effective and can contribute to xerosis. Solutions can be used on the scalp or other hirsute areas, although the alcohol in them can be quite irritating when used on inflamed or excoriated lesions. Ingredients used to formulate the different bases may be irritating to individual patients and may cause sensitization. In addition, it is worth remembering that the corticosteroid molecule itself can induce allergic contact dermatitis (41). The diagnosis is often difficult to make on clinical grounds since it can present as a chronic or acute eczema, or even an id-like reaction with an erythema multiforme–type rash occuring at sites distant from the contact (reviewed in Ref. 42). Patch testing has been done primarily with tixocortol pivalate and budesonide. However, this approach may miss allergic reactions to some corticosteroid compounds (43). Unfortunately, expanded testing is associated with both false-positive and false-negative reactions.

Inadequate prescription size often contributes to suboptimally controlled AD, especially when patients have widespread, chronic disease. Patients may become frustrated with the need to refill prescriptions frequently, leading to decreased adherence with the prescribed treatment regimen. In addition, dispensing the prescribed medication in half pound or pound quantities can result in substantial financial savings for the patient. It is worth remembering that approximately 30 g of medication are needed to cover the entire body of an average adult. The fingertip unit (FTU) has been proposed as a measure for applying topical corticosteroids and has been studied in children with AD (44). This is the amount of topical medication that extends from the tip to the first joint on the palmar aspect of the index finger. It takes approximately one FTU to cover the hand or groin, 2 FTUs for the face or foot, 3 FTUs for an arm, 6 FTUs for the leg, and 14 FTUs for the trunk.

Patients should be instructed in the appropriate use of topical corticosteroids. Application of topical corticosteroids more than twice daily increases the chance of side effects, makes the therapy more costly, and usually does not increase efficacy. As the dermatitis improves, the frequency of use may be decreased or a less potent topical corticosteroid can be substituted. Once-daily treatment has been shown to be effective for certain corticosteroid preparations, including fluticasone propionate, a molecule with an increased binding affinity for the corticosteroid receptor (45). Topical mometasone has also been studied in children with AD and is approved for use once daily (46). Once-daily application may also help with adherence with the treatment regimen.

When the inflammatory process resolves, the topical corticosteroid can be discontinued, but hydration and moisturizer therapy need to be continued. However, since even normal-appearing skin in AD has immunological abnormalities, the use of topical corticosteroids as "maintenance therapy" may be of benefit. Unfortunately, there is a paucity of information on this approach. In a recent study, Van Der Meer et al. (47) showed that once control of AD with a once daily regimen is achieved, long-term control can be maintained with twice-weekly therapy. In this study, the topical therapy was applied to areas that appeared to have healed during the maintenance phase of the study, which resulted in delayed relapses of AD compared with placebo therapy.

In addition to their anti-inflammatory properties, topical corticosteroids may have an effect on bacterial colonization in AD. Nilsson et al. showed that the density of $S.$ $aureus$ on the skin could be reduced by topical corticosteroid therapy (48). Furthermore, in a double-blind, randomized trial the bacteriological and clinical effects of desonide were compared with its excipient in 40 children with AD (49). Before treatment, no differences in clinical score or $S.$ $aureus$ colonization were noted between the two groups. After 7 days of once-daily topical treatment, the clinical score improved ($p < 0.001$) in the desonide group, and $S.$ $aureus$ density decreased dramatically ($p < 0.001$). In the excipient group, no significant differences in clinical score or $S.$ $aureus$ density were noted. A comparison of the two groups demonstrated statistically significant differences with regard to clinical score ($p < 0.001$) and *S. aureus* density ($p < 0.05$). These results show the efficacy of topical corticosteroid treatment alone on *S. aureus* colonization in atopic skin and suggest a role for inflammation in bacterial colonization.

Finally, a number of patients with AD may not respond appropriately to their topical corticosteroid. Reasons for this may include complication by superinfection or inadequate potency of the preparation used, as discussed above. However, as discussed in Chapter 8, allergen-induced immune activation can alter the T-cell response to glucocorticoids by inducing cytokine-dependent abnormalities in glucocorticoid receptor binding affinity. Of note, PBMCs from patients with chronic AD also have reduced glucocorticoid receptor-binding affinity, which can be sustained with the combination of IL-2 and IL-4. In addition, corticosteroid unresponsiveness may contribute to treatment failure in some patients (50). Endogenous cortisol levels have been found to control the magnitude of cutaneous allergic inflammatory responses, suggesting that impaired response to steroids could contribute to chronic AD (51). Alternatively, Blotta et al. (52) have suggested that chronic corticosteroid therapy can have deleterious albeit insidious effects in allergic patients. The results, however, are based on in vitro data and thus may not recreate the complex milieu in allergic inflammation. A much more practical reason for failure of corticosteroid therapy is nonadherence with the treatment regimen. As with any chronic disease, patients or parents often expect a quick and permanent resolution of the problem and become disillusioned by the lack of cure with topical corticosteroids. In addition, a significant number of patients or caregivers admit to nonadherence with topical corticosteroids to fear of using this class of medications (53). These findings point to the need for both education and alternative therapies.

VI. TAR PREPARATIONS

Prior to the advent of topical steroids, crude coal tar extracts were used to reduce skin inflammation. The anti-inflammatory properties of tars are not as pronounced as those of topical corticosteroids, but they are long-lasting and side effects are fewer. Tar preparations may be useful in reducing the need for topical corticosteroids in chronic maintenance therapy of AD. In a recent comparison with a moderate-potency topical corticosteroid, tar therapy was found to be similar in its ability to inhibit the influx of a number of pro-inflammatory cells as well as in the expression of adhesion molecules in response to epicutaneous allergen challenge (54).

Tars are currently used primarily in shampoo form for scalp inflammation (T/Gel®, Ionil T®) and as bath additives (Balnetar®). Newer coal tar products have been developed which are better tolerated with respect to odor and staining of clothes. A moisturizer applied over the tar product will decrease the drying effect on the skin. Some patients prefer a tar compounded in an ointment or cream base such as 5% LCD (Liquor Carbonis detergents) in Aquaphor® ointment to avoid need for multiple layers. Tar preparations may be used primarily at bedtime to increase compliance. This regimen allows the patient to remove the preparation by washing in the morning, thus eliminating the concern about odor during the day and limiting staining to a few pairs of pajamas and bed sheets. Tar preparations should not be used on acutely inflamed skin, since this may result in skin irritation. Side effects associated with tars include inflammation of hair follicles and occasionally photosensitivity.

VII. WET WRAPS

Wet-wrap dressing therapy acts as a barrier from trauma associated with scratching, reduces pruritus and inflammation by cooling of the skin, and improves penetration of topical corticosteroids. One form of this treatment modality involves using tubular bandages applied over diluted topical corticosteroids. In a recent study, children with severe AD showed significant clinical improvement after one week of treatment (55). Of note, there was no significant difference noted using several dilutions of the mid-potency topical corticosteroid. This would suggest that clinical benefit can be obtained with this treatment in more severe patients even with the use of lower-potency corticosteroids. Long-term studies with this therapy are lacking, although most of the improvement in the latter study occurred in the first week. An alternative approach used for many years with success at National Jewish Medical and Research Center in Denver employs wet clothing, such as long underwear and cotton socks, applied over an undiluted layer of topical corticosteroids with a dry layer of clothing on top (56). Alternatively, the face, trunk, or extremities can be covered by wet, followed by dry, gauze and secured in place with a variety of dressings like Spandage®, elastic bandages, or by pieces of tube socks (Fig. 1). Wraps may be removed when they dry out or may be rewet. However, it is often practical to apply them at bedtime, and most patients are able to sleep with them on. Overuse of wet wraps may result in chilling or maceration of the skin and may be complicated by secondary infection. Given the cumbersome nature of this therapy, it is probably best reserved for acute exacerbations of atopic dermatitis, although it can also be used selectively to limited areas of resistant dermatitis with minimal inconvenience.

VIII. ANTI-INFECTIVE THERAPY

Patients with AD have an increased tendency for the development of bacterial and fungal skin infections (see Chapters 19 and 20). *S. aureus* is found in more

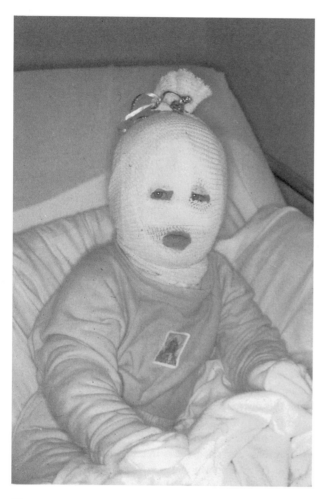

Figure 1   Wet wrap therapy.

than 90% of AD skin lesions. In contrast, only 5% of healthy subjects harbor this organism (57). The density of *S. aureus* on inflamed AD lesions without clinical superinfection can reach up to 10^7 colony-forming units (CFU) per square centimeter on lesional skin. The importance of *S. aureus* is supported by the observation that even AD patients without superinfection show a reduction in severity of skin disease when treated with a combination of antistaphylococcal antibiotics and topical corticosteroids (58,59). Fusidic acid in a topical combination with a corticosteroid has been shown to be effective in AD, and resistance has apparently not been a limiting factor (60). On the other hand, use of neomycin topically can result in development of allergic contact dermatitis as neomycin is among the more common allergens causing contact dermatitis (61).

Williams et al. (62) showed that a higher rate of *S. aureus* colonization in AD lesions compared to lesions from other skin disorders may be associated with colonization of the nares. In addition, this study pointed to the importance of *S. aureus* carriage on the hands, suggesting that this may be the vector for transmitting these bacteria from the nasal reservoir to lesional skin and in addition to close contacts of patients. Of interest, treatment for nasal carriage with an intranasal antibiotic showed a trend for reduction in *S. aureus* carriage and hand carriage was significantly reduced in the treated group compared with controls (63). In addition, mupirocin (Bactroban®) applied three times daily to affected areas for 7–10 days may be effective for localized areas of acute infection with *S. aureus* (64).

Although antibacterial cleansers have been shown to be effective in reducing bacterial skin flora (65), they may be too irritating to use on inflamed skin in AD. The antiseptic gentian violet has been shown to decrease *S. aureus* density significantly in lesional ($p < 0.001$) and uninvolved skin ($p < 0.001$) (66). This treatment also reduced the clinical severity of AD. Use of a 10% povidone-iodine solution also resulted in a 10- to 100-fold decrease in the density of *S. aureus* in patients with an initial density of >1000 CFU/10 cm^2 (67). Erythema and exudation also decreased after povidone-iodine treatment in patients colonized with high levels of *S. aureus*. Of interest, the authors found that *S. aureus* may produce biofilm-like structures in AD patients that may help the organisms colonizing these patients resist the disinfectant therapy. Ultimately, treatment may need to be directed at eliminating or neutralizing the exotoxins secreted by *S. aureus* that contribute to the chronic inflammation and severity of AD (as discussed in Chapter 19). There has also been some interest in the role of fungi, particularly *Malassezia furfur* (*Pityrosporum ovale*/*Pityrosporum orbiculare*) as pathogens in AD. *M. furfur* is a lipophilic yeast, and IgE antibodies against *M. furfur* are commonly found in AD patients and most frequently in patients with head and neck dermatitis (68). In contrast, IgE sensitization to *M. furfur* is rarely observed in healthy control subjects or asthmatic patients. Positive allergen patch test reactions to this yeast have also been demonstrated. The potential importance of *M. furfur* as well as other dermatophyte infections is further supported by the reduction in AD skin severity in patients treated with antifungal agents (69). Other studies have not shown a clear association between AD and lipophilic yeasts. In one study, approximately 50% of patients with antifungal IgE failed to show specific functional activity as assessed by basophil histamine release or skin testing (70). Most likely, this was due to nonspecific interaction of fungal elements with IgE. Thus, the clinical significance of fungi in AD remains unresolved. In fact, many patients with a head and neck type eczematous dermatitis, even with IgE antibodies to *M. furfur*, respond better to topical steroids than to topical antifungal therapy.

IX. ANTIHISTAMINES AND ANTIPRURITICS

Pruritus is the hallmark of AD, and an itch-scratch cycle often complicates the course of AD. Despite this, the pathophysiology of itch in AD is still incompletely understood (71). Treatment of AD with topical antihistamines and local anesthetics has generally been avoided because of potential sensitization. These drugs can cause cutaneous hypersensitivity reactions, and contact allergy could preclude systemic use of these drugs. However, in a multicenter, double-blind, vehicle-controlled study, treatment with topical 5% doxepin cream resulted in a significant reduction of pruritus (72). In this one-week study, sensitization was not reported, although rechallenge with the drug after the original course of therapy has not been evaluated. In a randomized, double-blind, controlled trial, pruritus relief and lessening of pruritus severity were significantly greater with the use of combination topical doxepin/topical corticosteroid than topical doxepin alone (73). In more recent studies, however, patients with AD treated in a double-blind study with 5% doxepin cream or vehicle ointment had a similar antipruritic response, possibly due to the antipruritic effects of using a moisturizer alone (74). Finally, topical 5% doxepin cream has been associated with marked sedation in patients with AD, which may limit its usefulness in certain patients (75).

It is important to remember that the role of histamine in the pruritus of AD has been called into question. In a study with topically applied capsaicin 0.05% as pretreatment, the pruritogenic and wheal-and-flare reactions to histamine iontophoresis were evaluated in normals and patients with AD (76). In control subjects, but not in AD patients, capsaicin pretreatment significantly reduced the flare area. Compared with control subjects, AD patients showed a lack of alloknesis or significantly smaller areas of alloknesis in pretreated and nonpretreated skin. In control subjects, capsaicin pretreatment significantly reduced itch sensations compared with nonpretreated skin, whereas in AD patients no differences were seen. Itch sensations in capsaicin-pretreated skin were significantly lower in control subjects than in AD patients. The authors concluded that capsaicin does effectively suppress histamine-induced itching in healthy skin but has less effect in AD. The diminished itch sensations and the absence of alloknesis in atopic individuals suggest that histamine is not the key factor in the pruritus of AD. The importance of other mediators was confirmed in a more recent study using a dermal microdialysis technique (77). Of interest, cutaneous field stimulation is a treatment modality that can mimic beneficial effects of scratching without inducing skin damage and has been shown to be of benefit in patients with AD (78).

X. TOPICAL TYPE 4 PHOSPHODIESTERASE INHIBITORS

Monocytes from AD patients have an abnormal increase in PDE (phosphodiesterase) enzyme activity, and PDE inhibitors such as Ro 20-1724 have been shown to decrease IgE synthesis (79) and basophil histamine release in vitro (80). Culture of AD monocytes with Ro 20-1724 also results in significant reduction of abnormal levels of IL-4, IL-10, and PGE_2 (81). In addition, Essayan et al. (82) reported that a PDE inhibitor could inhibit antigen-induced proliferation and cytokine production. In a recent study, the authors looked at the effects of the PDE4 inhibitor rolipram on toxin-mediated IL-12 production and CLA+ T-cell induction (83). They showed that the PDE4 inhibitor, but not the PDE3 or PDE5 inhibitors, reduced staphylococcal enterotoxin B–mediated CLA+ CD3+ induction. In addition, they showed that this effect was due to inhibition of IL-12 production and could be reverted by adding exogenous IL-12. Of practical relevance, AD patients treated with CP80,633, a potent inhibitor of PDE4 applied topically in a blinded, placebo-controlled paired-lesion study, showed significant clinical improvement with the active drug (81).

XI. OTHER TOPICAL THERAPIES

A. Topical Immunomodulators

Calcineurin inhibitors are discussed in depth in Chapter 27. These immunomodulators including cyclosporin (Cs) A, tacrolimus, and ascomycin derivatives act by binding to specific cytoplasmic proteins and interfering with gene transcription (84). Topical administration of CsA in a 3-week, double-blind, vehicle-controlled study with 10% CsA gel and 10% CsA ointment failed to show significant clinical improvement (85). On the other hand, randomized, multicentered, blinded, vehicle-controlled trials with tacrolimus 0.03% and 0.1% ointment in both children and adults with moderate-severe AD demonstrated both efficacy and safety in 3-week trials (86,87). These results were confirmed in phase 3 trials, and long-term safety and efficacy have also been reported (88). Of note, tacrolimus ointment has recently been approved in the United States for use in patients with AD 2 years of age and older. Ascomycin derivatives have also been studied in topical formulations. Twice-daily application of 1% SDZ ASM 981 cream in a randomized, double-blind, vehicle-controlled, right-and-left comparison trial in adult patients with moderate AD has been shown to be significantly more effective than vehicle over a 21-day period (89). No clinically relevant drug-related adverse effects were noted. Pharmakokinetic studies have been done in children with AD down to 3 months of age with this compound. In addition, multicenter phase 3 pediatric trials have been completed, and 1% SDZ ASM 981 cream is undergoing FDA review for approval in AD.

Burek-Kozlowska et al. (90) applied intravenous gammaglobulin (IVGG) topically to an affected area of AD on one extremity and a halogenated corticosteroid to a corresponding control area on the opposite extremity in six patients. Treated areas were covered by nonocclusive dressings. After once-daily treatment for 9 days, the IVGG-treated areas showed significant improvement in five of six patients and was superior to topical corticosteroids in two of these patients and equivalent in three.

An 8-amino-acid peptide encoding a sequence of the transmembrane region of the T-cell receptor alpha chain was recently shown to result in clinical improvement when applied topically to AD skin in a controlled study (91). These data suggest that T-cell receptor mimic peptides or cDNA might be effective in T-cell–mediated dermatoses.

Two recent uncontrolled studies showed that repeated application of the contact sensitizer dinitrochlorobenzene resulted in clinical improvement in refractory AD (92,93). The authors of both studies concluded that the beneficial effect observed was the result of immunomodulation by the dinitrochlorobenzene, possibly by effecting the T helper 1 versus T helper 2 imbalance.

B. Herbal Products and Dietary Supplements

Herbal treatments are being used with increased frequency to treat dermatological conditions, including AD (reviewed in Ref. 94). Unfortunately, among the most prevalent adulterants in topical herbal preparations are corticosteroids, including potent ones, especially in Chinese herbal creams (95,96). In a recent study from London, chromatographic analysis showed that 8 of 11 samples of Chinese herbal creams contained dexamethasone in significant concentrations (97).

Essential fatty acids are also used in AD in oral as well as topical forms. An ointment containing docosahexaenoic and eicosapentaenoic acids was studied in 64 patients with AD aged 2 months to 29 years who had a poor response to conventional therapy (98). The authors found significant improvement with the use of these essential fatty acids. In another study, topical oil of evening primrose was studied in two different vehicles (99). The authors concluded that a beneficial effect was seen only with a water-in-oil, not amphiphilic emulsion. Of note, controlled trials with an oral preparation of essential fatty acids have not shown clinical benefit in AD (100).

In a partially double-blind, randomized study carried out as a half-side comparison, Kamillosan® cream containing chamomile extract was tested vs. 0.5% hydrocortisone cream and the vehicle cream as placebo in patients with moderate AD (101). After 2 weeks of treatment, the active chamomile-containing cream showed a mild benefit over the low-potency corticosteroid and vehicle. Unfortunately, topical use of chamomile, as well as a number of other plant and herbal products, has been associated with allergic contact dermatitis (94).

Topical application of nicotinamide, a B vitamin, has been shown to increase ceramide and free fatty acid levels in the stratum corneum and decrease transepidermal water loss in dry skin (102). Nicotinamide was shown in vitro to improve the permeability barrier by stimulating de novo synthesis of ceramides with upregulation of serine palmitoyltransferase, the rate-limiting enzyme in sphingolipid synthesis. In addition, nicotinamide increased not only ceramide synthesis but also free fatty acid and cholesterol synthesis.

C. Other Topical Therapy

Cromolyn in a water-soluble emollient cream in a final concentration of 0.21% was studied in moderate-to-severe AD in a double-blind, placebo-controlled study (103). Treatment with topical cromolyn in the hydrophilic emollient resulted in significant clinical improvement compared to therapy with vehicle alone.

Massage therapy can be considered a topical adjunct treatment for AD. In one study, young children with AD were treated with standard topical care and massaged by their parents 20 minutes daily for a 1-month period while a control group received standard topical care only (104). The children's affect and activity levels significantly improved, and their parents' anxiety decreased immediately after the massage therapy sessions. Over the one-month period, parents of children in the massaged group reported lower anxiety levels in their children and the children improved significantly on all clinical measures including redness, scaling, lichenification, excoriation, and pruritus. The control group showed significant improvement only in scaling. These data suggest that massage therapy may be a cost-effective adjunct treatment for AD.

XII. CONCLUSIONS

Conventional topical therapy is effective for most patients with AD. Key elements include patient education, recognition and avoidance of irritants and proven allergens, appropriate use of hydration and emollients, and treatment of inflammation with topical corticosteroids. Adjunctive therapy includes judicious use of antibiotics, although in topical form these are used primarily to areas of limited involvement or for treatment of S. aureus colonization of the nares. Topical antihistamine therapy is of limited value, and as a rule topical antipruritic agents should be avoided due to the possibility of sensitization. New topical agents such as type 4 phosphodiesterase inhibitors may be steroid-sparing, although at the present time there are none pending approval. The most promising new topical immunomodulators are the calcineurin inhibitors (discussed in Chapter 27).

REFERENCES

1. Broberg A, Kalimo K, Lindblad B, Swanbeck G. Parental education in the treatment of childhood atopic eczema. Acta Derm Venereol 1990; 70(6):495–499.
2. Nassif A, Chan SC, Storrs FJ, Hanifin JM. Abnormal skin irritancy in atopic dermatitis and in atopy without dermatitis. Arch Dermatol 1994; 130(11):1402–1407.
3. Tabata N, Tagami H, Kligman AM. A twenty-four-hour occlusive exposure to 1% sodium lauryl sulfate induces a unique histopathologic inflammatory response in the xerotic skin of atopic dermatitis patients. Acta Derm Venereol (Stockh) 1998; 78:244–247.
4. Forsch PJ, Kligman AM. The soap chamber test, a new method for assessing the irritancy of soaps. J Am Acad Dermatol 1979; 1:35–41.
5. Breneman DL, Hanifin JM, Berge CA, Keswick BH, Neumann PB. The effect of antibacterial soap with 1.5% triclocarban on *Staphylococcus aureus* in patients with atopic dermatitis. Cutis 2000; 66(4):296–300.
6. Langeveld-Wildschut EG, Reidl H, Thepen T, et al. Clinical and immunologic variables in skin of patients with atopic eczema and either positive or negative atopy patch test reactions. J Allergy Clin Immunol 2000; 105:1008–1016.
7. Fischer B, Yawalkar N, Brander KA, Pichler WJ, Helbling A. Coprinus comatus (shaggy cap) is a potential source of aeroallergen that may provoke atopic dermatitis. J Allergy Clin Immunol 1999; 104:836–841.
8. Scalabrin DM, Bavbek S, Perzanowski MS, Wilson BB, Platts-Mills TA, Wheatley LM. Use of specific IgE in assessing the relevance of fungal and dust mite allergens to atopic dermatitis: a comparison with asthmatic and nonasthmatic control subjects. J Allergy Clin Immunol 1999; 104:1273–1279.
9. Schafer T, Heinrich J, Wjst M, Adam Heinrich, Ring J, Wichmann H-E. Association between severity of atopic eczema and degree of sensitization to aeroallergens in schoolchildren. J Allergy Clin Immunol 1999; 104:1280–1284.
10. van Reijsen FC, Bruijnzeel-Koomen CA, Kalthoff FS, Maggi E, Romagnani S, Westland JK, et al. Skin-derived aeroallergen-specific T-cell clones of Th2 phenotype in patients with atopic dermatitis. J Allergy Clin Immunol 1992; 90:184–193.
11. Tan BB, Weald D, Strickland I, Friedmann PS. Double-blind controlled trial of effect of house dust-mite allergen avoidance on atopic dermatitis. Lancet 1996; 347:15–18.
12. Holm L, Ohman S, Bengtsson A, van Hage-Hamsten M, Scheynius A. Effectiveness of occlusive bedding in the treatment of atopic dermatitis—a placebo-controlled trial of 12 months' duration. Allergy 2001; 56:152–158.
13. Wood RA, et al. A placebo-controlled trial of a HEPA air cleaner in the treatment of cat allergy. Am J Respir Crit Care Med 1998; 158:115–120.
14. Werner Y, Lindberg M. Transepidermal water loss in dry and clinically normal skin in patients with atopic dermatitis. Acta Derm Venereol (Stockh) 1985; 65:102–105.
15. Werner Y. The water content of the stratum corneum in patients with atopic dermatitis. Acta Derm Venereol (Stockh) 1986; 66:281–284.
16. Fartasch M, Diepgen T. The barrier function in atopic dry skin. Disturbance of

membrane-coating granule exocytosis and formation of epidermal lipids? Acta Derm Venereol Suppl (Stockh) 1992; 176:26–31.

17. Linde Y. Dry skin in atopic dermatitis. Acta Derm Venereol Suppl (Stockh) 1992; 177:9–13.

18. Imokawa G, Abe A, Jin K, Higaki Y, Kawashima M, Hidano A. Decreased level of ceramides in stratum corneum of atopic dermatitis: an etiologic factor in atopic dry skin? J Invest Dermatol 1991; 96:523–526.

19. Kubota K, Machida I, Tamura K, et al. Treatment of refractory cases of atopic dermatitis with acidic hot-spring bathing. Acta Derm Venereol 1997; 77:452–454.

20. Inoue T, Inoue S, Kubota K. Bactericidal activity of manganese and iodide ions against *Staphylococcus aureus*: a possible treatment for acute atopic dermatitis. Acta Derm Venereol 1999; 79:360–362.

21. Loden M. Biophysical properties of dry atopic and normal skin with special reference to effects of skin care products. Acta Derm Venereol Suppl (Stockh) 1995; 192:1–48.

22. Lucky AW, Leach AD, Laskarzewski P, Wenck H. Use of an emollient as a steroid-sparing agent in the treatment of mild to moderate atopic dermatitis in children. Pediatr Dermatol 1997; 14(4):321–324.

23. Tabata N, O'Goshi K, Zhen YX, Kligman AM, Tagami H. Biophysical assessment of persistent effects of moisturizers after their daily applications: evaluation of corneotherapy. Dermatology 2000; 200(4):308–313.

24. Loden M, Andersson AC, Lindberg M. Improvement in skin barrier function in patients with atopic dermatitis after treatment with a moisturizing cream (Canoderm). Br J Dermatol 1999; 140(2):264–267.

25. Hagstromer L, Nyren M, Emtestam L. Do urea and sodium chloride together increase the efficacy of moisturisers for atopic dermatitis skin? A comparative, double-blind and randomised study. Skin Pharmacol Appl Skin Physiol 2001; 14(1):27–33.

26. Vilaplana J, Coll J, Trullas C, Azon A, Pelejero C. Clinical and non-invasive evaluation of 12% ammonium lactate emulsion for the treatment of dry skin in atopic and non-atopic subjects. Acta Derm Venereol 1992; 72(1):28–33.

27. Lavker RM, Kaidbey K, Leyden J. Effects of topical ammonium lactate on cutaneous atrophy from a potent topical corticosteroid. J Am Acad Dermatol 1992; 26: 535–544.

28. Di Nardo A, Wertz P, Giannetti A, Seidenari S. Ceramide and cholesterol composition of the skin of patients with atopic dermatitis. Acta Derm Venereol 1998; 78(1): 27–30.

29. Bleck O, Abeck D, Ring J, Hoppe U, Vietzke JP, Wolber R, Brandt O, Schreiner V. Two ceramide subfractions detectable in Cer(AS) position by HPTLC in skin surface lipids of non-lesional skin of atopic eczema. J Invest Dermatol 1999; 113(6):894–900.

30. Hara J, Higuchi K, Okamoto R, Kawashima M, Imokawa G. High-expression of sphingomyelin deacylase is an important determinant of ceramide deficiency leading to barrier disruption in atopic dermatitis. J Invest Dermatol 2000; 115(3):406–413.

31. Man MQ M, Feingold KR, Thornfeldt CR, Elias PM. Optimization of physiological lipid mixtures for barrier repair. J Invest Dermatol 1996; 106(5):1096–1101.
32. Barnes PJ. New directions in allergic diseases: mechanism-based anti-inflammatory therapies. J Allergy Clin Immunol 2000; 106(1 Pt 1):5–16.
33. Yawalkar N, Karlen S, Egli F, Brand CU, Graber HU, Pichler WJ, Braathen LR. Down-regulation of IL-12 by topical corticosteroids in chronic atopic dermatitis. J Allergy Clin Immunol 2000; 106(5):941–947.
34. Stoughton RB. Vasoconstrictor assay-specific applications. In: Maibach HI, Surber C, eds. Topical Corticosteroids. Basel: Karger, 1992:42–53.
35. Stoughton RB. The vasoconstrictor assay in bioequivalence testing: practical concerns and recent developments. Int J Dermatol 1992; 31:26–28.
36. Volden G. Successful treatment of therapy-resistant atopic dermatitis with clobetasol propionate and a hydrocolloid occlusive dressing. Acta Derm Venereol Suppl (Stockh) 1992; 176:126–128.
37. Vernon HJ, Lane AT, Weston W. Comparison of mometasone furoate 0.1% cream and hydrocortisone 1.0% cream in treatment of childhood atopic dermatitis. J Am Acad Dermatol 1991; 24:603–607.
38. Kligman AM, Frosch PJ. Steroid addiction. J Int J Dermatol 1979; 18:23–31.
39. Rapaport MJ Rapaport V. Eyelid dermatitis to red face syndrome to cure: clinical experience in 100 cases. J Am Acad Dermatol 1999; 41(3 Pt 1):435–442.
40. McLean C, Lobo R, Brazier D. Cataracts, glaucoma, femoral avascular necrosis caused by topical corticosteroid ointment. Lancet 1995; 345:3330.
41. Dooms-Goossens A, Morren M. Results of routine patch testing with corticosteroid series in 2073 patients. Contact Dermatitis 1992; 26:182–191.
42. Matura M, Goossens A. Contact allergy to corticosteroids. Allergy 2000; 55:698–704.
43. Seukeran DC, et al. Patch testing to detect corticosteroid allergy: Is it adequate? Contact Dermatitis 1997; 36:127–130.
44. Long CC, Mills CM, Finlay AY. A practical guide to topical therapy in children. Br J Dermatol 1998; 138(2):293–296.
45. Wolkerstorfer A, et al. Fluticasone propionate 0.05% cream once daily versus clobetasone butyrate 0.05% cream twice daily in children with atopic dermatitis. J Am Acad Dermatol 1998; 39:226–231.
46. Lebwohl M. A comparison of once-daily application of mometasone furoate 0.1% cream compared with twice-daily hydrocortisone valerate 0.2% cream in pediatric atopic dermatitis patients who failed to respond to hydrocortisone: mometasone furoate study group. Int J Dermatol 1999; 38(8):604–606.
47. Van Der Meer JB, Glazenburg EJ, Mulder PG, Eggink HF, Coenraads PJ. The management of moderate to severe atopic dermatitis in adults with topical fluticasone propionate. Br J Dermatol 1999; 140:1114–1121.
48. Nilsson EJ, Henning CG, Magnusson J. Topical corticosteroids and *Staphylococcus aureus* in atopic dermatitis. J Am Acad Dermatol 1992; 27:29–34.
49. Stalder JF, Fleury M, Sourisse M, Rostin M, Pheline F, Litoux P. Local steroid therapy and bacterial skin flora in atopic dermatitis. Br J Dermatol 1994; 131:536–540.

50. Clayton MH, Leung DYM, Surs W, Szefler SJ. Altered glucocorticoid binding in atopic dermatitis. J Allergy Clin Immunol 1995; 96:421–423.

51. Herrscher RF, Kasper C, Sullivan TJ. Endogenous cortisol regulates immunoglobulin E–dependent late phase reaction. J Clin Invest 1992; 90:596–603.

52. Blotta MH, DeKruyff RH, Umetsu DT. Corticosteroids inhibit IL-12 production in human monocytes and enhance their capacity to induce IL-4 synthesis in CD4+ lymphocytes. J Immunol 1997; 158:5589–5595.

53. Charman CR, Morris AD, Williams HC. Topical corticosteroid phobia in patients with atopic eczema. Br J Dermatol 2000; 142:931–936.

54. Langeveld-Wildschut EG, et al. Modulation of the atopy patch test reaction by topical corticosteroids and tar. J Allergy Clin Immunol 2000; 106:737–43.

55. Wolkerstorfer A, et al. Efficacy and safety of wet-wrap dressings in children with severe atopic dermatitis: influence of corticosteroid dilution. Br J Dermatol 2000; 143:999–1004.

56. Nicol NH. Atopic dermatitis: the (wet) wrap-up. Am J Nurs 1987; 87(12):1560–1563.

57. Leyden JE, Marples RR, Kligman AM. *Staphylococcus aureus* in the lesions of atopic dermatitis. Br J Dermatol 1974; 90:525–530.

58. Leyden J, Kligman A. The case for steroid-antibiotic combinations. Br J Dermatol 1977; 96:179–187.

59. Lever R, Hadley K, Downey D, Mackie R. Staphylococcal colonization in atopic dermatitis and the effect of topical mupirocin therapy. Br J Dermatol 1988; 119: 189–198.

60. Abeck D, Mempel M. *Staphylococcus aureus* colonization in atopic dermatitis and its therapeutic implications. Br J Dermatol 1998; 139(suppl 53):13–16.

61. Albert MR, Gonzalez S, Gonzalez E. Patch testing reactions to a standard series in 608 patients tested from 1990 to 1997 at Massachusetts General Hospital. Am J Contact Dermat 1998; 9(4):207–211.

62. Williams JV, et al. S. aureus isolation from the lesions, the hands, and the anterior nares of patients with atopic dermatitis. Ped Dermatol 1998; 15:194–198.

63. Doebeling BN, et al. Long-term efficacy of intranasal mupirocin ointment. A prospective cohort study of *Staphylococcus aureus* carriage. Arch Intern Med 1994; 154:1505–1508.

64. Luber H, Amornsiripanitch S, Lucky AW. Mupirocin and the eradication of *Staphylococcus aureus* in atopic dermatitis. Arch Dermatol 1988; 124:853–854.

65. Stalder JF, Fleury M, Sourisse M, et al. Comparative effects of two topical antiseptics (chlorhexidine vs KMnO$_4$) on bacterial skin flora in atopic dermatitis. Acta Derm Venereol Suppl (Stockh) 1992; 176:132–134.

66. Brockow K, Grabenhorst P, Abeck D, Traupe B, Ring J, Hoppe U, Wolf F. Effect of gentian violet, corticosteroid and tar preparations in *Staphylococcus aureus*-colonized atopic eczema. Dermatology 1999; 199(3):231–236.

67. Akiyama H, Tada J, Toi J, Kanzaki H, Arata J. Changes in *Staphylococcus aureus* density and lesion severity after topical application of povidone-iodine in cases of atopic dermatitis. J Dermatol Sci 1997; 16(1):23–30.

68. Jensen-Jarolim E, Poulsen L, With H, Kieffer M, Ottevanger V, Skov P. Atopic

dermatitis of the face, scalp and neck: type I reaction to the yeast *Pityrosporum ovale*? J Allergy Clin Immunol 1992; 89:44–51.

69. Back O, Scheynius A, Johansson SG. Ketoconazole in atopic dermatitis: therapeutic response is correlated with decrease in serum IgE. Arch Dermatol Res 1995; 287: 448–451.

70. Nissen D. et al. IgE-sensitization to cellular and culture filtrates of fungal extracts in patients with atopic dermatitis. Ann Allergy Asthma Immunol 1998; 81:247–255.

71. Wahlgren CF. Itch and atopic dermatitis: an overview. J Dermatol 1999; 26(11): 770–779.

72. Drake LA, Fallon JD, Sober A, Group DS. Relief of pruritus in patients with atopic dermatitis after treatment with topical doxepin cream. J Am Acad Dermatol 1994; 31(4):613–616.

73. Drake LA, Cohen L, Gillies R, Flood JG, Riordan AT, Phillips SB, Stiller MJ. Pharmacokinetics of doxepin in subjects with pruritic atopic dermatitis. J Am Acad Dermatol 1999; 41(2 Pt 1):209–214.

74. Groene D, Martus P, Heyer G. Doxepin affects acetylcholine induced cutaneous reactions in atopic eczema. Exp Dermatol 2001; 10(2):110–117.

75. Sabroe RA, Kennedy CT, Archer CB. The effects of topical doxepin on responses to histamine, substance P and prostaglandin E2 in human skin. Br J Dermatol 1997; 137(3):386–390.

76. Weisshaar E, Heyer G, Forster C, Handwerker HO. Effect of topical capsaicin on the cutaneous reactions and itching to histamine in atopic eczema compared to healthy skin. Arch Dermatol Res 1998; 290(6):306–311.

77. Rukwied R, et al. Mast cell mediators other than histamine induce pruritus in atopic dermatitis patients: a dermal microdialysis study. Br J Dermatol 2000; 142:1114–1120.

78. Nilsson H-J, Levinsson A, Schouenborg, J. Cutaneous field stimulation (CFS): a new powerful method to combat itch. Pain 1997; 71:49–55.

79. Cooper KD, Kang K, Chan SC, Hanifin JM. Phosphodiesterase inhibition by Ro 20-1724 reduces hyper-IgE synthesis by atopic dermatitis cells in vitro. J Invest Dermatol 1985; 84:477–482.

80. Butler JM, Chan SC, Stevens S, Hanifin JM. Increased leukocyte histamine release with elevated cyclic AMP-phosphodiesterase activity in atopic dermatitis. J Allergy Clin Immunol 1983; 71:490–497.

81. Hanifin JM, et al. Type 4 phosphodiesterase inhibitors have clinical and in vitro anti-inflammatory effects in atopic dermatitis. J Invest Dermatol 1996; 107:51–56.

82. Essayan DM, Huang S, Kagey-Sobotka A, et al. Differential efficacy of lymphocyte- and monocyte- selective pretreatment with a Type 4 phosphodiesterase inhibitor on antigen-driven proliferation and cytokine gene expression. J Allergy Clin Immunol 1997; 99:28–37.

83. Santamaria LF, et al. Rolipram inhibits staphylococcal enterotoxin B-mediated induction of the human skin-homing receptor on T lymphocytes. J Invest Dermatol 1999; 113:82–86.

84. Liu J, Farmer JD, Lane WS, Friedman J, Weissman I, Schreiber SL. Calcineurin

is a common target of cyclophilin-cyclosporin A and FKBP-FK506 complexes. Cell 1991; 66:807–815.

85. De Rie MA, Meinardi MHM, Bos JD. Lack of efficacy of topical cyclosporin A in atopic dermatitis and allergic contact dermatitis. Acta Derm Venereol 1991; 71(5):452–454.

86. Boguniewicz M, Fiedler VC, Raimer S, Lawrence ID, Leung DYM, Hanifin JM, Pediatric Tacrolimus Study Group. A randomized, vehicle-controlled trial of tacrolimus ointment for treatment of atopic dermatitis in children. J Allergy Clin Immunol 1998; 102:637–644.

87. Ruzicka T, Bieber T, Schopf E, Rubins A, Dobozy A, Bos JD, Jablonska S, Ahmed I, Thestrup-Pedersen K, Daniel F, Finzi A, Reitamo S, European Tacrolimus Multicenter Atopic Dermatitis Study Group. A short-term trial of tacrolimus ointment for atopic dermatitis. N Engl J Med 1997; 337(12):816–821.

88. Hanifin JM. Tacrolimus ointment: Advancing the treatment of atopic dermatitis. J Am Acad Dermatol 2001; 44(1 suppl):S1–72.

89. Van Leent EJ, Graber M, Thurston M, Wagenaar A, Spuls PI, Bos JD. Effectiveness of the ascomycin macrolactam SDZ ASM 981 in the topical treatment of atopic dermatitis. Arch Dermatol 1998; 134(7):805–809.

90. Burek-Kozlowska A, Morell A, Hunziker T. Topical immunoglobulin G in atopic dermatitis. Int Arch Allergy Immunol 1994; 104(1):104–106.

91. Gollner GP, Muller G, Alt R, Knop J, Enk AH. Therapeutic application of T cell receptor mimic peptides or cDNA in the treatment of T cell-mediated skin diseases. Gene Ther 2000; 7(12):1000–1004.

92. Yoshizawa Y, Matsui H, Izaki S, Kitamura K, Maibach HI. Topical dinitrochlorobenzene therapy in the treatment of refractory atopic dermatitis: systemic immunotherapy. J Am Acad Dermatol 2000; 42(2 Pt 1):258–262.

93. Mills LB, Mordan LJ, Roth HL, Winger EE, Epstein WL. Treatment of severe atopic dermatitis by topical immune modulation using dinitrochlorobenzene. J Am Acad Dermatol 2000; 42(4):687–689.

94. Ernst E. Adverse effects of herbal drugs in dermatology. Br J Dermatol 2000; 143(5):923–929.

95. Wood B, Wishart J. Potent topical steroid in a Chinese herbal cream. NZ Med J 1997; 110:420–421.

96. Allen BR, Parkinson R. Chinese herbs for eczema. Lancet 1990; 336:177.

97. Keane FM, Munn SE, du Vivier AWP, et al. Analysis of Chinese herbal creams prescribed for dermatological conditions. Br Med J 1999; 318:563–567.

98. Watanabe T, Kuroda Y. The effect of a newly developed ointment containing eicosapentaenoic acid and docosahexaenoic acid in the treatment of atopic dermatitis. J Med Invest 1999; 46(3–4):173–177.

99. Gehring W, Bopp R, Rippke F, Gloor M. Effect of topically applied evening primrose oil on epidermal barrier function in atopic dermatitis as a function of vehicle. Arzneimittelforschung 1999; 49(7):635–642.

100. Berth-Jones J, Graham-Brown RA. Placebo-controlled trial of essential fatty acid supplementation in atopic dermatitis. Lancet 1993; 341(8860):1557–1560.

101. Patzelt-Wenczler R, Ponce-Poschl E. Proof of efficacy of Kamillosan(R) cream in atopic eczema. Eur J Med Res 2000; 5(4):171–175.

102. Tanno O, Ota Y, Kitamura N, Katsube T, Inoue S. Nicotinamide increases biosynthesis of ceramides as well as other stratum corneum lipids to improve the epidermal permeability barrier. Br J Dermatol 2000; 143(3):524–531.

103. Moore C, Ehlayel MS, Junprasert J, Sorensen RU. Topical sodium cromoglycate in the treatment of moderate-to-severe atopic dermatitis. Ann Allergy Asthma Immunol 1998; 81(5 Pt 1):452–458.

104. Schachner L, Field T, Hernandez-Reif M, Duarte AM, Krasnegor J. Atopic dermatitis symptoms decreased in children following massage therapy. Pediatr Dermatol 1998; 15(5):390–395.

23
Special Aspects in Pediatric Patients

Christine Bodemer and Yves de Prost
Hôpital Necker Enfants Malades, Paris, France

An important aspect of the treatment of pediatric atopic dermatitis (AD) is to develop a trusting relationship with the patient's parents, who must be well informed of the aim of the treatment. Indeed, it is particularly important to explain that the aim of the treatment is to control pruritus and eczematous lesions, but that cure is not possible. The chronic course of the disease is very worrying for the family, and the psychological impact of the disease has to be well considered. It is important to explain that the disease is not caused by stress, but that the child may be stressed or manipulative because of the disease itself. The education of the child and the family very often requires a lot of time because of preconceived ideas about AD, but this step of discussion and explanation is required for the good management and efficacy of home treatment.

I. EDUCATION OF THE FAMILY

Many parents will claim that stress or allergies trigger AD in their child. Physicians have to explain the multifactorial etiology of AD and put allergy and stress in their rightful place. The disease itself is stressful because of itch, with—in severe form—a lack of sleep. Moreover, a parent's anxiety and numerous exacerbating factors (e.g., sweat-producing activities, swimming, foods, pets) are very disturbing for a child and are very often not justified. Parents must understand that each case of AD has to be considered individually, and they must be careful not to interpret too quickly confusing disinformation. The physician should listen and understand the family's expectations of the treatment. The abundance of preconceived ideas is classic for such chronic and stressful diseases. Doctors have to keep in mind that the best treatment is the treatment agreed upon with the family and the child, taking into account their own history, difficulties, and expectations. The first consultation must be sufficiently thorough to establish a trusting relationship with the family. No management can be effective without this essential step.

II. GENERAL ADVICE

The life of a child with AD should be as normal as possible. Itch is probably the most distressing symptom for the child, and it is important to reduce factors that could increase the scratching process.

One should reduce the conditions that make the children hot and sweaty (e.g., no central heating in the bedroom; light and large night clothes; air conditioning in hot climates; lukewarm water for the bath). Sport activities should not be arbitrarily prohibited, as is sometimes done. Parents should discuss with their child what is important for his or her well-being.

One should reduce the conditions that enhance dryness and irritation of the skin (e.g., a humidifier in the child's bedroom, cotton clothes—synthetics and wool are irritating). Swimming in pools or the ocean should not be systematically forbidden. Swimming in chlorinated pools is well tolerated by most children with AD. Emollients can be applied just before swimming. Afterwards the child should rinse off completely and reapply emollients.

Allergen avoidance must not dominate the lives of atopic patients and their families. Potential allergens should be identified by taking a very careful patient history and carrying out selective prick tests. Avoidance of foods should not lead to special diets without a strict medical analysis (see Sec. IV.A). In dust mite–allergic patients, avoidance measures include use of dust mite–proof casings on pillows and mattresses, removal of bedroom carpeting, and decreasing indoor humidity levels with air conditioning. Families should keep in mind that there is no way to totally eradicate dust mites, and that avoidance measures are laborious and expensive. Household pets should be avoided if at all possible.

III. PARTICULARITIES OF CONVENTIONAL TREATMENT OF AD IN PEDIATRIC PATIENTS

The same conventional topical treatment (emollients, topical corticosteroids)— and antibiotic treatment if necessary—is used in pediatric patients as with adults.

However, some special aspects of disease management in pediatric patients should be emphasized.

A. Topical Corticosteroids

Local side effects in pediatric cases are the same as in adults. Children are at higher risk for systemic side effects because they have a greater surface-to-body ratio. These theoretical systemic side effects consist of adrenal suppression, failure to thrive, Cushing's syndrome, glaucoma, and benign cephalic hypertension (1–3). Topical corticosteroids are safe in AD pediatric cases when used correctly. Factors that enhance the risk of systemic side effects include which anatomical area is being treated (body fold areas as the napkin area provide a natural occlusive phenomenon), the size of the skin surface treated, the frequency of application, the length of the treatment, and the potency of the glucocorticoid (4–6). When topical corticosteroids are correctly used well on children there are no deleterious effects. Even when cortisol levels are depressed, they return to normal as soon as the skin inflammation is under control. Growth delay in some children with severe AD and long periods of topical corticosteroid treatment is a difficult problem to understand and resolve. But the topical treatment—if judiciously used—is rarely the cause of this delay (7,8). We completely agree with the conclusions of David (9) that the combined use of inhaled and oral corticosteroids for asthma, some particular regimes, and loss of sleep are contributing factors to short stature. However, severe AD can lead to a chronic, inadequate daily use of high-potency corticosteroids because of the lack of disease-free periods. In these cases of inadequate response, alternative therapies should be discussed.

To be safe, topical corticosteroids should be used for brief periods on limited areas without occlusion. We propose several general recommendations for treatment.

It is important to choose a good potency level (low to medium)—not too high but also not too low. The best way of limiting percutaneous absorption is to quickly control the inflammation. The more potent the steroid, the shorter the treatment and the better the compliance and safety. High-potency steroids need not be prohibited, even in pediatric patients, if in some special cases they are required. However, because of the chronic course of atopic dermatitis, it is better in children to begin with weaker steroids. The location of the eczema is important in choosing the potency of topical steroids. For instance, the face must be treated carefully. No more than 1% hydrocortisone should be applied on the eyelids, even if the risk of developing glaucoma remains theoretical.

A sufficient amount of medication should be prescribed. Very often too little medicine is applied because the right number of tubes is not specified on the prescription or because the family is afraid of steroids. Less frequently, excessive use of strong steroids is suspected. Clear explanations and clear prescriptions are essential. The exact role of the topical steroid in the management of the AD must be explained as often as necessary, and doctors should address at each visit the family's fears of the treatment's side effects.

It is very difficult to define the appropriate quantity of steroid medicament. Long et al. (4) developed a finger-type unit technique to determine the quantity of cream necessary to cover each area (e.g., hand, arm, leg) (Table 1): two adult fingertip units = 1 g of cream or ointment. The number of tubes necessary must be clearly prescribed.

Treatment regimen is not standardized (10,11). In our experience, if a correct potency of steroid is chosen (not too high or low), once-per-day application is sufficient. We recommend this regimen for 7–10 days, progressively reducing the regimen (1-0-1-0; 1-0-0-1-0-0-1) during 7–10 days. For the diaper area topical steroid should be chosen from a lower-potency group and not applied for more than 10 days because percutaneous absorption is greatly enhanced due to moisture from occlusion in this region. In adolescents the risk of striae at the breasts and thighs requires careful of steroids in these areas (i.e., low potency and short periods). The patients and families should be clearly instructed in proper steroid use, and the quantity of topical steroid (number of tubes) utilized by the parents should be evaluated at each visit.

B. Infections

Secondary infection, particularly bacterial infections (staphylococcal or streptococcal) are frequent in pediatric patients. Infections can delay response to topical steroids. Herpes simplex virus (HSV) infections are special complications of childhood atopic dermatitis.

Herpes simplex infections can lead to the acute disseminated viral infection, *eczema herpeticum* (EH). EH is usually a primary HSV infection in atopic children. The reason some atopic children (a minority) are susceptible to developing EH is not known. The highest incidence occurs in 2- to 3-year-olds. Rarely, the response to steroids is delay with a sudden deterioration of the child's eczema. Vesicles are the most common lesions, but the presenting lesions may also be pustules, papules, and crusts. Clinical diagnosis is difficult when vesicles are absent, and it is sometimes difficult to distinguish viral vesicles or pustules from bacterial lesions. A Tzanck smear may be helpful.

Widespread dissemination of the virus may occur, leading to multisystem involvement. The child should in such a case be quickly hospitalized, and most such patients require intravenous aciclovir, 500 mg/m^2, three times daily (12,13). Children with poor extensive lesions usually respond well to oral aciclovir (14,15). Some children with EH have recurrent localized cutaneous HSV infections, occurring usually within a few months of EH. During the acute phase of

Table 1 Guidelines to Management of Atopic Dermatitis

Location	6 months	1 year	5 years	10 years
Hand × 2	0.5	0.5	1	2
Arm × 2	0.5	1	2	3
Leg × 2	1	1.5	4	5
Foot × 2	0.5	0.5	2	2
Trunk (front)	1	1.5	3	4
Trunk (back)	1	1.5	3	4
Face and neck	0.25	0.5	0.5	1
Total FTU per treatment	4.75	7	15.5	21

Source: Ref. 4.

EH, treatment of secondary bacterial infections with antibiotics, and parenteral fluids to correct dehydration and electrolyte disorders are often necessary, and topical steroid treatment is stopped.

Parents should be informed of the risk of contact with cold sores for children with atopic dermatitis.

Smallpox vaccination is contraindicated in patients with atopic dermatitis unless there is a real risk due to the possibility of a widespread viral infection (*eczema vaccinatum*) that has a similar appearance to EH. In this regard, vaccination of family members should also take into consideration the potential of *eczema vaccinatum* in household contacts.

C. Emollients

This conventional topical treatment is discussed in Chapter 22. Such treatment is usually easy in small children and infants, but older children may tire of or rebel against it. It is therefore important to involve children as soon as possible in their own treatment and to let them apply the cream and choose the emollient that is cosmetically most acceptable to them (even if it is less greasy).

D. Antihistamines

Non-sedating antihistamines are usually of little benefit. Sedating antihistamines are more useful for children who wake regularly during the night or who scratch while asleep. Unfortunately some children hyperreact to antihistamines and are more worked up with the treatment. The best treatment for itching is certainly to cure quickly the relapse of the dermatitis with topical treatment and to reduce the conditions that enhance dryness and irritation of the skin.

E. Psychological Management

Physiological stress responses may influence inflammatory and immune mechanisms and exacerbate inflammatory dermatoses in genetically predisposed patients. Although emotional stress does not cause AD, it often exacerbates the illness. AD children often respond to stressful events with increased pruritus and scratching, and excessive scratching may be a form of attention seeking. Scratching is not, of course, always associated with significant secondary gain. The question remains the same: Does the atopic dermatitis cause particularly dependent, fragile, anxious and emotional personalities or vice versa? In fact it appears that there is no atopic dermatitis–specific personality (16–18), but the effect of itching, disturbed sleep, difficult chronic topical treatment, unattractive appearance in the severe forms, anxiety of the mother, and parenting distress can generate important psychological and relational problems for the child and the family. Failure in affective modulation and dysfunctional familial behavior, enhance anxiety and promote emotional stress through somatic pathways. Therefore, when conventional therapies fail in severe forms of atopic dermatitis, a psychological approach may be considered for the quality of life of the whole family, with sometimes beneficial effects on the dermatitis.

F. Hospitalization

It is remarkable to observe that some children fairing poorly at home become quickly better when hospitalized, even with the same apparent treatment (e.g., steroid potency). Three reasons for this are possible: (1) the topical steroid treatment had not been applied as prescribed, in which case the education of the family has to be reconsidered; (2) the treatment was well conducted, but the hospital pediatric environment, the modalities of steroids and emollients applications, and the psychological approach to the child are different; or (3) secondary infections delayed response time to topical steroids. Thus it is very important to observe the child hospitalized for untreated atopic dermatitis for several days before changing the treatment and to consider second-line therapies.

IV. SECOND-LINE THERAPIES IN REFRACTORY PEDIATRIC ATOPIC DERMATITIS

A. Diet

The role of food hypersensitivity in the pathogenesis of AD has been debated for years, and dietary management is still controversial. Most specialists agree that certain food allergens can cause cutaneous manifestations in atopic dermatitis. The frequency of these manifestations varies from 5 to 30% in the different series. The lesions consist mainly of contact urticaria, edema, and pruritus usually situated around the mouth or on the fingers or nonspecific erythematous rash. They occur very rapidly after ingestion of the incriminated foodstuff (19). Parents are generally aware of such reactions when they first consult and often avoid giving the suspect food to their children. Manifestations are not specific to atopic dermatitis and resemble food intolerance reactions in nonatopic children. Do food allergens aggravate atopic dermatitis? It is far more difficult to answer this question, as aggravations occur late after introduction of the allergen. In addition, the gravity of atopic dermatitis is hard to measure, and most studies have not been based on precise criteria. Mothers are often convinced that certain foods, such as cow's milk, are responsible for a child's AD, but this may simply reflect the fact that the disease begins at around 3 months of age, i.e., when solid foods are introduced. Sampson reviewed the data on this subject (20) and found manifestations of late hypersensitivity in one third of cases in a series of 300 patients aged from 6 months to 25 years and monitored for 10 years. The diagnostic criteria for atopic dermatitis were poorly defined. Tests were generally challenge tests with food allergens in the form of dried powders. Skin lesions in 75% of cases took the form of a morbiliform rash and pruritus, but not truly specific signs of atopic dermatitis were described. Onset was rapid, from a few minutes to 2 hours after ingestion. The most frequently accused foods were eggs, milk, peanuts, soy, flour, and fish. Some patients had later reactions with pruritus and an erythematous rash. These results must be interpreted with the utmost care: the author himself pointed out that the study population was not representative, as it comprised children who already had suspected aggravations of cutaneous or gastrointestinal manifestations by food allergens. Atherton et al. (21,22) have published several studies in the area. Their conclusions are less affirmative, but rechallenge studies suggested the possibility that food allergens could aggravate atopic dermatitis in a very small number of cases. They stressed the difficulties inherent in these studies given the enormous number of potential food allergens and the difficulty of carrying out placebo-controlled studies.

Avoidance diets have generally been tested in the hospital setting, but this introduces a bias, as hospitalization itself can improve atopic dermatitis. To avoid such artifacts, Devlin et al. studied the effect of an avoidance diet in the home environment in 63 children with AD (23,24). They observed an improvement in the group on the diet at the beginning of the study, but at the end of 12 months there was no longer any difference between the two groups. Other studies support the findings of Mankvad et al. (25), who reported no effect of a 3-week diet in 33 patients with severe AD, and those of Van Asperin et al. (26), who found no benefit of a strict diet in children of between 2 and 12 years with severe AD. As yet, there are no tests capable of predicting the effect of a given avoidance diet. Even specialists who support such diets admit that neither the specific IgE titer nor the results of prick tests correlate with a beneficial effect.

Avoidance diets can be dangerous, especially when prescribed for long periods, leading to weight loss, growth retardation, and even malnutrition with hypoalbuminemia or rickets. It should also be remembered that these avoidance diets are expensive and have a negative impact on the children's and parents day-to-day life (19,22,26).

The clinical impact of the early introduction of cow's milk has been extensively studied, but the results have been conflicting. Children with a family history of atopic disease have been shown to run a greater risk of developing atopic symptoms when exposed to cow's milk protein (28). Furthermore, atopic dermatitis is not infrequent in children who are exclusively breast-fed, so any protective effect of such feeding would be limited. Few studies have focused on the very early introduction of cow's milk formula. Kramer and Moroz conducted a retrospective study on 636 children and found that neither breast feeding nor the time of the introduction of solid foods influenced the risk of AD (29). Indeed, 36% of breast-fed infants developed AD, compared with only 26% of bottle-fed infants. The risk of developing atopic disease after early feeding with cow's milk–based formulas was studied by Gustafsson et al. (30), who studied 736 healthy full-term children exposed to cow's milk formula and breast milk from donors on the maternity ward. The children were divided into three groups: group 1 received only their mother's milk, group 2 received their mother's and human donor milk, and group 3 received their mother's milk, donor milk, and cow's milk–based formulas. No significant differences were found in the cumulative incidence of atopic diseases between the three groups. Children with a family history of allergy ran the same risk of developing atopic disease whether they were fed formula or breast milk alone, and the authors concluded that cow's milk–based formula did not seem to increase the risk of atopic disease. Kay et al., in a prevalence study of childhood atopic dermatitis, interviewed 1077 parents or guardians in the outskirts of Birmingham (31). The lifetime prevalence of atopic dermatitis was 20% in boys and 19% in girls. Prevalence in the previous year was 10–14% in boys aged 3–11 years. Atopic dermatitis developed in the first year of life in 60% of the children and in the first 6 months in three quarters of cases. The proportion of breast-fed children who had atopic dermatitis was 21%, compared to 19.5% in those breast-fed for 6 months or more and 18.5% in children who were exclusively bottle-fed. These data, recently confirmed by Nakamura et al. (32), clearly showed that breast feeding, even for 6 months or more, had no protective effect in this population.

B. Phototherapy

Phototherapy may be used in pediatric atopic dermatitis, but only for children over 10 years. Narrow-band UVB (TLO) appeared better for children than PUVA because it is safer (see Chapter 25).

C. Immunosuppressive Treatments

Better knowledge about the pathophysiology of atopic dermatitis has led to a better understanding of certain underlying immunological mechanisms and to proposing immunosuppressive therapy. Oral immunosuppressive drugs have been used mainly in the treatment of adults. Oral cyclosporine treatment was studied in children in severe recalcitrant cases of childhood AD. The dosage was the same (5 mg/kg/day) with very good efficacy, but frequent relapse occurred after reducing the dose (33). The side effects of systemic immunosuppressive therapy have stimulated research into topical treatments. The discovery of an immunosuppressive drug acting after local application is an old idea that is starting to appear feasible. Such local immunosuppressors should eventually replace dermocorticoids. The first to be studied in this context, more than 10 years ago, was local cyclosporine. Its poor efficacy in this use led to a loss of interest, and efforts are now being focused on new derivatives of macrolide antibiotics such as Tacrolimus (FK506) and Pimecrolimus (SDZ ASM 981). FK506 is a new immunosuppressive antibiotic of the macrolide family discovered by the Fujisawa Pharmaceutical Company. Tacrolimus was introduced in the early 1990s for the prevention of allograft rejection following liver transplantation. The systemic use of FK506 may be associated with adverse effects such as nephrotoxicity and hypertension. Tacrolimus has a similar mechanism of action as cyclosporine, but seems to be more potent and has a lower molecular weight. In vitro, the effects of Tacrolimus are inhibition of histamine release from mast cells and basophils and inhibition of IL-2, -3, -4, -5 and interferon-γ production from T lymphocytes. Reitamo et al. reported good results after application of 0.1% Tacrolimus ointment on atopic lesions in a study of 316 adult patients (34). Boguniewicz et al. confirmed these results in a study of 180 children (35) with concentrations of 0.1 and 0.3%, as did Paller et al. in a 12-week study (36). The other topical drug recently tested in atopic dermatitis is the Pimecrolimus or SDZ ASM 981. It is a novel macrolactam derived from ascomycin. It inhibits degranulation of mast cells and suppresses the production of tumor necrosis factor (TNF) in murine cell line. It does not induce skin atrophy when applied to normal skin for 4 weeks (37). The first pediatric study was designed to measure systemic exposure in children 1–4 years of age with atopic dermatitis treated twice daily for 3 weeks with 1% SDZ ASM 981 cream. Blood concentrations were consistently low, leading to larger studies in children (38).

V. CONCLUSION

Careful recommendations for the use of local steroid therapy and prevention based on allergological investigations as well as against infections have substantially improved the management of AD in childhood. However, specifically dedicated programs are urgently needed to improve the education of parents and patients. Programs for atopic dermatitis in a concerted action of physicians and patient organizations have been created in many countries and should considerably help to effectively involve the parents in the management of AD in children. In the future, networks involving pediatric dermatologists, allergists, pediatricians, and general practitioners should assure a better survey and provide disease management programs necessary for the control of this paradigmatic chronic skin disease.

REFERENCES

1. Dandine M, Lavaud J, Besson-Leaud M, Limal JM. Insuffisance surrénale et syndrome de Cushing iatrogène par absorption cutanée de corticoïdes chez un nourrisson de 8 mois. Ann Dermatol Venereol 1980; 107:191–195.

2. Patel L, Clayton PE, Addison GM, Price DA, David TJ. Adrenal function following topical steroid treatment in children with atopic dermatitis. Br J Dermatol 1995; 132:950–955.

3. Kristmundsdottir F, David TJ. Growth impairment in children with atopic dermatitis. J Roy Soc Med 1987; 80:9–12.

4. Long CC, Mills CM, Finlay AY. A practical guide to topical therapy in children. Br J Dermatol 1998; 138:293–296.

5. Turpeinen M, Salo OP, Leisti S. Effects of percutaneous absorption of hydrocortisone on adrenocortical responsiveness in infants with severe skin disease. Br J Dermatol 1986; 115 : 475–484.

6. Turpeinen M. Absorption of hydrocortisone from the skin reservoir in atopic dermatitis. Br J Dermatol 1991; 358–360.

7. Patel L, Clayton PE, Jenney ME, Fergusson JE, David TJ. Adult height in patients with childhood onset atopic dermatitis. Arch Dis Child 1997; 76:505–508.

8. Massarano AA, Hollis S, Devlin, David TJ. Growth in atopic eczema. Arch Child Dis 1993; 68:677–679.

9. David TL. Short stature in children with atopic dermatitis. Acta Derm Venereol (Stockh) 1989; 144 (suppl):41–44.

10. Lagos BR, Maibach HI. Frequency of application of topical corticosteroids: an overview. Br J Dermatol 1998; 139:763–766.

11. Aalto-Korte, Turpeinen M. Pharmacokinetics of topical hydrocortisone at plasma level after applications once or twice daily in patients with widespread dermatitis. Br J Dermatol 1995; 133:259–263.

12. Atherton DJ, Harper JL. Management of eczema herpeticum. J Am Acad Dermatol 1988; 18:757–758.

13. Taieb A, Fontan I, Maleville J. Oral acyclovir in eczema herpeticum. Br Med J 1984; 288:531–532.

14. Woolfson H. Oral acyclovir in eczema herpeticum. Br Med J 1984; 288:531–532.

15. Muelleman PJ, Doyle JA, House RF. Eczema herpaticum treated with oral acyclovir. J Am Acad Dermatol 1986; 15:716–717.

16. Musgrove K, Morgan J. Infantile eczema: a long-term follow-up study. Br J Dermatol 1976; 95:365.

17. Fritz G. Psychological aspects of atopic dermatitis: a viewpoint. Clin Pediatr 1979; 18:360–364.

18. Kuypers B. Atopic dermatitis: some observations from a psychological viewpoint. Dermatologica 1967; 136:387–394.

19. Esterly NB. Significance of food hypersensitivity in children with atopic dermatitis. Pediatr Dermatol 1986; 3:167–174.

20. Sampson HA. The immuno pathogenic role of food hypersensitivity in atopic dermatitis. Acta Derm Venereol (Stock) 1992; (suppl 176):34–37.

21. Pike MG, Carter C, Boulton P, Turner M, Soothill JF, Atherton DJ. Few food diets in the treatment of atopic eczema. Arch Dis Child 1989; 64:1691–1698.

22. Atherton DJ, Seurell M, Soothill JF, Wells RS, Chilvers C. A double blind controlled crossover trial of an antigen avoidance diet in atopic eczema. Lancet 1978; 1:401–403.

23. Devlin J, David TJ, Stanton RHJ. Elemental diet for refractory atopic eczema. Arch Dis Child 1991; 66:93–99.

24. Devlin J, David TJ, Stanton RHJ. Six food diet for childhood atopic dermatitis. Acta Derm Venereol 1991; 71:20–24.

25. Mankvad M, Danielson L, Hoj L. Antigen-free diet in adult patients with atopic dermatitis. Acta Derm Venereol (Stock) 1984; 64:524–528.

26. Van Asperin PP, Lewis M, Rogers M, Kemp AS, Thompsar S. Experience with an elimination diet in children with atopic dermatitis. Clin Allergy 1983; 13:479–485.

27. Stifler WC, Sedlis E. Some challenge studies with foods. J Pediatr 1965; 66:235–241.

28. Chandra RK. Influence of maternal diet during lactation and use of formula feeds on development of atopic eczema in high risk infants. Br Med J 1989; 299:228–231.

29. Kramer MS, Moroz B. Do breast feeding and delayed introduction of solid foods protect against subsequent atopic eczema? J Pediatr 1981; 98:546–550.

30. Gustafsson D, Lowhagen T, Andersson K. Risk of developing atopic dermatitis after early feeding with cow's milk based formula. Arch Dis Child 1992; 67:1008–1010.

31. Kay J, Gaxkrodger DJ, Mortimer MJ, Jaron AG. The prevalence of childhood atopic eczema in a general population. J Am Acad Dermatol 1994; 30:35–39.

32. Nakamura Y, Oki I, Tanihara S, et al. Relationship between breast milk feeding and atopic dermatitis in children. J Epidemiol 2000; 10(2):74–78.

33. Harper J, Ahmed I, Barclay G, et al. Cyclosporin for severe childhood atopic dermatitis: short course versus continuous therapy. Br J Dermatol 2000; 142(1):52–58.

34. Reitamo S, Wollenberg A, Schöpf, et al. Safety and efficacy of 1 year tacrolimus ointment monotherapy in adults with atopic dermatitis. Arch Dermatol 2000; 136:999–1006.

35. Boguniewicz M, Fiedler VC, Raimer S, Lawrence ID, Leung DYM, Hanifin JM. A randomized vehicle-controlled trial of tacrolimus ointment for treatment of atopic dermatitis in children. J Allergy Clin Immunol 1998; 102:637–644.

36. Paller A, Eichenfield LF, Leung DY, Stewart D, Appell M. A 12 week study of tacrolimus ointment for the treatment of atopic dermatitis in pediatric patients. J Am Acad Dermatol 2001; 44:S47–57.

37. Quenille-Roussel C, Paul C, Duteil L, et al. The new topical ascomycin derivative SDZ ASM 981 does not induce skin atrophy when applied to normal skin for 4 weeks: A randomized double blind controlled study. Br J Dermatol 2001; 144:507–513.

38. Harper J, Green A, Scott G, et al. First experience of topical SDZ ASM 981 in children with atopic dermatitis. Br J Dermatol 2001; 144:781–787.

24

Role of Cyclic Nucleotide Phosphodiesterases in Atopic Dermatitis

Luis F. Santamaria
Almirall Prodesfarma S.A., Barcelona, Spain

The role of the cyclic nucleotide phosphodiesterases (PDE) in the pathogenesis of atopic dermatitis (AD) was proposed more than 20 years ago as a possible explanation for the rapid enzymatic breakdown of cAMP found in leukocytes from atopic dermatitis patients when compared to leukocytes from healthy controls (1). Based on these findings, inhibition of PDE enzymes was proposed as an approach to correct the biochemical abnormality found in AD.

PDE enzymes are responsible for the hydrolysis of cAMP and cGMP to AMP and GMP, respectively. So far, 11 different families of PDE enzymes have been identified (2). Tissue expression of the PDE isoenzymes varies according to the PDE subfamily. PDE isoenzymes present in inflammatory cells belong to the PDE 3, 4, and 7 subfamilies (3,4).

Different in vitro inhibition studies with Ro-1724, a selective PDE 4 inhibitor, have shown a reduction in spontaneous IgE production (5), histamine release (6), and IL-4 production (7) by AD leukocytes. Cellular localization studies with different leukocyte populations demonstrated that the abnormal PDE activity in AD patients was found in monocytes (8). Further studies with monocytes from AD patients showed spontaneous PGE_2 (9) and IL-10 (10) production. Interestingly, the abnormal PDE activity found in monocytes correlated with such spontaneous cytokine production. Based on the inhibitory effects of PGE_2 and IL-10 on IFN-γ production (11,12), it was proposed that the low levels of IFN-γ, induced by PGE_2 and IL-10, would modify the Th1/Th2 balance towards the Th2 cytokine profile found in AD (9). However, in the last few years, various studies on the immunopathology of AD have shown that besides a predominant Th2 cytokine profile, other pathological mechanisms should be taken into consideration. Some of these include IFN-γ, which has been detected in the chronic phase, and bacterial infections, which through the production of superantigens may play a role in AD pathogenesis (13).

For this reason, the effect of PDE 4 inhibitors as a treatment for AD may be considered not only from the abnormal PDE 4 activity point of view, but also in the context of the new findings in AD pathogenesis. The objective of this chapter is to consider the possible role for PDE 4 inhibition in the treatment of AD in the current scenario of AD.

I. ANTI-INFLAMMATORY EFFECTS OF PDE INHIBITORS

PDE inhibitors are cAMP-elevating agents as they block the PDE enzymes that convert cAMP to 5'AMP, leading to the intracellular accumulation of cAMP (Fig. 1). This is a relevant point to consider when proposing the possible role of PDE 4 inhibitors in AD treatment. It has been known for a long time that intracellular elevation of cAMP has anti-inflammatory properties (14,15). PDE 4 inhibitors may therefore act as anti-inflammatory agents by increasing cAMP and at the same time blocking the increased PDE activity found in AD. PDE 4 inhibitors have been shown to block a number of leukocyte functions in vitro (see Table 1).

PDE 4 inhibitors affect most relevant inflammatory cells, including mast cells, eosinophils, lymphocytes, monocytes, and dendritic cells, since all these express the PDE 4 family of enzymes. The anti-inflammatory activity of PDE 4 inhibitors has also been documented in animal models of inflammatory diseases. Thus, PDE 4 inhibitors block antigen-induced bronchoconstriction, hyperreactivity and airway inflammation (3), collagen-induced arthritis (16), as well as experimental autoimmune encephalomyelitis (17).

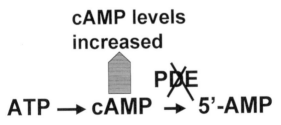

Figure 1   In inflammatory cells where the PDE 4 family is preferentially found, inhibition of the cAMP degradation pathway produces intracellular increases of cAMP. Such cAMP elevation interferes with many different inflammatory capacities of those cells.

Table 1 PDE 4 Effects on Inflammatory Cells

Inflammatory cell type	PDE isoform expressed	Inhibition
Basophil	3, 4	Histamine release
B cell	3, 4	Spontaneous IgE production
Dendritic cell	3, 4	TNF-α release
Eosinophil	3, 4	Activation, chemotaxis
Mast cell	3, 4	Histamine release
Monocyte/macrophage	3, 4	TNF-α production
Neutrophil	4	Activation
T cell	3, 4 (CD45R0>RA) 7	Proliferation, cytokine production

The fact that PDE 4 inhibitors can reduce inflammatory processes in leukocytes from healthy donors and animals, where no PDE abnormality is present, indicates that the spectrum of anti-inflammatory activity of such compounds for AD may involve other mechanisms than blocking increased PDE 4 activity.

II. PDE INHIBITORS IN AD TREATMENT

The anti-inflammatory activity of PDE 4 inhibitors has been documented in models of cutaneous inflammation in guinea pig and mouse (18,19).

Recently a double-blind, placebo-controlled, right/left paired-comparison clinical trial was performed in 20 AD patients with a topically administered selective PDE 4 inhibitor (20). Results indicate clinically significant anti-inflammatory activity in AD patients with a reduction in all inflammatory parameters (20). This was the first clinical assessment of this new class of anti-inflammatory compounds for AD treatment and can be considered as the proof of concept for this mechanism in this indication.

Pruritus is an early and important symptom in AD and may also be susceptible to treatment via PDE 4 inhibition. There is to date only limited information regarding PDE inhibitors as antipruritic compounds except for theophylline, as mentioned in Ref. 21. PDE 4 inhibitors have recently been shown to have anti–skin irritant activity in a clinical trial where Balsam of Peru was the irritant agent (22). The assay was performed with a sensitized individual, and the anti-irritant activity of PDE 4 inhibitors was found to correlate with their in vitro capacity to inhibit the PDE 4 enzyme (22).

III. POSSIBLE ANTI-INFLAMMATORY EFFECTS OF PDE 4
INHIBITORS IN DISTINCT PHASES OF AD

Recent advances in understanding the pathogenesis of AD suggest how PDE 4 inhibitors could work in the different phases of AD. In vitro data relating PDE 4 inhibitors with the mechanisms involved in the acute phase, chronic phase, and bacterial infection present in AD may support the anti-inflammatory activity of PDE 4 inhibitors in a more complete scenario of AD.

A. Acute Phase

The acute phase is characterized by spongiosis with a Th2 cytokine profile, sparse perivascular infiltrate of CD4+ CD45RO+ T cells, Langerhans cells, and macrophages exhibiting surface bound IgE (13).

Langerhans cells bearing allergen-specific IgE bound to the FcεRI on their surface may play an important role in initiating the cascade of inflammatory events, as has recently been suggested in vivo (23). Langerhans cells may present allergen to Th2 cells through an IgE-facilitated uptake mechanism. Moreover, engagement of FcεRI can also induce Langerhans cell activation followed by NF-κB activation and TNF-α production (24,25). Thus, Langerhans cells may initiate production of pro-inflammatory cytokines that activate endothelial cells and other cutaneous cells to produce chemokines and adhesion molecules involved in the recruitment of various leukocyte populations. One of these circulating could be skin-homing activated T cells (Fas ligand+) which may induce apoptosis of Fas receptor+ keratinocytes and generate spongiosis and subsequent eczema (26).

Different studies indicate that PDE 4 inhibitors may be affecting some of the inflammatory mechanisms present in the acute phase of AD described above. With respect to Langerhans cell function, PDE inhibitors have been shown to block TNF-α production by in vitro generated human dendritic cells (27) and NF-κB mediated transcription in monocytes and endothelial cells (28,29).

Most of the T lymphocytes present in cutaneous inflammation are memory (CD45RO+) T cells. Interestingly, human CD45RO+ T cells express higher levels of PDE 4 than CD45RA T cells (30) and could therefore be more susceptible to PDE 4 inhibitors. Studies have shown that PDE 4 inhibitors can interfere with allergen-induced T-cell activation, proliferation, and Th1 and Th2 cytokine production (31,32) by targeting the responder T-lymphocyte population (32). With respect to the mechanism of Fas ligand–induced keratinocyte apoptosis, it has been shown recently that cAMP inhibits TCR-coupled Fas ligand expression on T cells (33).

B. Chronic Phase

In the chronic phase of AD, IgE-bearing macrophages and eosinophils are the most relevant cells in the dermal infiltrate, together with Th1 cytokine expression. IL-12 has been proposed to play a role in the Th2-to-Th1 shift present in the chronic phase of AD. Sources of IL-12 might be eosinophils and macrophages (34). On the other hand, eosinophils might be attracted to the cutaneous lesion by IL-5 produced by Th2 lymphocytes together with eotaxin. In fact, eotaxin has been shown to be associated with CCR3 expression and eosinophil infiltration in AD (35).

The role for PDE 4 inhibitors in treatment of the chronic phase is supported by some recent reports. The selective PDE 4 inhibitor rolipram suppresses human eosinophil activation and eotaxin-mediated transendothelial cell layer migration (36). It has also been shown that superantigen enterotoxin B (SEB)–induced IL-12 production by PBMCs is inhibited by rolipram (37). Interestingly, PDE 4 inhibitors also reduce IL-12 production by mouse macrophages (16).

PDE 4 inhibitors are effective inhibitors of TNF-α production by macrophages. TNF-α plays a role in FcεRI-mediated prolonged survival of monocytes and possibly macrophages and dendritic cells (38). Thus, it may be suggested that PDE 4 inhibitors may affect such inflammatory mechanism.

C. Superantigens and Bacterial Infection

Bacterial infections are involved in chronic cutaneous inflammatory diseases such as AD. *Staphylococcus aureus* is present in more than 90% of cutaneous lesions in AD. The relevance of superantigens, in particular SEB, in the induction of dermatitis in AD patients has recently been underlined (39). Disease severity has been associated with the presence of *S. aureus* in the skin of children with AD (40,41) and with the presence of IgE to superantigens (42). The contribution of bacterial infections to AD inflammation is highlighted by the reduction in clinical severity obtained when applying a simultaneous topical treatment of corticosteroids and antibiotics (43).

Since AD is an allergic, T-cell–mediated inflammatory disease of the skin, we looked at whether T cells related to the cutaneous immune system in AD presented an increased percentage of staphylococcal-related T-cell-receptor variable segments (Vβ). Since skin-homing T cells bearing the CLA antigen on their surface have been shown to be associated to AD pathogenesis (44), we studied the Vβ expression on circulating CLA+ T cells from patients with AD. An increased percentage of cells bearing TCR Vβ segments related to *S. aureus* was found in circulating CLA+ T cells from children (45) with active AD. Similar results were found in an adult AD population (12).

Superantigens have been shown to induce CLA expression on activated T lymphocytes by a mechanism involving IL-12 produced by antigen-presenting cells (46). Based on these data it has been proposed that *S. aureus* infection may induce an amplification of T-cell–mediated inflammation in AD.

Regarding the role of PDE 4 inhibitors in the influence of superantigens in AD inflammation, we have recently shown that PDE 4 inhibition affects SEB-induced CLA antigen expression on human T lymphocytes (37). IL-12 was suppressed by the PDE 4 inhibitor rolipram but not by PDE 3 or PDE 5 selective inhibitors (37). These data indicate that PDE 4 inhibition of SEB-mediated CLA+ T-lymphocyte generation may interfere with the effect of bacterial superantigens on the cutaneous T cells involved in AD.

IV. CONCLUSION

The current understanding of AD pathology suggests an expanding role for PDE 4 inhibitors in AD treatment. Besides blocking the abnormal PDE activity found in AD patients, PDE 4 inhibitors may interfere with the most relevant features of AD immunopathogenesis: acute phase, chronic phase, and bacterial superantigen-mediated effects. Several in vivo and in vitro data support the relevance of the anti-inflammatory effects of PDE 4 inhibitors, through increased cAMP levels, in cutaneous inflammation.

Future clinical studies will certainly clarify the role of this new type of anti-inflammatory agent in the management of AD.

REFERENCES

1. SR Grewe, SC Chan, JM Hanifin. Elevated leukocyte cyclic AMP-phosphodiesterase in atopic disease: a possible mechanism for cyclic AMP-agonist hyporesponsiveness. J Allergy Clin Immunol 70:452–457, 1982.
2. L Fawcett, R Baxendale, P Stacey, C McGrouther, I Harrow, S Soderling, J Hetman, JA Beavo, SC Phillips. Molecular cloning and characterization of a distinct human phosphodiesterase gene family: PDE11A. Proc Natl Acad Sci USA 97:3702–3707, 2000.
3. TJ Torphy. Phosphodiesterase isozymes: molecular targets for novel antiasthma agents. Am J Respir Crit Care Med 157:351–370, 1998.
4. DM Essayan. Cyclic nucleotide phosphodiesterase (PDE) inhibitors and immuno-modulation. Biochem Pharmacol 57:965–973, 1999.
5. KD Cooper, K Kang, SC Chan, JM Hanifin. Phosphodiesterase inhibition by Ro 20–1724 reduces hyper-IgE synthesis by atopic dermatitis cells in vitro. J Invest Dermatol 84:477–482, 1985.
6. JM Butler, SC Chan, S Stevens, JM Hanifin. Increased leukocyte histamine release

with elevated cyclic AMP-phosphodiesterase activity in atopic dermatitis. J Allergy Clin Immunol 71:490–497, 1983.

7. SC Chan, SH Li, JM Hanifin. Increased interleukin-4 production by atopic mononuclear leukocytes correlates with increased cyclic adenosine monophosphate-phosphodiesterase activity and is reversible by phosphodiesterase inhibition. J Invest Dermatol 100:681–684, 1993.

8. CA Holden, SC Chan, JM Hanifin. Monocyte localization of elevated cAMP phosphodiesterase activity in atopic dermatitis. J Invest Dermatol 87:372–376, 1986.

9. JM Hanifin, SC Chan. Monocyte phosphodiesterase abnormalities and dysregulation of lymphocyte function in atopic dermatitis. J Invest Dermatol 105:84S–88S, 1995.

10. JD Ohmen, JM Hanifin, BJ Nickoloff, TH Rea, R Wyzykowski, J Kim, D Jullien, T McHugh, AS Nassif, SC Chan. Overexpression of IL-10 in atopic dermatitis. Contrasting cytokine patterns with delayed-type hypersensitivity reactions. J Immunol 154:1956–1963, 1995.

11. SC Chan, JW Kim, WR Henderson, Jr., JM Hanifin. Altered prostaglandin E2 regulation of cytokine production in atopic dermatitis. J Immunol 151:3345–3352, 1993.

12. KW Moore, A O'Garra, R de Waal Malefyt, P Vieira, TR Mosmann. Interleukin-10. Annu Rev Immunol 11:165–190, 1993.

13. DY Leung. Atopic dermatitis: new insights and opportunities for therapeutic intervention. J Allergy Clin Immunol 105:860–876, 2000.

14. HR Bourne, LM Lichtenstein, KL Melmon, CS Henney, Y Weinstein, GM Shearer. Modulation of inflammation and immunity by cyclic AMP. Science 184:19–28, 1974.

15. CS Henney, LM Lichtenstein. The role of cyclic AMP in the cytolytic activity of lymphocytes. J Immunol 107:610–612, 1971.

16. SE Ross, RO Williams, LJ Mason, C Mauri, L Marinova-Mutafchieva, AM Malfait, RN Maini, M Feldmann. Suppression of TNF-alpha expression, inhibition of Th1 activity, and amelioration of collagen-induced arthritis by rolipram. J Immunol 159: 6253–6259, 1997.

17. H Dinter, J Tse, M Halks-Miller, D Asarnow, J Onuffer, D Faulds, B Mitrovic, G Kirsch, H Laurent, P Esperling, et al. The type IV phosphodiesterase specific inhibitor mesopram inhibits experimental autoimmune encephalomyelitis in rodents. J Neuroimmunol 108:136–146, 2000.

18. MM Teixeira, AG Rossi, TJ Williams, PG Hellewell. Effects of phosphodiesterase isoenzyme inhibitors on cutaneous inflammation in the guinea-pig. Br J Pharmacol 112:332–340, 1994.

19. AM Ehinger, G Gorr, J Hoppmann, E Telser, B Ehinger, M Kietzmann. Effects of the phosphodiesterase 4 inhibitor RPR 73401 in a model of immunological inflammation. Eur J Pharmacol 392:93–99, 2000.

20. JM Hanifin, SC Chan, JB Cheng, SJ Tofte, WR Henderson, Jr., DS Kirby, ES Weiner. Type 4 phosphodiesterase inhibitors have clinical and in vitro anti-inflammatory effects in atopic dermatitis. J Invest Dermatol 107:51–56, 1996.

21. R Sidbury, JM Hanifin. Old, new, and emerging therapies for atopic dermatitis. Dermatol Clin 18:1–11, 2000.

22. E Goyarts, T Mammone, N Muizzuddin, K Marenus, D Maes. Correlation between

in vitro cyclic adenosine monophosphate phosphodiesterase inhibition and in vivo anti-inflammatory effect. Skin Pharmacol Appl Skin Physiol 13:86–92, 2000.

23. EG Langeveld-Wildschut, PL Bruijnzeel, GC Mudde, C Versluis, AG Van Ieperen-Van Dijk, IC Bihari, EF Knol, T Thepen, CA Bruijnzeel-Koomen, FC van Reijsen. Clinical and immunologic variables in skin of patients with atopic eczema and either positive or negative atopy patch test reactions. J Allergy Clin Immunol 105:1008–1016, 2000.

24. M Jurgens, A Wollenberg, D Hanau, H de la Salle, T Bieber. Activation of human epidermal Langerhans cells by engagement of the high affinity receptor for IgE, Fc epsilon RI. J Immunol 155:5184–5189, 1995.

25. Bieber T, Katoh N, Koch S, et al. FcεRI on antigen presenting cells: more than just antigen focusing. 23rd CIA Symposium, May 18–23, Hakone, Japan.

26. A Trautmann, M Akdis, D Kleemann, F Altznauer, HU Simon, T Graeve, M Noll, EB Brocker, K Blaser, CA Akdis. T cell-mediated Fas-induced keratinocyte apoptosis plays a key pathogenetic role in eczematous dermatitis. J Clin Invest 106: 25–35, 2000.

27. F Gantner, C Schudt, A Wendel, A Hatzelmann. Characterization of the phosphodiesterase (PDE) pattern of in vitro-generated human dendritic cells (DC) and the influence of PDE inhibitors on DC function. Pulm Pharmacol Ther 12:377–386, 1999.

28. V Ollivier, GCN Parry, RR Cobb, D de Prost, N Mackman. Elevated cyclic AMP inhibits NF-kappaB-mediated transcription in human monocytic cells and endothelial cells. J Biol Chem 271:20828–20835, 1996.

29. GC Parry, N Mackman. Role of cyclic AMP response element-binding protein in cyclic AMP inhibition of NF-kappaB-mediated transcription. J Immunol 159:5450–5456, 1997.

30. Y Sun, L Li, F Lau, JA Beavo, EA Clark. Infection of CD4+ memory T cells by HIV-1 requires expression of phosphodiesterase 4. J Immunol 165:1755–1761, 2000.

31. DM Essayan, SK Huang, BJ Undem, A Kagey-Sobotka, LM Lichtenstein. Modulation of antigen- and mitogen-induced proliferative responses of peripheral blood mononuclear cells by nonselective and isozyme selective cyclic nucleotide phosphodiesterase inhibitors. J Immunol 153:3408–3416, 1994.

32. DM Essayan, SK Huang, A Kagey-Sobotka, LM Lichtenstein. Differential efficacy of lymphocyte- and monocyte-selective pretreatment with a type 4 phosphodiesterase inhibitor on antigen-driven proliferation and cytokine gene expression. J Allergy Clin Immunol 99:28–37, 1997.

33. SC Hsu, MA Gavrilin, HH Lee, CC Wu, SH Han, MZ Lai. NF-kappa B-dependent Fas ligand expression. Eur J Immunol 29:2948–2956, 1999.

34. M Grewe, CA Bruijnzeel-Koomen, E Schopf, T Thepen, AG Langeveld-Wildschut, T Ruzicka, and J Krutmann. A role for Th1 and Th2 cells in the immunopathogenesis of atopic dermatitis. Immunol Today 19:359–361, 1998.

35. N Yawalkar, M Uguccioni, J Scharer, J Braunwalder, S Karlen, B Dewald, LR Braathen, M Baggiolini. Enhanced expression of eotaxin and CCR3 in atopic dermatitis. J Invest Dermatol 113:43–48, 1999.

36. LF Santamaria, JM Palacios, J Beleta. Inhibition of eotaxin-mediated human eosino-

phil activation and migration by the selective cyclic nucleotide phosphodiesterase type 4 inhibitor rolipram. Br J Pharmacol 121:1150–1154, 1997.

37. LF Santamaria, R Torres, AM Gimenez-Arnau, JM Gimenez-Camarasa, H Ryder, JM Palacios, J Beleta. Rolipram inhibits staphylococcal enterotoxin B-mediated induction of the human skin-homing receptor on T lymphocytes. J Invest Dermatol 113:82–86, 1999.

38. N Katoh, S Kraft, JHM weßendorf, and T Bieber. The high-affinity IgE receptor (FcεRI) blocks apoptosis in normal human monocytes. J Clin Invest 105:183–190, 2000.

39. L Skov, JV Olsen, R Giorno, PM Schlievert, O Baadsgaard, DY Leung. Application of staphylococcal enterotoxin B on normal and atopic skin induces up-regulation of T cells by a superantigen-mediated mechanism. J Allergy Clin Immunol 105:820–826, 2000.

40. R Bunikowski, ME Mielke, H Skarabis, M Worm, I Anagnostopoulos, G Kolde, U Wahn, H Renz. Evidence for a disease-promoting effect of *Staphylococcus aureus*-derived exotoxins in atopic dermatitis. J Allergy Clin Immunol 105:814–819, 2000.

41. TM Zollner, TA Wichelhaus, A Hartung, C Von Mallinckrodt, TO Wagner, V Brade, R Kaufmann. Colonization with superantigen-producing *Staphylococcus aureus* is associated with increased severity of atopic dermatitis. Clin Exp Allergy 30:994–1000, 2000.

42. R Bunikowski, M Mielke, H Skarabis, U Herz, RL Bergmann, U Wahn, H Renz. Prevalence and role of serum IgE antibodies to the *Staphylococcus aureus*-derived superantigens SEA and SEB in children with atopic dermatitis. J Allergy Clin Immunol 103:119–124, 1999.

43. R Lever, K Hadley, D Downey, R Mackie. Staphylococcal colonization in atopic dermatitis and the effect of topical mupirocin therapy. Br J Dermatol 119:189–198, 1988.

44. LF Santamaria Babi, LJ Picker, MT Perez Soler, K Drzimalla, P Flohr, K Blaser, C Hauser. Circulating allergen-reactive T cells from patients with atopic dermatitis and allergic contact dermatitis express the skin-selective homing receptor, the cutaneous lymphocyte-associated antigen. J Exp Med 181:1935–1940, 1995.

45. MJ Torres, FJ Gonzalez, JL Corzo, MD Giron, MJ Carvajal, V Garcia, A Pinedo, A Martinez-Valverde, M Blanca, LF Santamaria. Circulating CLA+ lymphocytes from children with atopic dermatitis contain an increased percentage of cells bearing staphylococcal-related T-cell receptor variable segments. Clin Exp Allergy 28:1264–1272, 1998.

46. DY Leung, M Gately, A Trumble, B Ferguson-Darnell, PM Schlievert, LJ Picker. Bacterial superantigens induce T cell expression of the skin-selective homing receptor, the cutaneous lymphocyte-associated antigen, via stimulation of interleukin 12 production. J Exp Med 181:747–753, 1995.

25
Phototherapy for Atopic Dermatitis

Jean Thomas Krutmann
Heinrich Heine University Düsseldorf, Düsseldorf, Germany

Akimichi Morita
Nagoya City University Medical School, Nagoya, Japan

I. FROM HELIOTHERAPY TO MODERN PHOTOTHERAPY OF ATOPIC DERMATITIS

It has been appreciated for decades that ultraviolet (UV) radiation may be beneficial for patients with atopic dermatitis (reviewed in Ref. 1). In 1929 the German dermatologist Buschke stated that the effect of sea climate on atopic dermatitis was "simply surprising," and in the 1940s Lomhold and Norrlind concluded that most patients with atopic dermatitis improved during the summer season (2). Nexman in 1948 was the first to systematically assess the beneficial effects of phototherapy in atopic dermatitis patients, which in his study were exposed to radiation from a carbon arc lamp (3). Modern fluorescent lamps with defined emission spectra for phototherapy of atopic dermatitis have been continously used from the end of the 1970s until today. During the last 5 years, several new phototherapeutic modalities, including UVA-1 therapy (4,5) as well as 311 nm UVB therapy (6), have been introduced. As a consequence, dermatologists may now select from a diversified spectrum of distinct phototherapeutic modalities the phototherapy of choice for their particular patient.

During the same time period, substantial progress has been made in advancing our knowledge about the pathogenesis of atopic dermatitis. A modern approach to phototherapy of atopic dermatitis has to reflect treatment decisions on the background of recent pathogenetic concepts (7). This chapter will therefore briefly summarize current knowledge about the pathogenesis of atopic dermatitis.

II. THE PATHOGENESIS OF ATOPIC DERMATITIS

It is now generally believed that atopic dermatitis represents a T-cell–mediated immune response directed against inhalant allergens (8). This concept is supported by the fact that the major clinical, histological, and immunohistochemical features of atopic dermatitis strongly resemble those observed in allergic contact dermatitis. Lesional skin of patients with atopic dermatitis contains an inflammatory infiltrate, which predominately consists of T-helper (Th) lymphocytes. Cytokines, which are produced in situ by these helper T cells, considerably contribute to the generation and maintenance of skin lesions in atopic dermatitis patients. It has been learned that the quality of the cytokine profile expressed in lesional skin of patients with atopic dermatitis critically depends on the stage of this disease (9). Biopsies taken either from acute atopic dermatitis or from eczematous skin lesions, which had been initiated under standardized conditions in atopic dermatitis patients by epicutaneous application of inhalant allergens and were analyzed at an early stage during their development (24 hours after allergen application), revealed a preponderance of the Th2-like cytokine interleukin-4 (IL-4), whereas at the same time point expression of the Th1-like cytokine interferon-γ (IFN-γ) was decreased below background levels. At later time points, that is, either in chronic, lichenified lesions of spontaneously evolving atopic eczema or in 48-hour inhalant allergen patch test–induced skin lesions, this cytokine pattern was reversed. At these later time points, expression of the Th1-like cytokine IFN-γ predominated, whereas IL-4 expression was decreased (10–12). Increased expression of IFN-γ appears to be responsible for the generation and maintenance of clinically apparent skin lesions in atopic dermatitis, since a close correlation between the clinical course of atopic dermatitis and in situ expression of IFN-γ in lesional atopic skin was observed. These findings may best be described by a two-phase model of the pathogenesis of atopic dermatitis, in which an initiation phase, which represents a Th2-like inflammatory response and develops without clinically apparent skin lesions, is switched into a second, eczematous phase, which is dominated by the Th1-like cytokine IFN-γ and clinically presents as eczema (9). Recent studies indicate that the observed switch from a Th2-like into a Th1-like cytokine pattern may be caused by an increased expression of the cytokine IL-12.

III. CONCEPT LINKED PHOTOTHERAPY FOR ATOPIC DERMATITIS

Based on this two-phase model, it is now possible to discriminate phototherapeutic strategies, which are directed at the initiation phase of atopic dermatitis and, thus, in a more general sense may be regarded as prophylactic, from photothera-

Table 1 Phototherapy for Atopic Dermatitis

Indication	Modality	Comment	Mode of action
Acute, severe	High-dose UVA-1 PUVA Extracorporeal Photopheresis	Monotherapy, alternative to glucocorticosteroids	Symptomatic, antieczematous
Chronic, moderate	311 nm UVB UVA-UVB Low-dose UVA-1 Broadband UVB Broadband UVA	Combination therapy, to save glucocorticosteroids	Symptomatic, antieczematous, maintenance therapy

pies, which are directed at the eczematous phase of this disease and which provide symptomatic relief by downregulating IFN-γ expression in lesional atopic skin (7). Symptomatic phototherapy of atopic dermatitis needs to be differentiated further into very potent phototherapeutic modalities, which may be used as a monotherapy for short periods of time to effectively treat patients with acute, severe exacerbation of atopic dermatitis, and less effective forms of phototherapy, which may be successfully employed as combination regimens over longer periods of time to treat patients with chronic forms of atopic dermatitis (Table 1). Current phototherapy of atopic dermatitis as conducted in daily practice is identical with symptomatic phototherapy.

A. Photo(chemo)therapy for Acute, Severe Atopic Dermatitis

In general, symptomatic phototherapy of acute, severe exacerbation of atopic dermatitis may be achieved with UVA-1, systemic psoralen plus UVA radiation (PUVA), and extracorporeal photochemotherapy, whereas conventional UVA/UVB and narrow-band UVB therapy represent phototherapeutic modalities, which are primarily indicated for treatment of chronic stages of this disease (Table 1).

1. UVA-1 Phototherapy

The rational for employing UVA-1 radiation, that is, long wavelength UVA radiation (340–400 nm), in the treatment of patients with atopic dermatitis was based on immunological studies in which it was demonstrated that exposure of human skin to a single dose of 130 J/cm^2 UVA-1 radiation was associated with abrogation of epidermal Langerhans cell function to activate alloreactive T cells (13).

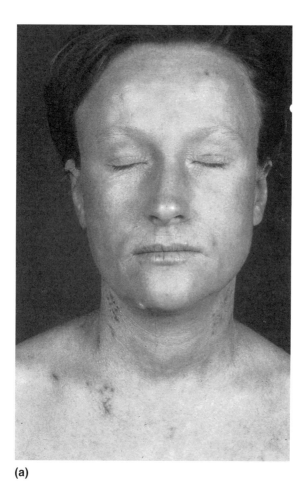

(a)

Figure 1   A patient with severe, acute exacerbation of atopic dermatitis before (a) and after (b) UVA-1 phototherapy (10×130 J/cm^2).

At the same time, evidence was accumulating that epidermal Langerhans cells, by virtue of their capacity to bind IgE molecules, may play an important role in inhalant allergen–mediated T-cell activation and thus be of critical importance for the pathogenesis of atopic dermatitis (14). In addition, clinical studies comparing the efficacy of broadband UVB therapy versus UVA/UVB therapy in the management of patients with atopic dermatitis indicated that the therapeutic effectiveness of conventional UVB therapy may be significantly improved by increasing the UVA portion of the action spectrum (UVA/UVB therapy) (15).

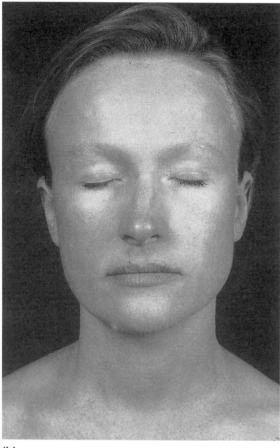

(b)

The therapeutic effectiveness of UVA-1 irradiation in the management of patients with atopic dermatitis was first assessed in a pilot study, in which patients with acute, severe exacerbation of atopic dermatitis were exposed one time per day to a single dose of 130 J/cm^2 UVA-1 (high-dose UVA-1 therapy) for 15 consecutive days (5). The therapeutic effectiveness of UVA-1 therapy was compared to that of a conventional UVA/UVB therapy by employing both modalities as a monotherapy, that is, additional treatment was restricted in both groups to the use of emollients. Therapeutic effectiveness was assessed by two means: (1) an established clinical scoring system originally developed by Costa et al. (16), consisting of a severity and a topographical score and (2) monitoring of serum levels of eosinophil cationic protein. Serum levels of eosinophil cationic protein previously had been identified as sensitive parameters that reflect disease activity in atopic dermatitis, and therefore they were used as objective parameters to evaluate the therapeutic effectiveness of UVA-1 irradiation (17). Assessment of clinical scores demonstrated that UVA-1 therapy was efficient in promptly inducing an improvement in clinical symptoms of patients with atopic dermatitis, and that in comparison to conventional UVA/UVB therapy, significant differences in favor of UVA-1 therapy were observed after 6 and 15 exposures (Fig. 1). Similarly, elevated serum levels of eosinophil cationic protein in patients with atopic dermatitis were significantly decreased by UVA-1 therapy, but remained essentially unaltered in patients undergoing UVA/UVB therapy.

These preliminary but promising results indicated that UVA-1 therapy may represent a novel phototherapeutic modality, which could be employed as a monotherapeutic approach to treat patients with acute, severe exacerbation of atopic dermatitis. During subsequent years, these original observations were confirmed by numerous reports, which mainly represent uncontrolled, open, and sometimes not even comparative studies (18–22). The pilot study by Krutmann et al. (5) failed to provide a direct comparison of UVA-1 therapy with the gold standard in the management of patients with acute, severe exacerbation of atopic dermatitis—the topical use of glucocorticosteroids. In a subsequent multicenter trial, a total of 53 patients were therefore randomly assigned to either UVA-1 therapy (once daily 130 J/cm^2, total of 10 days) or conventional UVA/UVB therapy (once daily, MED-dependent, total of 10 days) or topical treatment with fluocortolone (once daily for 10 days) (23). To this very day, this study is the only one to provide a multicentric evaluation of the efficacy of UVA-1 therapy in a controlled randomized fashion. It was observed that after 10 treatments, patients in all three groups had improved, but the decrease in total clinical scores and thus clinical improvement was significantly greater in patients receiving glucocorticosteroid or UVA-1 therapy, as compared to UVA/UVB therapy. Under these conditions, UVA-1 therapy, as compared to glucocorticosteroid treatment, was significantly better at day 10 of therapy in reducing the total clinical score. These clinical observations were corroborated by laboratory assessments, in which serum levels of eosinophil cationic protein as well as peripheral blood eosinophilia were compared before and after therapy between the three treatment groups. In aggregate, the multicenter trial results indicate that UVA-1 therapy and glucocorticosteroid treatment are superior to conventional UVA/UVB therapy in the management of patients with acute, severe exacerbation of atopic dermatitis. UVA-1 therapy may thus be used as an alternative to glucocorticosteroids to treat severe atopic dermatitis.

UVA-1 therapy may not be performed in atopic dermatitis patients with UVA-1–sensitive atopic dermatitis or photodermatoses such as polymorphic light eruption (24). It is necessary to exclude these diseases prior to initiation of UVA-1 therapy. This can easily be accomplished by photoprovocation testing. Except for eczema herpeticatum, no acute side effects have been observed in any of the atopic dermatitis patients treated with UVA-1. No other side effects have been observed, although potential carcinogenic risk is a theoretical concern (24). Exposure of hairless, albino Skh-hr1 mice to UVA-1 radiation has been shown to induce squamous cell carcinoma. The actual contribution of UVA-1 radiation to the development of malignant melanoma in humans is currently under debate and at this point cannot be excluded. Until more is known about UVA-1 therapy, its use should be limited to periods of severe, acute exacerbation, and, in general, one treatment cycle should not exceed 10–15 continously applied exposures and should not be repeated more than once a year. Under no circumstances should UVA-1 phototherapy be used for children (<18 years) with atopic dermatitis (24). In order to assess potential long-term side effects of UVA-1 photoherapy in a systematic manner, in Europe a prospective longitudinal study has been started to monitor patients treated with UVA-1 phototherapy for the development of skin cancer and photoaging.

There is an ongoing debate as to whether the therapeutic effectiveness of UVA-1 therapy is dose-dependent. Similar to a high-dose regimen with 130 J/cm^2, a medium UVA-1 dosage schedule seems to be superior to UVA/UVB (19). A direct comparison between low-dose versus high-dose UVA-1 regimen has been performed by Dittmar et al. (unpublished). In this open study, a high-dose protocol (130 J/cm^2) was superior to a medium-dose regimen (50 J/cm^2), which was more efficient than a low-dose schedule (20 J/cm^2). The latter observation is consistent with previous reports suggesting that a medium-dose regimen (50 J/cm^2) is superior to a low-dose regimen (20 J/cm^2) (24). Also, UVA/UVB therapy was reported to be superior to a low-dose regimen (20 J/cm^2). It thus appears that a low-dose regimen does not offer any advantage over conventional phototherapeutic modalities. This is in contrast to medium- and high-dose UVA-1 phototherapy. In order to achieve an optimal and long-lasting therapeutic response, however, a high-dose regimen might be necessary (18).

Substantial progress has been made in understanding the photoimmunological mechanisms responsible for the therapeutic effectiveness of UVA-1 therapy in atopic dermatitis (25). From these studies it appears that UVA-1 therapy is capable of downregulating in situ expression of IFN-γ in lesional skin of patients with atopic dermatitis. This inhibitory effect was relatively specific since in the same biopsies expression of neither the housekeeping gene β-actin nor the cytokine IL-4 was reduced. Inhibition of IFN-γ expression in atopic eczema may not only be achieved by UVA-1 therapy, but could also be seen after topical application of glucocorticosteroids and most likely represents a general mechanism by which various treatment forms induce symptomatic relief in atopic dermatitis (10).

Downregulation of IFN-γ expression in atopic eczema is the consequence of direct effects of UVA-1 radiation on Th1 cells present within the dermal infil-

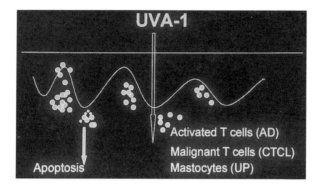

Figure 2   Scheme of the proposed mode of action of UVA-1 phototherapy.

trate (26,27) (Fig. 2). In vitro UVA-1 irradiation was found to be highly efficient in inducing apoptosis (programmed cell death) in human T cells. In vivo studies have revealed that UVA-1 phototherapy induced apoptosis in skin-infiltrating T cells and thereby caused a gradual reduction of the inflammatory infiltrate and a concomitant improvement of patients' skin disease (28). These observations have stimulated interest in the use of UVA-1 phototherapy for other T-cell–mediated skin diseases as well (29).

In addition to directly affecting epidermal and dermal T cells, UVA-1 radiation may alter Th1 cell IFN-γ expression via indirect mechanisms, e.g. by inducing the production of anti-inflammatory cytokines such as IL-10 by epidermal keratinocytes, which in turn may act on T cells in a paracrine manner. In keeping with this concept are in vitro studies demonstrating increased expression of IL-10 mRNA and secretion of IL-10 protein by cultured human keratinocytes following UVA-1 radiation exposure (30).

Immunohistochemical studies employing biopsies obtained from patients with atopic dermatitis undergoing UVA-1 therapy indicate that in addition to T cells and keratinocytes, epidermal Langerhans cells as well as dermal mast cells represent target cells for UVA-1 radiation (10). UVA-1 therapy, in contrast to UVA/UVB therapy, reduced not only the relative number of IgE-bearing Langerhans cells in the epidermis, but also the number of dermal CD1a+ Langerhans cells and mast cells. The latter observation prompted the use of UVA-1 therapy in the treatment of patients with urticaria pigmentosa, in which immediate and long-lasting remissions from cutaneous and systemic symptoms could be achieved (31).

2. PUVA Therapy

Systemic photochemotherapy combines the oral administration of psoralens with UVA radiation. Since its introduction into dermatological phototherapy some thirty years ago, PUVA has been found to be highly effective for the treatment of a variety of skin diseases (reviewed in Ref. 32), including atopic dermatitis. Although there is no doubt that PUVA therapy may be successfully used not only for moderate but also severe and even erythrodermic forms of atopic dermatitis, it has to be realized that PUVA therapy for this disease is associated with significant disadvantages (33–39). Compared to PUVA therapy for psoriasis, the actual number of treatments to clear atopic dermatitis was found to be relatively high. Even more important, cessation of PUVA therapy was associated with the occurrence of rebound phenomena in a high percentage of patients if photochemotherapy was not combined with systemic glucocorticosteroids or if maintenance therapy was not continued for longer time intervals extending over several years (40). Long-term use of PUVA is of particular concern in view of the relatively low age of patients with atopic dermatitis, and recent reports indicate that long-term PUVA may be associated with an increased risk of developing skin cancer, including malignant melanoma (41,42). Further disadvantages result from prolonged photosensitivity requiring protection by sunglasses to prevent cataract formation and the occurence of systemic side effects such as nausea in a relatively high percentage of patients (up to 20%). PUVA therapy is thus of limited use for the treatment of patients with atopic dermatitis and does not represent an equivalent alternative to glucocorticosteroids or UVA-1 therapy in the management of severe exacerbation of atopic dermatitis.

3. Extracorporeal Photochemotherapy

Evidence exists that extracorporeal photopheresis may be of benefit for the management of patients with severe atopic dermatitis. Extracorporeal photopheresis consists of the passage of freshly drawn blood that contains photoactivatable psoralen (8-methoxypsoralen) through an extracorporeal UVA exposure system (43). It is generally assumed that UVA radiation activates pharmacologically inactive 8-methoxypsoralen, which then is thought to affect the lymphocytes within the blood preparation, and subsequently these "modulated" lymphocytes are reinfused into the patient.

Extracorporeal photopheresis has been used with some success in the treatment of patients with Sézary syndrome. There are also some indications that it might be used with benefit for the treatment of several immunologically based skin diseases such as graft-versus-host disease (44). Prinz et al. were the first to successfully use extracorporeal photochemotherapy for patients with atopic dermatitis (45). They reported on three patients with severe atopic dermatitis with a life-long history of atopic dermatitis. Because their disease had finally become resistant to conventional therapies, extracorporeal photopheresis was started in these patients at 4-week intervals and found to induce clinical improvement of skin lesions associated with a reduction in serum levels of total IgE. Extracorporeal photopheresis was not used as a monotherapeutic approach but was combined with external use of topical prednicarbat, which by itself was insufficient to control disease activity in these patients. These studies have been confirmed in an independent study in which three patients with previously intractable atopic dermatitis were subjected to extracorporeal photochemotherapy in a monotherapeutic design (46). All patients showed prompt improvement which was dependent on the frequency of treatment cycles (Fig. 3). When extracorporeal photochemotherapy was given at 2-week intervals, a rapid decrease in the overall skin score

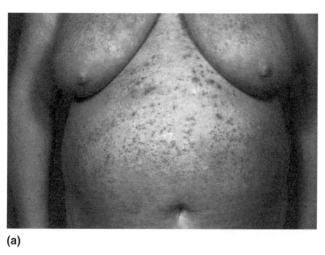

(a)

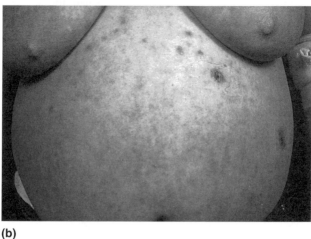

(b)

Figure 3   A patient with previously intractable atopic dermatitis before (a) and after (b) extracorporeal photochemotherapy (4 treatment cycles).

and in serum levels of eosinophil cationic protein and total IgE was observed. Upon extention of treatment-free intervals from 2 to 4 weeks, however, these beneficial effects were rapidly lost, but they were reachieved after reinstatement of the 2 week treatment schedule. In aggregate these studies suggest that extracorporeal photopheresis is effective for the treatment of patients with atopic dermatitis, but controlled randomized studies with larger patient cohorts are required to confirm these preliminary observations. Also, this modality is expensive and time-consuming, and therefore its use should be limited to atopic dermatitis patients in which other modalities have proven to be ineffective.

B. Photo(chemo)therapy for Chronic, Moderate Atopic Dermatitis

Broadband UVB therapy, combined UVA/UVB therapy, 311 nm UVB therapy, broadband UVA therapy, or low-dose UVA1 therapy, are effective treatments in mild and moderate atopic eczema, but are not effective in patients with acute severe excacerbation of their disease (1,4,6,15,18,20,24,36,47–54). These forms of UV phototherapy are usually not employed as monotherapeutic approaches but rather are used in combination with topical glucocorticosteroids in order to reduce the need for corticosteroid application.

1. UVA/UVB Phototherapy

Recent studies indicate that combinations of UVB irradiation with UVA irradiation, i.e., UVA/UVB therapy, are superior to conventional broadband UVB, conventional UVA, and low-dose UVA-1 therapy in the management of chronic, moderate atopic dermatitis. In two paired-comparison studies, Jekler and Larkö showed UVB therapy to be superior to placebo and UVB in high doses (0.8 MED) to be equipotent to UVB in moderate doses (0.4 MED) (24). The same authors, employing a clinical scoring system, demonstrated in a paired-comparison study statistically significant differences in favor of UVA-UVB therapy, as compared to broadband UVB therapy (15). In this trial, patients were allowed to continue use of topical glucocorticosteroids and, in addition, were irradiated three times per week for a maximum of 8 weeks in a UVB-MED–dependent manner. These careful observations further prove the concept that UVA-UVB therapy is superior to UVB therapy in the management of patients with atopic dermatitis (7).

2. Narrow-Band UVB Phototherapy

The patients most frequent complaint of patients undergoing phototherapy for atopic dermatitis relates to worsening of itch and induction of sweating by heat, which may be associated with UV, in particular UVA, therapy. In a recent study,

George et al. incorporated air-conditioning into a 311 nm UVB irradiation unit (6). By employing 50 100 W-W TL 01 lamps equippped with reflectors, a UVB output of 5 mW/cm^2 was achieved, which resulted in maximum treatment times of less than 10 minutes. In this well-designed study, steroid use by patients with moderate, chronic atopic dermatitis was monitored 12 weeks prior to phototherapy, during 12 weeks of phototherapy, and followed up for 24 weeks after cessation of phototherapy. Start of 311 nm UVB therapy not only decreased the total clinical score, but also substantially reduced the use of potent steroids. These beneficial effects were still present in the majority of patients 6 months after cessation of phototherapy.

These studies indicate that 311 nm UVB therapy may represent the phototherapeutic modality of choice to induce long-term improvement in patients with atopic dermatitis. They have recently been confirmed by an independent report, which suggested that no special cooling system is required in order to achieve the excellent therapeutic effects reported by George et al. (6).

In our hands, 311 nm UVB therapy has been found to be ideal in following UVA-1 therapy, which is used in the initial phase of treatment in order to manage acute, severe exacerbation of atopic dermatitis. UVA-1 therapy is then replaced by 311 nm UVB therapy, which is employed as an effective and presumably safe modality for maintenance therapy (55). Because of the latter argument, it has also been advocated to be used for children (47).

C. Photo(chemo)therapy for Chronic Vesicular Hand and Foot Eczema

Vesicular eczema of palms and soles is a common manifestation of atopic dermatitis, which often runs a chronic course. Since clinical symptoms are limited to defined areas of the skin, whole body UV irradiation would seem inappropriate. The recent development of cream-PUVA therapy offers the possibility to treat single, defined skin areas such as palms and soles without exposing nonlesional skin to UV radiation (56). In addition, partial body UVA-1 irradiation has been proposed for this indication (57).

1. Cream-PUVA Photochemotherapy

For cream-PUVA, a water-in-oil ointment containing 0.0006% 8-methoxypsoralen is applied to the skin area to be treated 1 hour prior to UVA irradiation. Optimal phototoxicity is given 1–3 hours after cream application and then rapidly falls off. In a first report, cream-PUVA therapy was found to be extremely beneficial for patients with chronic hand and foot eczema (56). After an average of 40 treatments, complete remission was observed in 7 of 10 patients. These observations have recently been confirmed in an independent study, in which cream-

PUVA was reported to be superior to bath-PUVA for this indication (30). This might be due to the fact that the repetitive use of cream-PUVA, in contrast to bath-PUVA, does not cause desiccation of eczematous skin. In addition cream-PUVA, as compared with bath-PUVA, is easier, cheaper, and safer to perform.

2. Partial Body UVA-1 Phototherapy

In a recent study, palms and backs of 12 patients with chronic dyshidrotic eczema were exposed to local UVA-1 phototherapy at a single dose of 40 J/cm^2 (57). Local UVA-1 phototherapy was given as a monotherapy. After 15 treatments, there was a gradual improvement in 10 out of 12 patients. There was no relapse over a 3-month follow-up period. It has been suggested that the latter might be an advantage of UVA-1 phototherapy in comparison with local PUVA therapy. Controlled, comparative studies to prove this point, however, are currently not available.

IV. PERSPECTIVES

In most instances photo(chemo)therapy for atopic dermatitis, in contrast to psoriasis, has been assessed in a monotherapeutic setting. Since atopic dermatitis, similar to psoriasis, is a chronic disease for which no curative treatment is available, therapeutic safety has to be a major concern. In this regard combination regimens are of great interest because theoretically they allow to combine modalities with different modes of action in order to enhance efficacy and safety at the same time. Controlled, randomized, comparative studies to assess the value of combining topical steroid treatment with new phototherapeutic modalities such as 311 nm UVB or UVA-1 phototherapy are therefore of significant practical relevance. The recent introduction of topical immunosuppressants for the management of patients with atopic dermatitis provides a completely new perspective for the symptomatic therapy of this disease. In this regard, combination regimens pose a major safety concern because immunosuppressive substances such as tacrolimus might increase the risk to develop skin cancer, in particular when used in combination with UV radiation. For a fair evaluation of this problem, safety studies are an indispensable prerequisite.

Little is currently known about the possibility of using phototherapy in the prophylaxis of atopic eczema. A prophylactic phototherapeutic approach would be based on the capacity of ultraviolet radiation to specifically interfere with the initiation phase of this disease. In this regard it is of particular interest that repeated exposures of human skin to high doses of UVA-1 radiation is capable of suppressing the development of positive skin reactions in inhalant allergen patch tests of patients with atopic dermatitis (58). Epicutaneous application of inhalant allergens such as house dust mite allergen on nonlesional skin of patients with atopic dermatitis and proven sensitization against the allergen tested has been found to induce eczematous skin lesions within 48 hours after allergen application in about 45–50% of patients tested (59–61). Numerous immunohistochemical and, in particular, immunological studies have clearly established that the skin lesions induced are specifically caused by the inhalant allergen applied to the skin, and not merely represent an unspecific, i.e., irritant reaction. As a consequence, the inhalant allergen patch test may be regarded as a model for the initiation phase of atopic dermatitis, which, by definition, comprises the time point at which the skin is hit by the aeroallergen to the time point at which eczematous skin lesions start to develop. Within the same patient, i.e., intraindividually, the induction of positive inhalant allergen patch test reactions has been a highly reproducible event, and this observation enabled us to ask whether UV radiation may have any effects on this system (62). We have found that exposure of human skin to UVA-1 radiation is highly effective in completely suppressing the development of positive inhalant allergen patch tests. This inhibitory effect was relatively specific, since in the same patients, preirradiation of human skin with an equivalent dose of UVA-1 radiation failed to suppress the development of positive patch test reactions which were provoced by epicutaneous application of the irritant sodium lauryl sulfate. These preliminary observations indicate that repeated exposure of human skin to UVA-1 radiation may provide protection against initiation of atopic dermatitis lesions by inhalant allergens. This view is consistant with the clinical observation that cessation of high-dose UVA-1 therapy is not associated with rebound or immediate relapse of eczema in atopic dermatitis patients. Further studies are required to assess the underlying mechanisms responsible for the UVA-1 radiation–induced suppression of inhalant allergen patch test reactions. It will also be of interest to determine whether similar effects may be achieved by other wavelengths such as 311 nm UVB therapy. These studies may ultimately allow the development of phototherapeutic regimens in which patients with atopic dermatitis are irradiated at given intervals in order to provide maximal prophylaxis against reexacerbation of their disease.

REFERENCES

1. J Jekler. Phototherapy of atopic dermatitis with ultraviolet radiation. MD thesis, Graphics Systems AB, University of Göteborg, Göteborg, 1992.
2. S Lomhold. Hudsygdommene og deres Behandling. 2nd ed., Copenhagen: 1927, p. 425.
3. P-H Nexman. Clinical studies of Besnier's prurigo. MD thesis, Rosenkilde and Bagger Publishers, Copenhagen, 1947.
4. J Krutmann, E Schöpf. High-dose UVA1 therapy: a novel and highly effective ap-

proach for the treatment of patients with acute exacerbation of atopic dermatitis. Acta Derm Venereol (Stockh) 1992; 76:120–122.

5. J Krutmann, W Czech, T Diepgen, R Niedner, A Kapp, E Schöpf. High-dose UVA1 therapy in the treatment of patients with atopic dermatitis. J Am Acad Dermatol 1992; 26:225–230.

6. SA George, DJ Bilsland, BE Johnson, J Fergusson. Narrow-band (TL01) UVB air-conditioned phototherapy for chronic severe adult atopic dermatitis. Br J Dermatol 1993; 128:49–56.

7. J Krutmann. Phototherapy for atopic dermatitis. Dermatol Ther 1996; 1:24–31.

8. JD Bos, EA Wierenga, JHS Smitt, FL van der Heijden, ML Kapsenberg. Immune dysregulation in atopic eczema. Arch Dermatol Res 1992; 128:1509–1514.

9. M Grewe, CAFM Bruijnzeel-Koomen, E Schöpf, T Thepen, GA Langeveld-Wildschuh, T Ruzicka, J Krutmann. A role for Th1 and Th2 cells in the immunopathogenesis of atopic dermatitis. Immunol Today 1998; 19:359–361.

10. M Grewe, K Gyufko, E Schöpf, J Krutmann. Lesional expression of interferon-γ in atopic eczema. Lancet 1994; 343:25–26.

11. M Grewe, S Walther, K Gyufko, W Czech, E Schöpf, J Krutmann. Analysis of the cytokine pattern expressed in situ in inhalant allergen patch test reactions of atopic dermatitis patients. J Invest Dermatol 1995; 105:407–410.

12. Q Hamid, M Boguniewicz, DYM Leung. Differential in situ cytokine gene expression in acute versus chronic atopic dermatitis. J Clin Invest 1994; 94:870–876.

13. O Baadsgard, S Lisby, G Lange-Wantzin, HC Wulf, KD Cooper. Rapid recovery of Langerhans cell alloreactivity, without induction of autoreactivity, after in vivo ultraviolet A, but not ultraviolet B exposure of human skin. J Immunol 1989; 142:4213–4217.

14. C Bruynzeel-Koomen. IgE on Langerhans cells: new insights into the pathogenesis of atopic dermatitis. Dermatologica 1986;172:181–184.

15. J Jekler, O Larkö. Combined UV-A-UV-B versus UVB phototherapy for atopic dermatitis. J Am Acad Dermatol 1990; 22:49–53.

16. C Costa, A Rillet, M Nicolet, JH Saurat. Scoring atopic dermatitis: the simpler the better. Acta Derm Venereol (Stockh) 1989; 69:41–47.

17. W Czech, J Krutmann, E Schöpf, A Kapp. Serum eosinophil cationic protein is a sensitive measure for disease activity in atopic dermatitis. Br J Dermatol 1992; 126:351–355.

18. D Abeck, et al. Long-term efficacy of medium dose UVA-1 phototherapy in atopic dermatitis. J Am Acad Dermatol 2000; 42:254–257.

19. G Kobyletzki, C Pieck, K Hoffmann, M Freitag, P Altmeyer. Medium-dose UVA1 cold-light phototherapy in the treatment of severe atopic dermatitis. J Am Acad Dermatol 1999; 41:931–937.

20. L Kowalzick, A Kleinhenz, M Weichenthal, J Ring. Low dose versus medium dose UVA-1 treatment in severe atopic dermatitis. Acta Derm Venereol (Stockh) 1995; 75:43–45.

21. H Meffert, N Sönnichsen, M Herzog, A Hutschenreuther. UVA-1 cold light therapy of severe atopic dermatitis. Dermatol Monatsschr 1992; 78:291–296.

22. F von Bohlen, J Kallusky, R Woll. The UVA1 cold light treatment of atopic dermatitis. Allergologie 1994; 17:382–384.

23. J Krutmann, TL Diepgen, TA Luger, S Grabbe, H Meffert, N Sönnichsen, W Czech, A Kapp, H Stege, M Grewe, E Schöpf. High-dose UVA1 therapy for atopic dermatitis: results of a multicenter trial. J Am Acad Dermatol 1998; 38:589–593.

24. J Krutmann. Therapeutic photomedicine: Phototherapy. In: IM Freedberg, AZ Eisen, K Wolff, KF Austen, LA Goldsmith, SI Katz, TB Fitzpatrick, eds. Fitzpatrick's Dermatology in General Medicine. 5th ed. New York: McGraw-Hill, 1999, pp. 2870–2879.

25. J Krutmann. UVA1-induced immunomodulation. In: J Krutmann, CA Elmets, eds. Photoimmunology. Oxford: Blackwell Scientific, 1995, pp. 246–256.

26. DE Godar. Preprogrammed and programmed cell death mechanisms of apoptosis: UV-induced immediate and delayed apoptosis. Photochem Photobiol 1996; 63:825–830.

27. DE Godar. UVA 1 radiation mediates singlet-oxygen and superoxide-anion production which trigger two different final apoptotic pathways: the S and P site of mitochondria. J Invest Dermatol 1999; 112:3–12.

28. A Morita, T Werfel, H Stege, C Ahrens, K Karmann, M Grewe, S Grether-Beck, T Ruzicka, A Kapp, LO Klotz, H Sies, J Krutmann. Evidence that singlet oxygen-induced human T-helper cell apoptosis is the basic mechanism of ultraviolet-A radiation phototherapy. J Exp Med 1997; 186:1763–1768.

29. H Plettenberg, H Stege, M Megahed, T Ruzicka, Y Hosokawa, T Tsuji, A Morita, J Krutmann. Ultraviolet A1 (340–400 nm) phototherapy for cutaneous T-cell lymphoma. J Am Acad Dermatol 1999; 41:47–50.

30. M Grewe, K Gyufko, J Krutmann. Interleukin-10 production by cultured human keratinocytes: regulation by ultraviolet B and A1 radiation. J Invest Dermatol 1995; 104:3–6.

31. H Stege, T Ruzicka, E Schöpf, J Krutmann. High-dose UVA1 for urticaria pigmentosa. Lancet 1996; 347:64.

32. WL Morison. Phototherapy and Photochemotherapy of Skin Disease. 2nd ed. New York: Raven Press, 1985, pp. 148–152.

33. DJ Atherton, F Carabott, MT Glover, JM Hawk. The role of psoralen photochemotherapy (PUVA) in the treatment of severe atopic eczema in adolescents. Br J Dermatol 1988; 118:791–795.

34. O Binet, C Aron-Brunetiere, M Cuneo, M-J Cesaro. Photochimiotherapie par voie orale et dermatite atopique. Ann Dermatol Venereol 1982; 109:589–590.

35. WL Morison, JA Parrish, TB Fitzpatrick. Oral psoralen photochemotherapy of atopic eczema. Br J Dermatol 1978; 98:25–30.

36. O Salo, A Lassus, T Juvaksoski, L Kanerva, J Lauharanta. Behandlung der Dermatitis atopica und der Dermatitis seborrhoica mit selektiver UV-Phototherapie und PUVA. Dermatol Monatsschr 1983; 169:371–375.

37. C Sannwald, JP Ortonne, J Thivolet. La photochimiotherapie orale de l'eczema atopique. Dermatologica 1979; 159:71–77.

38. E Soppi, M Viander, A-M Soppi, CT Jansen. Cell-mediated immunity in untreated and PUVA-treated atopic dermatitis. J Invest Dermatol 1982; 79:213–217.

40. G Rajka. Recent therapeutic events: cimetidine and PUVA. Acta Derm Venereol (Stockh) suppl 1980; 92:117–118.

41. RS Stern, Members of the Photochemotherapy Follow-Up Study. Genital tumors

among men with psoriasis exposed to psoralen and ultraviolet A radiation (PUVA) and ultraviolet B radiation. N Engl J Med 1990; 322:1093–1096.

42. RS Stern RS, et al. Malignant melanoma in patients treated for psoriasis with methoxsalen (psoralen) and ultraviolet A radiation (PUVA). N Engl J Med 1997; 336: 1041–1045.

43. F Gasparro, RL Edelson. Extracorporeal photochemotherapy. In: J Krutmann, CA Elmets, ed. Photoimmunology. Oxford: Blackwell Scientific, 1995, pp. 231–245.

44. B Volcz-Platzer, H Hönigsmann. Photoimmunology of PUVA and UVB therapy. In: J Krutmann, CA Elmets, eds. Photoimmunology. Oxford: Blackwell Scientific, 1995, pp. 265–273.

45. B Prinz, F Nachbar, G Plewig. Treatment of severe atopic dermatitis with extracorporeal photopheresis. Arch Dermatol Res 1994; 287:48–52.

46. H Richter, C Billmann-Eberwein, M Grewe, H Stege, M Berneburg, T Ruzicka, J Krutmann. Successful monotherapy of severe and intractable atopic dermatitis by photopheresis. J Am Acad Dermatol 1998; 38:585–588.

47. P Collins, J Ferguson. Narrowband (TLO1) UVB air-conditioned phototherapy for atopic eczema in children. Br J Dermatol 1995; 133:653–654.

48. ES Falk. UV-light therapies in atopic dermatitis. Photodermatol Photoimmunol Photomed 1985; 2:241–246.

49. M Hannuksela, J Karvonen, M Husa, R Jokela, L Katajamäki, M Leppisaari. Ultraviolet light therapy in atopic dermatitis. Acta Derm Venereol (Stockh) 1985; 114:137–139.

50. MJ Hudson-Peacock, BL Diffey, PM Farr. Narrow-band UVB phototherapy for severe atopic dermatitis. Br J Dermatol 1996; 135:332.

51. J Jekler, O Larkö. UVB phototherapy of atopic eczema. Br J Dermatol 1988; 119: 697–705.

52. K Midelfart, S-E Stenvold, G Volden. Combined UVB and UVA phototherapy of atopic eczema. Dermatologica 1985; 171:95–98.

53. NS Potekaev, LY Sevidova, VV Vladimirov, NG Kochergin, NN Shinaev. Selective phototherapy and dimociphon immunocorrective therapy in atopic dermatitis. Vestn Dermatol Venereol 1987; 9:39–42.

54. H Pullmann, E Möres, S Reinbach. Wirkungen von Infrarot- und UVA-Strahlen auf die menschliche Haut und ihre Wirksamkeit bei der Behandlung des endogenen Ekzems. Z Hautkr 1985; 60:171–177.

55. AR Young. Carcinogenicity of UVB phototherapy assessed. Lancet 1995; 345: 1431–1432.

56. H Stege, M Berneburg, T Ruzicka, J Krutmann. Cream-PUVA-Photochemotherapy. Hautarzt 1997; 48:89–93.

57. T Schmidt, D Abeck, K Boeck, M Mempel, J Ring. UVA1 irradiation is effective in treatment of chronic vesicular dyshidrotic hand eczema. Acta Derm Venereol (Stockh) 1998; 78:318–319.

59. CH Ramb-Lindhauer, A Feldmann, M Rotte, CH Neumann. Characterization of grass pollen reactive T-cell lines derived from lesional atopic skin. Arch Dermatol Res 1991; 283:71–76.

60. S Reitamo, K Visa, K Kähönen, S Stubb, OP Salo. Eczematous reactions in atopic

patients caused by epicutaneous testing with inhalant allergens. Br J Dermatol 1986; 114:303–308.

61. N Sager, A Feldmann, G Schilling, P Kreitsch, C Neumann. House dust-mite specific T cells in the skin of subjects with atopic dermatitis: frequency and lymphokine profile in the allergen patch test. J Allergy Clin Immunol 1992; 89: 801–807.

62. S Walter, M Grewe, K Gyufko, W Czech, A Kapp, H Stege, E Schöpf, J Krutmann. Inhalant allergen patch tests as a model for the induction of atopic dermatitis: analysis of the in situ cytokine pattern and modulation by UVA1 (abstr). Arch Dermatol Res 1994; 286:220.

26

The Psychological Aspects
of Atopic Dermatitis

Caroline S. Koblenzer
*University of Pennsylvania and Philadelphia Association for
Psychoanalysis, Philadelphia, Pennsylvania*

I. INTRODUCTION

Perhaps no other disease has stimulated so much interest in the complexities of psychosomatic interaction, or generated as many theories, as has atopic dermatitis. The synonym—neurodermatitis—speaks to this; as early as 1892 (1), papers began to appear in the literature that tentatively explored the interface between skin and psyche in this condition. The middle of the nineteenth century, a time of great interest in psychosomatics, produced numerous publications about atopy and the emotions. These have been ably summarized by Obermayer (2), Wittkower and Russell (3), and others (4–6). More recently, advances in psychoneuroimmunology (7) and in our understanding of both emotional development (8–11) and the emotional impact of physical illness on patient and family (12) have led to a renewed interest in this very important aspect of atopic dermatitis, to which genetic predisposition, emotional environment, and developmental influences all contribute.

II. NORMAL EMOTIONAL DEVELOPMENT AND THE IMPORTANCE OF EMPATHIC TACTILE EXPERIENCE FOR HEALTHY DEVELOPMENT

There is much evidence to support the belief that patients who exhibit strong psychosomatic interactions have experienced predisposing difficulties in very early life. These difficulties have to do with certain aspects of the very earliest relationships (12,13). The quality of tactile stimulation experienced by the infant and the emotional environment in which that experience takes place have a major impact on the development of three very important emotional functions, each of which plays a role in the life of the atopic individual because of the inherent qualities of the atopic skin. These functions are the evolution of physical and emotional boundaries that determine the integrity of the body image, the level of self-esteem that is engendered, and the capacity of the individual to master the modulation of emotion effectively (5,8–11). This latter, as we shall see, is of crucial importance if the individual is to be protected in later life from expressing emotional distress in the form of physical symptoms.

A. Body Image and Self-Esteem

Already in utero there is progressive development of tactile perceptive function in fetal skin. This can be demonstrated over the entire body surface by 32 weeks of gestation (14) and is crucial both for development of the body image and as a source of sensual gratification and self-esteem (8–11,14,15). Through cutaneous and kinesthetic stimulation, the physical boundaries of the self begin to be defined and a body image laid down, first by contact with the uterine wall and later, after delivery, through the empathic touch of loving caregivers. It can be shown that the greater the amount of touch an infant receives in a loving and stable environment during the early months of life—touch that is in tune with the infant's own specific tactile and emotional needs—the closer that internal image will be to objective reality (8–11,14–16), the more stable will also be the physical and emotional boundaries, and the more secure the personal and sexual identity, as the individual matures. In addition, loving touch is a source of emotional gratification and of self-esteem; the more empathic it is, the more attractive the individual feels, the more he will like himself, and the closer he will feel to others (14). In the atopic patient, for reasons that will be addressed below, it is not unusual to find self-esteem diminished, relationships suboptimal, and boundaries ill-defined. Thus, the integrity of the body image, the level of self-esteem, and the capacity to relate to others are all intimately entwined, and are largely determined by the quality of the early cutaneous experience and the emotional environment in which it takes place.

B. The Capacity to Modulate Emotion

In early infancy, all tension is released through physical pathways. Anxiety, frustration, and pain are expressed in physical movement, crying, and autonomic discharge. Initially this discharge is modulated by a two-way, nonverbal communication that takes place through close physical contact with the mother or primary caregiver. As she soothes her infant, her calming presence modulates his autonomic discharge until self-regulation is established. She also transmits to him a full range of her own emotional expression (14,17,18). Thus, the negative feelings of an anxious, angry, or hostile mother are picked up and mirrored by the infant, escalating his distress, while the relaxed, confident, and loving mother has a calming influence, helping her infant to learn to modulate anxiety, which is the infantile precursor of mature emotional experience (18). If these regulatory mechanisms are not internalized in infancy, at a later time, after the development of speech, tension will not be discharged optimally through the medium of dreams, fantasy, and play (19), words may not be developed to describe emotion (20,21), and the discharge of tension will continue through physical pathways (19), with associated physical symptoms.

III. THE SIGNIFICANCE OF EARLY DEVELOPMENTAL FACTORS IN ATOPIC DERMATITIS

For the atopic infant, vulnerable and abnormal-looking skin creates many vicissitudes along the developmental path described above. Inherently itchy and uncomfortable (13,23), the infant cannot readily be soothed, while the mother, unable to calm her increasingly frantic infant, herself becomes anxious, frustrated, and perhaps angry. Her distress is readily picked up by the infant, serving only to increase his anxiety and escalate the tension between the two. The quality of this interaction reduces the opportunity for the infant to internalize the capacity to modulate emotion, creates an ongoing cycle of discomfort for both, and increases the likelihood of later somatization (24–28). The higher than normal levels of anxiety characteristic of atopic individuals are most likely related to this early experience.

In terms of the developing body image, the part played by the altered sensory function of atopic skin is not fully understood, but in clinical practice we find that in the atopic patient, physical and emotional boundaries are frequently blurred. Scratching may then become a means of defining the physical boundaries of the self and a way to express feelings with which the individual may not be in touch, and for which no words can develop (29). Interference in the normal passage through this developmental phase may permit the skin to retain its early phase-appropriate significance as a primary source of sensual gratification and self-esteem, with a parallel arrest of other aspects of the personality. Alternatively, a fixation point may develop to which regression may occur at times of stress in an individual whose development has otherwise been uneventful (30). In practical terms, this emotional fixation, or regression, is expressed in terms of increased cutaneous reactivity and emotional immaturity.

IV. THE PROCESS OF SOMATIZATION

The concept of a developmental failure in the capacity to express and process feelings through the medium of words and fantasy, or a regression to that state at times of stress, provides a working hypotheses for the "why" of somatization, which is supported by psychoanalytic studies (10,19–22). These studies show that, in addition to expressing emotional content through physiological pathways in a way that may lead to physical symptom, such an individual is usually immature in other ways, showing a tendency towards dependent behaviors and having poorly developed psychological coping mechanisms—personality characteristics that are shown to affect disease susceptibility (31,32). Patients with severe atopic dermatitis frequently fit this profile (27,33). Although it is not yet possible to outline exactly the "how" of somatization, the rapidly expanding field of psychoneuroimmunology is providing many exciting clues as to the ways in which psychosocial and developmental factors contribute to a complex bi-directional system of intercommunication between the central nervous, neurohormonal, and immune systems, which can, in turn, lead to peripheral immunological and inflammatory changes (34–39).

A detailed discussion of the information currently available in this area is beyond the scope of this chapter, but in simple terms, centers in the cortical and limbic forebrain, which mediate cognitive and affective processes, respond to stress, to affective states, and to sensory input from both the outside and the inner worlds. Through connections with the hypothalamus, these centers activate both arms of the stress response and stimulate the release of pituitary hormones that mediate immunological and inflammatory reactions peripherally. These same cortical and limbic centers can also respond to immunological change with altered neuronal activity or monoamine metabolism (35,37). Autonomic nerves supply immunological tissues, and while lymphocytes, monocytes, and macrophages carry neurohormone receptors, they can also synthesize neurohormones, such as adrenocorticotropic hormone (ACTH), melatonin, and endorphins, which regulate cutaneous inflammation, and cell proliferation (38). Thus, it is clear that pathways exist whereby cognitive and affective material can be processed and translated into physiological transactions that result in physical change peripherally, and physical change can alter cognitive and affective processes in the central nervous system.

What constitutes a stressor may be quite obvious and external, or stress may be engendered by activation of old memories or the reinterpretation of seemingly inconsequential events in the light of past experience. Response is individual, and what is stressful to one may be exciting and stimulating to another. Acute and chronic stress (or strain) affect immune mechanisms by influencing the redistribution of immunoreactive cells and the release of cytokines (35–41). Gender differences in response to stress may implicate other neuroendocrine pathways, such as the hypothalamic-pituitary-gonadal pathway, since female hormones generally enhance inflammation (42). These mechanisms have been studied intensively in certain infective processes (37,42), and in autoimmune disease (37,42).

A particularly fruitful area of research in recent years has been the study of neuropeptides, more than 40 of which have so far been identified. These agents are ubiquitous throughout the body, acting as neurotransmitters, as vasoactive agents, and as mediators in numerous other interactions, including immune regulation (34,39). As part of the stress response, they are released centrally and peripherally. Relevant to cutaneous function, neuropeptide receptors have been identified on B cells, T cells, monocytes, Langerhans cells, keratinocytes, fibroblasts, and endothelial cells (22,34,36,38–41). They have also been identified on autonomic and sensory nerve fibers, particularly the cutaneous nociceptive C-fibers. In the skin, neuropeptides act directly on the vessel walls to produce vasodilation and also, by release of cytokines from mast cells and endothelial cells, as mediators of inflammation; via corticotropin-releasing hormone (CRH) and pro-opiomelanocortin they take part in immune modulation. Substance P, vasoactive intestinal peptide (VIP), and calcitonin gene–related peptide (CGRP), in particular, have been associated with the wheal-and-flare response (23,44) and— of special significance in atopic dermatitis, since it is such a cardinal feature of the disease—with itching (42). The endogenous opioids and serotonin have also been associated with itching and may be released as part of the stress response. Depression and anxiety, with or without overt skin disease, are also associated with itching, and there is evidence to suggest that the release of endogenous opioids may occur in response to stressful situations in which the individual feels helpless, a state particularly common in those who are depressed (49). Thus, although exact pathways and mechanisms have not yet been worked out, there are numerous connections between the cognitive and affective areas of the brain, the stress response, the immune system, and a variety of inflammatory mediators, which can help to explain what has long been recognized clinically—that inflammatory skin disease can be precipitated or exacerbated by situations that are experienced as stressful.

Another psychological phenomenon that may play a part in atopic dermatitis is that of conditioning. As with animals, human subjects can be conditioned to carry out mechanical acts, and evidence suggests that the act of scratching may in some cases be the result of conditioning (50).

V. PSYCHOSOMATIC FINDINGS IN ATOPIC INDIVIDUALS

As we know, genetic, developmental and environmental factors all play a part in the genesis and perpetuation of severe atopic dermatitis. Early studies showed that infants who subsequently developed the disorder demonstrated at birth greater cutaneous excitability than did nonaffected children, as measured by the cremasteric and rooting reflexes (13). From a developmental perspective, the earliest relationships clearly play a crucial role (see Sec. II). Early work in this area focused on the inability of emotionally immature, impoverished, and covertly hostile mothers to meet the needs, specifically the tactile needs, of their inherently itchy infants (13,51–56). More recently clinical observation shows that even mature and emotionally healthy mothers may have difficulties. That the child is visibly flawed arouses ambivalent and conflicting emotions in the mother, of which she may not be consciously aware. Disappointment, shame, and guilt may intrude on her loving acceptance and may make her either reject the child emotionally or, in defense against unacceptable negative feelings, fail to set appropriate limits so as not to frustrate him. These responses, inevitably reinforced by the child's restlessness and discomfort, impact negatively upon the child in the ways described earlier. Unable to comfort the child, and exhausted from lack of sleep, the mother feels inadequate and insecure in her parenting skills. She becomes increasingly anxious, and frustration and anger foment the negative side of the ambivalence, leading to a constellation of behaviors that we see over and over again in clinical practice (12,24,56). Fearful of upsetting him further and empathic to his distress, the mother allows herself to be manipulated by the tiny tyrant, whose needs soon rule the household. Frequently the child is nightly taken into the parental bed, to the detriment of the parental relationship (24).

Certainly cultural factors influence attitudes towards co-sleeping (58), but in the United States, where it is not customary, psychoanalytic studies show that this environment provides more emotional stimulation than the young child can tolerate, leading to increased anxiety (24,30,58,59). From the parental perspective, it is our experience that the mother commonly gives her full attention to preventing her child from scratching, while the father may be relegated to sleeping on the couch, which understandably increases emotional tension within the family. This level of emotional gratification deprives the infant of incentive to give up the manipulative and sensually satisfying scratching behavior, which soon becomes a conditioned response (50) and which, by releasing inflammatory mediators locally, serves to perpetuate the disease.

Though findings are inconsistent, a number of studies support the clinical observations described above. Higher levels of state and trait anxiety and depression (60) can be demonstrated in atopic individuals (61), in whom perceived itch may be enhanced in response to stress (62), while increased environmental stress within the family is associated with more severe disease (63). Conditioned responses can more easily be achieved in those with higher levels of anxiety (60), and in many patients scratching has the quality of a conditioned response. Another study showed that the failure of mothers of preschool children to set limits for fear of confrontation and increased scratching was reflected in psychosocial and motor delay in the children and increased stress and feelings of insecurity in the mothers (64)—findings that are entirely consistent with our own clinical observation. While as many as 81% of patients with atopic dermatitis report their condition to be aggravated by stress (23), there are some who respond to stressful situations by scratching, without conscious awareness of the cause.

Much has been written about the role of conscious or unconscious unexpressed anger as a precipitant of atopic dermatitis (46,65–67), and recent work suggests that, although in one study more than half of the patients were aware of their anger and of its source, there are many who, by the psychological defense mechanisms of denial and repression, avoid experiencing hostile feelings and their attendant itching (24). Reportedly there are patients who experience frustration in situations where they feel helpless, a feeling that is associated with release of endogenous opioids, neuropeptides that are associated with itching. One recent study supports this finding and confirms that adult atopic patients are more anxious and show greater psychophysiological reactivity than patients with psoriasis or control subjects. These patients were more likely to feel angry, but less likely to express it or to act assertively (45). While aggressive feelings usually cause distress, some patients achieve sensual gratification and tension release by scratching. Much has been written about this erotic component of the itch-scratch cycle in the older literature (2,3), and in clinical practice there are patients who will confirm it.

VI. THE IMPACT OF SEVERE ATOPIC DERMATITIS ON THE QUALITY OF LIFE

Any chronic illness inevitably has an impact on patient and family. When the onset is in infancy, and when the demands in time and money are as great as for patients with atopic dermatitis, the impact is that much more profound. A recent study has shown the social and financial cost to the family, for the care of a child with moderately severe atopic dermatitis, to be greater than that for insulin-dependent diabetes mellitus (68). Apart from the ambivalent feelings engendered in the mother and the dysfunctional nature of the mother-child relationship so often seen in these families, and discussed above, there are many practical considerations that affect the parents and siblings of the atopic child that, even under the most favorable circumstances, may generate resentment and conflict (12).

Topical treatments are expensive and time-consuming, often straining the family budget, limiting clothing, and taking the mother's attention away from her husband and her other children. Activities for the family may be restricted, not only because of financial restraints, but in order to avoid situations in which the itching may be aggravated (69). Social interaction for the parents is often limited because of anxiety about leaving the patient and because it is hard to find anyone willing to baby-sit the afflicted child (63). Siblings, feeling left out and unimportant, may resort to attention-seeking behaviors, which may further disrupt the family (24), while for the patient so much attention focused on the body may be experienced as intrusive, an assault, particularly if the genitals are involved (70). Alternatively, the body may become overvalued and the focus of later hypochondriacal concerns.

The parents must constantly be on guard to protect the patient from stigmatization (71,72), ready to reassure others that the condition is not infectious or contagious. Once the child reaches school age, difficulties may arise because his physical appearance, and the attention that his condition has demanded may already have caused him to view himself as defective or different at a time when "sameness" is crucial. Not only does the rash make him different, but he is likely to be smaller than the norm and behind in his motor and psychosocial development (24,61,63,64), his behavior dependent and clinging, and his performance impaired by sleep deprivation (73–75). As a result, his self-esteem is likely to be diminished. Both his appearance and his constant scratching may arouse anxiety in his peers, in defense against which they may make the patient the butt of teasing and aggressive behavior. Aware of the negative response he has generated, the patient may withdraw socially, becoming isolated, and function suboptimally in all areas of his life. Alternatively, in reaction to the feelings of rejection, he may become pushy and aggressive, driving people away and further increasing his isolation. When exudates, crusts, or odor are part of the picture, the situation is even more distressing, and many adult patients movingly describe their childhood confusion about causation and the pain of feeling contaminated, dirty, and unlovable—and often also guilty, as though the rash were punishment for some unnamed and terrible hidden crime (24,61,63).

Adolescence is particularly difficult for patients because of increased peer pressure and because the age-related consolidation of personal and gender identity imposes an additional stress. If body image and self-esteem are already fragile, the pressures may lead to real psychological difficulties, particularly if the face or genitals are involved (76–79). In adult life, though perhaps recognized as illogical, the childhood worries and beliefs often still persist at some level. The constant itching and persistent rash are now an integral part of the body image, and in their inner lives, many patients continue to feel guilty and flawed or damaged, perceiving themselves as unlovely and unlovable (79).

Because of the physical appearance, or because of the need to avoid contact with irritants, employment and recreational opportunities are often limited, as are clothing choices (69,71). Patients are resentful and angry about these limitations and about the time and money that they must expend on skin care that is often messy and uncomfortable (69,71). This expenditure may also occasion guilt, particularly if it puts a strain on a family budget or deprives a child of a wished-for opportunity (68). The characteristic high levels of anxiety, dependent personality, difficulty in handling anger (45,46,61,62), and feelings of ineffectiveness all contribute to interpersonal difficulties for these patients, who may develop rather passive, self-defeating modes of relating (45).

Surprisingly, it is only in the past decade that serious attention has been paid to the quality of life for the patient with chronic skin disease. This very important aspect of dermatology, as we have seen, has implications not only for the patient, but also for the family and the community. Attempts have been made to develop indices that will quantify, reliably and reproducibly, the impact of a number of different skin diseases on the physical and psychosocial aspects of the patient's life (80,81). These measures have some importance in validating the very real disability caused by skin disease, as compared with the more commonly recognized systemic diseases. They are important also in providing a patient-oriented means of clinical monitoring, in assessing the effectiveness of different treatment modalities (82) and the effectiveness and availability of clinical services (83).

Though much of the early work in this area concerned psoriasis and acne, the Dermatology Quality of Life Index (DQLI) and the Children's Quality of Life Index (CDQLI) (85) reflect many aspects of the physical social and emotional life of patients with a number of skin diseases and confirm that for the patient with atopic dermatitis, the toll is very heavy indeed (68,86,87).

VII. PSYCHOLOGICAL TREATMENT OF PATIENTS WITH ATOPIC DERMATITIS

A. The Psychotherapies

In the treatment of any chronic disease, the power of the doctor-patient relationship, as a therapeutic tool, is something we cannot afford to lose sight of. This is especially the case in atopic dermatitis because of the specific nature of the disease and the impact on patient and family. Unless the doctor, the patient, and the parents can forge a trusting relationship, even the latest scientific advances are likely to be of little benefit. Strong feelings of anger, frustration, and guilt, though perhaps hidden, are prevalent in all the involved parties, while the anxiety so characteristic of these patients may be heightened still further by lack of information about the causation, common triggers, and implications of the disease (5,24).

It is important for the doctor to allow the patient to know that he or she can empathize with the feelings of patient and family and with the burdens imposed by the illness and its treatment. The patient and family should know that these feelings are understandable and allowable and that, if they can be freely verbalized, they are less likely to be acted out in counter-productive ways (24). Education, at a level that the patient or parent can readily understand, is central to establishing rapport and should address our current knowledge, possible exacerbating factors, and expectable course of the disease. This information will help to temper anxiety, enhance compliance (24,27,88,89), and provide a basis for helping the patient to develop optimal coping skills. Another aspect of the doctor-patient relationship is the doctor's own emotional response to the other players in the drama. Exacerbating or unresponsive disease, noncompliance, or overly dependent, demanding, or entitled behavior may arouse frustration, anger, and anxiety in the doctor, with a resulting breakdown in empathy. This is a not uncommon reason for patients to "doctor-shop."

The parents of infants and small children need education about the importance of empathic but not excessive touch and about the potential risks of ongoing genital manipulation (24,70), which should become the domain of the patient as soon as he or she is able to handle the responsibility. Parents need help with limit-setting, with interfamily relationships, with understanding the potential problems due to sleep deprivation, and with control of the manipulative use of scratching (24,63,64,73,74,89). Massage therapy has been found helpful in small children (90), and counseling services for mothers and support groups have a place in the overall management.

In the treatment of adults, early work described the benefits of psychoanalytic (91) and insight-oriented psychotherapies, and there is still a place for these treatment modalities (10,22,24,33,92–94). Supportive (95), behavioral (96), and group therapies (97,98), stress-reduction techniques (97,98), and hypnotherapies (99–101) are also reportedly effective, while attention has recently been turned to alternative therapies in dermatology (102). Many parents find support groups helpful, not only for emotional support, but for the exchange of information about coping strategies and the availability of resources (98,103). An interesting emergent phenomenon is topical steroid phobia in atopic eczema, and patients must be helped to approach this concern rationally (104).

B. The Use of Psychotropic Drugs in Atopic Dermatitis

1. Anxiolytic Drugs

Anxiety, depression, itching, and sleep difficulties are all characteristic of atopic dermatitis, and all may be treated with psychotropic drugs (105,106). Anxiety is characterized by autonomic arousal, edginess, motor restlessness, apprehension and dread, fearing the worst, irritability, insomnia, increased or decreased appetite, and fatigue. In the atopic patient, anxiety may also be characterized by scratching, and when itching is regularly exacerbated by stress, with or without any or all of the other symptoms mentioned, anxiolytic drugs are indicated. The benzodiazepines and buspirone are the anxiolytics most frequently prescribed, but doxepin at bedtime is helpful if itching disturbs sleep. If there is a compulsive quality to the scratching, the serotonin antagonist antidepressants or certain of the atypical antipsychotics may be indicated.

The benzodiazepines have an immediate effect, but they are sedating, habit-forming, and subject to tachyphylaxis. It is recommended, therefore, that these drugs be reserved for acute anxiety or the stress associated with physical illness. The characteristics and dosage schedules for these drugs are listed in Table 1. Alprazolam (Xanax) has the advantage that it also has some antidepressant action and may therefore be helpful in situations where both anxiety and depression pertain. For chronic anxiety, a better drug is buspirone (BuSpar), which is neither habit-forming nor sedating and is not subject to tachyphylaxis. Buspirone is usually well tolerated, but takes up to three weeks to take effect. It is advisable to start with a low dose and increase gradually to therapeutic levels to minimize side effects. It is acceptable to prescribe one of the short-acting benzodiazepines along with the buspirone until the latter takes effect. The characteristics of buspirone are listed in Table 1. In childhood, promethazine (Phenergan) is still a particularly useful agent because of sedative and antihistamine effects.

2. Antidepressants

Depression is characterized by changes in sleep or appetite, decreased sex drive, irritability, poor concentration, "always tired," anxiety and worry, social withdrawal, loss of interest in former pursuits, and feelings of helplessness and hopelessness. Unexplained physical symptoms are often part of the picture as well as, in atopic dermatitis, intractable itching. Two groups of antidepressant drugs are commonly used in dermatology (105,106): tricyclics and specific serotonin reuptake inhibitors (SSRIs). The characteristics and dose schedules for these drugs are listed in Table 2. The tricyclics, though tried and true, are less well accepted because of a less favorable side effect profile. However, because of the advantage of sedative and strong antihistamine effects, doxepin, in a small dose at bedtime, may be a useful addition to the treatment regimen.

The SSRIs act almost exclusively on serotonin receptors and therefore have few of the cholinergic side effects of the cyclic drugs. Though in terms of antidepressant effect, all in the group are reportedly equally effective, as with any psychotropic drug, individual response is unpredictable, and it may be necessary to try another in the group if the desired response is not achieved. In recent years, several of these drugs have been approved for treatment of anxiety states, and paroxetine may be a good choice if, along with depression, anxiety is a prominent part of the picture.

3. Atypical Antipsychotics

When itching is wholly intractable and unresponsive to any of the usual dermatological or psychiatric approaches, pimoside (Orap) or olanzepine (Zyprexa), in very low doses, may be tried (105,106). In addition to dopamine pathways, pimoside's association with opioid receptors (105) may account for its very powerful

Table 1 Anxiolytic Drugs

Drug	Onset of action	Dose	Drug interactions	Advantages	Common disadvantages	Withdrawal symptoms
Alprazolam (Xanax)	Peak in 2 hours	0.25–1.0 mg once daily at bedtime, to four times daily, prn, anxiety; taper slowly on discontinuing	Itraconazole Fluconazole Erythromycin CNS depressants Alcohol (decrease the dose of Alprazolam)	Immediate onset Some antidepressive action	Sedation Possible dependency CNS depression Impaired coordination and cognition	Headache Insomnia Motor restlessness Depression Confusion
Buspirone (Buspar)	2–4 weeks	5 mg twice daily, increasing by increments of 5 mgm daily to a total of 10–15 mg × 3, daily	MAO inhibitors Nefazodone (Serzone) Erythromycin Itraconazole Fluconazole (decrease the dose of Buspirone)	Nonsedating Non–habit-forming Little interation with alcohol Long-term use in chronic conditions not contraindicated	Delayed onset of action (may use alprazolam, until buspirone takes effect) Headache, nausea, dizziness if dose increased too quickly	None
Promethazine (Phenergan)	20 minutes –6 hours	6.25–25 mg once daily at bedtime, to four times daily as needed for itching, or anxiety.	CNS depressants Alcohol	Antihistamine Antipruritic Sedative	Drowsiness Lowers seizure threshold Cholinergic effect Possible extrapyramidal effect	None

Table 2 Antidepressant Drugs

1. SSRIs—In order to reduce side effects to a minimum, dosing should start with half the lowest dose available. This should be raised only once weekly by increments of the same amount until the desired effect is achieved. The drug is given once daily, with food. The time of day is determined by whether or not the patient experiences somnolence.

Drug	Dose (mg)	Onset of action	Drug interactions	Advantages	Disadvantages
Fluoxetine (Prozac)	5–60	1–4 weeks	MAO inhibitors Alcohol Tryptophan Warfarin Sumatriptin (Imitrex)	No antihistamine, cholinergic, or α-adrenergic action	GI distress Insomnia Jitteriness Restlessness Headache Increased perspiration Decreased libido Delayed orgasm
Paroxetine (Paxil)	5–50	—	Drugs metabolized by cytochrome		
Sertraline (Zoloft)	25–200	—	p450 enzymes, including tricyclics		

2. Venlafaxin (Effexor)—This antidepressant combines serotonergic with adrenergic effects. It has a more rapid onset of action than the SSRIs, and is less likely to interact with the other drugs listed. The side effect profile is similar to that of SSRIs, but blood pressure should be monitored initially because of occasional treatment emergent hypertension. In some patients it has an antipruritic effect. Dosing starts with 18.75 mg twice daily and is increased by 18.75 mg every 3 days to a dose of 75 mg twice daily.

3. Doxepin—This tricyclic antidepressant has a powerful antihistamine effect and is useful as a sedative and antipruritic, in doses of 10–25 mg at bedtime. The sedative and cholinergic effects limit its usefulness as an antidepressant.

Table 3 Atypical Antipsychotic Drugs

Drug	Onset of action	Dose	Drug interactions	Advantages	Common disadvantages
Pimozide (Orap)	Peak antipruritic action 4–12 hours	0.5–2.0 mg once daily, given at bedtime, unless it causes insomnia (then give in AM)	Drugs that prolong Q-T interval Macrolide antibiotics Itraconazole Fluconazole	Potent antipruritic Some anticompulsive and impulsive effect on scratching	Impaired coordination Anticholinergic effect May lower convulsive threshold Reversible extrapyramidal symptoms at start of treatment (tardive dyskinesia not reported in dermatology patients, to date) Drowsiness Sedation Insomnia Motor restlessness
Olanzepine (Zyprexa)	6 hours Steady state in 1 week	2.5 mg once daily, or alternate days, at bedtime	Carbamazepine (decrease dose of Olanzepine) Alcohol	Sedative Some anticompulsive and anti-impulsive effect on scratching	Orthostatic hypotension Drowsiness Impaired cognitive and motor function (dose-related) Hyperprolactinemia Headache Cholinergic effect Antihistamine effect

Note: In the doses recommended for dermatology patients, side effects have been minimal.

Table 4 Hypnotic Drugs

Drug	Dose (mg)	Drug interaction	Advantages	Disadvantages
Diphenhydramine (Benadryl) antihistamine	25–50	Alcohol	Antihistamine Antipruritic Non–habit forming No tachyphyllaxis	Oversedation Dry mouth and mucous membranes
Doxepin (Sinequan), antidepressant[a]	10–25	MAO inhibitors; alcohol; drugs metabolized by cytochrome p450; SSRI antidepressants (unlikely to cause problems in low-dose schedules)	Antihistamine Antipruritic Non–habit forming No tacchyphyllaxis	Cholinergic effect
Trazadone (Desyrel), antidepressant	50–100 (with food)	Alcohol	Non–habit forming No tachyphyllaxis Safe in patients taking M.A.O.I.'s	Dry mouth Priapism (rare) Orthostatic hypotension
Zolpidem (Ambien), non-benzodiazepine	5–10	None reported	Probably not habit forming No rebound insomnia No tachyphyllaxis No ante-retrograde amnesia Rapid onset of action	Lacks muscle relaxant properties
Flurazepam (Dalmane), benzodiazepine[b]	15–30	Alcohol	Rapid onset of action	Habit forming Rebound insomnia Daytime sedation Withdrawal reactions

[a] Doxepin is a tricyclic antidepressant, with powerful antihistamine, antipruritic, and sedative effects—useful as a hypnotic.
[b] Flurazepam is a short-acting benzodiazepine auxiolytic with sedative action that makes it a useful hypnotic.

antipruritic effect. The action of olanzepine in this regard is not fully understood. The characteristics and dose range for these drugs is listed in Table 3.

4. Hypnotics

Sleep deprivation due to itching is a major problem for many atopic patients. Doxepin and trazadone (Desyrel), another antidepressant, in a low-dose regimen (see Table 4) may be used for sleep without fear of dependency. Hypnotics, such as zelpidem (Ambien), like the benzodiazepines, should be reserved for short-term use.

5. Psychiatric Referral

Characteristically, even when there is a strong psychological component, dermatology patients tend to resist psychiatric referral, but when things are not going well, despite adequate trials of all the above approaches, referral is indicated (5). Once rapport is established, it is often possible to help the patient to identify situations and patterns of behavior, or dysfunctional modes of relating, that are stressful and that trigger flares. Once these are established and the patient can see that the quality of life is impaired, the patient may be encouraged to accept psychiatric referral.

REFERENCES

1. Brocq L, Jacquet L. Notes pour servir à l'histoir des neurodermaties: on lichen circumscriptus des anciens auters, on lichen simplex chronique de M. le Dr. E. Vidal. Ann Dermatol Syphie (Paris) 1891; 2:634.
2. Obermayer ME. Psychocutaneous Medicine. Springfield, IL: Charles C Thomas, 1955, pp. 200–266.
3. Wittkower E, Russell B. Emotional Factors in Skin Disease. New York: Paul B. Hoeber, Inc., 1953, pp. 11–25.
4. Panconesi E. Stress and Skin Diseases, Psychosomatic Dermatology. Philadelphia: J.B. Lippincott, 1984, pp. 107–125.
5. Koblenzer, CS. Psychocutaneous Disease. Orlando, FL: Grune and Stratton, 1987, pp. 1–9, 59–80, 281–310.
6. Gieler U. Atopic dermatitis. In: Paulley JD, Delser HE, eds. Psychological Management for Psychosomatic Disorders. New York: Springer-Verlag, 1989, pp. 257–269.
7. Ader R, Felten DL, Cohen N, eds. Psychoneuroimmunology. 2nd ed. New York: Academic Press, 1991.
8. Greenspan SI. The Development of the Ego. Madison, CT: International Universities Press, 1989, pp. 1–53, 117–130.

9. Greenacre P. Emotional Growth. New York: International Universities Press, Inc., 1971, pp. 22–25.
10. Anzieu D. The Skin Ego. New Haven, CT: Yale University Press, 1989, pp. 55–113.
11. Mahler MS, Pine F, Bergman A. The Psychological Birth of the Human Infant. New York: Basic Books, 1975, pp. 52–64.
12. Koblenzer CS. The psychological and social impact of skin disease. In: Pierini AM, Garcia-Diaz de Pierini R, Bustamente RE, eds. Pediatric Dermatology. New York: Elsevier, 1995, pp. 3–12.
13. Spitz RA. The First Year of Life. New York: International Universities Press, Inc., 1965, pp. 224–242.
14. Weiss SJ. Parental touching. In: Barnard KE, Brazelton B, eds. Touch, the Foundation of Experience. Madison, CT: International Universities Press, 1990, pp. 425–459.
15. Weiss SJ. Parental touch and the child's body image. In: Brown CC, ed. The Many Facets of Touch. Pediatric Round Table 10. Skillman, NJ: Johnson & Johnson, 1984, pp. 130–139.
16. Hoffer W. Development of the Body Ego. In: Eissler RS, Freud A, Hartman H, Uris E, eds. Psychoanalytic Study of the Child. Vol 5. New York: International Universities Press, 1950, pp. 18–23.
17. Pines D. A Woman's Unconscious Use of Her Body. New Haven, CT: Yale University Press, 1994, pp. 8–25.
18. Hofer MA. The mother-infant interaction as a regulator of infant physiology and behavior. In: Plutchnik R, ed. Emotion, Theory, Research & Experience. Vol II. Orlando, FL: Academic Press, 1983, p. 74.
19. Taylor GJ. Psychosomatic Medicine and Contemporary Psychoanalysis. New York: International Universities Press, 1987, pp. 123–125.
20. Nemiah JC, Freyberger H, Sifneos PE. Alexithymia: a view of the psychosomatic process. In: Hill OW, ed. Modern Trends in Psychosomatic Medicine. Vol 3. London: Butterworth, 1976, pp. 430–439.
21. Nemiah J. Alexithymia and Psychosomatic Illness. J Contin Ed Psychiatry 1978; 39:25–37.
22. McDougall J. Theaters of the Body. A Psychoanalytic Approach to Psychosomatic Illness. New York: W.W. Norton & Co, 1989, pp. 24–25, 81–85.
23. Wahlgren CF. Pathophysiology of itching in urticaria and atopic dermatitis. Allergy 1992; 47:65–75.
24. Koblenzer CS, Koblenzer PJ. Chronic intractable atopic eczema: its occurrence as a sign of impaired parent-child relationships and psychological developmental arrest: improvement through parent insight and education. Arch Dermatol 1988; 124: 1673–1677.
25. Rogerson CH. Psychological factors in skin disorders. Br J Dermatol 1947; 59: 6–13.
26. Ring J, Palos E, Zimmermann F. Psychosomatic aspects of parent-child relations in atopic eczema. Hautarzt 1986; 37:560–567.
27. Cotterill JA. Psychophysiologic aspects of eczema. Semin Dermatol 1990; 9:216–219.

28. Cohen DJ. Psychosomatic models of development. In: Anthony EJ, ed. Explorations in Child Psychiatry. New York: Plenum Press, 1975, pp. 197–212.
29. Tantam D, Kalucy R, Brown DE. Sleep, scratching and dreams in eczema, a new approach to alexithymia. Psychother Psychosom 1982; 37:26–35.
30. Freud A. The writings of Anna Freud: Normality and Pathology in Childhood. Vol. 6. New York: International Universities Press, Inc., 1965, pp. 66–67, 93–99, 148–159.
31. Pennebaker JW, Watson D. The psychology of somatic symptoms. In: Kirmayer LJ, Robbins JM, eds. Current Concepts in Somatization. Research and Clinical Perspectives. Washington, DC: American Psychiatric Press, 1991, pp. 21–35.
32. Robbins JM, Kirmayer LJ. Cognitive and social factors in somatization. In Kirmayer LJ, Robbins JM, eds. Current Concepts in Somatization. Research and Clinical Perspectives. Washington, DC: American Psychiatric Press, 1991, pp. 107–141.
33. Koblenzer CS. Psychotherapy for intractable inflammatory dermatoses. J Am Acad Dermatol 1995; 32:609–612.
34. Panconesi E, Hautmann G. Psychophysiology of stress in dermatology. Dermatol Clin 1996; 14:399–421.
35. Miller AH. Neuroendocrine and immune system interactions in stress and depression. Psychiatr Clin North Am 1998; 21:443–463.
36. Tobin D, Nabarro G, Baart de la Faille H, van Vloten WA, van der Pulte SCJ, Schuurman H-J. Increased numbers of immunoreactive nerve fibers in atopic dermatitis. J Allergy Clin Immunol 1992; 90:613–622.
37. O'Leary A. Stress, emotion and human immune function. Psychol Bull 1990; 108:363–382.
38. Luger TA, Sholzen T, Grabbe S. The role of α-melanocyte-stimulating hormone in cutaneous biology. J Invest Dermatol Symp Prog 1997; 2:87–93.
39. Eedy DJ. Neuropeptides in skin. Br J Dermatol 1993; 128:597–605.
40. Hagermark O. Peripheral and central mediators of itch. Skin Pharmacol 1992; 5:1–8.
41. Georgala S, Schulpis KH, Papacoustantinou E, Varelzidis A. Raised serum levels of β-endorphin in chronic urticaria. J Eur Acad Dermatol Venereol 1994; 3:27–30.
42. Sternberg EM. Neuroendocrine factors in susceptibility to inflammatory disease: focus on the hypothalamic-pituitary adrenal axis. Horm Res 1995; 43:159–161.
43. Scholtzen T, Armstrong CA, Bunnett NW, Luger TA, Olerud JE, Ansel JC. Neuropeptides in the skin: interactions between the neuro-endocrine and the skin immune sytems. Exp Dermatol 1998; 7:81–96.
44. Ansel JC, Armstring CA, Song IS, Quinlan KL, Olerud JE, Caughman SW, Bunnett NW. Interactions of the skin and nervous systems. J Invest Dermatol 1997; 2:23–26.
45. Whitlock FA. Psychophysiologic Aspects of Skin Disease. Philadelphia: Saunders, 1976, pp. 110–114.
46. Ginsburg IH, Prystowsky JH, Kornfeld DS, Wolland H. Role of emotional factors in adults with atopic dermatitis. Int J Dermatol 1993; 32:656–660.
47. Edwards KCS. Pruritus in melancholia. Br Med J 1954; II:1527–1529.

48. Prange AJ, Loosen PT. Peptides in depression. In: Ustin E, ed. Frontiers in Biochemical and Pharmacologic Research. New York: Raven Press, 1984, p. 137.

49. Gupta MA, Gupta AK, Schork NJ, Ellis CN. Depression modulates pruritus perception: a study of pruritus in psoriasis, atopic dermatitis, and chronic idiopathic urticaria. Psychosom Med 1994; 56:36–40.

50. Jordan JM, Whitlock FA. Emotions and the skin: the conditioning of scratch responses, in cases of atopic dermatitis. Br J Dermatol 1972; 86:574–585.

51. Williams DH. Management of atopic dermatitis in children. Control of the maternal rejection factor. Arch Dermatol Syphylol 1951; 63:545–560.

52. Marmor J, Ashley M, Tabachnick N, Storkan M, McDonald F. The mother-child relationship in the genesis of neurodermatitis. Arch Dermatol 1956; 74:599–605.

53. Vaughan VC. Emotional undertones in eczema in children. J Asthma Res 1966; 3:193–197.

54. Rosenthal MJ. A psychosomatic study of infantile eczema I, the mother-child relationship. Pediatrics 1952; 10:581–591.

55. Miller H, Baruch DW. Psychosomatic studies of children with allergic manifestation. I. Maternal rejection: a study of 63 cases. Psychosom Med 1948; 10:275–278.

56. Gil KM, Sampson HA. Psychological and social factors of atopic dermatitis. Allergy 1989; 44 (suppl 9):84–89.

57. Ehlers A, Osen A, Wenniger K, Gieler U. Atopic Dermatitis and stress: possible role of negative communication with significant others. Int J Behav Med 1994; 1: 107–121.

58. Latz S, Wolf AW, Lozoff B. Co-sleeping in context. Sleep practice and problems in young children in Japan, and the United States. Arch Pediatr Adolesc Med 1999; 153:339–346.

59. Furman E. Toddlers and their mothers. A study in early personality development. Madison, CT: International Universities Press, 1992, pp. 168–175, 226.

60. Gupta MA, Gupta AK. Depression and suicidal ideation in dermatology patients with acne, alopecia areata, atopic dermatitis and psoriasis. Br J Dermatol 1998; 139:846–850.

61. Faulstich ME, Williamson DA, Duchmann EG, Conerly SC, Brantley PJ. Psychophysiological analysis of atopic dermatitis. J Psychosom Res 1985; 29:415–417.

62. Faulstich ME, Williamson DA. An overview of atopic dermatitis: towards a biobehavioral integration. J Psychosom Res 1985; 29:647–654.

63. Gil KM, Keefe FJ, Sampson HA, McCaskill CC, Rodin J, Krisson JE. The relation of stress and family environment to atopic dermatitis symptoms in children. J Psychosom Res 1987; 31:673–684.

64. Daud LR, Garraldu ME, David TJ. Psychosocial adjustment in pre-school children with atopic eczema. Arch Dis Child 1993; 69:670–676.

65. Miller H, Baruch DW. A study of hostility in allergic children. Am J Orthopsychiatry 1950; 20:506–519.

66. Brown DG. Emotional disturbance in eczema: a study of symptom-reporting behavior. J Psychosom Res 1967; 11:27–40.

67. White A, Horn DJ de L, Varigos GA. Psychological profile of the atopic eczema patient. Australas J Dermatol 1990; 31:13–16.

68. Kemp AS. Atopic eczema: It's social and financial costs. J Pediatr Child Health 1999; 35:229–231.
69. Morren MA, Przybilla B, Bamehs M, Hykants B, Reynaer A, Degreef H. Atopic dermatitis: triggering factors. J Am Acad Dermatol 1994; 31:467–473.
70. Herman-Giddens ME. Harmful genital care practices in children. A type of child abuse. J Am Med Assoc 1989; 261:577–579.
71. Ginsburg IH, Link BG. Feelings of stigmatization in patients with psoriasis. J Am Acad Dermatol 1989; 20:53–63.
72. Eun HC, Finlay AY. Measurement of atopic dermatitis disability. Ann Dermatol 1990; 2:9–12.
73. Absolon CM, Cottrell D, Eldridge SM, Glover MT. Psychologic disturbances in atopic eczema: the extent of the problem in school-aged children. Br J Dermatol 1997; 137:241–245.
74. Dahl RE, Bernhisel-Broadbent J, Scanlon-Holdford S, Sampson HA, Lupo M. Sleep disturbances in children with atopic dermatitis. Arch Pediatr Adolesc Med 1995; 149:846–860.
75. Stores G, Burrows A, Crawford C. Physiological sleep disturbance in children with atopic dermatitis: a case control study. Pediat Dermatol 1998; 15:264–268.
76. Kaplan EH. Adolescence age 15–18. A psychoanalytic developmental view. In: Greenspan SI, Pollock GE, eds. The Course of Life. Vol. IV, Adolescence. Madison, CT: International Universities Press, 1991, p. 205.
77. Blos P. The adolescent passage. Developmental issues. New York: International Universities Press, 1979, pp. 141–170.
78. Blos P. On adolescence. A psychoanalytic interpretation. New York: Free Press, 1962.
79. Koblenzer CS. Psychodermatology of women. Clin Dermatol 1997; 15:127–141.
80. Morgan M, McCreedy R, Simpson J, Hay RJ. Dermatology quality of life scales—a measure of the impact of skin disease. Br J Dermatol 1997; 136:202–206.
81. Finlay AY. Quality of life measurement in dermatology: a practical guide. Br J Dermatol 1997; 136:305–314.
82. Salek MS, Finlay AY, Luscombe DK, Allen BR, Berth-Jones J, Camp RDR, Graham-Brown RAC, Khan GK, Marks R, Motley RJ, Ross JS, Sowden JM. Cyclosporin greatly improves the quality of life of adults with severe atopic dermatitis. Br J Dermatol 1993; 129:422–430.
83. Jemec GBE, Wulf HC. Patient-Physician consensus on quality of life in dermatology. Clin and Exp Dermatol 1996; 21:177–179.
84. Finlay AY, Khan GK. Dermatology Life Quality Index (DLQI)—a simple practical measure for routine clinical use. Clin and Exp Dermatol 1994; 19:210–216.
85. Lewis-Jones MS, Finlay AY. The Children's Dermatology Life Quality Index (CDLQI): initial validation and practical use. Br J Dermatol 1995; 132:942–949.
86. Finlay AY. Measures of the effect of adult severe atopic eczema on quality of life. J Eur Acad Dermatol Venereol 1996; 7:149–154.
87. Lawson V, Lewis-Jones MS, Finlay AY, Reid P, Owens RG. The family impact of childhood atopic dermatitis: The Dermatitis Family Impact Questionnaire. Br J Dermatol 1998; 138:107–113.

88. Yamamoto K. How doctor's advice is followed by mothers of atopic children. Acta Derm Venereol (Stockh) 1989; (suppl 144):31–33.

89. Friman PC, Hoff KE, Schnoes MA, Freeman KA, Woods DW, Blum M. The bedtime pass. An approach to crying, and leaving the room. Arch Pediatr Adolesc Med 1999; 153:1027–1029.

90. Schachner L, Field T, Hernandez-Reif M, Duarte AM, Krasnegor J. Atopic dermatitis symptoms decreased, in children following massage therapy. Pediatric Dermatol 1998; 15:390–395.

91. Schecter M. Psychoanalysis of a latency boy with neurodermatitis. In: Eissler RS, ed. Psychoanalytic Study of the Child, Vol. 26. New York: Quadrangle Books, 1973, pp. 529–564.

92. Rogerson CH. The role of psychotherapy in the treatment of the asthma-eczema-prurigo complex in children. Br J Dermatol 1934; 46:368–378.

93. Schoenberg B, Carr AC. An investigation of criteria for brief psychotherapy of neurodermatitis. Psychosom Med 1963; 253–263.

94. Brown DG, Beltley FR. Psychiatric treatment of eczema: a controlled trial. Br Med J 1971; 2:729–734.

95. Ehlers A, Stangier G, Gieler U. Treatment of atopic dermatitis: a comparison of psychologic and dermatologic approaches to relapse prevention. J Consult Clin Psychol 1995; 63:624–635.

96. Noren P, Melin L. The effect of combined topical steroids, and habit-reversal treatment in patients with atopic dermatitis. Br J Dermatol 1989; 121:359–366.

97. Cole WC, Roth HL, Sachs LB. Group psychotherapy as an aid in the medical treatment of eczema. J Am Acad Dermatol 1988; 18:286–291.

98. McSkimming J, Gleeson L, Sinclair M. A pilot study of a support group for parents of children with eczema. Aust J Dermatol 1984; 25:8–11.

99. McManamy CJ, Katz RC, Gipson M. Treatment of eczema by EMG biofeedback and relaxation training: A multiple baseline analysis. J Behav Ther Exp Psychiatry 1988; 19:221–227.

100. Smyth JM, Stone AA, Hurewitz A, Krell A. Effects of writing about stressful experiences on symptom reduction, in patients with asthma and rheumatoid arthritis. J Am Med Assoc 1999; 281:1304–1309.

101. Stewart AC, Thomas SE. Hypnotherapy as a treatment for atopic dermatitis in adults and children. Br J Dermatol 1995; 132:778–783.

102. Eisenberg D. Alternative therapies for cutaneous disorders (editorial). Arch Dermatol 1997; 133:379–380.

103. Ardil L. The National Eczema Society. The Practitioner 1984; 228:1059–1062.

104. Charman CR, Morris AD, Williams HC. Topical corticosteroid phobia in patients with atopic eczema. Br J Dermatol 2000; 142:931–936.

105. Koblenzer CS. Psychotropic drugs in dermatology. In: Advances in Dermatology, Vol. 15. James WD, Cockerell CJ, Dzubow LM, Paller AS, Yancey KB, eds. New York: Mosby, 1999, pp. 183–201.

106. Gupta MA, Gupta AK. Psychodermatology: an update. J Am Acad Dermatol 1996; 34:1030–1046.

27
Topical Macrolide Immunomodulators for Therapy of Atopic Dermatitis

Sakari Reitamo
University of Helsinki, Helsinki, Finland

I. INTRODUCTION

To date, tacrolimus (FK 506) and the ascomycin derivative pimecrolimus (SDZ ASM 981) are the most studied topical macrolide immunomodulators. Both of these drugs have a high specificity for inhibiting the expression of inflammatory T-cell cytokines and have shown promising results in the treatment of atopic dermatitis (AD) when applied topically. This chapter will review the pharmacology and clinical findings for these agents.

II. ORIGINS

Tacrolimus was discovered, using the mixed lymphocyte reaction as a screening method, by T. Goto and colleagues in 1984 from a strain of *Streptomyces* isolated from a soil sample from Mount Tsukuba in Japan. They named this strain *Streptomyces tsukubaensis* after Mount Tsukuba (1). Pimecrolimus is a derivative of ascomycin, the latter being discovered in a screen for antifungal agents from the strain *Streptomyces hygroscopicus* var. *ascomyceticus* and later assessed for activity in the mixed lymphocyte reaction (2,3). Both ascomycin and tacrolimus have antifungal activity (2,4). Ascomycin differs from tacrolimus at a single site with an ethyl group instead of the propenyl side chain residue (Fig. 1). Tacrolimus and pimecrolimus have similar molecular weights (822.05 for tacrolimus and

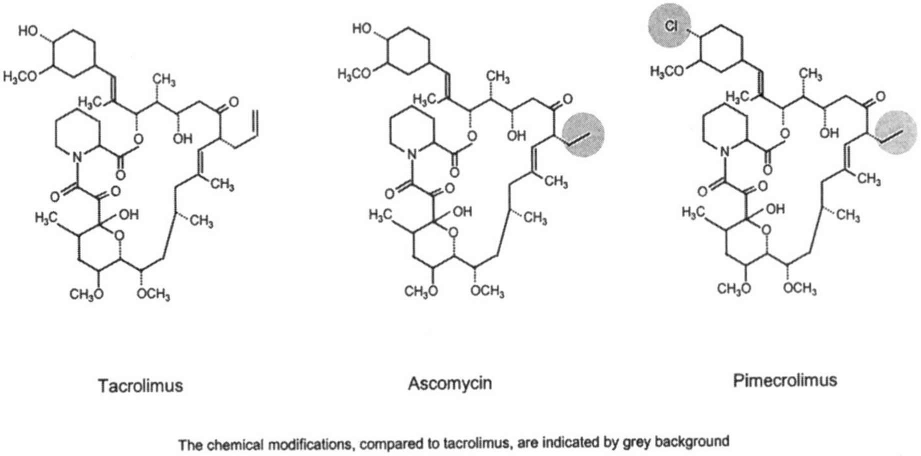

Tacrolimus   Ascomycin   Pimecrolimus

The chemical modifications, compared to tacrolimus, are indicated by grey background

Figure 1 Molecular structures of tacrolimus, ascomycin, and pimecrolimus/SDZ ASM 981. (Adapted from Refs. 1, 3, and 24, respectively.)

810.48 for pimecrolimus) and similar structures, the differences being the above-mentioned ethyl group of ascomycin in pimecrolimus instead of the propenyl side chain residue and an exchange of a hydroxyl group in tacrolimus for chlorine in pimecrolimus to make pimecrolimus more lipophilic (Fig. 1).

III. MECHANISM OF ACTION

Tacrolimus and pimecrolimus have similar modes of action (Fig. 2). Both drugs bind to the FK506-binding protein (FKBP-12), a 12 kDa macrophilin. The FKBP-12/tacrolimus (or pimecrolimus) complex inhibits the phosphatase activity of calcineurin and thereby the dephosphorylation of the nuclear factor of activated

Figure 2 T cells and Langerhans cells in atopic dermatitis. FcεRI: high-affinity IgE receptor; FKBP: FK-binding protein; IMP3: inositol-3-phosphate; IL-2R: interleukin-2 receptor; NF-ATp: nuclear factor for activated T-cell protein; PKC: protein kinase C; LC: Langerhans cell. (a) Antigen presentation by Langerhans cell (LC) to T_{HELPER} cell. (b) Effect of tacrolimus/pimecrolimus on antigen-presentation by LC and activation of T_{HELPER} cells. Tacrolimus downregulates the expression of FcεRI in LC. The effect of pimecrolimus on LC has not been studied. In T_{HELPER} cells, tacrolimus/pimecrolimus inhibits the expression of inflammatory cytokines by blocking the dephosphorylation of NF-ATp. (From Ref. 10.)

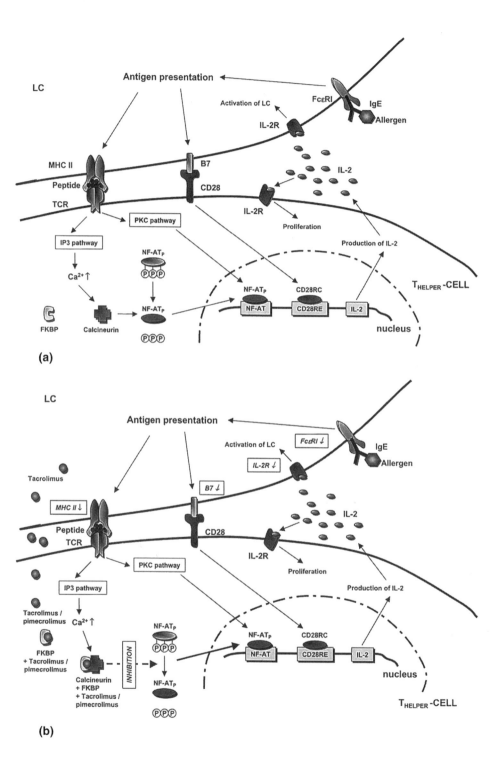

(a)

(b)

T-cell protein (NF-ATp), a transcription factor necessary for the expression of inflammatory cytokines. Inhibition of T-cell proliferation in the mixed lymphocyte reaction by tacrolimus (1) and pimecrolimus (5) principally reflects downregulation of the expression of the cytokine interleukin-2 (IL-2). Tacrolimus also inhibits the expression of the T-cell cytokines IL-3, IL-4, IL-5, granulocyte-macrophage colony-stimulating factor (GM-CSF), interferon-γ (INF-γ), and tumor necrosis factor-α (TNF-α) (6). Pimecrolimus has been shown to inhibit in T cells the expression of IL-2, IL-4, IL-10, and INF-γ (5). In the immune pathology of AD, type-2 T-helper (Th2) cell cytokines (principally IL-4 and IL-5) mediate the early inflammatory response and eosinophil proliferation, and Th1 cell cytokines (principally INF-γ) mediate the late and chronic phases of the inflammatory response (7,8). IL-3, GM-CSF, and TNF-α, in addition to IL-4 and IL-5, are important in the eosinophil inflammatory response in AD (8).

In addition to T cells, Langerhans cells as antigen-presenting cells seem to play an important role in AD (9,10) (Fig. 2a). AD is characterized by strong expression of the high-affinity receptor for IgE (FcϵRI) on antigen-presenting epidermal dendritic cells, i.e., Langerhans cells and related CD1a+ dendritic cells (9). Thus, FcϵRI is a potential target in AD therapy. In vitro, tacrolimus downregulated the expression of FcϵRI (Fig. 2b), whereas betamethasone upregulated its expression (11,12). The effect of pimecrolimus on FcϵRI expression has not been assessed.

Cutaneous mast cells and basophils are involved in the pathophysiology of cutaneous inflammation and in the mediation of itch in AD. In human skin mast cells activated with anti-IgE, tacrolimus inhibited the release of histamine and de novo synthesis of prostaglandin D_2 (13). The release of histamine and de novo synthesized peptide leukotriene C_4 from activated human basophils was also inhibited by tacrolimus (14). In an in vitro mouse system, tacrolimus inhibited cytokine release of stimulated mast cells but not their proliferation (15,16). Pimecrolimus shares a specificity for mast cells. Pimecrolimus inhibited the release of the preformed pro-inflammatory mediator hexosaminidase from stimulated mouse mast cells (5). In rat basophilic leukemia cells, pimecrolimus inhibited FcϵRI-mediated release of the preformed mediators serotonin and β-hexosaminidase and of the transcription and release of TNF-α (17). Pimecrolimus has also been shown to inhibit anti-IgE–stimulated mediator release in human dermal mast cells (18).

AD has features in common with type I and type IV hypersensitivity. In in vivo studies, topical tacrolimus had no effect on the immediate phase of type I hypersensitivity but inhibited the late phase of this biphasic reaction and inhibited type IV delayed hypersensitivity. In mice, tacrolimus ointment (0.01%, 0.1%, 1%) did not inhibit egg albumin–induced passive cutaneous anaphylaxis or ear edema in the immediate phase of the biphasic reaction. However, it did inhibit ear edema in the late phase reaction (19,20). T cells in the late phase reaction have a cytokine expression pattern similar to that of Th2 cells (IL-3, IL-4, IL-5, and GM-CSF, but no IFN-γ) (21), and Th2 cells are implicated in the acute inflammatory response of AD. Thus, it seems that tacrolimus blocks the late phase reaction of type I hypersensitivity and the acute inflammatory reaction of AD by inhibiting the expression of Th2-specific cytokines. Tacrolimus ointment also inhibited delayed (type IV) hypersensitivity (allergic contact dermatitis/ACD) in tuberculin-sensitized mice and rats (20), suggesting downregulation of the expression of cytokines involved in the activation of antigen-specific memory T cells. Inhibition of delayed hypersensitivity by topically applied tacrolimus has also been demonstrated in dinitrofluorobenzene-sensitized domestic pigs (22), in oxazolone-sensitized mice (19), and in dinitrochlorobenzene-sensitized human volunteers (23).

Topical pimecrolimus inhibited delayed hypersensitivity reactions in dinitrofluorobenzene-sensitized domestic pigs, in dinitrofluorobenzene-sensitized rats, and in oxazolone-sensitized mice (24). The effect of topical pimecrolimus on type I hypersensitivity seems not to have been assessed.

Tacrolimus has an approximately threefold higher affinity to the FK-binding protein than pimecrolimus and consequently a higher calcineurin-inhibiting potency (25). The greater calcineurin-inhibiting activity of tacrolimus may be relevant in vivo. When applied topically, tacrolimus was more effective than pimecrolimus in inhibiting delayed hypersensitivity reactions in dinitrofluorobenzene-sensitized pigs; an inhibition of gross lesions of approximately 55% was observed with 0.04% tacrolimus, whereas a concentration of 0.13% pimecrolimus was required to reach a 48% inhibition under similar conditions (22,24). However, comparison of these two studies may not be valid as they were conducted 5 years apart, with a change in the source of animals and a possible change in the subjective assessment of the clinical scores (A. Stuetz, personal communication). Oral doses required to inhibit delayed hypersensitivity reactions in oxazolone-sensitized mice were similar for tacrolimus and pimecrolimus (30 mg/kg, 2 h before and immediately after challenge) (24,26). In contrast, orally administered tacrolimus but not pimecrolimus inhibited the sensitization phase in this murine allergic contact dermatitis model (26). Further studies are needed to find out whether these differences are truly qualitative in nature or depend on the doses used for tacrolimus and pimecrolimus, respectively.

Both tacrolimus and pimecrolimus were effective in animal models of AD. In NC/Nga mice, tacrolimus ointment (0.1%) suppressed the development of dermatitis, was effective against established dermatitis, and suppressed increases in T cells, mast cells, eosinophils, IL-4, IL-5, and IgE (27). Similarly, oral (12.5 mg/kg) and topical administration of pimecrolimus (0.4% in a ethanol/glycol solution) prevented or inhibited AD-like symptoms in hypomagnesaemic hairless rats and reduced histaminemia, leucocytosis, eosinophilia, and serum nitric oxide levels (28). In terms of models of systemic immunosuppression, both tacrolimus and pimecrolimus prevented kidney allograft rejection and graft-versus-host disease in rats (24,26,29,30).

As the mode of action of tacrolimus and pimecrolimus is different from corticosteroids, these agents do not have the potential for causing skin atrophy. For tacrolimus ointment, this was confirmed in a rat study (31) and in a randomized, double-blind clinical study with AD patients ($n = 14$) and healthy volunteers ($n = 12$) (32). In the clinical study, subjects were treated for one week under occlusion, and the carboxy- and amino-terminal propeptides of procollagen I (PICP, PINP) and the amino-terminal propeptide of procollagen III (PIIINP) were measured from suction blister fluid with specific radioimmunoassays. Sites treated with 0.1% betamethasone-valerate ointment showed median PICP, PINP, and PIIINP concentrations of 17.0%, 17.6%, and 39.5% of the vehicle control, respectively, whereas 0.1% and 0.3% tacrolimus-treated sites showed median concentrations comparable to the vehicle control ($\cong 100\%$) ($p < 0.001$) (see Fig. 3). Betamethasone-valerate ointment was also the only treatment to reduce skin thickness. The median decrease in skin thickness was 7.4% relative to 0.1% tacrolimus, 7.1% relative to 0.3% tacrolimus, and 8.8% relative to the vehicle control ($p < 0.01$ in pairwise comparisons).

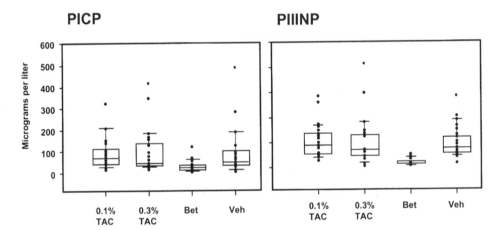

Figure 3 Concentrations of PICP, PINP, and PIIINP after 1 week of treatment with 0.1% tacrolimus, 0.3% tacrolimus, 0.1% betamethasone, or a vehicle control ($n = 25$). The middle line of each box represents the median value. The top and bottom lines of each box represent the upper and lower quartiles, respectively, and the upper and lower bars represent the 90% and 10% limits. The closed circles are individual values. 0.1% Tac, 0.1% tacrolimus; 0.3% Tac, 0.3% tacrolimus; Bet, 0.1% betamethasone; Veh, vehicle (the tacrolimus ointment base). (From Ref. 32.)

Similarly, a safety pharmacology study in pigs (24) and a clinical 4-week, randomized, double-blind study with healthy volunteers showed pimecrolimus not to induce skin atrophy (33,34). In the latter study four different preparations—pimecrolimus 1% cream, the corresponding vehicle of pimecrolimus cream, betamethasone-17-valerate 0.1% cream, and triamcinolone acetonide 0.1% cream—were applied to the volar aspect of the forearms of 16 healthy volunteers, twice daily, 6 days a week, for 4 weeks (33,34). Skin thickness was evaluated by echography, clinical signs of atrophy by stereomicroscopy, and epidermal thickness was assessed by histology. Both topical corticosteroids induced a significant reduction in skin thickness, as compared to pimecrolimus 1% cream and vehicle, which were shown to be equivalent. The difference in skin thickness (measured by echography) between patients treated with pimecrolimus 1% cream and those receiving either of the two topical steroids was significant from day 8 onwards. Histological analysis performed at day 29 showed significant epidermal thinning with topical steroids compared to pimecrolimus 1% cream or the vehicle.

IV. PHARMACOKINETICS

All studies to date indicate that systemic absorption of topically applied tacrolimus and pimecrolimus is minimal.

In a pharmacokinetic study in which 0.3% tacrolimus (a 10-fold higher concentration than the lowest commercial dose) was applied to 100 cm^2 ($n = 21$), 500 cm^2 ($n = 6$), 1000 cm^2 ($n = 6$), or 5000 cm^2 ($n = 6$) of skin in patients with moderate to severe AD, systemic exposure was low but tended to increase with increasing treatment areas (35). In adults ($n = 31$, with treatment areas up to 500 cm^2), the C_{max} ranged from 0.2 to 3.5 $\pm$ 3.1 ng/mL and the area under the curve at 0–24 hours (AUC_{0-24}) ranged from 2.2 $\pm$ 0.8 to 42.5 $\pm$ 37.1 ng.h/mL. In children (1–12 years old, $n = 8$, with 100 cm^2 treatment area), the C_{max} ranged from 0.1 $\pm$ 0.1 to 1.9 $\pm$ 1.3 ng/mL and the AUC_{0-24} ranged from 0.9 $\pm$ 1.0 to 17.3 $\pm$ 10.7 ng.h/mL. Compared with historical AUC data following intravenous administration of tacrolimus, the bioavailability of topical tacrolimus was <0.5% (35). Systemic exposure (AUC_{0-24}) was lower on day 8 than on day 1, supporting the lack of systemic accumulation.

Twelve clinical studies, which included a total of 2015 adult and pediatric AD patients treated with 0.03–0.3% tacrolimus ointment, included assessments of tacrolimus concentrations in whole blood. Treatment areas were up to 100% of the total body surface area, with treatment periods of up to 1 week ($n = 40$), 3 weeks ($n = 659$), 12 weeks ($n = 443$), and 12 months ($n = 873$). Of these 2015 patients, the maximum tacrolimus concentration was below 0.5 ng/mL for 60.5% of patients, 0.5–<1 ng/mL for 20.6% of patients, 1–<2 ng/mL for 10.9% of patients, 2–<5 ng/mL for 6.7% of patients, with only 1.3% of patients having a concentration over 5 ng/mL at any time during the study (N. Undre, personal communication, 2000). For patients who experienced a measurable tacrolimus determination, systemic exposure was transient, decreasing as skin healed. By comparison, daily trough (predosing) concentrations of 5–20 ng/mL, maintained for the lifetime of a transplant recipient, are recommended for prevention of allograft rejection (package insert for Prograf®, Fujisawa). Thus, the systemic exposure with tacrolimus ointment observed in these studies can be considered minimal and unlikely to be of clinical significance. The only cases of systemic exposure of potential clinical systemic significance were two patients in a Japanese pharmacokinetic study, who experienced a transient level of 20 ng/mL after whole body application of 0.1% tacrolimus (36). These two patients (0.1% of the total treated population) represent the maximum levels reported worldwide.

In a pharmacokinetic study in which 1% pimecrolimus cream was applied to 15–59% of the total body surface in 12 adult patients, the majority of the blood samples (78%) provided nonquantifiable (below the assay limit of quantitation of 0.5 ng/mL) concentrations (38). The maximum area under the curve at 0–12 hours (AUC_{0-12}) was 11.4 h.ng/mL (37). Maximum concentrations were 1.1, 1.4, and 4.6 ng/mL, with the latter value having been excluded from pharmacokinetic analysis because it was suspected to have been associated with contamination during venipuncture. In 40 patients treated for up to 1 year on an as-needed basis on up to 62% of their body surface area, the maximal blood concentration was 0.8 ng/mL and 98% of the blood concentrations were below 0.5% ng/mL. There was no evidence of systemic accumulation with repeated dosing. In pediatric pharmacokinetic studies involving a total of 58 AD patients aged 3 months to <2 years ($n = 35$), 2–4 years ($n = 13$), and 8–14 years ($n = 19$) treated on up to 92% of their total body surface area, blood concentrations were consistently low (38), typically <1 ng/mL (39). The maximum blood concentration in infants was 2.26 ng/mL (39). The range of blood concentration measured in infants was comparable to that measured in children and adults. In all these patients, systemic exposure was low. There is limited clinical experience from only one study with orally administered pimecrolimus (40); thus, the significance of any dose-related systemic exposure is mainly from a maximum tolerated dose study in patients with psoriasis (40). In this study the clinical tolerability was good at all dose levels of pimecrolimus observed up to the highest dose tested (30 mg b.i.d.). On the basis of the low blood levels of pimecrolimus observed after topical use and their relationship to the levels associated with no toxicity in animal toxicology studies and in the human oral study, there is a considerable safety factor for the 1% pimecrolimus cream.

Molecules larger than 500 daltons are usually unable to penetrate the epidermis of healthy skin (41). Thus, tacrolimus (822.05 daltons) and pimecrolimus (810.48 daltons) could be self-regulatory, with no penetration through healthy skin and low absorption through skin having a compromised barrier function, such as in AD. The much larger calcineurin inhibitor cyclosporin (1202.6 daltons) is not effective when applied topically (42,43), although it is effective when administered orally (see Chapter 29).

V. CLINICAL EFFICACY AND SAFETY IN ADULTS

A. Tacrolimus Ointment

Early pilot studies in Japan showed promising results for tacrolimus ointment in the treatment of adult patients with AD (44,45). In a phase I study conducted in the United States with patients who had moderate to severe AD, 17 of 31 adult patients (54%) reported excellent improvement or clearance after 8 days of treatment with 0.3% tacrolimus ointment, and no safety concerns were identified (35).

In Europe, a randomized, double-blind, multicenter phase II study compared ointments containing 0.03% ($n = 54$), 0.1% ($n = 54$), and 0.3% tacrolimus ($n = 51$) with a vehicle control ($n = 54$) in adult patients (13–60 years old) with moderate to severe atopic dermatitis (46). The treatment area was restricted to 1000 cm^2. The primary endpoint was a combined score for erythema, edema, and pruritus (each graded on a scale of 0–3) after 3 weeks of treatment. Only 13–14% of patients withdrew from the tacrolimus treatment groups, whereas 39% of patients on vehicle prematurely withdrew from the study. After 3 weeks of treatment, median decreases of 66.7%, 83.3%, and 75.0% in the combined score were observed on the trunk and extremities for 0.03%, 0.1%, and 0.3% tacrolimus ointment, respectively, whereas only a 22.5% decrease was observed for the vehicle control group ($p < 0.001$). Differences among the three tacrolimus treatment groups were not statistically significant. A separate analysis of efficacy for face and neck regions showed similar results. Burning sensation of the skin was the only adverse event that showed a higher incidence with tacrolimus ointment compared with the vehicle control ($p < 0.001$).

Two phase III multicenter, randomized, double-blind, vehicle-controlled studies in the United States demonstrated the efficacy and safety of 0.03% and 0.1% tacrolimus ointment in adult patients with moderate to severe AD (47,48). In these two studies combined, patients received 0.03% tacrolimus ($n = 211$), 0.1% tacrolimus ($n = 209$), or vehicle ($n = 212$) twice daily for up to 12 weeks. At baseline, the mean affected BSA was approximately 45% across treatment groups. The drop-out rate was high in the vehicle group (68.4%) compared with the 0.03% tacrolimus (28.9%) and 0.1% tacrolimus (24.9%) groups. Most withdrawals in the vehicle group were attributed to lack of efficacy. All efficacy assessments showed significantly greater improvement for patients who received 0.03% or 0.1% tacrolimus compared with those who received vehicle. Treatment success [defined as excellent (90–99%) improvement or cleared (100% improvement)] was observed in 6.6% of patients who received vehicle compared with

27.5% and 36.8% of patients who received 0.03% and 0.1% tacrolimus, respectively; differences between vehicle and both tacrolimus treatment groups ($p <$ 0.001) and between the 0.03% and 0.1% tacrolimus groups ($p = 0.041$) were statistically significant. Moderate or better improvement was observed for 19.8%, 61.6%, and 72.7% of patients, respectively (Fig. 4). The Eczema Area and Severity Index, total score, pruritus, and percent affected BSA also showed statistically significant greater improvement with tacrolimus ointment compared with vehicle. Findings for the two individual studies were consistent with the combined analysis. Tacrolimus ointment, 0.03% and 0.1%, was also shown to be safe. Skin burning and pruritus were common but tended to occur only during the first few days of treatment. Flu-like symptoms (investigator terms were upper respiratory tract infection, cold, head cold, flu, flu symptoms, stomach flu, etc.) were common and showed a higher incidence rate in the 0.1% tacrolimus group than in the vehicle group. Other adverse events showing a higher incidence rate in the 0.03% or 0.1% tacrolimus group were headache, skin tingling, acne, alcohol intolerance (skin/facial flushing, redness, heat sensation after alcohol consumption), hyperesthesia (sensitive skin, skin sensitive to temperature changes), folliculitis (inflamed, swollen, or infected hair follicles), rash, sinusitis, cyst, myalgia, and back pain. Some of these differences may have occurred by chance. Laboratory profiles during the study were unremarkable.

The safety and efficacy of up to one year of 0.1% tacrolimus ointment monotherapy in adults with moderate to severe atopic dermatitis was demonstrated in a multicenter, open-label phase III study conducted in Europe (49). Three hundred and sixteen patients were enrolled and received treatment; 200 patients were assigned to 6 months of treatment and 116 to 12 months. In total, 245 patients (77.5%) completed the study; 246 patients completed at least 6 months of therapy and 68 completed at least 12 months of therapy. Reasons for withdrawal were administrative (withdrawal of consent, noncompliance, lost to follow-up, pregnancy, 23/316, 7.3%), lack of efficacy (19/316, 6.0%), prohibited therapy (13/316, 4.1%), adverse events (13/316, 4.1%), and other (3/316, 0.9%). At baseline, a median of approximately one third of the total body surface area was affected with AD. During treatment initiation, local irritation, including such adverse events as burning sensation (47% of patients), pruritus (24%), and erythema (12%), was common. There was no evidence of an increased risk of any

---

Figure 4 Physician's global evaluation of clinical response in adult and pediatric 12-week studies comparing 0.03% and 0.1% tacrolimus ointment with a vehicle control. Cumulative percentage of patients with ratings of cleared (100% improvement), excellent (90–99% improvement), marked (75–89% improvement), or moderate (50–74% improvement) at the end of treatment. (Adapted from Refs. 47 and 59.)

Adult patients (N = 632)

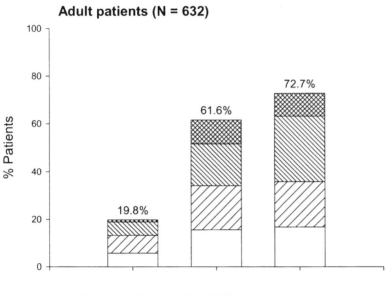

Pediatric patients (N = 351)

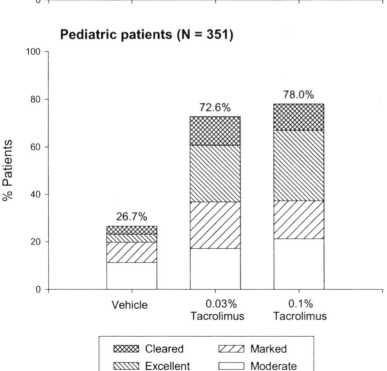

type of infection compared with historical data from the literature. All efficacy endpoints showed improvement within one week of starting treatment and continued improvement with long-term treatment. The mean SD modified Eczema Area and Severity Index Score was 23.7 ± 12.6 at day 1, 13.5 ± 11.3 at week 1, 6.1 ± 9.2 at month 6, and 6.1 ± 8.1 at month 12. Excellent (90–99%) improvement or clearance (100% improvement) was observed in 17% of patients at week 1 and approximately 60% of patients at months 6 and 12. Daily ointment use decreased by about one half from week 1 (median of 3.9 g) to month 6 or 12 (median, 2.1 and 2.3 g, respectively). The size of the treated area decreased by about two thirds from week 1 (median, 29.2%) to month 6 or 12 (median, 7.0 and 9.0%, respectively). During this study, some patients experienced several months during which no treatment was necessary. It would be of interest to assess this prospectively. Long periods of clearance in which treatment would be unnecessary would be a great advantage over conventional treatment with topical corticosteroid preparations.

Staphylococcus aureus is found in more than 90% of AD skin lesions (50). At our center ($n = 19$), we found that staphylococcal colonization of AD lesions significantly decreased after 1 week ($p = 0.012$), 6 months ($p < 0.001$), and 12 months ($p = 0.008$) of treatment with 0.1% tacrolimus ointment compared with baseline (51). These decreases followed clinical improvement. Tacrolimus has no inhibitory effect on bacteria, including *S. aureus* (52); thus, decreases in colonization probably reflect improvement of skin barrier function.

B. Pimecrolimus Cream

In a proof-of-concept study, 1% pimecrolimus cream and the cream vehicle were applied to the same patient on two target lesions (right vs. left) (53). The size of the target lesions was 1–2% of the total body surface area. Adult patients with moderate AD were enrolled in this study. In the 16 patients who received twice-daily treatment, lesions treated with pimecrolimus cream showed significantly greater decreases in the Atopic Dermatitis Severity Index than lesions treated with the vehicle control ($p < 0.001$). Once-daily treatment ($n = 18$) was not as effective as twice-daily treatment. No clinically relevant drug-related adverse events were noted.

In a randomized, double-blind multicenter phase II study with 260 adult AD patients with at least 5% body surface area involved, pimecrolimus cream (0.05, 0.2, 0.6, and 1%) was compared with vehicle and 0.1% betamethasone-17-valerate cream. Betamethasone-17-valerate cream, with an average improvement of 78%, was more effective than 1% pimecrolimus cream, with an average improvement of 46.7% (Fig. 5). However, with the exception of the lowest concentration of pimecrolimus cream, all others were more effective than vehicle

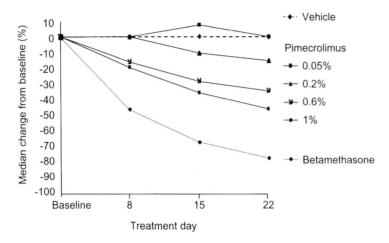

Figure 5 Median changes in Atopic Dermatitis Severity Index in patients treated with vehicle, pimecrolimus/SDZ ASM 981, or betamethasone. (From Ref. 56.)

(Fig. 5) (54–56). No clinically relevant drug-related adverse events were reported.

Preliminary findings have been reported for a phase III adult AD study which compared pimecrolimus with a corticosteroid cream over a one-year study period (57). This was a multicenter, parallel group, double-blind, active-controlled study that was conducted in Europe and Canada. A total of 658 patients were randomized to receive 1% pimecrolimus cream or corticosteroid cream (0.1% triamcinolone acetonide for trunk and extremities and 1% hydrocortisone for face, neck, and intertriginous areas). Treatment was twice daily according to need on all affected lesions. Few patients in the pimecrolimus treatment group completed the study (41% of patients) compared with the corticosteroid group (71% of patients). The safety profiles were similar for both treatment groups. In an analysis that excluded treatment failures (early withdrawals), efficacy was similar for the two treatment groups.

VI. CLINICAL EFFICACY AND SAFETY IN CHILDREN

A. Tacrolimus Ointment

In a phase I study conducted in the United States with patients who had moderate to severe AD, six of eight children (75%) reported excellent improvement or clearance after 8 days of treatment with 0.3% tacrolimus ointment, and no safety concerns were identified (35).

A randomized, double-blind, multicenter phase II study in the United States compared twice-daily application of ointments containing 0.03% ($n = 43$), 0.1% ($n = 49$), and 0.3% tacrolimus ($n = 44$) with a vehicle control ($n = 44$) in children, 7–16 years old, with moderate to severe atopic dermatitis for a treatment period of 22 days (58). The drop-out rate was higher in the vehicle control group (15.9% of patients) than in the three tacrolimus treatment groups (4.6, 10.2, and 9.1% of patients, respectively). In the physician's global evaluation of clinical response, 69%, 67% and 70% of patients who received 0.03%, 0.1% and 0.3% tacrolimus ointment, respectively, had marked to excellent (75%) improvement or clearing of their AD, compared with 38% of patients in the vehicle control group ($p = 0.005, 0.007$, and 0.004, respectively, for the three tacrolimus groups compared with the vehicle group). The mean percent improvement in the modified Eczema Area and Severity Index at the end of treatment was also significantly better in the tacrolimus treatment groups (0.03%, 72%; 0.1%, 77%; 0.3%, 81%) than in the vehicle group (26%) ($p < 0.001$). No serious systemic side effects were observed.

The results of a phase III comparative study in the United States, which included children (2–15 years old) with moderate to severe AD, demonstrated the efficacy and safety of 0.03% and 0.1% tacrolimus ointment in the pediatric population (59). This was a randomized, double-blind, vehicle-controlled multicenter study. Patients received 0.03% tacrolimus ($n = 117$), 0.1% tacrolimus ($n = 118$), or vehicle ($n = 116$) twice daily for up to 12 weeks. At baseline, the mean affected body surface area was approximately 50% across treatment groups. The drop-out rate was high in the vehicle group (56.0%) compared with the 0.03% tacrolimus (19.7%) and 0.1% tacrolimus (14.4%) groups. Lack of efficacy was the main reason for withdrawal in the vehicle group. All assessments showed significantly greater improvement for patients who received 0.03% or 0.1% tacrolimus compared with those who received vehicle. Treatment success [defined as excellent (90–99%) improvement or cleared (100% improvement)] was observed in 6.9% of patients who received vehicle compared with 35.9% and 40.7% of patients who received 0.03% and 0.1% tacrolimus, respectively ($p < 0.001$). Moderate or better improvement was observed for 26.7, 72.6 and 78.0% of patients, respectively (Fig. 4). Differences between 0.03% and 0.1% tacrolimus were not statistically significant. The Eczema Area and Severity Index, total score, pruritus, and percent affected BSA also showed statistically significant greater improvement with either concentration of tacrolimus compared with vehicle. Tacrolimus ointment, 0.03% and 0.1%, was also shown to be safe. Compared with vehicle, a higher rate of skin burning, pruritus, chickenpox, and vesiculobullous rash (''blisters'' on a nonapplication site) was observed with 0.03% tacrolimus but not with the higher (0.1%) concentration. Skin burning and pruritus were common (27–43% of patients) but tended to occur only during treatment initiation. The incidence of chickenpox was low (<5%), and it occurred only in younger children (<8 years old), for whom it is generally common; thus, the higher incidence in the 0.03% tacrolimus group probably occurred by chance; the clinical course of these episodes was normal. Laboratory profiles during the study were unremarkable.

The safety and efficacy of up to one year of 0.1% tacrolimus ointment monotherapy in children (2–15 years old) with moderate to severe atopic dermatitis were demonstrated in a multicenter, open-label phase III study in the United States (60). Application was twice daily for up to 12 months. Of the 255 patients enrolled, 189 (74.1%) completed the study. On average, patients were treated with 0.1% tacrolimus for 279 days or 87% of study days. Withdrawal was attributed to administrative causes, such as loss to follow-up and noncompliance (18.8%), adverse events (3.9%), and lack of efficacy (3.1%). At baseline, a mean of approximately 40% of the total body surface area was covered with AD lesions. Local irritation, including such adverse events as burning sensation (25.9% of patients) and pruritus (23.1%), were common but tended to occur only when initiating treatment (Fig. 6). There was no increased risk of nonapplication site

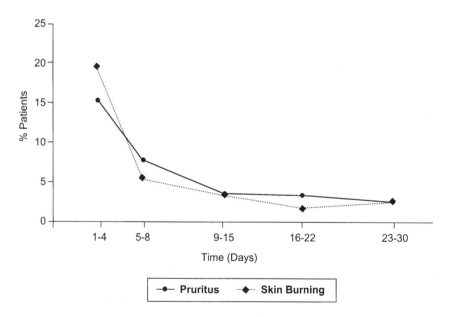

Figure 6 Prevalence of application-site adverse events pruritus and skin burning during first month of the study in a 12-month noncomparative pediatric study with 0.1% tacrolimus ointment. (From Ref. 60.)

adverse events, including infection, with cumulative drug use or duration of exposure. In addition, the incidence of infections was comparable to or lower than historical data from the literature; flu-like symptoms (investigator terms were cold, common cold, influenza, etc.) were reported by 34.5% of patients, fever by 17.6%, cough increased by 14.5%, and an application site skin infection by 11.4%. The incidence of asthma (16.1%), headache (18.0%), and allergic reaction, for example food allergies, allergies to grass, cats, dogs, etc. (15.3%), over the 12-month treatment period were consistent with what would be expected in a pediatric population with atopic diathesis. All efficacy endpoints, the Eczema Area and Severity Index, total score, pruritus score, and affected BSA showed improvement after one week of therapy and continued to show improvement over the 12-month study period.

B. Pimecrolimus Cream

The phase III comparative pediatric study for 1% pimecrolimus cream was a multicenter, vehicle-controlled, randomized, double-blind trial, with 2- to 17-year-old children who had mild to moderate AD (61). The drop-out rate was low; 88% of patients (236/267) in the pimecrolimus group and 75% of patients (102/136) in the vehicle group completed 6 weeks of twice-daily treatment. The mean affected body surface area was approximately 26% for both treatment groups. According to the investigator's global assessment (IGA) at baseline, 30.5% of patients had mild, 59.3% had moderate, 8.4% had severe, and 1.7% had very severe symptoms. Treatment success as defined by IGA, clear or almost clear at the end of the 6-week treatment period, was experienced by 34.8% of patients who received pimecrolimus compared with 18.4% of patients who received vehicle ($p < 0.001$). Common adverse events ($>10\%$ of patients) were application site burning, skin infection, upper respiratory tract infection, nasopharyngitis, pyrexia, cough, and headache, but incidences were similar for patients who received pimecrolimus or vehicle.

To assess long-term safety and efficacy in children (2 to <18 years of age), a multicenter parallel group, double-blind, controlled 1-year study was performed (62). A total of 713 patients with mild to severe atopic dermatitis were randomized to either 1% pimecrolimus cream or corresponding vehicle (2:1), to be applied b.i.d. according to need. Emollients were allowed, as were medium-high-potency topical corticosteroids for flares not controlled by study medication. The control treatment, vehicle cream, and corticosteroids can be considered to be equivalent to current standard care. The vehicle treatment was included in order to maintain the study blind. In total, 75.9% of the 1% pimecrolimus cream and 51.9% of the control-treated patients completed 6 months of treatment. The main reason for discontinuation in the control group was unsatisfactory therapeutic effect.

A flare was defined as an investigator's global assessment (IGA) of severe or very severe. Primary efficacy analysis was conducted on the incidence of flares observed in 6 months, adjusting for discontinuations. Pimecrolimus cream (1%) reduced the incidence of flares compared to the control group ($p < 0.001$). Sixty-one percent of patients in the pimecrolimus group completed 6 months without a flare compared to 35% in the control group (62). The incidence of adverse events was comparable in both study groups.

VII. IMMUNE MODULATION OR IMMUNE SUPPRESSION?

The etiology of AD is an enigma. As assessed by the proportion of patients with elevated IgE, environmental allergens play an important role in approximately 80% of AD patients (63). This suggests an overreactivity of the immune system to otherwise harmless environmental substances. An irony is that AD patients tend to have a compromised cell-mediated immunity (64). Thus, it seems that the burden of the skin's hyperreactivity to house dust mites and grass pollen, for example, has compromised the immune system's ability to protect against infectious agents such as herpes simplex virus.

Approximately 20% of patients have an intrinsic (non–IgE-related) form of the disease. One proposed explanation for the etiology of AD in these patients is that endotoxins released by *S. aureus* act as superantigens, which, independently of IgE, promote the release of proinflammatory molecules such as IL-1 and TNF-α from monocytes and dendritic cells and activate T cells (discussed in Ref. 10). There is also evidence indicating that allergen-specific T cells, independently of IgE, play a role in the immune pathology of AD (63,65). T cells are equally important in extrinsic AD. Increased IL-13 expression by T cells from lesions of patients with extrinsic AD is considered to account for increased IgE production via stimulation of B cells (65). Thus, T-cell activation, whether by IgE-bound antigens or other means, is a critical feature of both intrinsic and extrinsic AD. Inhibition of the expression of T-cell inflammatory cytokines by tacrolimus or pimecrolimus directly targets this immune pathology. This was recently demonstrated in an in vitro study with cells isolated from AD patients and healthy volunteers, in which tacrolimus specifically blocked *S. aureus* super-antigen–induced T-cell proliferation (66). This pathway seems to be corticosteroid resistant (64,65). Thus, tacrolimus ointment potentially has a great advantage in patients with AD who have therapeutic resistance to corticosteroids (Fig. 7).

The difference between immune modulation and immune suppression is subtle. In AD there is an immune pathology in which skin lesions have infiltrates of inflammatory immune cells (i.e., T cells, macrophages, basophils, eosinophils). In this instance, application of a drug that blocks the activation of these cells at the site of the lesion reverses the immune pathology and thus can be considered

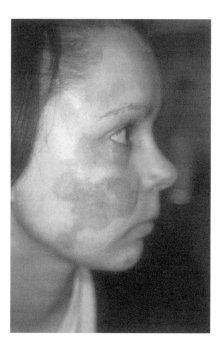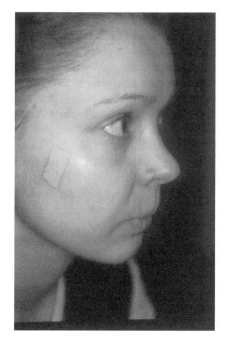

Figure 7 A 23-year-old patient who was insensitive to topical corticosteroid therapy quickly responded to 0.1% tacrolimus ointment. (Left) Before treatment with 0.1% tacrolimus; (right) 7 days after application of 0.1% tacrolimus. Histology from biopsy taken prior to treatment revealed an eczema; immunohistology remained negative.

to modify the local immune response. On the other hand, systemic immune suppression with such drugs as tacrolimus (Prograf®) and cyclosporin (Neoral®) was developed to suppress a normal immune response to the nonself antigens of an allograft. In doing so, it also suppresses normal immune responses to infectious agents and decreases immune surveillance in the protection against cancer.

Tacrolimus ointment and pimecrolimus cream are considered to be immune modulators because they target a specific immune pathology and because their action seems to be limited to the site of the immune pathology. The absence of a systemic effect is supported by the minimal systemic exposure observed with tacrolimus ointment and pimecrolimus cream in AD patients and by clinical findings, which show no apparent increased risk of cutaneous or systemic infections. It is also of interest to note that long-term use of tacrolimus ointment in adult patients with AD did not reduce cell-mediated immunity as assessed in the Recall

Antigen Test (49) and was associated with a decrease in staphylococcal colonization of the skin (51).

VIII. STATUS OF MARKETING APPROVALS

Tacrolimus ointment 0.1% has been on the market in Japan for treatment of moderate to severe AD in adults since November 1999 under the trade name Protopic®. In December 2000, the U.S. Food and Drug Administration approved Protopic (0.03% and 0.1%) ointment for adults and Protopic 0.03% ointment for children with moderate to severe AD. A marketing authorization application for tacrolimus ointment, 0.03% and 0.1%, was filed with the European Agency for the Evaluation of Medicinal Products (EMEA) in July 2000.

Pimecrolimus cream 1% is being developed for chronic AD, for which Novartis submitted a new drug application to the U.S. Food and Drug Administration in December 2000, which has now been approved. A marketing authorization application for pimecrolimus 1% cream has been filed with some European countries.

IX. CONCLUSIONS

Patients with AD and parents of children with AD have long awaited an alternative to topical corticosteroid therapy. A fear of using topical corticosteroids has developed among many patients and parents of patients, and some patients (e.g., those with corticosteroid resistance) are truly not helped by standard therapy. Also, skin atrophy and other side effects resulting from misuse of topical corticosteroids is not uncommon in daily medical practice. Tacrolimus (Protopic) ointment, 0.03% and 0.1%, offers the first alternative treatment for patients with moderate to severe AD, and 1% pimecrolimus cream may soon offer an alternative to AD patients as well.

Once both drugs have entered the postmarketing phase, it would be of interest to compare the efficacy and safety of tacrolimus ointment and pimecrolimus cream in patients with moderate AD (the common patient population, as tacrolimus ointment was developed for patients with moderate to severe AD, and pimecrolimus for patients with mild to moderate AD). Findings for studies comparing tacrolimus with topical corticosteroid reference therapies will be reported soon.

Any serious safety concerns about these drugs are theoretical. The clinical data collected so far indicate that there is no increased risk of skin cancer, infection, or other undesirable immunosuppressive effects. However, in terms of mode of action, topical tacrolimus and pimecrolimus may decrease immune surveillance of treated skin, and thus, over a period of many years, increase the risk of basal cell or squamous cell carcinoma. Thus, patients receiving therapy with a topical immunomodulator should be educated about adequate measures of sun protection, and an important aim of postmarketing research should be long-term safety.

ACKNOWLEDGMENTS

I would like to thank the following individuals for supplying information and/ or critical review of the manuscript: Connie Grogan, MA, and Nas Undre, MD (both Fujisawa GmbH, Munich), Ira Lawrence, MD (Fujisawa Healthcare, Inc., Deerfield, IL), Ari Heinonen, MSc (Fujisawa GmbH, Finland), Michael Gräber, MD, and Friedrich Mayer, PhD (both Novartis Pharma AG, Basle), Anton Stuetz, PhD (Novartis Research Institute, Vienna), and my coworkers Anita Remitz, MD, PhD, Haokan Granlund, MD, PhD, Hannele Kyllönen, MD, and Johanna Saarikko, MD (all from Department of Dermatology, University of Helsinki).

REFERENCES

1. T Goto, T Kino, H Hatanaka, N Nishiyama, M Okuhara, M Kohsaka, H Aoki, H Imanaka. Discovery of FK-506, a novel immunosuppressant isolated from *Streptomyces tsukubaensis*. Transpl Proc 19(suppl 6):4–8, 1987.
2. T Arai, Y Koyama, T Suenaga, H Honda. Ascomycin, an antifungal antibiotic. J Antibiot Ser A 15:231–232, 1962.
3. H Hatanaka, T Kino, S Miyata, N Inamura, A Kuroda, T Goto, H Tanaka, M Okuhara. FR-900520 and FR-900523, novel immunosuppressants isolated from a streptomyces II. Fermentation, isolation and physico-chemical and biological characteristics. J Antibiot 41:1592–1601, 1988.
4. H Nakagawa, T Etoh, Y Yokota, F Ikeda, K Hatano, N Teratani, K Shimomura, Y Mine, T Amaya. Tacrolimus has antifungal activities against *Malassezia furfur* isolated from healthy adults and patient with atopic dermatitis. Clin Drug Invest 12: 244–250, 1996.
5. M Grassberger, T Baumruker, A Enz, P Hiestand, H Hultsch, F Kalthoff, W Schuler, M Schulz, F-J Werner, A Winiski, B Wolff, G Zenke. A novel anti-inflammatory drug, SDZ ASM 981, for the treatment of skin diseases: in vitro pharmacology. Br J Dermatol 141:264–273, 1999.
6. MJ Tocci, DA Markovich, KA Collier, P Kwok, F Dumont, S Lin, S Degudicibus, JJ Siekierka, J Chin, NI Hutchinson. The immunosuppressant FK506 selectively inhibits expression of early T cell activation genes. J Immunol 143:718–726, 1989.
7. Thepen T, Langeveld-Wildschut EG, Bihari IC, van Wichen DF, van Reijsen FC, Mudde GC, Bruijnzeel-Koomen FM. Biphasic response against aeroallergen in atopic dermatitis showing a switch from an initial Th2 response into a Th1 response

in situ: an immunocytochemical study. J Allergy Clin Immunol 97:828–837, 1996.

8. EA Wierenga, B Backx, M Snoek, L Koenderman, ML Kapsenberg. Relative contributions of human types 1 and 2 T-helper cell-derived eosinophilotrophic cytokines to development of eosinophilia. Blood 82:1471–1479, 1993.

9. A Wollenberg, S Kraft, D Hanau, T Bieber. Immunomorphological and ultrastructural characterization of Langerhans cells and a novel, inflammatory dendritic epidermal cell (IDEC) population in lesional skin of atopic eczema. J Invest Dermatol 106:446–453, 1996.

10. S Reitamo. Tacrolimus: a new topical immunomodulatory therapy for atopic dermatitis. J Allergy Clin Immunol 107:445–448, 2001.

11. A Panhans-Groβ, N Novak, S Kraft, T Bieber. Human epidermal Langerhans cells are targets for the immunosuppressive macrolide tacrolimus (FK506). J Allergy Clin Immunol 107:345–352, 2001.

12. A Wollenberg, S Sharma, D von Bubnoff, E Geiger, J Haberstok, T Bieber. Topical tacrolimus (FK506) leads to profound phenotypic and functional alterations of epidermal antigen presenting dendritic cells in atopic dermatitis. J Allergy Clin Immunol 107:519–525, 2001.

13. A De Paulis, C Stellato, R Cirillo, A Ciccarelli, A Oriente, G Marone. Anti-inflammatory effect of FK-506 on human skin mast cells. J Invest Dermatol 99:723–728, 1992.

14. A De Paulis, R Cirillo, A Ciccarelli, M Condorelli, G Marone. FK-506, a potent novel inhibitor of the release of proinflammatory mediators from human FcεRI+ cells. J Immunol 146:2374–2381, 1991.

15. SM Hatfield, NW Roehm. Cyclosporine and FK506 inhibition of murine mast cell cytokine production. J Pharmacol Exp Ther 260:680–688, 1992.

16. SM Hatfield, JS Mynderse, NW Roehm. Rapamycin and FK506 differentially inhibit mast cell cytokine production and cytokine-induced proliferation and act as reciprocal antagonists. J Pharmacol Exp Ther 261:970–976, 1992.

17. T Hultsch, KD Mueller, JG Meingassner, M Grassberger, RE Schopf, J Knop. Ascomycin macrolactam derivative SDZ ASM 981 inhibits the release of granule-associated mediators and of newly synthesised cytokines in RBL 2H3 mast cells in an immunophilin-dependent manner. Arch Dermatol Res 290:501–507, 1998.

18. T Zuberbier, S Chong, S Guhl, P Welker, BM Henz, M Grassberger. SDZ ASM 981 inhibits anti-IgE stimulated mediator release in human dermal mast cells (abstr). J Invest Dermatol 112:608, 1999.

19. T Sengoku, K Morita, S Sato, S Sakuma, T Ogawa, J Hiroi, T Fujii, T Goto. Effects of tacrolimus ointment on type I (immediate and late) and IV (delayed) cutaneous allergic reactions in mice. Nippon Yakarigaku Zasshi 112:221–232, 1998.

20. T Sengoku, K Morita, S Sakuma, Y Motoyama, T Goto. Possible inhibitory mechanism of FK506 (tacrolimus hydrate) ointment for atopic dermatitis based on animal models. Eur J Pharmacol 379:183–189, 1999.

21. AB Kay, S Ying, V Varney, M Gaga, SR Durham, R Moqbel, et al. Messenger RNA expression of cytokine gene cluster, interleukin 3 (IL-3), IL-5, and granulocyte/macrophage colony-stimulating factor, in allergen-induced late-phase cutaneous reactions in atopic subjects. J Exp Med 173:775–778, 1991.

22. JG Meingassner, A Stütz. Immunosuppressive macrolides of the type FK 506: a novel class of topical agents for treatment of skin diseases? J Invest Dermatol 98: 851–855, 1992.

23. AI Lauerma, HI Maibach, H Granlund, P Erkko, M Kartamaa, S Stubb. Inhibition of contact allergy reaction by topical FK 506 (letter). Lancet 340:556, 1992.

24. JG Meingassner, M Grassberger, H Fahrngruber, HD Moore, H Schuurman, A Stütz. A novel anti-inflammatory drug, SDZ ASM 981, for the topical and oral treatment of skin diseases: in vivo pharmacology. Br J Dermatol 137:568–576, 1997.

25. D Bochelen, M Rudin, A Sauter. Calcineurin inhibitors FK506 and SDZ ASM 981 alleviate the outcome of focal cerebral ischemic/reperfusion injury. J Pharmacol Exp Ther 288:653–659, 1999.

26. A Bavandi, H Fahrngruber, JG Meingassner. SDZ ASM 981 is different from FK 506 and cyclosporin A in pharmacodynamic profile based on a murine allergic contact dermatitis model. Poster presented at the 9th Congress of the European Academy of Dermatology and Venereology, October 11–15, 2000, Geneva, Switzerland.

27. J Hiroi, T Sengoku, K Morita, S Kishi, S Sato, T Ogawa, M Tsudzuki, H Matsuda, A Wada, K Esaka. Effect of tacrolimus hydrate (FK506) ointment on spontaneous dermatitis in NC/Nga mice. Jpn J Pharmacol 76:175–183, 1998.

28. G Neckermann, A Bavandi, J Meingassner. Atopic dermatitis-like symptoms in hypomagnesaemic hairless rats are prevented and inhibited by systemic or topical SDZ ASM 981. Br J Dermatol. 142:669–679, 2000.

29. H Jiang, S Sakuma, Y Fujii, Y Akizama, T Ogawa, K Tamura, M Kobayashi, T Fujitsu. Tacrolimus versus cyclosporin A: a comparative study on rat renal allograft survival. Transpl Int 12:92–99, 1999.

30. N Murase, AJ Demetris, J Woo, M Tanabe, T Furaya, S Todo, TE Starzl. Graft-versus-host disease after brown Norway-to-Lewis and Lewis-to-brown Norway rat intestinal transplantation under FK506. Transplantation 58:1–7, 1993.

31. A Hisatomi, T Mitamura, M Kimura, Y Oishi, T Fujii, K Ohara. Comparison of FK506 (tacrolimus) and glucocorticoid ointment on dermal atrophogenicity in rats. J Toxicol Pathol 10:97–102, 1997.

32. S Reitamo, J Rissanen, A Remitz, H Granlund, P Erkko, P Elg, P Autio, AI Lauerma. Tacrolimus ointment does not affect collagen synthesis: results of a single-center randomized trial. J Invest Dermatol 111:396–398, 1998.

33. JP Ortonne. SDZ ASM 981 does not induce skin atrophy: a randomised, double-blind controlled study (abstr). J Eur Acad Dermatol Venereol 12(suppl 2):S140, 1999.

34. C Queille-Roussel, C Paul, L Duteil, MC Lefebvre, G Raptz, M Zagula, JP Ortonne. The new topical ascomycin derivative SDZ ASM 981 does not induce skin atrophy when applied to normal skin for four weeks: a randomised, double-blind controlled study. Br J Dermatol 144:507–513, 2001.

35. S Alaiti, S Kang, VC Fiedler, CN Ellis, DV Spurlin, D Fader, G Ulyanov, SD Gadgil, A Tanase, I Lawrence, P Scotellaro, K Raye, I Bekersky. Tacrolimus (FK506) 0.3% ointment for atopic dermatitis; a phase I study in adults and children. J Am Acad Dermatol 38:69–76, 1998.

36. M Kawashima, H Nakagawa, M Ohtsuji, K Tamaki, Y Ishibashi. Tacrolimus concen-

trations in blood during topical treatment of atopic dermatitis (letter). Lancet 348: 1240–1241, 1996.

37. M Graeber, EJM Van Leent, P Burtin, ME Ebelin, B Dorobek, JD Bos. Profiling SDZ ASM 981: evaluation of local tolerability and safety in the treatment of atopic dermatitis (abstr). Ann Dermatol Venereol 125(suppl 1):214–215, 1998.

38. R Allen, T Davies, JD Bos, EJM Van Leent, J Harper, A Green, M Cardno, G Scott, ME Ebelin. Pharmacokinetics of SDZ ASM 981 cream 1% in adults and children. Poster presented at the 9th Congress of the European Academy of Dermatology and Venereology, October 11–15, 2000, Geneva, Switzerland.

39. U Wahn, D Pariser, AB Gottlieb, R Kaufmann, L Eichenfeld, R Langley, M Ebelin, M Bueche, D Barilla, G Scott, P Burtin. Low blood concentrations of SDZ ASM 981 in infants with extensive atopic dermatitis treated with cream 1%. Poster presented at the 59th Annual Meeting of the American Academy of Dermatology, March 2–7, 2001, Washington, DC.

40. K Rappersberger, M Komar, ME Ebelin, G Scott, P Burtin, A Stuetz, K Wolff. Clinical experience with oral SDZ ASM 981 in psoriasis. Poster presented at the 9th Congress of the European Academy of Dermatology and Venereology, October 11–15, 2000, Geneva, Switzerland.

41. JD Bos, MMHM Meinardi. The 500 Dalton rule for the skin penetration of chemical compounds and drugs. Exp Dermatol 9:165–169, 2000.

42. Y de Prost, C Bodemer, D Teillac. Double-blind randomized placebo-controlled trial of local cyclosporine in atopic dermatitis. Arch Dermatol 125:570, 1989.

43. MA de Rie, MMHM Meinardi, JD Bos. Lack of efficacy of topical cyclosporin in atopic dermatitis and allergic contact dermatitis. Acta Derm Venereol 71:452–454, 1991.

44. H Nakagawa, T Etoh, Y Ishibashi, Y Higaki, M Kawashima, H Torii, S Harada. Tacrolimus ointment for atopic dermatitis (letter). Lancet 344:883, 1994.

45. H Aoyama, N Tabata, M Tanaka, Y Uesugi, H Tagami. Successful treatment of resistant facial lesions of atopic dermatitis with 0.1% FK506 ointment (letter). Br J Dermatol 133:494–496, 1995.

46. T Ruzicka, T Bieber, E Schöpf, A Rubins, A Dobozy, JD Bos, S Jablonska, I Ahmed, K Thestrup-Pedersen, F Daniel, A Finzi, S Reitamo. A short-term trial of tacrolimus ointment for atopic dermatitis. N Engl J Med 337:816–821, 1997.

47. JM Hanifin, MR Ling, R Langley, D Breneman, E Rafal and the Tacrolimus Ointment Study Group. Tacrolimus ointment for the treatment of atopic dermatitis in adult patients: Part I, Efficacy. J Am Acad Dermatol 44:S28–38, 2001.

48. NA Soter, AB Fleischer, GF Webster, E Monroe, I Lawrence and the Tacrolimus Ointment Study Group. Tacrolimus ointment for the treatment of atopic dermatitis in adult patients: Part II, Safety. J Am Acad Dermatol 44:S39–46, 2001.

49. S Reitamo, A Wollenberg, E Schöpf, JL Perrot, R Marks, T Ruzicka, E Christophers, A Kapp, M Lahfa, A Rubins, S Jablonska, M Rustin. Safety and efficacy of 1 year of tacrolimus ointment monotherapy in adults with atopic dermatitis. Arch Dermatol 136:999–1006, 2000.

50. R Aly. Bacteriology of atopic dermatitis. Acta Dermatol Venereol 92:16–18, 1980.

51. A Remitz, H Kyllönen, H Granlund, S Reitamo. Tacrolimus ointment reduces staph-

ylococcal colonization of atopic dermatitis lesions (letter). J Allergy Clin Immunol 107:196–197, 2001.

52. T Kino, H Hatanaka, M Hashimoto, M Nishiyama, T Goto, M Okuhara, M Kohsaka, H Aoki, T Ochiai. FK 506, a novel immunosuppressant isolated from a streptomyces. I. Fermentation, isolation, and physio-chemical and biological characteristics. J Antibiot (Tokyo) 49:1249–1255, 1987.

53. EJM Van Leent, M Gräber, M Thurston, A Wagenaar, PI Spuls, J Bos. Effectiveness of the ascomycin macrolactam SDZ ASM 981 in the topical treatment of atopic dermatitis. Arch Dermatol 134:805–809, 1998.

54. T Luger, EJM van Leent, M Graeber, S Hedgecock, M Thurston, A Kandra, J Berth-Jones, J Bjerke, E Christophers, J Knop, AC Knulst, M Morren, A Morris, S Reitamo, J Roed-Petersen, E Schoepf, K Thestrup-Pedersen, PGM van der Valk, JD Bos. SDZ ASM 981: An emerging safe and effective treatment for atopic dermatitis. Br J Dermatol 144:788–794, 2001.

55. EJM Van Leent, M Graeber, ME Ebelin, P Burtin, HJC de Vries, JD Bos. Efficacy and safety of SDZ ASM 981 cream in atopic dermatitis (abstr). J Eur Acad Dermatol Venereol 12:51, 1999.

56. M Graeber, EJM van Leent, M Thurston, JD Bos. SDZ ASM 981 cream: an emerging new drug for treatment of atopic dermatitis. Poster presented at the Clinical Dermatology 2000 Congress, June 18–20, 1998, Singapore.

57. JD Bos, K Meyer, HJC de Vries, S Molloy, A Kandra, M Graeber on behalf of the European/Canadian Study Group. Long-term safety and efficacy of SDZ ASM 981 cream in adult patients with atopic dermatitis (abstr). Br J Dermatol 143:S34, 2000.

58. M Boguniewicz, VC Fiedler, S Raimer, ID Lawrence, DYM Leung, JN Hanifin for the Pediatric Tacrolimus Study Group. A randomized, vehicle-controlled trial of tacrolimus ointment for treatment of atopic dermatitis in children. J Allergy Clin Immunol 102:637–644, 1998.

59. A Paller, LF Eichenfield, DYM Leung, D Steward, M Appell and the Tacrolimus Ointment Study Group. A 12-week study of tacrolimus ointment for the treatment of atopic dermatitis in pediatric patients. J Am Acad Dermatol 44:S47–57, 2001.

60. S Kang, AW Lucky, D Pariser, I Lawrence, JM Hanifin and the Tacrolimus Ointment Study Group. Long-term safety and efficacy of tacrolimus ointment for the treatment of atopic dermatitis in children. J Am Acad Dermatol 44:S58–64, 2001.

61. J Hanifin, K Marshal, C Bush, M Thurston, M Graeber, R Cherill. SDZ ASM 981 cream 1% effective in the treatment of pediatric atopic dermatitis: two 6-week, randomized, double-blind, vehicle-controlled, multi-center studies with 20-week open-label phases. Poster presented at the 9th Congress of the European Academy of Dermatology and Venereology, October 11–15, 2000, Geneva, Switzerland.

62. U Wahn, S Molloy, M Graeber, M Thurston, R Cherill, Y de Prost. Long-term management with SDZ ASM 981 cream 1% in atopic dermatitis patients. Poster presented at the 59th Annual Meeting of the American Academy of Dermatology, March 2–7, 2001, Washington DC.

63. T Werfel, A Kapp. What do we know about the etiopathology of the intrinsic type of atopic dermatitis. In: B Wüthrich, ed. The Atopy Syndrome in the Third Millennium. Basel: Karger, 1999, pp. 29–36.

64. Ö Strannegård, I-L Strannegård. Changes in cell-mediated immunity in atopic ec-

zema. In: T Ruzicka, J Ring, B Przybilla, eds. Handbook of Atopic Eczema. Berlin: Springer-Verlag, 1991, pp. 221–231.

65. CA Akdis, M Akdis, D Simon, B Dibbert, M Weber, S Gratzl, O Kreyden, R Disch, B Wüthrich, K Blaser, H-U Simon. Role of T cells and cytokines in the intrinsic form of atopic dermatitis. In: B Wüthrich, ed. The Atopy Syndrome in the Third Millennium. Basel: Karger, 1999, pp. 37–44.

66. PJ Hauk, DYM Leung. Tacrolimus (FK506): new treatment approach in superantigen-associated diseases like atopic dermatitis? J Allergy Clin Immunol 107:391, 2001.

67. PJ Hauk, QA Hamid, GP Chrousos, DYM Leung. Induction of corticosteroid insensitivity in human peripheral blood mononuclear cells by microbial superantigens. J Allergy Clin Immunol 105:782–787, 2000.

28

Chinese Herbal Therapy in Atopic Dermatitis

John R. Reed and Malcolm H. A. Rustin
Royal Free Hospital, London, United Kingdom

I. INTRODUCTION

Atopic dermatitis is an increasingly prevalent chronic pruritic inflammatory skin condition that is thought to have an immune and genetic basis influenced by environmental factors. The inflammatory infiltrate shows similar characteristics to a delayed-type hypersensitivity reaction with increased CD4+, CD45RO+ T lymphocytes, RFD7+ macrophages, RFD1+ dendritic cells, and CD1+ Langerhans cells (1,2). Additionally, aberrant expression of the low-affinity receptor for IgE (FcεRII/CD23) (3) and constitutive expression of the high-affinity IgE receptor (FcεRI) on antigen-presenting cells within the infiltrate is recognized (4,5). This suggests that the pathogenesis of atopic dermatitis represents a delayed-type hypersensitivity response to environmental allergens and antigens, triggered by IgE receptor–bearing antigen-presenting cells. In support of this, it is increasingly recognized that the induction of lesional atopic dermatitis is associated with a biphasic pattern of cytokine expression. In situ hybridization studies have shown increased numbers of cells expressing mRNA for interleukins (IL)-4, IL-5, and IL-13 in atopic dermatitis (6). Chronic eczematous lesions had significantly fewer IL-4 and IL-13 positive cells compared to acute lesions, but there were increased numbers of cells expressing interferon (IFN)-γ and IL-5 mRNA. This biphasic pattern has also been demonstrated in atopic patch test reactions with a peak of IL-12 mRNA expression preceding the increased IFN-γ expression (7). It, therefore, appears that the initiation of atopic dermatitis is driven by Th2 polarized cytokine expression and this switches to a Th1 polarized pattern, which drives the chronic inflammatory phase of the disease. Additionally leukocytes, particularly monocytes, in atopic dermatitis have increased cyclic AMP phosphodiesterase enzyme activity, which contributes to the increased secretion of IL-10 and prostaglandin E_2. This inhibits IFN-γ production by T cells and appears to contribute to increased IL-4 production by T cells (8).

The basic treatment of atopic dermatitis has remained unchanged for several decades. Topical emollients are used to improve skin hydration and corticosteroids to reduce the inflammation. A minority of patients respond poorly to these measures and may require treatment with systemic corticosteroids, narrowband ultraviolet B (UVB) (9) or psoralen photochemotherapy (PUVA) (10). Other treatments that have been reported to be effective include cyclosporine (11), azathioprine (12), type IV phosphodiesterase inhibitors (8) and IFN-γ (13). The use of topical tacrolimus ointment has also recently been shown to be efficacious (14). These treatments can be associated with significant side effects, and a minority of patients are even recalcitrant to these measures. This often leads patients to try alternative therapies, of which Chinese herbal therapy is one of the most commonly used. Five million patients consulted a complementary practitioner in 1999, and the retail sale of herbal, homeopathic and aromatherapy preparations is predicted to total $180 million by 2002 (15). There are now three double-blind, placebo-controlled studies on Chinese herbal therapy in atopic dermatitis in the English-language medical literature in conjunction with follow-up data. Much of this work, particularly in adults, was undertaken in our hospital in collaboration with other centers.

II. PRINCIPLES OF CHINESE HERBAL THERAPY

Medical and pharmaceutical literature has existed in China for more than 5000 years. The earliest pharmacopeia of Chinese herbs, known as the *Herbal Classic of the Divine Plowman*, was written in approximately 100 B.C. Traditional Chinese medicine seeks to treat the whole person rather than one specific disease entity. The first principle of Chinese medicine is based upon the interpretation of signs and symptoms in conjunction with the philosophy of yin and yang, the two opposing and complementary sides of nature. Literally, the words mean two banks of a river: yin indicates the shady side and yang the sunny side. In a healthy body they are balanced, but in illness there is an imbalance between the two. The clinical manifestations of yin and yang can be better understood by the following examples (Table 1).

Another fundamental concept in Chinese medicine is qi (pronounced chi). To the Chinese, the human body is a miniature cosmos. As the world is air, sea, and land, so the body is qi, blood, and body fluids. Just as nature is governed by the weather so the body is affected by internal weather. Qi has been variously

Table 1 Features of Yin
and Yang

Yin	Yang
Cold	Hot
Quiet	Restless
Wet	Dry
Soft	Hard
Slow	Rapid

translated as energy, material force, matter, matter-energy, vital power, and subtle breath. The reason for the difficulty in giving a specific definition is its fluid nature. Maciocia explains that qi is an energy that manifests simultaneously on the physical and spiritual level and is in a constant state of flux and varying states of aggregation (16,17).

Traditional Chinese physicians perceive skin disease as a breakdown in the essential relationship between the yin nourishment and yang activity. This allows the subsequent invasion of the body by pathogenic factors such as wind, heat, and dampness, which exacerbate the disease further by damaging the qi, blood, and body fluids. Chinese herbal therapy seeks to realign the fundamental yin and yang balance. Since most skin diseases are seen to be the result of internal disharmony, the majority of skin treatments involve systemic treatments rather than topical treatments. These are called decoctions, a "tea" that results from the boiling down of a herbal prescription so as to extract the essence. It is not unusual to prescribe 10–12 herbs at a time, and the prescription is designed along traditional lines having 1 or 2 major ingredients (emperor herbs), a further 1 or more minister herbs, which aid the emperor, 1 or more assistant herbs, and a harmonizing or guide herb to direct the prescription to its target and to enable it to be better assimilated. The herbs are believed to work synergistically, some enhancing the role of others, while others check possible side effects of other constituents.

According to traditional Chinese medicine theory, there appear to be two basic forms of dermatitis. One kind is caused by damp heat, where the skin is weeping and there is oozing, heat, and itching. The other is characterized by wind heat, producing red, dry, itchy dermatitis. This fundamental difference underlies the individualized prescription of herbs for each patient, which is also based on an evaluation of the nature of the pulse and appearance of the tongue. This makes scientific assessment of Chinese herbal therapy seriously difficult. A standardized formulation has been designed for a particular type of atopic dermatitis with the help of Dr. Luo, a Chinese herbal therapist working in London. This is called

Zemaphyte and was produced in collaboration with Phytopharm Ltd, Godmanchester, Cambridgeshire, England. Although it is a modern formulation, it is arranged along traditional lines, in particular aiming to eliminate the pathogenic factors of wind heat from the body through the skin and urine. Thus, the prescription contains four herbs (*Rehmannia glutinosa, Lophatherum gracile, Clematis armandii, Glycyrrhiza glabra*), which themselves constitute an ancient prescription [Lead the Red Powder (Dou Chi San) originally formulated by Qian Yi in 1119 in the Craft of Medicinal Treatment for Childhood Disease Patterns (Xiao Er Yao Zheng Zhi)]. This removes heat from the heart and blood by urination. Other herbs, such as *Ledebouriella seseloides* and *Schizonepeta tenuifolia*, have been used since ancient times to vent heat and wind through the skin by sweating, whereas others such as *Paeonia suffruticosa* and *Potentilla chinensis* are famed for cooling the blood. The 10 herbs can be ranked in the hierarchy as discussed above (Table 2).

By collaborating with the pharmaceutical company Phytopharm Ltd, quality control procedures could be undertaken. The herbs were all grown in mainland China, and top-grade ingredients were obtained from a single supplier of medicinal herbs (OPTEC, Shanghai, China) or herbs of equivalent quality from U.K. brokers. All batches of herbs were screened for microbial contaminants, aflatoxins, and heavy metals such as lead, mercury, cadmium, selenium, and chromium.

Table 2   Herbs Used in the Chinese Herbal Therapy of Atopic Dermatitis

Herb[a]	Category	Chinese name	Mode of action
Rehmannia glutinosa	Emperor	Sheng di huang	Clears heat, cools blood
Paeonia suffruticosa/ **Paeonia chinensis**	Minister	Mu dan pi	Clears heat, cools blood
Potentilla chinensis	Minister	Wie ling cai	Clears heat, cools blood
Schizonepta tenuifolia	Minister	Jing jie	Cools blood, releases wind, causes sweating
Ledebouriella seseloides	Minister	Fang feng	Clears wind-damp, causes sweating
Tribulus terrestris	Assistant	Bai ji li	Allays wind
Dictamnus dasycarpus	Assistant	Bai xian pi	Clears wind, damp-heat, and fire-poison
Clematis armandii	Assistant	Mu tong	Clears heat via urination
Lophatherum gracile	Assistant	Dan zhu ye	Clears heat through the kidneys
Glycyrrhiza uralensis/ **G. glabra**	Guide	Gan cao	Harmonizes the prescription

[a] Herbs in boldface are contained in Zemaphyte.

Thin-layer chromatography was performed to fingerprint the herbs and ensure that different batches were comparable to standard herbs identified by botanists at Kew Gardens. Batches were rejected if they differed substantially from the reference material. The herbs were finely ground in a hammer mill until they passed through a 1 mm screen and were then packaged as 10 g sealed porous sachets containing the herbs *Rehmannia glutinosa*, *Lophatherum gracile*, *Clematis armandii*, *Glycyrrhiza glabra*, *Ledebouriella seseloides*, *Paeonia suffruticosa*, *Tributis terrestris*, *Dictamnus dasycarpus,* and *Potentilla chinensis*. The herb *Schizonepeta tenuifolia* contains volatile oils and was therefore packaged in separate sachets.

III. DOUBLE-BLIND CLINICAL TRIALS

Two randomized, double-blind, placebo-controlled, crossover studies of children and adults have been carried out in the United Kingdom using Zemaphyte (18,19). In both studies patients had atopic dermatitis determined by Hanifin and Rajka criteria, which was refractory to conventional therapy. Extensive (>20% of body surface area) lichenified or urticated papular and plaque-like atopic dermatitis with no evidence of exudation or infection was required for entry into the studies. All patients were required to have a normal full blood count and renal and hepatic function tests before commencing the study. Patients who had received systemic corticosteroids, antibiotics, PUVA, or other immunosuppressive treatment within the preceding 2 months were excluded. Other exclusion criteria included serious concomitant illness, pregnancy, breastfeeding, or intention to become pregnant. All women of child-bearing age were required to take appropriate contraceptive precautions. Patients were asked not to change their diet or dermatological treatments. In the adult study, patients were instructed not to increase the potency or frequency of their topical corticosteroid usage during the trial. In the child study, patients agreed not to use any topical corticosteroids during the run-up period or throughout the study to avoid possible interference with urinary steroid analyses.

Double-blind, placebo-controlled, crossover studies lasting 5 months were employed. Each patient was randomly allocated to receive either active treatment for 8 weeks then a 4-week washout period followed by an identically packaged placebo for 8 weeks or the same treatment in reverse. The placebo comprised *Humulus lupulus*, *Hordeum distichon*, *Hordeum distichon ustum*, baker's bran, sucrose, *Salvia* spp., *Thymus vulgaris*, *Rosmarinus officianalis*, *Mentha piperita*, and *Oleum caryophylli*. This mixture has no known benefit in atopic dermatitis, but the smell and taste are similar to the active treatment. The treatment was freshly prepared each day as a decoction. Four of the large sachets were boiled in 800 mL of tap water, and after 90 minutes of simmering four of the smaller sachets containing *S. tenuifolia* were added for 3 minutes. The decoction measured approximately 200 mL and was drunk while still warm. Patients were also asked to not eat anything for 1 hour.

In the double-blind and follow-up studies, the same standardized scoring system was used. Patients were assessed at 4-week intervals and a quantitative assessment of erythema and surface damage (papulation, vesiculation, scaling, excoriation and lichenification) was made. The body was divided into 20 roughly equal areas and within each area a score of 0 (none) to 3 (severe) was made for the degree of erythema and surface damage. For each clinical feature an estimate of the percentage area in each zone was made. A score of 1 was given where the area affected was <33%, 2 where the area was between 34 and 66%, and 3 where the area was >67%. The severity and area scores were multiplied then added together to provide a total body score with a maximum of 180. Investigations undertaken at baseline and at the end of each treatment period included full blood count, liver function tests, urea and electrolytes, creatinine, calcium and phosphate, glucose, creatinine phosphokinase, and creatinine clearance. Blood pressure and weight were checked at each visit.

Forty patients entered the adult study with 20 in each arm (18). Of the patients selected, 35 were Caucasian, 4 Afro Caribbean, and 1 Chinese. Thirty-one patients completed the study (mean age 30.8 years, range 17–57). Nine patients were excluded from the analysis: 8 were withdrawn because of noncompliance due to unpalatability of the decoction and 1 patient became pregnant. Of those patients selected for the placebo Chinese herb therapy sequence, 1 did not complete the placebo period and 2 did not complete the active period. In the other sequence, 3 did not complete the active period and 3 did not complete the placebo period.

Patients in the active Chinese herbal therapy phase of either sequence showed significant improvement of both erythema and surface damage scores (Fig. 1). The geometric mean for erythema at the end of the active therapy was 12.6 [95% confidence interval (CI) 5.9–22] compared to 113 (95% CI 65–180) at the end of the placebo phase. Similarly, the geometric mean for surface damage scores at the end of the active therapy was 11.3 (95% CI 5.8–21.8) compared to 111 (95% CI 68–182) at the end of the placebo phase. Based on logarithmic values, the mean proportional change between the end of the placebo phase and end of the active phase for erythema was 46% (95% CI 25.2–67%). Similarly the mean proportional change for surface damage was 49% (95% CI 27–71%). There was no evidence of an order effect or carry-over effect of the treatments in that there was no significant difference in the clinical scores between the sequences at the end of the washout period. Of the 31 patients who completed the study, 14 said that they itched less during the active phase compared to 1 in the placebo phase. Fifteen patients said that they slept better in the active phase compared to 6 in the placebo phase. No change in asthma symptoms was noted. When asked to express a preference, 20 indicated the active phase compared to

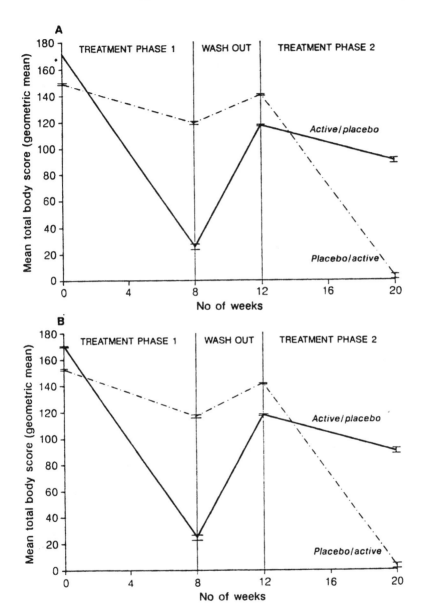

Figure 1 Sequential body scores (geometric means) for (A) erythema and (B) surface damage. (Kindly reproduced by the permission of The Lancet, Elsevier Scientific Publishing.)

4 patients who preferred the placebo. Adverse effects were rare. Two patients reported mild abdominal distension and headaches while taking the active phase. One patient developed three episodes of facial herpes and another noted loss of taste while on placebo. Apart from eosinophilia noted in 24 patients at baseline and at the end of the study, no other abnormalities were detected.

In the children's trial, 47 patients were enrolled and 37 completed the 5-month study (19). The number of sachets used in the preparation of the decoction varied depending on the age of the child: 1–7 years, 2 large and 2 small sachets/day; 8–13 years, 3 large and 3 small sachets/day; and ≥14 years, adult dose. Five were excluded because of noncompliance due to unpalatability, two others received systemic corticosteroids for asthma, and the other three had been prescribed antibiotics for skin infections. Most improvement was noted during the first 4 weeks of the active phase. The median percentage decrease in erythema scores during the active phase was 51.0 (95% CI 34.5, 72.6) compared to 6.1 (95% CI −25.2, 30.7) during the placebo phase (95% CI for the difference 13.4, 89.7). The median percentage decrease in surface damage scores during the active phase was 63.1 (95% CI 34.5, 72.6) compared to 6.2 (95% CI −25.2, 30.7) during the placebo phase (95% CI for the difference 19.2, 97.9). No significant order or carry-over effect was noted. Nineteen children reported an improved ability to sleep during the active phase compared to 3 in the placebo phase. Parents indicated a preference for the active phase in 27 cases and the placebo phase in 2 cases. No abnormalities in hepatic or renal function were noted, and no adverse events were recorded.

IV. LONG-TERM STUDIES

Patients who had completed the double-blind studies were offered continued Chinese herbal therapy for up to 1 year. Of the 31 adult patients who completed the original study, 21 chose to continue with therapy (20). This involved a 2-month washout period, then after 2 months of further treatment the follow-up treatment period began. Two patients left the study within 2 months, because of the cumbersome preparation and unpalatability of the decoction. Two other patients became pregnant at 5 and 10 months into follow-up having stopped the treatment 2 months earlier. Seventeen patients, therefore, completed the year (group 1). Of the 10 other patients who did not wish to continue treatment, 1 was lost to follow-up. It was decided to include the 2 patients who had failed to complete the induction phase in this control group (group 2). At the end of the year 12 patients in group 1 had a greater than 90% reduction, and the remaining 5 had greater than 60% reduction in clinical scores compared with baseline values. The clinical scores of patients in group 2 gradually deteriorated so that by the end of the year the difference between groups 1 and 2 was highly significant ($p = 0.005$ for erythema and $p = 0.0002$ for surface damage). There was no difference between the groups at the start of follow-up.

All patients remained on daily treatment for the first 3 months. Eight patients were on an alternate day regimen by 6 months and remained on this until the end of the year and 7 were able to control their eczema with a 1 in every 3 days treatment regimen. The remaining 2 patients remained on daily treatments. No biochemical abnormalities arose during the study. Eosinophilia was detected in all patients at baseline; it had resolved in all group 1 patients and 6 of the group 2 patients by the end of the study. No significant differences in IgE levels or peripheral blood lymphocyte subsets were detected. Transient nausea and abdominal distension were often reported after drinking the decoction and a mild laxative effect was noted in approximately one third of patients in group 1.

All 37 children who completed the double-blind study elected to continue with the active treatment (21). Ten withdrew during the first 3 months due to lack of response. Four other children withdrew despite clinical improvement, because of unpalatability or difficulty in preparing the decoction. Twenty-three children completed the study, and at the end of the year, 18 had at least 90% reductions in the eczema scores and the other 5 showed reductions ranging between 30 and 89%. Seven children were able to discontinue therapy without relapse, and of the other 16 only 4 were requiring daily treatment by the end of the year of follow-up. A mild laxative effect was noted in about one-third of patients. Two children did develop asymptomatic raised aspartate transaminase levels to 7–14 times the normal values after 6 months of treatment when their eczema was clear. Liver function tests normalized after discontinuation of Chinese herbal therapy with no relapse of their eczema. Peripheral eosinophilia was noted in 19 of the 23 patients, and all had normalized by the end of the trial.

These studies have shown that Chinese herbal therapy can produce a sustained remission in disease activity in patients with atopic eczema, which has been unresponsive to conventional measures. Furthermore, remission can be achieved in some patients allowing discontinuation of treatment, and in others whose eczema has responded withdrawal of treatment produces a gradual relapse, but to a severity less than pretreatment levels.

V. OTHER CLINICAL STUDIES OF CHINESE HERBAL THERAPY

The results of a randomized double-blind, placebo-controlled, crossover study using Zemaphyte® among Chinese patients with recalcitrant atopic dermatitis have recently been published (22). The study design was very similar, except that children and adults were combined in the one study, the treatment periods involved 4 weeks of daily treatment then 4 weeks of alternate day treatment, and the clinical signs, particularly surface damage, lichenification, and scaling, were assessed independently. Additionally, smaller dosages were prescribed taking into account the lower average body weight of Chinese patients, i.e., age ≥ 14 years: three small and three large sachets/treatment. Thirty-seven out of 40 recruited patients completed the study. There was a general trend of improvement in both patient sequences, but there was no significant difference between Zemaphyte and placebo, except for lichenification at 4 weeks. No abnormality of renal or hepatic function was noted. One patient noted increased hair loss, two transient dizziness, four gastrointestinal symptoms, and one developed a lichenoid eruption. The authors speculated that better compliance and greater use of topical corticosteroid treatment combined with reduction in psychological stress from more intensive medical attention during the trial might have contributed to the lack of significant benefit. They also felt that from the standpoint of traditional Chinese medicine, the use of a standardized preparation was likely to produce disappointing results.

In another open study using a similar herbal decoction, 6 out of 10 patients dropped out of the study in the first week because of an exacerbation of their dermatitis (23). Two other patients reported less itching and slept better in the first 2 weeks, but then withdrew when their symptoms worsened. Unfortunately some of these patients had active exudation and infection. The two remaining patients, who had moderate atopic dermatitis, responded favorably and were able to discontinue topical corticosteroids. The herbal decoction contained lower doses of herbs and omitted *P chinensis*, which is known to have anti-inflammatory and antibacterial actions against *Staphylococcus aureus*. Clearly further corroborative studies are required, but these must be well designed and are awaited with interest.

A major complaint encountered during the clinical trials was of the unpleasant taste and smell the decoction of herbs produced. Phytopharm Ltd has formulated a freeze-dried preparation of the decoction, the resulting powder of which was compressed into mini-tablets coated with a flavorless lacquer. An open randomized study of the two preparations showed no significant difference in efficacy (24). Twenty-two patients took the decoction and 20 the new tablet preparation for 2 months. There was a 69% and 74% improvement in erythema and surface damage, respectively, for the tablet preparation compared to a 65% and 66% improvement for the decoction. Most patients taking the decoction commented on the unpalatability compared to those receiving the tablets.

VI. PHARMACOLOGY

The active ingredients that may account for the therapeutic efficacy of Chinese herbal therapy have not been identified. However, several pharmacologically active compounds are known to exist in the herbs used in the double-blind trials.

P. suffruticosa contains the monoterpene glycoside paeoniflorin (25). Paeoniflorin has anti-inflammatory, smooth muscle relaxant, peripheral vasodilatory, and immunostimulant properties (26,27). Paeoniflorin has also been shown to inhibit the binding of steroids to their receptors in rabbits and may positively or negatively influence steroid levels through their receptors (28). Paeonol is also a constituent of *P. suffruticosa* and has antimicrobial activity against *S. aureus*

Table 3 Major Constituents and Pharmacological Actions of Herbs in Chinese Herbal Therapy Used in Atopic Dermatitis

Herb[a]	Major chemical components and pharmacological effects
Rehmannia glutinosa	Sterol, campesterol, catalpol, rehmannin, acetoside, iridoids Antibacterial, immunosuppressive, anti-inflammatory
Paeonia suffruticosa/***Paeonia lactiflora***	Paeonolide, paeonoside, paeoniflorin, astragalin, pelargonin Antimicrobial, analgesic, sedative, antipyretic, anti-inflammatory
Potentilla chinensis	Tannin Antibacterial, smooth muscle relaxant
Schizonepta tenuifolia	D-Menthone, D-limonene, flavenoids Lowers body temperature by diaphoresis, antibacterial
Ledebouriella sesloides	Monoterpenoids, coumarins, diterpenes Antipyretic, analgesic, antibacterial
Tribulus terrestris	Tribuloside, astragalin, harmane, harmine, steroidal saponins Hypotensive, diuretic
Dictamnus dasycarpus	Dictamnine, skimmianine, fragarine, preskimmanine, isomaculosindine, limonin, obakinone, fraxinellone, psoralens, aurapfen, bergapten, saponins, essential oils Antipyretic, antifungal
Clematis armandii	Akebin, hederagonin, oleanolic acid Diuretic, antibacterial
Lophatherum gracile	Arundoin, cylindrin, friedelin, triterpenoids Antibacterial, antipyretic
Glycyrrhiza uralensis/***G. glabra***	Glycyrrhizin, glycyrrhetinic acid, liquiritin, isoliquiritin, neoliquiritin, licorione Glucocorticoid, mineralocorticoid, anti-inflammatory, analgesic, antipyretic

[a] Herbs in boldface are contained in Zemaphyte.

as well as anti-inflammatory properties. It has been proposed as one of the active components in the Chinese herbal therapy used to treat atopic dermatitis (29).

Another likely active agent is glycyrrhetinic acid. This is a constituent of licorice, which is derived from the root of *Glycyrrhiza uralensis* and *G. glabra*. Glycyrrhetinic acid inhibits the enzyme 11-β-hydroxysteroid dehydrogenase, which metabolizes the conversion of active cortisol to inactive cortisone. It, therefore, enhances corticosteroid effects indirectly (30). Glycyrrhetinic acid also inhibits 15-hydroxyprostaglandin dehydrogenase and Δ^3-prostaglandin reductase, two enzymes that are important in the metabolism of prostaglandins E_2 and F_2 (31). Furthermore, it is additionally a potent inhibitor of the classical complement pathway, which would confer anti-inflammatory properties (32). On the other hand, however, glycyrrhetinic acid has been shown to augment IL-2 and IL-2 receptor expression (33), and polysaccharide fractions obtained from *Glycyrrhiza uralensis* and *G. glabra* can activate murine macrophages (34). Extracts from *Schizonepeta tenuifolia* were able to inhibit compound 48/80 and substance P–induced immediate-type reactions in rats and mice (35,36).

Two major references were used to provide information on the major components in the formulation and their pharmacological effects (37,38) (Table 3). From the current knowledge at our disposal, the compounds present in Chinese herbal therapy for eczema may perform one or more of the following: (1) modulate cortisol release by adrenocortical stimulation, (2) potentiate the action of endogenous corticosteroids by inhibiting metabolizing enzymes or receptors, (3) contain compounds that have corticosteroid-like activity, (4) interfere with the generation of inflammatory mediators, (5) have a central or peripheral antipruritic effect, (6) have antimicrobial activity, or (7) have immunomodulatory cellular and/or cytokine activity.

VII. SIDE EFFECTS

It is a common misconception that natural medications are a safer mode of therapy because of their presumed lack of adverse side effects. Significant concern, however, has been expressed in the medical literature regarding the safety of Chinese herbal therapy, particularly with regard to hepatotoxicity and nephrotoxicity. Most of the side effects recorded in patients during the English trials were minor, but two children did develop abnormal liver function tests after 6 months of long-term treatment, with raised aspartate transaminase levels and elevated bilirubin in one. These normalized after discontinuation of Chinese herbal therapy. It was, however, not possible to establish a definitive causal relationship, because viral serology was not checked and one patient was also taking amoxycillin and theophylline (21).

The Medical Toxicology Unit at Guy's Hospital in London have reported on 11 cases of hepatitis following the use of Chinese herbal medicine for skin conditions and highlighted other cases reported in the literature (39,40). Four of the cases demonstrated substantial evidence for a causal association, and in particular 2 cases developed recurrent hepatitis on rechallenge. All patients recovered, except for one patient who restarted therapy and developed fatal acute liver failure. In this case, however, doubt has been raised over the exact identification of herbs ingested, since *Eurysolen gracilis* and *Cocculus tribolus*, listed as being taken by the patient, have been reported as not usually being exported or not for use in Chinese medicine (41). The authors were unable to incriminate a common ingredient(s) responsible for the episodes of hepatitis. Additionally they were unable to identify a dose-response or time-course effect and concluded that the problem may be idiosyncratic (40). One other case of fatal hepatitis has been reported associated with an herbal slimming medicine taken in conjunction with dexfenfluramine. In this case *Teucrium chamaedrys* (wild germander) was incriminated since this has previously been associated with cases of hepatitis (42). A number of other cases have additionally highlighted the possible hepatotoxic effect of herbal medicines (11,43–45).

There have also been reports of rapidly progressive interstitial renal fibrosis with Chinese herbal medicine. An outbreak has been reported in Belgium associated with a weight loss regimen prescribed by one clinic. This consisted of a low-calorie diet, psychological support, an intradermal injection of artichoke extract and euphyllin, capsules containing a mixture of cascara powder, acetazolamide, belladonna extract, *Stephania tetrandra*, and *Magnolia officinalis*, and a second set of capsules containing fenfluramine, diethylpropion, and meprobamate. The original report identified 9 patients with end-stage renal failure, but subsequently more than 100 cases were reported, at least 30 of which had end-stage renal failure (46–48). One of these cases was additionally associated with extensive progressive ureteric fibrosis (49). The problem arose after a new formulation was introduced, which included *Stephania tetrandra* and *Magnolia officinalis*. The possibility of contamination or adulteration with a heavy metal, diuretic, anti-inflammatory drug, or fungal nephrotoxin, e.g., ochratoxin A produced by *Penicillin verrucosum*, was considered but excluded on clinical grounds and after chemical analysis (46). It was subsequently demonstrated that aristolochic acid was present in 11 out of 12 batches of herbs distributed as powders under the name of *Stephania tetrandra*. Aristolochic acid is potentially nephrotoxic and carcinogenic, especially in the setting of Chinese herb–induced nephropathy (50,51). It is a constituent of *Aristolochia fangchi* and not *Stephania tetrandra*. The Chinese name for *Aristolochia fangchi* is *Fangchi*, which is very similar to *Fangji*, the name for *Stephania tetrandra* (47). Two cases of aristolochic acid–induced nephropathy following Chinese herbal medication for eczema have additionally been reported in the United Kingdom (52).

This emphasizes the need for strict quality-control measures in the preparation of herbal medicines (53) but succinctly highlights the ease with which mis-identification can occur and the subsequent effects that this can have. There are four ways to name a herb: the English common name, transliteration of the herb name, the Latinized pharmaceutical name, and the scientific name. For example, the corresponding names for ginseng are ginseng, ren-shen, radix ginseng, and *Panax ginseng* (Oriental ginseng). The name ginseng is also applied to *P. quinquefolium* (American ginseng) and *Eleutherococcus senticosus* (Siberian ginseng) (41). Thus, the scientific name is the most specific and acceptable name to use in preparing a prescription or reporting in the literature.

There has been one report of facial herpes simplex developing within 2 weeks of commencing Chinese herbal therapy. The patient had been affected by a similar episode 2 weeks after starting azathioprine, but he had also had 6 other episodes over the course of the preceding 2 years while on conventional therapy, making it difficult to establish a causal relationship (54). There has also been a report of reversible dilated cardiomyopathy following a 2-week course of herbal therapy for atopic eczema; in this case, more than 30 herbal components were identified (55). Aconitum poisoning from Chinese herbal medicines is a recognized cause of cardiotoxicity (56). One case of photosensitivity has been reported following the ingestion of Chinese herbal therapy for vitiligo, which contained powdered seeds of *Psoralea corylifolia* (57).

Finally, there have been concerns raised regarding the illegal supply of prescription-only corticosteroids peddled as topical herbal therapies (58,59) and the adulteration of herbal creams with corticosteroids. In a recent study, out of 11 herbal creams from 5 different suppliers in South London, 8 were found to contain dexamethasone (60).

The problems highlighted above can be minimized in the setting of a rigorously prepared product, which has an extensive toxicological pedigree and is manufactured by a pharmaceutical company that can institute quality control combined with careful pretreatment and maintenance monitoring of laboratory investigations. It is encouraging that the House of Lords Select Committee on Science and Technology in the United Kingdom has recently recommended proper regulation and increased research in the complementary sector (15).

VIII. IMMUNOLOGICAL STUDIES ON THE POSSIBLE MECHANISM OF ACTION

The exact mode of action of Chinese herbal therapy in atopic dermatitis is unknown, but studies have been undertaken to investigate the mechanisms by which Zemaphyte may improve atopic dermatitis. Data from the original adult follow-up trial showed no difference in IgE levels, absolute lymphocyte numbers, or the ratio of CD4 and CD8 subsets despite significant clinical improvement (20). Initial in vitro studies looked at the effect of the herbal medicine on monocytes collected from nonatopic individuals and the level of IL-4–induced CD23 expression. Chinese herbal therapy inhibited CD23 expression by up to 60% in a dose-dependent fashion as compared with placebo, which had no significant effect (Fig. 2). Cell death or loss of functionality was not responsible for this effect (61).

In contrast, patients treated with Chinese herbal therapy for 8 weeks showed no significant difference in CD23 expression on peripheral blood monocytes despite significant clinical improvement. However, when peripheral blood monocytes from these patients were cultured in the presence of IL-4, CD23 expression was significantly diminished. Therapy led to decreased levels of soluble IL-2 receptor, soluble vascular cell adhesion molecule, and serum IgE complexes, but not total IgE or soluble intracellular adhesion molecule levels (62). When immunohistochemical studies were carried out on lesional skin from patients with atopic dermatitis before and after treatment, the overall number of CD23+ cells decreased significantly. This was associated with significant decreases in the number of CD23+ RFD1+ dendritic cells, RFD7+ tissue macrophages, and

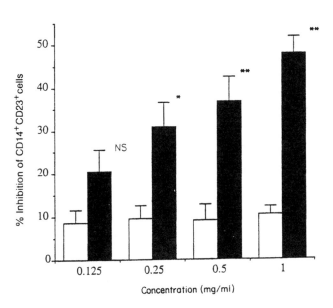

Figure 2 Inhibition of CD23 on monocytes by Chinese herbal therapy extract (■) and placebo extract (□) in 12 control subjects. Chinese herbal therapy inhibits in a dose-dependent manner, and the inhibition is still significant at a dose of 250 µg/mL. (Kindly reproduced by the permission of British Journal of Dermatology, Blackwell Science Ltd.)

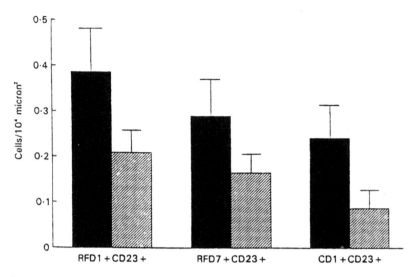

Figure 3 Mean (±SD) number of cells expressing double phenotypic markers within lesional skin taken before and after treatment with Chinese herbal therapy. The data are from eight subjects. ■, before treatment; ▨, after treatment (Kindly reproduced by the permission of British Journal of Dermatology, Blackwell Science Ltd.)

CD1+ Langerhans cells (Fig. 3). Significant differences in the number of these cells in lesional compared to nonlesional skin became nonsignificant following treatment. Additionally the number of cells expressing FcεRI remained unchanged and no change in cell numbers in nonlesional skin was seen (63). Further studies confirmed that the Chinese herbal treatment had no effect on CD23 expression on peripheral blood monocytes, but that a significant reduction in positive tissue macrophages occurred in lesional skin (64). This suggests that the effects of the Chinese herbal medicine modulate CD23 expression in the microenvironment of lesional skin rather than systemically.

Studies have also been carried out looking at the effects of Zemaphyte on allergic contact sensitivity in guinea pigs using equivalent doses to those given to humans. Chinese herbal therapy had no effect on the induction of sensitization to DNCB (1-chloro-2,4-dinitrobenzene) as measured by skin thickness on the flank, but recall reactions were significantly reduced by therapy (control animal reaction 2.6 mm, treated animal reaction 1.5 mm, $p < 0.01$). Two weeks of treatment was required as a minimum to achieve a significant reduction in recall skin reactions, and no cumulative effect was seen after 4 weeks of treatment. No consistent dose-response effect was observed, but if a threefold increase over the human equivalent dose was given, more sustained suppression of the recall reactions was observed (X.-J. Xu, M. H. A. Rustin, L. W. Poulter, unpublished).

IX. CONCLUSION

Clinical studies have shown that a particular formulation of Chinese herbal therapy, Zemaphyte, is an effective treatment for severe atopic dermatitis that is not exudative or infected. Corroborative studies are needed, and these should be designed to allow comparison with existing data. The possibility of side effects is real, but with proper manufacturing, quality control, and monitoring of treatment, the risk can be minimized. Regulation, improved training, and increased scientific research in the complementary medicine sector are all required. This can be partly solved by increased cooperation between practitioners of orthodox and complementary medicine, as shown by the clinical studies carried out in London. Without this, doubts and suspicions will remain regarding safety and efficacy. Ongoing research is trying to identify the active ingredients in Chinese herbal therapy, but one has to be aware that individual chemicals may not produce clinical benefit, since Chinese herbal therapy is based upon the treatment of a number of contributory factors with a combination of herbs containing a multitude of different chemicals that may act in concert.

REFERENCES

1. CC Buckley, C Ivison, LW Poulter, MHA Rustin. Fc epsilon RII/CD23 receptor distribution in patch test reactions to aeroallergens in atopic dermatitis. J Invest Dermatol 99:184–188, 1992.
2. CH Orteu, MHA Rustin, E O'Toole, C Sabin, M Salmon, LW Poulter, AN Akbar. The inhibition of cutaneous T cell apoptosis may prevent resolution of inflammation in atopic eczema. Clin Exp Immunol 122:150–156, 2000.
3. CC Buckley, C Ivison, LW Poulter, MHA Rustin. CD23/Fc epsilon RII expression in contact sensitivity reactions: a comparison between aeroallergen patch test reactions in atopic dermatitis and the nickel patch test reaction in non-atopic individuals. Clin Exp Immunol 91:357–361, 1993.
4. D Maurer, G Stingl. Immunoglobulin E-binding structures on antigen-presenting cells present in skin and blood. J Invest Dermatol 104:707–710, 1995.
5. T Bieber. Fc epsilon RI-expressing antigen-presenting cells: new players in the atopic game. Immunol Today 18:311–313, 1997.
6. Q Hamid, M Boguniewicz, DY Leung. Differential in situ cytokine gene expression in acute versus chronic atopic dermatitis. J Clin Invest 94:870–876, 1994.
7. M Grewe, CA Bruijnzeel-Koomen, E Schopf, T Thepen, AG Langeveld-Wildschut,

T Ruzicka, J Krutmann. A role for Th1 and Th2 cells in the immunopathogenesis of atopic dermatitis. Immunol Today 19:359–361, 1998.

8. JM Hanifin, SC Chan, JB Cheng, SJ Tofte, WRJ Henderson, DS Kirby, ES Weiner. Type 4 phosphodiesterase inhibitors have clinical and in vitro anti-inflammatory effects in atopic dermatitis. J Invest Dermatol 107:51–56, 1996.

9. SA George, DJ Bilsland, BE Johnson, J Ferguson. Narrow-band (TL-01) UVB air-conditioned phototherapy for chronic severe adult atopic dermatitis. Br J Dermatol 128:49–56, 1993.

10. WL Morison, J Parrish, TB Fitzpatrick. Oral psoralen photochemotherapy of atopic eczema. Br J Dermatol 98:25–30, 1978.

11. JM Sowden, J Berth-Jones, JS Ross, RJ Motley, R Marks, AY Finlay, MS Salek, RA Graham-Brown, BR Allen, RD Camp. Double-blind, controlled, crossover study of cyclosporin in adults with severe refractory atopic dermatitis. Lancet 338:137–140, 1991.

12. JG Morrison, EJ Schulz. Treatment of eczema with cyclophosphamide and azathioprine. Br J Dermatol 98:203–207, 1978.

13. U Reinhold, S Kukel, J Brzoska, HW Kreysel. Systemic interferon gamma treatment in severe atopic dermatitis. J Am Acad Dermatol 29:58–63, 1993.

14. S Reitamo, A Wollenberg, E Schopf, JL Perrot, R Marks, T Ruzicka, E Christophers, A Kapp, M Lahfa, A Rubins, S Jablonska, MHA Rustin. Safety and efficacy of 1 year of tacrolimus ointment monotherapy in adults with atopic dermatitis. The European Tacrolimus Ointment Study Group. Arch Dermatol 136:999–1006, 2000.

15. J O'Neale Roach. Lords call for regulation of complementary medicine. Br Med J 321:1365, 2000.

16. G Maciocia. The Foundations of Chinese Medicine. Edinburgh: Churchill Livingstone, 1989, pp. 1–65.

17. G Maciocia. The Practice of Chinese medicine. Edinburgh: Churchill Livingstone, 1994, pp. 128–138.

18. MP Sheehan, MHA Rustin, DJ Atherton, C Buckley, DW Harris, J Brostoff, L Ostlere, A Dawson, DJ Harris. Efficacy of traditional Chinese herbal therapy in adult atopic dermatitis. Lancet 340:13–17, 1992.

19. MP Sheehan, DJ Atherton. A controlled trial of traditional Chinese medicinal plants in widespread non-exudative atopic eczema. Br J Dermatol 126:179–184, 1992.

20. MP Sheehan, H Stevens, LS Ostlere, DJ Atherton, J Brostoff, MHA Rustin. Follow-up of adult patients with atopic eczema treated with Chinese herbal therapy for 1 year. Clin Exp Dermatol 20:136–140, 1995.

21. MP Sheehan, DJ Atherton. One-year follow up of children treated with Chinese medicinal herbs for atopic eczema. Br J Dermatol 130:488–493, 1994.

22. AY Fung, PC Look, LY Chong, PP But, E Wong. A controlled trial of traditional Chinese herbal medicine in Chinese patients with recalcitrant atopic dermatitis. Int J Dermatol 38:387–392, 1999.

23. HN Liu, SK Jaw, CK Wong. Chinese herbs and atopic dermatitis. Lancet 342:1175–1176, 1993.

24. P Banerjee, MHA Rustin. Efficacy of a new palatable formulation of Chinese herbal therapy as a treatment of atopic eczema. Br J Dermatol 131(suppl 44):26, 1994.

25. J Yu, PG Xiao. Ontogenic chemical changes of the active constituents in mudan (*P. suffruticosa*) and shaoyao (*P. lactiflora*). Acta Pharmacol Sin 20:782–784, 1985.

26. W Tang, G Eisenbrand. Chinese Drugs of Plant Origin. Berlin: Springer-Verlag, 1992, pp. 1–1056.

27. H Hikino. Recent Research on Oriental Medicinal Plants in Economic and Medicinal Plant Research. London: Academic Press, 1985, pp. 53–85.

28. T Tamaya, S Sato, HH Okada. Possible mechanism of steroid action of the plant herb extracts glycyrrhizin, glycyrrhetenic acid and paeoniflorin: inhibition by plant herb extracts of steroid protein in the rabbit. Am J Obstet Gynecol 155:1134–1139, 1986.

29. JH Galloway, ID Marsh, SB Bittiner, AG Messenger, DJ Gawkrodger, R Glet, AR Forrest. Chinese herbs for eczema, the active compound? Lancet 337:566, 1991.

30. CR Edwards, S Teelucksingh. Glycyrrhetinic acid and potentiation of hydrocortisone activity in skin. Lancet 336:322–323, 1990.

31. ME Baker, DD Fanestil. Liquorice as a regulator of steroid and prostaglandin metabolism. Lancet 337:428–429, 1991.

32. BH Kroes, CJ Beukelman, AJ van den Berg, GJ Wolbink, H van Dijk, RP Labadie. Inhibition of human complement by beta-glycyrrhetinic acid. Immunology 90:115–120, 1997.

33. YH Zhang, K Isobe, F Nagase, T Lwin, M Kato, M Hamaguchi, T Yokochi, I Nakashima. Glycyrrhizin as a promoter of the late signal transduction for interleukin-2 production by splenic lymphocytes. Immunology 79:528–534, 1993.

34. M Nose, K Terawaki, K Oguri, Y Ogihara, K Yoshimatsu, K Shimomura. Activation of macrophages by crude polysaccharide fractions obtained from shoots of Glycyrrhiza glabra and hairy roots of Glycyrrhiza uralensis in vitro. Biol Pharm Bull 21:1110–1112, 1998.

35. TY Shin, HJ Jeong, SM Jun, HJ Chae, HR Kim, SH Baek, HM Kim. Effect of Schizonepeta tenuifolia extract on mast cell-mediated immediate-type hypersensitivity in rats. Immunopharmacol Immunotoxicol 21:705–715, 1999.

36. C Tohda, Y Kakihara, K Komatsu, Y Kuraishi. Inhibitory effects of methanol extracts of herbal medicines on substance P-induced itch-scratch response. Biol Pharm Bull 23:599–601, 2000.

37. HM Chang, PPH But. Pharmacology and Applications of Chinese Materia Medica. Singapore: World Scientific Publications, 1987, pp. 1-1320.

38. KC Huang. The Pharmacology of Chinese Herbs. Boca Raton, FL: CRC Press, 1993, pp. 1-388.

39. L Perharic-Walton, V Murray. Toxicity of Chinese herbal remedies. Lancet 340:674, 1992.

40. L Perharic, D Shaw, C Leon, PA De Smet, VS Murray. Possible association of liver damage with the use of Chinese herbal medicine for skin disease. Vet Hum Toxicol 37:562–566, 1995.

41. PP But. Need for correct identification of herbs in herbal poisoning. Lancet 341:637, 1993.

42. N Mostefa-Kara, A Pauwels, E Pines, M Biour, VG Levy. Fatal hepatitis after herbal tea. Lancet 340:674, 1992.

43. JA Kane, SP Kane, S Jain. Hepatitis induced by traditional Chinese herbs; possible toxic components. Gut 36:146–147, 1994.
44. EG Davies, I Pollock, HM Steel. Chinese herbs for eczema. Lancet 336:177, 1990.
45. FB MacGregor, VE Abernethy, S Dahabra, I Cobden, PC Hayes. Hepatotoxicity of herbal remedies. Br Med J 299:1156–1157, 1989.
46. L Vanherweghem, M Depierreux, C Tielemans, D Abramowicz, M Dratwa, M Jadoul, C Richard, D Vandervelde, D Verbeelen, R Vanhaelen-Fastre, M Vanhaelen. Rapidly progressive interstitial renal fibrosis in young women: association with slimming regimen including Chinese herbs. Lancet 341:387–391, 1993.
47. M Vanhaelen, R Vanhaelen-Fastre, P But, L Vanherweghem. Identification of aristolochic acid in Chinese herbs. Lancet 343:174, 1994.
48. L Vanherweghem. Misuse of herbal remedies: the case of an outbreak of terminal renal failure in Belgium (Chinese herbs nephropathy). J Altern Complement Med 4:9–13, 1998.
49. M Jadoul, J De Plaen, J Cosyns, C Van Ypersele De Strihou. Adverse effects from traditional Chinese medicine. Lancet 341:892–893, 1993.
50. RG Penn. Adverse reactions to herbal medicines. Adverse Drug Reaction Bull 376–379, 1983.
51. JP Cosyns, M Jadoul, JP Squifflet, FX Wese, C Van Ypersele De Strihou. Urothelial lesions in Chinese-herb nephropathy. Am J Kidney Dis 33:1011–1017, 1999.
52. GM Lord, R Tagore, T Cook, P Gower, CD Pusey. Nephropathy caused by Chinese herbs in the UK. Lancet 354:481–482, 1999.
53. DJ Atherton, MHA Rustin, J Brostoff. Need for correct identification of herbs in herbal poisoning. Lancet 341:637–638, 1993.
54. R Russell Jones. Recurrent facial herpes associated with Chinese herbal remedy. Lancet 338:55, 1991.
55. JE Ferguson, RJ Chalmers, DJ Rowlands. Reversible dilated cardiomyopathy following treatment of atopic eczema with Chinese herbal medicine. Br J Dermatol 136:592–593, 1997.
56. ST Kolev, P Leman, GC Kite, PC Stevenson, D Shaw, VS Murray. Toxicity following accidental ingestion of Aconitum containing Chinese remedy. Hum Exp Toxicol 15:839–842, 1996.
57. PD Maurice, JJ Cream. The dangers of herbalism. Br Med J 299:1204, 1989.
58. J O'Driscoll, AD Burden, TP Kingston. Potent topical steroid obtained from a Chinese herbalist. Br J Dermatol 127:543–544, 1992.
59. JR Hughes, EM Higgins, AC Pembroke. Oral dexamethasone masquerading as a Chinese herbal remedy. Br J Dermatol 130:261, 1994.
60. FM Keane, SE Munn, AWP du Vivier, NF Taylor, EM Higgins. Analysis of Chinese herbal creams prescribed for dermatological conditions. Br Med J 318:563–564, 1999.
61. Y Latchman, GA Bungy, DJ Atherton, MHA Rustin, J Brostoff. Efficacy of traditional Chinese herbal therapy in vitro. A model system for atopic eczema: inhibition of CD23 expression on blood monocytes. Br J Dermatol 132:592–598, 1995.
62. Y Latchman, P Banerjee, LW Poulter, MHA Rustin, J Brostoff. Association of immunological changes with clinical efficacy in atopic eczema patients treated with

traditional Chinese herbal therapy (Zemaphyte). Int Arch Allergy Immunol 109: 243–249, 1996.

63. XJ Xu, P Banerjee, MHA Rustin, LW Poulter. Modulation by Chinese herbal therapy of immune mechanisms in the skin of patients with atopic eczema. Br J Dermatol 136:54–59, 1997.

64. P Banerjee, XJ Xu, LW Poulter, MHA Rustin. Changes in CD23 expression of blood and skin in atopic eczema after Chinese herbal therapy. Clin Exp Allergy 28:306–314, 1998.

29
Systemic Pharmacotherapy

Werner Aberer
University of Graz, Graz, Austria

Klaus Wolff
University of Vienna, Vienna, Austria

I. INTRODUCTION

In the large majority of patients, atopic dermatitis can be managed by the use of emollients, hydration, topical corticosteroids, phototherapy, avoidance of irritants, and treatment of infection. Time-honored, systemic treatments include antihistamines to suppress pruritus, systemic corticosteroids for the control of inflammation and pruritus, and, more recently, cyclosporine to suppress ongoing T-cell activation in this chronically relapsing disorder. This review will focus on antihistamines, corticosteroids, and cyclosporine but will also briefly address other immunosuppressive and anti-inflammatory agents that have been employed to control atopic dermatitis or are presently being developed.

II. ANTIHISTAMINES

Antihistamines are among the most widely used drugs in the world and are "prescribed in large quantities by general practitioners not only for atopic eczema but seemingly for pruritus of any cause" (1). The rationale for their use in atopic dermatitis is to interrupt the itch-scratch-itch cycle. But even though early studies have reported increased histamine levels in normal and eczematous skin and that pruritus induced by intradermally administered histamine can be clinically sup-

589

pressed with H1 receptor antagonists (2), the mechanism of itch in atopic dermatitis is still largely unknown. It is undisputed that anthistamines are antipruritic in certain conditions such as insect bites or urticaria, and the ongoing controversy on their use in atopic dermatitis therefore rests on the issue whether they are also antipruritic in this disease (3).

Clinical trials of antihistamines have been criticized for being inadequate in terms of study designs and sample size, and the outcomes are contradictory. Current recommendations and practices are based largely on the individual experience of patients and physicians.

A. First-Generation Antihistamines

These include ethanolamines, clemastine, piperazine derivatives, meclizine, phenothiazine derivatives, trimeprazine, chlorpheniramine, ethylene diamines, and alkylamines. The drowsiness and decline in performance have been the primary limitations of their daytime use, and when given at night, there may be "hangover" effects the following day. Because itch intensity often increases at night, the soporific effect of sedating formulations can be quite useful. Sedating antihistamines are therefore frequently used, especially at bedtime, to facilitate peaceful sleep.

Should patients with atopic dermatitis use these sedating agents? The prime argument against their use is that they have not been proven to relieve pruritus, but in the experience of most authors they have been useful by virtue of their soporific effect. A disadvantage is that they can only be used for short periods because tolerance is thought to develop quite quickly (4). Any of the standard antihistamines are essentially equally effective (or not): all cause sedation, impairment of cognitive function, diminished alertness, and slow reaction times. These drugs may also cause fatigue, lassitude, drowsiness, somnolence, weakness, dizziness, ataxia, and even narcolepsy or coma. Occasionally, paradoxical stimulatory effects such as insomnia, hyperreflexia, irritability, headaches, muscle twisting, nervousness, tremor, dyskinesia, dystonia, or seizures may occur. Neuropsychiatric and neurological effects, dry mouth, and urinary retention have also been reported. Some first-generation H1 antagonists may cause gastrointestinal upset, appetite stimulation, and inappropriate weight gain. And pancytopenia and jaundice have been reported after ingestion of trimeprazine. Although occurring only sporadically, these are too many potential side effects for drugs with questionable efficacy in a non–life-threatening disease, where safer and better alternatives are available.

B. Second- and Third-Generation Antihistamines

These include piperidine derivatives (e.g., terfenadine and astemizole), loratadine, azelastine, fexofenadine, cetirizine, and others. They are generally less sedating and produce considerably less impairment of cognitive and motor function than their earlier chemical cousins. The drowsiness and dry mouth associated with older, first-generation antihistamines resulted from significant penetration of these agents into the central nervous system (CNS). The chemical structures of the second-generation agents differ in that these newer agents are less lipophilic and bind to proteins to a greater extent, properties that prevent substantial CNS penetration. They are also more specific for the histamine receptor and do not appreciably block cholinergic receptors (5).

Some second-generation antihistamines are also not completely devoid of adverse CNS effects. The low sedating property of terfenadine, astemizole, loratadine, and others is well established (6). Pooled data from placebo-controlled clinical trials of cetirizine have indicated that while the incidence of sedation by cetirizine is lower than with older antihistamines, it is higher than with the other second-generation antihistamines (6–8). As a result, the U.S. Food and Drug Administration (FDA) has classified cetirizine as ''sedating'' rather than nonsedating, and thus the full sedation precautions also apply to this drug. As terfenadine and astemizole were found to cause potentially serious arrhythmias (9), they have meanwhile been withdrawn from the market. The goal for the third generation of antihistamines was to develop therapeutically active metabolites that are devoid of cardiac toxicity. This group includes fexofenadine (the active metabolite of terfenadine), which was approved in 1996, norastemizole (the active metabolite of astemizole), and descarboethoxyloratadine (derived from loratadine).

Data on the clinical efficacy of the newer non-sedating agents are conflicting. Whereas several controlled clinical trials with cetirizine, loratadine, acrivastine, and terfenadine appear to support efficacy of these antihistamines in atopic dermatitis (3,8), an evidence-based review of the efficacy of antihistamines in relieving pruritus in atopic dermatitis (10) concluded that ''little objective evidence exists to demonstrate relief of pruritus. The majority of trials are flawed in terms of the sample size or study design. Based on the literature alone, the efficacy of antihistamines remains to be adequately investigated. . . .'' However, newer in vitro studies with some second- and third-generation antihistamines have revealed properties of some of these products that might broaden their spectrum for clinical use and also justify their administration to patients with atopic dermatitis.

Loratidine in vitro inhibits the release of histamine and leukotriene C_4 (LTC4) from rodent mast cells, histamine and LTC4 from human basophils, and histamine, leukotrienes, and prostaglandin D_2 from human skin tissue (11). It also has been shown to inhibit superoxide anion generation and eosinophil chemotaxis in vitro and eosinophil accumulation in nasal and bronchoalveolar lavage material after antigen challenge in vivo (11). In allergic subjects, blood flow to the skin was increased and late-phase reactions to both histamine and allergen skin-prick challenge were inhibited (11). Following these observations, loratadine 10 mg once daily has shown to reduce pruritus and rash more effectively than placebo and at least as well as hydroxyzine (12). Double-blind, randomized, placebo-controlled studies have meanwhile reproduced similar positive effects (13).

Cetirizine was shown in patients with severe reactions to insect bites to inhibit both the early and late inflammatory reaction as well as eosinophil infiltration and accumulation (8). In a double-blind, multicenter, placebo-controlled study, cetirizine gave a marked improvement of pruritus and the extent and activity of skin lesions. This was paralleled by a pronounced decrease in the number of blood eosinophils (14).

Diverse anti-inflammatory properties, such as the inhibition of mediator release and leukocyte chemotaxis, have been described for descarbethoxylorata-dine, the active metabolite of loratadine, including cytokine synthesis and secretion from mast cells (15). Proven antihistaminic, anti-inflammatory (Th2 cytokines, chemokines, and adhesion molecules), and antiallergic (inhibition of mast cell products) activity has an enormous potential for treating the systemic aspects of allergic disease (15).

IgE-mediated hypersensitivity reactions and positive skin-prick tests to allergens are common in patients with atopic dermatitis and have been implicated in the pathogenesis of this disease. Since treatment with antihistamines has convincing effects in IgE-mediated disease like allergic rhinitis or urticaria and in patients allergic to drugs or insect venoms, they should theoretically also exert effects in atopic dermatitis, where antigen exposure via the skin may induce local and systemic immune responses.

C. Conclusions

Critical reviews of the large body of clinical trials that refute or support the efficacy of antihistamines in relieving pruritus in patients with atopic dermatitis have summarized that there is no evidence to support the effectiveness of antihistamines in atopic dermatitis (10). An article by Henz et al. (3) on the effects of H1 receptor antagonists in pruritic dermatoses points to the differential effects on pruritus versus whealing and the low efficacy in atopic eczema as compared to urticaria. These authors suspect that different anti-inflammatory properties of H1 antagonists, such as the inhibition of mediator release and leukocyte chemotaxis, cytokine synthesis and secretion from mast cells, mediator release from leukocytes and others, "might have no impact on the chronic inflammatory processes in atopic dermatitis, where cytokines and growth factors may be more promising targets of itch therapy" (2).

On the other hand, there are millions of patients with atopic dermatitis who have tried to suppress their pruritus for years with antihistamines with supposedly good results, and many studies by renowned dermatologists claim to have proven efficacy of antihistamines in the treatment of atopic dermatitis (3). Can they all be wrong, and are we dealing with placebo effects? Juhlin (14) has analyzed the many problems of such studies and concluded that "taking all clinical reports together, there is now evidence that the non- or less-sedative antihistamines can reduce pruritus in patients with atopic dermatitis." However, high doses are required to reach substantial symptom relief (3).

Of course, evidence-based medicine certainly calls for new large, randomized, double-blind, placebo-controlled clinical trials to provide a definite answer. Such studies, however, may be difficult or even impossible to perform as most patients with atopic dermatitis take antihistamines because of associated IgE-mediated disease such as allergic rhinitis or asthma. In addition, the heterogeneity of atopic dermatitis with its many different provocative factors, like food allergy, infections, occupational irritants, and mite exposure, make it difficult to identify patient cohorts comparable with regard to the extent and severity of eczema, level of IgE-associated symptoms, and compliance to perform such studies. The severity of disease has to justify treatment for a prolonged period of time, but then these patients apply topical corticosteroids that also relieve pruritus. Do we really need such a study? It is interesting that most expert clinicians dealing with atopic dermatitis indeed use antihistamines in their daily practice.

III. SYSTEMIC GLUCOCORTICOSTEROIDS

Glucocorticosteroids exert a wide range of anti-inflammatory and immunosuppressive effects and thus effectively reduce inflammation and pruritus in atopic dermatitis. Their use in atopic dermatitis is time honored, but large-scale controlled studies have never been performed. However, in contrast to the antihistamines they have an undisputable, proven efficacy in atopic dermatitis. By understanding the properties and mechanisms of action, one can maximize their efficacy and safety as therapeutic agents, but it has to be noted that they should be employed only as a rescue treatment in this chronic disease.

A. Mode of Action

Systemic steroids decrease the synthesis of a number of proinflammatory molecules, including cytokines, interleukins (IL-1, IL-2, IL-6, and tumor necrosis factor), and proteases, largely through their effects on transcription. Some mediators of inflammation such as cyclooxygenase-2 are inhibited, some others such as lipocortin-1 are increased. Replication and movement of cells is suppressed resulting in monocytopenia, eosinopenia, and lymphocytopenia (T more than B cells). Apoptosis of lymphocytes is induced, whereas the increase in circulating polymorphonuclear leukocytes is related to demargination of cells from the bone marrow and inhibition of neutrophil apoptosis. Activation, proliferation, and differentiation of cells of the immune system is obtained either indirectly via modulation of mediator production or by direct suppression of cellular functions (16). Very high doses are needed to suppress antibody production of B lymphocytes and plasma cells, a disadvantage in atopic diseases where there is a high degree of IgE-mediated problems. On the other hand, granulomatous infectious diseases, such as tuberculosis, are prone to exacerbate and relapse during prolonged systemic treatment.

The multiplicity of biological effects produced by glucocorticosteroids explains why currently there is no unifying hypothesis to explain the therapeutic efficacy of these agents.

B. Use in Atopic Dermatitis

Any decision to employ systemic glucocorticosteroids in atopic dermatitis should weigh expected benefits against potential side effects. In the small proportion of patients who do not respond to optimal skin care and topical management or when during an acute flare of severe atopic dermatitis more than 20% of the skin is affected, a decision to administer steroids systemically may be made (17,18). Systemic administration in atopic dermatitis thus represents a rescue treatment. Initial use of high doses of prednisone or prednisolone (1 mg/kg/ day) maximize the anti-inflammatory/immunosuppressive effects and allow more rapid tapering or conversion to an alternate day regimen (19). One should not taper too rapidly so as to minimize the risk of a steroid rebound, i.e., a posttherapeutic exacerbation of disease to a more severe level. A simple approach, also easy for patients to follow, is to administer 60 mg daily for 5 days, to be followed by 40 and 20 mg for 5 days each. Treatment is continued by 20 mg on alternate days for another week and then stopped. A single daily dose given in the morning is preferable, as this regimen is thought to minimize hypothalamic-pituitary-adrenal suppression by mimicking the normal circadian rhythm of adrenal cortisol production. Topical glucocorticoids, ascomycins, or tacrolimus or other steroid-sparing agents should be continued during the taper to suppress rebound flaring, and hydration and moisturizers need to be continued or even intensified.

The literature is scarce on systemic steroid treatment in atopic dermatitis, and well controlled studies have not been performed, obviously because of its empirically proven dramatic efficacy. Now that other systemic drugs like azathioprine and cyclosporine have proven effectiveness in atopic dermatitis, the use of systemic steroids is restricted to rescue treatment where a rapid response is required. This approach requires chronic retreatment leading to tachyphylaxis, cumulative long-term toxicity, and "steroid-addictive" behavior (20). Maintenance systemic glucocorticosteroid therapy has to be avoided in all instances.

C. Side Effects

The list of side effects is imposing and includes all the adverse events of topical corticosteroid therapy and multiple more significant sequelae like hypertension, gastric ulcers, osteoporosis, aseptic bone necrosis, and cataracts. Side effects on skin include atrophy and striae formation, possibly related to the antianabolic properties of glucocorticoids through suppression of proline hydroxylation and cross-linking of collagen, purpura from increased vascular fragility, formation of stellate pseudoscars, steroid acne, rosacea, perioral dermatitis, facial hypertrichosis, and initial masking and then worsening of cutaneous or systemic bacterial, fungal, or viral infections. Hypertriglyceridemia, altered lipid metabolism, hyperglycemia, gastritis, gastric ulcers, pancreatitis, potassium wasting, myopathy, posterior subcapsular cataracts, Cushingoid appearance, psychosis, pseudotumor cerebri, and growth retardation in children are all possible sequelae of prolonged systemic glucocorticoid administration.

D. Conclusions

In general, systemic steroids should be avoided in the management of a chronic, relapsing disorder such as atopic dermatitis. As rescue treatments they are justified but should never be administered on a long-term basis. If patients or parents demand immediate improvement of the disease and find topical therapy ineffective or impossible to perform, they have to be appropriately informed of the potential side effects of steroids and of the fact that dramatic improvement observed with systemic steroids may be and is frequently associated with an equally dramatic flare of atopic dermatitis following their discontinuation. Some patients and physicians have in the past preferred the use of systemic steroids over topical therapy, but with the availability of new topical drugs such as tacrolimus or ascomycins, this may become obsolete.

IV. CYCLOSPORIN

Cyclosporin A (CsA) is a fungal peptide with powerful immunosuppressive activity. It effectively suppresses cell-mediated immune responses, particularly graft rejection, and the graft-versus-host reaction. A first report indicating the efficacy of this nonmyelosuppressive immunosuppressive agent in the management of severe atopic dermatitis was published in 1987 (21); several uncontrolled and placebo-controlled trials have been reported, studying the effects in children and adults, short- and long-term safety, questions of dosage and different formulations, maintenance therapy and remission time, quality of life, disease markers like E-selectin or sCD30 levels in blood, and many others. Several workshop and consensus reports have been published (22–24). CsA is thus a drug for atopic dermatitis that has been carefully and extensively studied.

Regular CsA (marketed as Sandimmun®) has proven useful as a second-line treatment for severe atopic dermatitis in patients who do not respond to or cannot tolerate treatment with topical steroids or other modalities (25). However, its use has been somewhat hampered by high inter- and intrapatient variability in its bioavailability (26) and dose-dependent side effects. The use of CsA as a microemulsion (Sandimmun Neoral; Neoral®) in the treatment of dermatological diseases was pioneered by Bourke et al. (27). Further investigations showed that Neoral has a better and more reproducible pharmacokinetic profile resulting in improved control of therapy and fewer adverse events. Data obtained in a randomized, double-blind, crossover study suggest that Neoral is an adequate replacement for Sandimmun thanks to its high efficacy, its faster onset of action, and its better tolerability (26). The pharmacokinetic properties of Neoral provide for greater ease in individualizing dosage and maintaining CsA concentration within the therapeutic window (28). For conversion from the original formulation to the microemulsion formulation, a 1:1 dose-conversion strategy is recommended. It then may be necessary to make subsequent dose reductions in poor absorbers of conventional CsA to ensure that they are receiving the lowest effective dose. Careful safety monitoring is mandatory postconversion to comply with the safety guidelines (29).

A. Mode of Action

Peripheral blood eosinophilia frequently occurs in atopic dermatitis, and there is an increase of eosinophils and their products, the eosinophil cationic protein and eosinophil major basic protein, in atopic skin. These eosinophils are thought to be preactivated in the circulation as a result of exposure to the T-cell–mediated cytokines IL-3, IL-5, and GM-CSF. CsA probably acts by downregulating Th2 cells, which decreases IL-4 and IL-5, thereby lowering peripheral blood eosinophilia. Treatment of atopic dermatitis with CsA has also been shown to significantly reduce adhesion molecules that regulate leukocyte migration (E-selectin) (30) and CD30 (31), an activation marker of Th2 cell clones. Reduction of these factors significantly correlated with changes in disease activity parameters such as severity and extent of disease.

B. Patient Selection

CsA should at present only be used in adults (24) and children (23) with severe atopic dermatitis that cannot be controlled by emollients, topical glucocorticosteroids, phototherapy, and/or photochemotherapy. The atopic dermatitis should be of sufficient severity in terms of extent of disease and/or effects on quality of life to justify the risks inherent in CsA treatment. These risks include nephrotoxicity, hypertension, and the consequences of immunosuppression. In children, CsA should be used with even more caution than in adults, in that only short-term treatment should be considered.

The treatment with CsA should only be installed by dermatologists having a large experience of managing atopic dermatitis in the specific age group, children or adults, respectively, and comprehensive knowledge in the use of CsA in general. Close cooperation with a pediatrician or with the general physician of the patient and vice versa is recommended.

Before starting CsA therapy, patients should be clearly advised that this treatment necessitates close monitoring, is only symptomatic, and, based on the present state of knowledge, continuous treatment should not go beyond 6 weeks in children and 1 year in adults. Patients should also undergo a full physical examination with particular attention to skin neoplasms and blood pressure. Screening for gynecological or prostate malignancy is strongly recommended according to published guidelines (24). Blood chemistry (blood count, serum bilirubin, liver enzymes, urea, creatinine on two occasions, potassium, uric acid, fasting lipids, and urinalysis for protein) should exclude potential contraindications for CsA therapy (Table 1) (32). Pregnancy and lactation constitute contraindications (unless the potential benefits of CsA therapy outweigh the potential risks for the fetus or the baby). Drug interactions are numerous, some of them increasing CsA blood levels (Ca antagonists, antimycotics and antibiotics, corticosteroids, antiemetics, etc.), some lowering CsA levels (antiepileptics, barbiturates, some antibiotics, and somatostatin analogs), some increasing the risk of nephrotoxicity (aminoglycosides, NSAID, antimycotics and antibiotics, alkylating agents). CsA may raise blood levels of antigout agents, NSAID, cardiac glycosides, and corticosteroids. Concomitant therapy with systemic corticosteroids, immunomodulating agents, or radiation therapy is contraindicated; concomitant

Table 1 Contraindications for Use of Cyclosporin A

Previous or current malignancy (except basal cell carcinoma)
Premalignant conditions
Primary or secondary immunodeficiency
Severe renal and hepatic dysfunction
Uncontrolled hypertension
Serious infection
Drug or alcohol abuse
Lack of compliance with regular monitoring

Source: Ref. 31.

use of topical corticosteroids is permitted and even encouraged in unstable situations.

C. Dosing and Treatment Regimens

There are still no conclusive data on the most appropriate starting dose of CsA. Whereas most authors use a starting dose in adults of 5 mg/kg/d, the guidelines edited by Concensus Conferences usually recommend to start at 2.5 mg/kg/d, to divide this dose into a morning and evening dose, and to adjust this dose by increasing with 1 mg/kg/d after every 2 weeks, up to a maximum dose of 5 mg/kg/d (23,24). This "hesitant" approach is not undisputed: 5 mg/kg/d will induce a more rapid remission, and short-term toxicity is normally a lesser problem than long-term toxicity, which is related to duration of therapy and cumulative dose and not to the initial dose, when given with recommended levels. Early dose-finding studies indicated the superiority of starting with a high dose in clearing atopic dermatitis, in contrast to the crescendo regimen that entails a delay of clearing and thus often reduces the patient's confidence and compliance (33).

CsA should be stopped if patients do not respond after 8 weeks of treatment, which is rarely the case when starting at 5 mg/kg/d. When skin lesions improve to an acceptable level, the CsA dose should be reduced in steps of 1 mg/kg every 2 weeks to the lowest effective dose. If clinical improvement continues, CsA should be discontinued to determine if therapy is still needed. However, present evidence indicates that the majority of patients will relapse after cessation of 2 months' treatment (34). Therefore, longer-term therapy will inevitably have to be contemplated.

Whereas some authors recommend long-term therapy—up to one year—with the lowest dose providing adequate disease control, others plead for short-term cycles and to make every reasonable effort to limit the duration of CsA therapy cycles by returning to conventional means of treatment in between two cycles (35). Such a regimen would avoid or delay adverse effects, e.g., nephrotoxicity and hypertension, and ultimately improve the long-term safety of CsA in the treatment of atopic dermatitis. Studies to prove the superiority of one approach over the other have not been performed.

In children, several studies were performed on an open basis with an initial dose of 5mg/kg/d. Treatment was in most cases stopped after 6 weeks, not because of side effects but for safety precautions, although (limited) evidence from its use in transplantation, connective tissue disease, and diabetes mellitus would suggest that CsA is tolerated at least as well by children as by adults (29).

Body weight–independent dosing regimens of CsA were shown to be promising in transplant patients. In a double-blind study by Czech et al. (36), a total of 106 adults with severe atopic dermatitis were enrolled to receive either 2.2 mg/kg/d (low) or 4.2 mg/kg/d (high) of cyclosporine microemulsion. The results of this study suggest that weight-independent treatment is feasible in atopic dermatitis.

D. Safety Monitoring

In view of the potential toxicity of CsA, its use in atopic dermatitis must be carefully considered, monitored, and controlled (24). Follow-up investigations, including blood pressure estimations, serum creatinine, urinalysis, urea, and potassium should be repeated every 2 weeks during short-term treatment and the dose reduction or withdrawal of CsA be considered, if adverse effects arise, depending on their severity. If serum creatinine rises to more than 30% above the patient's baseline on two consecutive occasions, CsA dose should be reduced by 25–50% for at least 1 month. Therapy can be continued if the serum creatinine level drops to less than 30% above the patient's baseline. Future therapy can only be started if serum creatinine values return to less than 10% above the patient's baseline. If the patient develops a mean diastolic blood pressure >95 mmHg on two consecutive occasions, the CsA dose should be reduced by 25– 50% or the hypertension should be treated with a calcium antagonist not interacting with CsA (e.g., nifedipine). Although continuous CsA treatment seems safe for up to 1 year, no renal biopsy studies are available as is the case in psoriasis patients.

Lymphadenopathy can develop in patients with severe atopic dermatitis. If it persists, lymphoma should be excluded by biopsy. Other side effects, like suspicious skin changes for tumors, skin infections including *Staphylococcus aureus* and herpes simplex, necessitate regular careful skin inspection. Tremor, hypertrichosis, gingival hyperplasia, or nausea should be recorded and treatment dose adapted or stopped. Patients on long-term CsA should be warned of the risk of cutaneous malignancy following overexposure to solar radiation. There are no data on the predictive value of routine measurements of drug blood levels in atopic dermatitis, although this may be useful in detecting possible drug interactions or noncompliance—the latter potentially explaining some nonresponders (22). When the traditional oral formulation (Sandimmun) is prescribed at levels below 5 mg/kg/d or Neoral below 4 mg/kg/d, peak-trough measurements provide limited useful clinical information.

E. Response to Treatment and Evaluation of Efficacy

Physicians treating patients with the most severe forms of atopic dermatitis should not so much consider clinical improvement as success but concentrate more on patient satisfaction. The goal therefore is not to achieve complete clearing but marked improvement of the patient's symptoms. Different scoring systems have been developed in an attempt to reproducibly measure the signs and symptoms of atopic dermatitis and to assess the efficacy of therapeutic intervention. Ideally such a scoring system should be quick, simple, and exhibit high inter- and intraobserver reproducibility. The two most popular systems are the SCORAD index and the SASSAD severity index, and patients on CsA should be regularly followed using such a system (37). In recent years more attention has been paid to the impact of dermatological disease and therapeutic interventions on the patient's quality of life. The specialty-specific Dermatology Life Quality Index is simple and rapid and allows to objectively assess the subject's satisfaction with treatment (34,36).

In a representative paper (35), 43 patients with severe atopic dermatitis were closely followed after a 6-week treatment period with CsA at 5 mg/kg/d. An almost maximal response to treatment was already apparent after 2 weeks of treatment. The overall efficacy of treatment was rated as very good or good by 37 of 42 patients after the first treatment cycle. Forty-two percent of the patients relapsed within 2 weeks and 71% 6 weeks after CsA was stopped. A second treatment period was performed, and the results were similar, most patients again responding favorably. But in contrast to the majority of patients who relapsed quickly, all 7 patients who did not relapse after the first or second treatment period were still in remission after 1 year. This study confirms many similar ones demonstrating the efficacy of CsA in atopic dermatitis (25). It also suggests that CsA treatment may improve the long-term outcome of atopic dermatitis, although most patients initially relapsed a few weeks after CsA was stopped (35). It is also established that CsA reduces the pruritus in a subgroup of patients within 2 or 3 days and that in over 50% of treated patients the skin improves within 1– 2 weeks. In this well-responding group, the mean remission rate at month 6 is 70% (38).

Studies in children (23) have shown that at 6 weeks there was significant improvement from baseline of severity scores, proportion of skin surface affected, mean symptom scores for pruritus, irritability and sleep disturbance, and topical steroid requirement in almost all of the children. Of 27 children treated, 22 had complete clearing or marked improvement after 6 weeks; only 1 child completing treatment was considered to have shown no response. Quality of life improved for both the children and their families. Long remission after withdrawal of treatment was seen in some children, although most relapsed within a few weeks (23).

F. Side Effects

The potential side effects of CsA are substantial (23,24), the major limiting side effect being nephrotoxicity. Monitoring serum creatinine level seems to be a practical method of evaluating renal function, being easier and less error-prone than determinations of creatinine clearance or glomerular filtration rates. While CsA nephrotoxicity is generally reversible if detected early, renal biopsies frequently show changes of interstitial fibrosis and less frequently irreversible glomerulo-sclerosis.

Cardiovascular side effects are of concern in patients receiving CsA for atopic dermatitis, and some patients have suffered myocardial infarction while ingesting the drug. CsA may worsen hypertension in those with preexisting blood pressure elevation, requiring alterations in antihypertensive regimens. It may also induce hypertension in normotensic individuals. Diet, exercise, and antihypertensive drug therapy may be necessary. CsA may also cause elevation of serum triglycerides and less frequently cholesterol (24). Among the most striking cutaneous side effects are hypertrichosis and gingival hyperplasia. Table 2 lists common adverse effects associated with CsA use (39).

One of the main concerns relates to possible long-term carcinogenicity. This concern is based on the general immunosuppressive activity of CsA and observations in long-term users such as graft recipients and psoriatic patients. In the latter, however, factors such as previous chemotherapy or long-term photochemotherapy may have played an important role as cocarcinogens (38), cofactors that are normally absent in atopic dermatitis patients.

CsA-induced carcinogenesis is of even greater importance in children. The effects of its prolonged administration are unknown in this age group, although considerable information is becoming available from its use in children after organ transplantation. There are almost no reports of CsA-related malignancies in children, and it is unlikely that short courses of the drug, as used in atopic dermatitis, could have a detrimental effect. In addition, patients receiving CsA following organ transplantation are much more intensely immunosuppressed (40). If, however, the patient with atopic dermatitis has signs of severe photodamage due to previous sunlight exposure, photo- or photochemotherapy, CsA therapy is to be avoided (24).

Table 2 Adverse Effects of Cyclosporine A

System	Effects
Renal/electrolyte	Increase in blood-urea nitrogen and creatinine; decrease in glomerulum filtration and serum magnesium
Hematological	Mild normocytic, normochromic anemia
Gastrointestinal	Nausea, vomiting, diarrhea, bloating
Hepatic	Elevated transaminases and alkaline phosphatase
Cardiovascular	Hypertension, hyperlipidemia
Mucocutaneous	Hypertrichosis, gingival hyperplasia
Constitutional	Fatigue, weight loss early in therapy
Neurological	Encephalitis, tremor, paresthesias

Source: Ref. 38.

G. Conclusions

CsA has gained a place in treating difficult cases of atopic dermatitis in adults (24) and in children (23). The available evidence suggests that short-term treatment with CsA is efficacious and safe in patients with recalcitrant disease not responding to classical treatment. Long-term treatment should only be considered in adults that do not respond to an 8-week therapeutic schedule. Quality of life measures improve significantly while patients are on the drug. Dermatologists are urged to use one of the available scoring systems (e.g., SCORAD) to assess extent, activity, and symptoms of atopic dermatitis before, during, and after therapeutic intervention with CsA.

Patients must be encouraged to maintain topical treatment with emollients and topical steroids during CsA therapy. It is also important to explain to the patient that a short course of CsA therapy is intended to induce a remission of the disease but that, at present, long-term remission, although reported in some patients, remains uncertain. There is no evidence for a rebound phenomenon after stoppping CsA.

V. OTHER SYSTEMIC DRUGS

Antimetabolites such as azathioprine, methotrexate, and cytotoxic drugs such as cyclophosphamide have been employed in patients with severe atopic dermatitis, and variable results have been reported. Azathioprine, because of its still widespread use in some countries, shall be dealt with in more detail below. However, with none of these agents have controlled studies been performed. This also holds true for thymopentine, which has been administered with some success to a small number of patients (41). A double-blind, placebo-controlled study revealed no significant improvement in patients' well-being or immunological parameters. The excellent efficacy of CsA and the fact that this drug has been studied very carefully and guidelines are available indicate that these drugs may become obsolete in the future. A few controlled studies have examined the effect of interferon-gamma in atopic dermatitis and efficacy was shown in a smaller proportion of patients; 45% of rIFN-gamma–treated patients, but also 21% of placebo-treated patients achieved greater than 50% improvement in physicians' overall response evaluations (42,43). Because interferon-gamma is not without side effects and its efficacy in no way matches that of CsA, this treatment probably also will not be used very often. The same holds true for interferon-alpha (44), high-dose immunoglobulins (45), and interleukin-2 (46), of which all have been tried in limited numbers of patients.

A. Azathioprine

More than half of the dermatologists in the United Kingdom use azathioprine to treat severe atopic dermatitis (47), yet there is not one randomized controlled trial available to support its use (25). Several studies were therefore recently initiated in order to prove its efficacy and safety as compared to other immunosuppressive drugs (47–49). Tan et al. (47) point to uncontrolled studies involving small numbers of patients and leading to contradictory results. Their conclusion from the literature survey is that cyclosporin has potentially more side effects than azathioprine, but the latter is more cost-effective and easier to monitor, emphasizing the need for double-blind trials. Other authors also argue that azathioprine is an effective and cheaper alternative to cyclosporine in the treatment of severe adult atopic eczema, but that long-term toxicity remains unclear (49). Lear et al. (48) point to bone marrow suppression and its oncogenic potential; regarding the latter, a study comparing the incidence of cutaneous malignancy in renal allograft recipients who received cyclosporine or azathioprine showed no differences between the two drugs (50). In summary, azathioprine seems to be effective and is on the list of recommended systemic treatment modalities in the guidelines of care for atopic dermatitis of the American Academy of Dermatology (51), but more studies are needed to better clarify the safety-efficacy ratio of this drug in atopic dermatitis.

B. Mycophenolate Mofetil

Mycophenolate mofetil (MMF), an immunosuppressive agent that blocks the proliferative responses of T and B lymphocytes and is currently used to prevent rejection in renal transplant patients, has been used in the treatment of psoriasis, pemphigus vulgaris, bullous pemphigoid, pyoderma gangrenosum, and pompholyx (52). Trials in small numbers of patients suggest that MMF therapy may be beneficial for patients with atopic dermatitis (53) but call for controlled trials (54). Recent observations of staphylococcal septicemia complicating treatment of atopic dermatitis with MMF (52), however, call for a reconsideration of its use in atopic dermatitis, and its relative inefficacy in a small series of atopic dermatitis patients caused Hansen et al. (55) to conclude that MMF cannot be advocated based on existing knowledge.

C. New Agents

Systemic macrolides such as pimecrolimus (ASM SDZ-981, Elidel®) which has shown dramatic efficacy and a high degree of tolerability in psoriatic patients (56), is presently being tested in a large international multicenter trial. If the initial impression of a low-toxicity and high-efficacy profile of pimecrolimus can be verified also for patients with atopic dermatitis, this drug is probably going to be the first-line systemic treatment modality of atopic dermatitis in the future. Publications have shown significant results in a mouse model of atopic dermatitis (57) and with topical treatment in short-term trials in patients with moderate atopic dermatitis (58). The promising clincial trial profiles of this new type of calcineurin inhibitor may result in alternative therapies providing potent anti-inflammatory activity without the adverse effects that limit corticosteroid use (59).

VI. SUMMARY

The list of recommended substances for systemic treatment of patients suffering from atopic dermatitis (51) is long, ranging from antihistamines, antibiotics, and corticosteroids to immunosuppressants and from dietary supplements to unsatu-rated fatty acids and Chinese herbs (see Chapter 28) and miscellaneous other treatment considerations. Many of them have been in traditional use for decades, several without having ever been tested in placebo-controlled trials as is the case for systemic corticosteroids. Others "like interferons and thymopentin have never left the level of a research tool rather than being a serious management option" (60). Others, like cyclosporine, a relatively expensive and potentially toxic pro-prietary drug, have undergone well-controlled trials for the treatment of atopic dermatitis (25) and have fulfilled expectations. Other substances, like gamma-linoleic acid, heavily recommended even in guidelines (51), but in the first double-blind, multicentre analysis was shown to be more or less ineffective (61), emphasizing that the efficacy of any substance being used for the treatment of this complex disease should first pass a critical review process (25).

REFERENCES

1. Berth-Jones J, Graham-Brown RAC. Treatment of itching in atopic eczema. Br Med J 298: 491–492, 1989.
2. Greaves MW, Wall PD. Pathophysiology of itching. Lancet 348:938–940, 1996.
3. Henz BM, Metzenauer P, O'Keefe E, Zuberbier T. Differential effects of new-gener-ation H1-receptor antagonists in pruritic dermatoses. Allergy 53:180–183, 1998.
4. Kemp JP. Tolerance induction to antihistamines: Is it a problem? Ann Allergy 63: 621–623, 1989.
5. Simons FER. A new classification of H1-receptor antagonists. Allergy 50:7–11, 1995.
6. Mann RD, Pearce GL, Dunn N, Shakir S. Sedation with "non-sedating" antihista-mines: four prescription-event monitoring studies in general practice. Br Med J 320: 1184–1186, 2000.

7. Spector SL, Altman R. Cetirizine: a novel antihistamine. Am J Rhinol 1:1479, 1987.
8. Tharp MD. The clinical efficacy of antihistamines in the skin. Allergy 55:11–16, 2000.
9. Woosley RL. Cardiac actions of antihistamines. Annu Rev Pharmacol Toxicol 36: 233–252, 1996.
10. Klein PA, Clark RAF. An evidence-based review of the efficacy of antihistamines in relieving pruritus in atopic dermatitis. Arch Dermatol 135:1522–1525, 1999.
11. Marshall GD Jr. Therapeutic options in allergic disease: antihistamines as systemic antiallergic agents. J Allergy Clin Immunol 106:S303–309, 2000.
12. Monroe E. Loratadine in chronic urticaria and atopic skin conditions: a review. Advances Ther 11:95–109, 1994.
13. Langeland T, Fagertun HE, Larsen S. Therapeutic effect of loratadine on pruritus in patients with atopic dermatitis. Allergy 49:22–26, 1994.
14. Juhlin L. Nonclassical clinical indications for H1-receptor antagonists in dermatology. Allergy 50:36–40, 1995.
15. Henz BM. The pharmacologic profile of desloratadine: a review. Allergy 56:S7–13, 2001.
16. Schleimer RP. Glucocorticosteroids. Their mechanisms of action and use in allergic disease. In: Middleteon E, et al., eds. Allergy, Principles and Practice. St. Louis: Mosby, 1993, pp. 893–925.
17. Raimer SS. Managing pediatric atopic dermatitis. Clin Pediatr 39:1–14, 2000.
18. Tay YK, Khoo BP, Goh CL. The profile of atopic dermatitis in a tertiary dermatology outpatient clinic in Singapore. Int J Dermatol 38:689–692, 1999.
19. Hanifin JM. Breaking the cycle. How I manage difficult cases of atopic dermatitis. Fitzpatrick's J Dermatol 1:13–26, 1994.
20. Tofte SJ, Hanifin JM. Current management and therapy of atopic dermatitis. J Am Acad Dermatol 44:S13–16, 2001.
21. Van Joost T, Stolz E, Heule F. Efficacy of low-dose cyclosporine in severe atopic skin disease. Arch Dermatol 123:166–167, 1987.
22. Camp RDR, Reitamo S, Friedman PS, Ho V, Heule F. Cyclosporin A in severe, therapy-resistant atopic dermatitis: report of an international workshop, April 1993. Br J Dermatol 129:217–220, 1993.
23. Berth-Jones J, Finlay AY, Zaki I, et al. Cyclosporine in severe childhood atopic dermatitis: a multicenter study. J Am Acad Dermatol 34:1016–1021, 1996.
24. Naeyaert JM, Lachapelle JM, Degreef H, de al Brassinne M, Heenen M, Lambert J. Cyclosporin in atopic dermatitis. Dermatology 198:145–152, 1999.
25. Williams H, Adetugbo K, Wan Po AL, Naldi L, Diepgen T, Murrell D. The Cochrane Skin Group. Preparing, maintaining, and disseminating systematic reviews of clinical interventions in dermatology. Arch Dermatol 134:1620–1626, 1998.
26. Zurbriggen B, Wüthrich B, Cachelin AB, Will PB, Kägi MK. Comparison of two formulations of cyclosporin A in the treatment of severe atopic dermatitis. Dermatology 198:56–60, 1999.
27. Bourke JF, Berth-Jones J, Holder J, Graham-Brown RAC. A new microemulsion formulation (Neoral) is effective in treatment of cyclosporin-resistant dermatoses. Br J Dermatol 134:777–779, 1996.
28. Atakan N, Erdem C. The efficacy, tolerability and safety of a new oral formulation

of Sandimmun®-Sandimmun Neoral® in refractory atopic dermatitis. JEADV 11: 240–246, 1998.

29. Berth-Jones J, Graham-Brown RAC, Marks R, et al. Long-term efficacy and safety of cyclosporin in severe adult atopic dermatitis. Br J Dermatol 136:76–81, 1997.

30. Kägi MK, Joller-Jemelka H, Wüthrich B. Soluble E-selectin correlates with disease activity in cyclosporin A-treated patients with atopic dermatitis. Allergy 54:57–63, 1999.

31. Bottari V, Frezzolini A, Ruffelli M, Puddu P, Fontana L, De Pità O. Cyclosporin A (CyA) reduces sCD30 serum levels in atopic dermatitis: a possible new immune intervention. Allergy 42:507–510, 1999.

32. Berth-Jones J, Voorhees JJ. Consensus conference on cyclosporin A microemulsion for psoriasis, June 1996. Br J Dermatol 135:775–777, 1996.

33. Zachariae H. Therapeutic timidity in dermatology. J Am Acad Dermatol 44:140–141, 2001.

34. Salek MS, Finlay AY, Luscombe DK, et al. Cyclosporin greatly improves the quality of life of adults with severe atopic dermatitis: a randomized, double-blind, placebo-controlled trial. Br J Dermatol 129:422–430, 1993.

35. Granlund H, Erkko P, Sinisalo M, Reitamo S. Cyclosporin A in atopic dermatitis: time to relapse and effect of intermittent therapy. Br J Dermatol 132:106–112, 1995.

36. Czech W, Bräutigam M, Weidinger G, Schöpf E. A body-weight-independent dosing regimen of cyclosporine microemulsion is effective in severe atopic dermatitis and improves the quality of life. J Am Acad Dermatol 42:653–659, 2000.

37. Kunz B, Oranje AP, Labrèze L, Stalder JF, Ring J, Taieb A. Clinical validation and guidelines for the SCORAD index: consensus report of the European task force on atopic dermatitis. Dermatology 195:10–19, 1997.

38. Meinardi MMHM, Zonneveld IM, deRie MA, Bos JD. Cyclosporin A: a new therapeutic modality in the treatment of severe atopic dermatitis. J Dermatol Treatm 5: S5–7, 1994.

39. Kauvar AB, Stiller MJ. Cyclosporine in dermatology: pharmacology and clinical use. Int J Dermatol 33:86–96, 1994.

40. Penn I. Cancers following cyclosporine therapy. Transplantation 43:32–35, 1987.

41. Harper JI, Mason UA, White TR, Staughton RCD, Hobbs JR. A double-blind placebo-controlled study of thymostimulin (TP-1) for the treatment of atopic eczema. Br J Dermatol 125:368–372, 1991.

42. Hanifin JM, Schneider LC, Leung DYM, et al. Recombinant interferon gamma therapy for atopic dermatitis. J Am Acad Dermatol 28:189–197, 1993.

43. Reinhold U, Kukel S, Brzoska J, Kreysel HW. Systemic interferon gamma treatment in severe atopic dermatitis. J Am Acad Dermatol 29:58–63, 1993.

44. Rothe MJ, Grant-Kels JM. Atopic dermatitis: an update. J Am Acad Dermatol 35: 1–13, 1996.

45. Kimata H. High dose gammaglobulin treatment for atopic dermatitis. Arch Dis Child 70:335–336, 1994

46. Hsieh KH, Chou CC, Huang SF. Interleukin-2 therapy in severe atopic dermatitis. J Clin Immunol 11:22–28, 1991.

47. Tan BB, Lear JT, Gawkrodger DJ, English JSC. Azathioprine in dermatology: a survey of current practice in the U.K. Br J Dermatol 136:351–355, 1997.

48. Lear JT, English JSC, Jones P, Smith AG. Retrospective review of the use of azathioprine in severe atopic dermatitis. J Am Acad Dermatol 35:642–643, 1996.
49. Buckley DA, Baldwin P, Rogers S. The use of azathioprine in severe adult atopic dermatitis. JEADV 11:137–140, 1998.
50. Bunney MH, Benton EC, Barr BB, et al. The prevalence of skin disorders in renal allograft recipients receiving cyclosporin compared to those receiving azathioprine. Nephrol Dial Transplant 5:379–382, 1990.
51. Drake LA, Ceilley RI, Cornelison RL, et al. Guidelines of care for atopic dermatitis. J Am Acad Dermatol 26:485- 488, 1992.
52. Satchell AC, Barnetson RSC. Staphylococcal septicaemia complicating treatment of atopic dermatitis with mycophenolate. Br J Dermatol 143:202–203, 2000.
53. Neuber N, Schwartz I, Itschert G, Dieck AD. Treatment of atopic eczema with oral mycophenolate mofetil. Br J Dermatol 143: 385–391, 2000.
54. Grundmann-Kollmann M, Korting HC, Behrens S, Leiter U, Krähn G, Kaufmann R, Peter RU, Kerscher M. Successful treatment of severe refractory atopic dermatitis with mycophenolate mofetil. Br J Dermatol 141:175–176, 1999.
55. Hansen ER, Buus S, Deleuran M, Andersen KE. Treatment of atopic dermatitis with mycophenolate mofetil. Br J Dermatol 143:1324–1326, 2000.
56. Rappersberger K, Komar M, Ebelin ME, Scott G, Burtin P, Greig G, Kehren J, Chibout SD, Holter W, Richter L, Stütz A, Wolff K. Pimecrolimus: an ascomycin macrolactam for the oral treatment of psoriasis. J Invest Dermatol, in press.
57. Neckermann G, Bavandi A, Meingassner JG. Atopic dermatitis-like symptoms in hypomagnesaemic hairless rats are prevented and inhibited by systemic or topical SDZ ASM 981. Br J Dermatol 142:669–679, 2000.
58. Van Leent EJ, Graber M, Thurston M, Wagenaar M, Spuls PI, Bos JD. Effectiveness of the ascomycin macrolactam SDZ ASM 981 in the topical treatment of atopic dermatitis. Arch Dermatol 134:805–809, 1998.
59. Hanifin JM, Chan S. Biochemical and immunologic mechanisms in atopic dermatitis: New targets for emerging therapies. J Am Acad Dermatol 41:72–77, 1999.
60. Friedmann PS, Tan BB, Musaba E, Strickland I. Pathogenesis and management of atopic dermatitis. Clin Exp Allergy 25:799–806, 1995.
61. Henz BM, Jablonska S, Van de Kerkhof PCM, Stingl G, Blaszczyk M, Vandervalk PGM, Veenhuizen R, Muggli R, Raederstorff D. Double-blind, multicentre analysis of the efficacy of borage oil in patients with atopic eczema. Br J Dermatol 140:685–688, 1999.

30
Future Perspectives in Atopic Dermatitis

Thomas Bieber
University of Bonn, Bonn, Germany

Donald Y. M. Leung
*National Jewish Medical and Research Center,
Denver, Colorado*

I. INTRODUCTION

Atopic dermatitis (AD) belongs to a family of chronic inflammatory skin diseases that have been known for more than 2000 years but recognized as an individual entity at the end of the nineteenth century. Despite the tremendous progress made in the field of immunology and allergology during the last 30 years, we still face a complex and fascinating disease which consistently offers new challenges for physicians and researchers. In this concluding chapter, we felt it was necessary to state some of the most important and remaining open questions that must be addressed since they will have a major impact on how research in the field of AD will progress in the future.

II. THE NEED FOR A CLEARCUT AND CONSENSUAL DEFINITION OF AD

During the twentieth century there was some debate, mainly in Europe, as to how this disease should be named. Approximately 15 different names were proposed, from neurodermatitis or endogenous eczema to atopic eczema or atopic dermatitis and constitutional eczema. In a world of globalization and common efforts in cooperation and research programs, there is an increasing need for consensus as how to define this disease. In 2001, after long and intensive debates among the participants, the European Academy of Allergy and Clinical Immunology (EAACI) proposed a new nomenclature, which at least has the advantage of acknowledging the diversity of AD (1). In line with this, there have also been efforts to refine the clinical criteria of this disease. Although they have been most helpful and considered as the gold standard over two decades, the need for a critical reconsideration of their own criteria under the light of the progress in epidemiology and pathophysiology has been acknowledged by Jon Hanifin and Georg Rajka (Third International Symposium on Atopic Dermatitis, September 2001, Portland, OR). The semantics of defining a disease is not a static but a dynamic process tightly related to the progress made in understanding its pathophysiology. Thus, physicians should be able to accompany this progress and to accept the new frames provided by the scientific progress in this field while keeping the interest of their patients in mind.

To afford further progress in this particularly sensitive area, the development of new techniques supplementing our diagnostic tools is essential to reach the goal of an ideal clinical and biological phenotype definition. These developments are mandatory for future studies in genetic epidemiology as well as in other areas of AD research such as gene profiling (see below).

III. GENETIC EPIDEMIOLOGY: CHASING THE GENES LEADING TO AD

In contrast to monogenic diseases, AD is a prototypical multifactorial disorder in which genetic complexity increasingly reflects the complexity of the clinical spectrum of this condition. Thus, it is not surprising that the various reports dealing with genome wide scans, linkage, and association analysis have currently revealed more than a dozen candidate genes (2). This highlights the concept of gene-gene and gene-environment interactions, which are likely to play a major role in the pathophysiology of AD. After having sequenced the human genome, the real challenge has now started in attempting to identify variants/polymorphisms (single nuclear polymorphisms, or SNPs) which may be of relevance to AD. Clear and accepted clinical criteria for the AD phenotype are mandatory for the success of such sophisticated studies and to allow comparative approaches between reports. The era of functional genomics has now been open and will absorb many scientists over the next years in chasing the relevant genes and their products. Obviously progress in this field will dictate the advances in understanding the immunoallergological network that is the basis of AD and other diseases like psoriasis. Interestingly, while these two chronic inflammatory skin disorders have long been considered different diseases, some authors have further suggested that they may be mutually exclusive. It would not be surprising that progress in immunogenetics will correct our current point of view in this regard and suggest that certain aspects of AD and psoriasis develop on the basis of common genetic variants (3). One may imagine that chronic inflammation in the epidermis or dermis may be the result of polymorphism(s) in gene(s) coding for molecules involved in the downregulation of inflammation in the skin, which would explain why both diseases, although clinically distinct, tend to become chronic or persistent. With this in mind, chasing the genetic background of the so-called intrinsic form of AD (IAD) (4) may represent a crucial step in unraveling putative genes involved in the regulation of inflammatory reactions in the skin. However, these kinds of genetic studies require a clear-cut definition of the clinical and biological phenotypes of intrinsic AD and will be extremely challenging for clinicians and genetical epidemiologists since these patients represent a minority among AD patients.

IV. IMMUNOALLERGOLOGY OF AD

Recently, the concept of a maturating immune system in the postnatal phase of life where the Th2 dominance switches to a Th1 dominance in early childhood has been largely accepted (5). However, the nature of the signals required for this maturation are still debated. According to the hygiene hypothesis recently supported by epidemiological studies and investigations in animal models, microorganisms and particularly the resident microflora of the gut have been recognized as major players in this complex scenario (6,7). Lipopolysaccharides or so-called CpG sequences derived from distinct bacteria have been shown to be strong inducers of Th1 immune responses via their ability to bind to so-called pattern recognition receptors of the innate immune system expressed on APC. Based on this concept, the use of probiotics, e.g., from *Lactobacillus rhamnosus* GG or *Bifidobacterium lactis* Bb-12 during early childhood has been proposed as a simple strategy to reinforce the normal healthy gut flora and promote the postnatal Th2-to-Th1 switch. In the near future this will be further explored by colonization of the GI tract using a probiotic approach (8–10). Whether this type of strategy is not only beneficial for early infancy but may also be applied for older individuals needs to be addressed in further controlled studies, ideally combined with exploration of the immunogenetical background.

Based on the genetic, clinical, histological, and allergological background, it is reasonable to conclude that AD results from an immunological alteration in which cell-mediated mechanisms play a crucial role. It is also generally accepted that this type of inflammatory skin reaction needs at least the interaction of antigen-presenting cells (APC), which present certain antigen-derived peptides to effector T cells. In this context, the notion of intrinsic and extrinsic forms of

AD is of crucial importance since they imply the putative role of exogenous allergens, i.e., aeroallergens or food allergens in the case of extrinsic form, where specific IgE and IgE receptors on APC represent the link between the atopic status (as defined by sensitization to environmental allergens and subsequent production of specific IgE) and the cellular events acknowledged above (11). In contrast, some yet-to-be-defined cutaneous autoantigens, which may not require specific IgE for recognition by APC, could be of importance in the intrinsic form. The degree of complexity is even greater when one considers the putative role of so-called autoallergens as Hom S1 (12), to which atopic patients with otherwise increased IgE levels obviously became sensitized in the course of their disease. Thus there is a great need to clarify these issues since they are of paramount importance for understanding the immunopathology of the wide clinical spectrum of AD and to design future prevention and therapeutic strategies.

Finally, the pronounced colonization of the skin and nose of patients with AD with *Staphylococcus aureus* is a well-known phenomenon, and several studies have highlighted the role of these bacteria in triggering/maintaining the cutaneous inflammatory reactions (13). Whether this colonization is mainly due to the underlying inflammation as a kind of "natural agar" and/or a defective control in the skin microflora of these patients is still unclear. Recent progress in understanding the mechanisms of innate immunity of the skin has demonstrated the presence of natural antimicrobial peptides, i.e., β-defensins, which are produced by keratinocytes upon local signals delivered by colonizing microorganisms (14–17). Whether keratinocytes for AD have an intrinsic defect in the control of bacterial colonization, e.g., by polymorphism/variants in genes encoding for defensins, is a fascinating new field of research.

V. NEUROIMMUNOLOGY OF AD

Atopic dermatitis is considered a paradigmatic dermatological condition in which the skin often acts as a mirror of psychological situations. Clinicians are well aware of the important impact of psychological factors as triggers of AD and their relevance in the management of this disease. These observations clearly suggest that many of the above-mentioned immunoallergological events may be under the tight control of signals emerging from the central nervous system (CNS). As these signals are virtually lacking under in vitro conditions, the majority of the immunological phenomenons observed in laboratory investigations provide only a partial picture since they have been placed outside their in vivo microenvironment where neuropeptides most probably act as major players in dictating the reactivity thresholds. As the biological links between the CNS and the immune system have been unraveled during the last decade, increasing interest has been focused on the mechanisms underlying the control of immune responses by neuropeptides, particularly in the skin. Future progress in this area should shed some light in the black box of the pathophysiology of pruritus in AD. Undoubtedly, academic investigators and industry-based research should focus on this fascinating field of dermatological aspects of psychoneuroimmunology since the potential for breakthrough discoveries and their therapeutic perspectives have been underestimated so far.

VI. GENE PROFILING AND PHARMACOGENETICS: THE BASIS FOR FUTURE THERAPEUTICAL STRATEGIES

Tremendous technological progress has been made in the last few years, providing new exciting research tools in genomics and proteomics. Microchips for gene and protein arrays combined to bioinformatics will yield tremendous amounts of data, which, after meticulous and accurate sorting, should enable investigators to better understand complex interactions and regulatory mechanisms occuring in tissues (18,19). Based on the information provided by the analysis gene profiles (using gene chips) obtained from normal and involved skin before and after therapy, we should gain more information about the mechanisms involved in the initiation, regulation, and normalization of the inflammatory reactions in the skin. Thus, genes and their products could be identified as potential new targets for future therapeutic strategies. This is of special interest when looking for those genes responsible for the signals that should physiologically downregulate an inflammatory reaction but are for some reason unable to perform this function and therefore lead to chronic inflammation.

On the other hand, increasing financial support has been invested in projects such as functional genomics aimed to identify putative functionally and pathophysiologically relevant single nucleotide polymorphisms. These efforts should provide important new information concerning the individual reactivity of a given patient treated with conventional or newly developed medications. In fact, we should be able to distinguish responsive and nonresponsive individuals. This could be of critical importance for the recruitment of patients for future clinical trials. Finally, this knowledge may also be helpful in understanding why some patients are prone to display known or unexpected side effects during therapy. The pharmaceutical industry has already recognized the benefit of these new technologies and is confident in their potential for designing new immunopharmacologically active compounds.

VII. CONCLUSION

At the beginning of the twenty-first century, biomedical research has access to new technologies that will considerably speed up the acquisition of information in many areas, particularly in common diseases such as AD. However, the value of the data obtained by investigations using these technologies is rather limited as long as the criteria used to recruit the patients are not better standardized and updated. This multifactorial disease remains an attractive challenge in terms of research and management. There is no doubt that the current efforts in understanding the pathomechanisms of AD will rapidly lead to the design of new compounds able to specifically target discrete but essential mechanisms contributing to this condition. In this regard, the beginning of this new century is quite promising, but there remains a long way to go before physicians will be able to effectively control the maturation of the immune system and to cure atopic dermatitis.

REFERENCES

1. Johansson SG, Hourihane JO, Bousquet J, Bruijnzeel-Koomen C, Dreborg S, Haahtela T, Kowalski ML, Mygind N, Ring J, van Cauwenberge P, van Hage-Hamsten M, Wuthrich B. A revised nomenclature for allergy. An EAACI position statement from the EAACI nomenclature task force. Allergy 2001; 56:813–824.

2. Cookson WO. The genetics of atopic dermatitis: strategies, candidate genes, and genome screens. J Am Acad Dermatol 2001; 45:S7–9.

3. Cookson WO, Ubhi B, Lawrence R, Abecasis GR, Walley AJ, Cox HE, Coleman R, Leaves I, Trembath RC, Moffatt MF, Harper JI. Genetic linkage of childhood atopic dermatitis to psoriasis susceptibility loci. Nat Genet 2001; 27:372–373.

4. Schmid-Grendelmeier P, Simon D, Simon HU, Akdis CA, Wuthrich B. Epidemiology, clinical features, and immunology of the "intrinsic" (non-IgE-mediated) type of atopic dermatitis (constitutional dermatitis). Allergy 2001; 56:841–849.

5. Holt PG, Jones CA. The development of the immune system during pregnancy and early life. Allergy 2000; 55:688–697.

6. Holt PG. Parasites, atopy, and the hygiene hypothesis: resolution of a paradox? Lancet 2000; 356:1699–1701.

7. Anderson WJ, Watson L. Asthma and the hygiene hypothesis. N Engl J Med 2001; 344:1643–1644.

8. Isolauri E, Arvola T, Sutas Y, Moilanen E, Salminen S. Probiotics in the management of atopic eczema. Clin Exp Allergy 2000; 30:1604–1610.

9. Isolauri E, Sutas Y, Kankaanpaa P, Arvilommi H, Salminen S. Probiotics: effects on immunity. Am J Clin Nutr 2001; 73:444S–450S.

10. Kalliomaki M, Salminen S, Arvilommi H, Kero P, Koskinen P, Isolauri E. Probiotics in primary prevention of atopic disease: a randomized placebo-controlled trial. Lancet 2001; 357:1076–1079.

11. Novak N, Kraft S, Bieber T. IgE receptors. Curr Op Immunol 2001; 13:721–726.

12. Valenta R, Natter S, Seiberler S, Wichlas S, Maurer D, Hess M, Pavelka M, Grote M, Ferreira F, Szepfalusi Z, Valent P, Stingl G. Molecular characterization of an autoallergen, Hom s 1, identified by serum IgE from atopic dermatitis patients. J Invest Dermatol 1998; 111:1178–1183.

13. Leung DY. Atopic dermatitis and the immune system: the role of superantigens and bacteria. J Am Acad Dermatol 2001; 45:S13–16.

14. Jia HP, Schutte BC, Schudy A, Linzmeier R, Guthmiller JM, Johnson GK, Tack BF, Mitros JP, Rosenthal A, Ganz T, McCray PB Jr. Discovery of new human beta-defensins using a genomics-based approach. Gene 2001; 263:211–218.

15. Yang D, Chertov O, Bykovskaia SN, Chen Q, Buffo MJ, Shogan J, Anderson M, Schroder JM, Wang JM, Howard OM, Oppenheim JJ. Beta-defensins: linking innate and adaptive immunity through dendritic and T cell CCR6. Science 1999; 286:525–528.

16. Harder J, Bartels J, Christophers E, Schroder JM. Isolation and characterization of human beta-defensin-3, a novel human inducible peptide antibiotic. J Biol Chem 2001; 276:5707–5713.

17. Ong PY, Strickland I, Boguniewicz M, Kisich KO, Leung DYM. Reduced expression of human beta defensin-2 (HBD-2) and CCR6 in atopic dermatitis (AD). J Allergy Clin Immunol 2001. in press.

18. Schulze A, Downward J. Navigating gene expression using microarrays—a technology review. Nat Cell Biol 2001; 3:190–195.

19. Cuzin M. DNA chips: a new tool for genetic analysis and diagnostics. Transfus Clin Biol 2001; 8:291–296.

Index